National Registry Paramedic
Prep

Third Edition

Also from Kaplan Medical

Print

EMS Dosage Calculation: Math Review and Practice for Paramedics
EMT Exam Prep
Anatomy Coloring Book
Anatomy Flashcards
ATI TEAS Prep Plus

Online

NREMT Qbank: *kaptest.com/nremt*

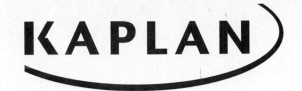

National Registry Paramedic

Prep

Third Edition

Our 80 years' expertise = Your competitive advantage

Practice + Proven Strategies

© 2022 by Kaplan North America, LLC

Published by Kaplan North America, LLC
1515 West Cypress Creek Road
Fort Lauderdale, Florida 33309

ISBN: 978-1-5062-7403-4
10 9 8 7 6 5 4

Kaplan Publishing print books are available at special quantity discounts to use for sales promotions, employee premiums, or educational purposes. For more information or to purchase books, please call the Simon & Schuster special sales department at 866-506-1949.

Table of Contents

Additional resources available at kaplanmedical.com/nremt

FOR TEST CHANGES OR LATE-BREAKING DEVELOPMENTS

kaptest.com/retail-book-corrections-and-updates

The material in this book is up-to-date at the time of publication. However, changes in the test may have been instituted after this book was published. Be sure to carefully read the materials you receive when you register for the test. If there are any important late-breaking developments—or any changes or corrections to the Kaplan test preparation materials in this book—we will post that information online at **kaptest.com/retail-book-corrections-and-updates**.

About the Author

Jason E. Konzelmann, BS, M.Ed., NR-P, CHSE

Mr. Konzelmann has been a paramedic for more than 20 years in eastern Pennsylvania. He is the coordinator of the Lehigh County EMT Program and EMT/paramedic adjunct instructor at Lehigh Carbon Community College in Allentown, Pennsylvania, and a PALS, ACLS, and CPR instructor with Lehigh Valley Health Network. He still finds time to work as a paramedic with Second Alarmers Rescue Squad in Montgomery County, Pennsylvania, and the City of Bethlehem EMS in the Lehigh Valley.

Earlier in his career, Mr. Konzelmann worked for 4 years as an administrative supervisor and simulation coordinator with the New York Simulation Center for the Health Sciences, a partnership between the New York University School of Medicine and the City University of New York. He is currently Assistant Director of the Healthcare Simulation Center with DeSales University in Center Valley, Pennsylvania. There, he helps design and implement simulation education experiences for learners in undergraduate and graduate nursing programs, physical therapy programs, and physician assistant studies. While with DeSales, he earned his Masters in Education and has become a Certified Healthcare Simulation Educator. He has a BS and secondary education certificate in chemistry from Muhlenberg College.

Physiology, Pathophysiology, and Shock

1

Learning Objectives

❑ Explain cellular chemistry.

❑ Explain dynamic equilibrium and its role in the body.

❑ Describe the acid-base buffer system in the body.

❑ Differentiate between metabolic and respiratory acidosis and alkalosis.

❑ Differentiate, assess, and treat different causes for shock.

To fully understand the disease processes and syndromes you may encounter in the field, it is important to have a working knowledge of cellular processes, i.e., what is happening at the cellular level to cause disease, organ failure, and eventually organism death. However, before any meaningful discussion on that level can happen, understanding what comprises *normal* is paramount. Disease processes and syndromes can then be looked at as a collection of deviations from normal, rather than as discrete and separate from each other. This chapter will cover normal cellular function, including cellular chemistry and metabolism, life cycles, and homeostasis, or how a cell maintains its steady internal equilibrium with its harsh surroundings. From there, the chapter will discuss what a disruption of these processes can do to the cell and, by extension, to the whole body in the general term known as *shock*.

CELLULAR CHEMISTRY

Although not often directly tested on any state or national paramedic examination, basic chemistry can subtly find its way into other questions. This section focuses on terminology, but references to cellular chemistry will occur in future chapters. A strong understanding of the basics can then be built into an improved understanding of physiology and anatomy.

Atomic Structure

All **matter**, anything that has mass or substance, at the most basic level is made up of at least one element but more likely a variety of elements. An element is a pure substance that is entirely comprised of the same atom, which is the smallest complete unit of an element that retains all the exclusive chemical properties of that element. **Atoms** are composed of discrete particles known as protons, neutrons, and electrons:

- **Protons** are located in the nucleus and carry a positive charge. The number of protons in the nucleus defines the atom in question. For example, all oxygen atoms have 8 protons in the nucleus, and all nitrogen atoms contain 7 protons. Finally, the atomic number of an element is indicated by the number of protons in the nucleus. Therefore, the atomic number of oxygen is 8, and for nitrogen it is 7.

- **Neutrons**, also found in the nucleus of the atom, are neutral in charge and serve to provide separation of the normally repellant positive charges of protons. Different isotopes of the same element (same number of protons) are caused by different numbers of neutrons in the nucleus. The sum of the neutrons and protons in the nucleus approximates the atomic weight of the element. Helium, for example, has 2 protons and 2 neutrons in its nucleus and thus has an atomic weight of 4.

- **Electrons** are substantially smaller in weight than either neutrons or protons and do not contribute materially to the weight of an atom. They carry a negative charge and are in constant motion around the nucleus. A neutral atom has the same number of electrons and protons; that is, the positive charges in the nucleus perfectly balance the negative charges surrounding it. The model shows an atom and the relative location of the subatomic particles.

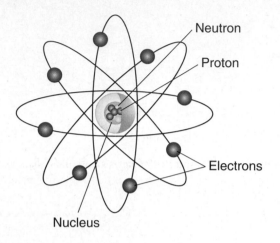

Figure 1-1. Atom Diagram
Simplified model of an atom showing relative locations of protons, neutrons, and electrons.

Ions are formed when an atom loses an electron or gains an extra one from another source. If electrons outnumber protons in an atom, the atom has an overall negative charge and is referred to as a negative ion or anion, whereas protons outnumbering electrons form a positive ion or cation. Because neutral is always more stable—less reactive— than charged ions, positively charged atoms often combine with negatively charged atoms to form molecules.

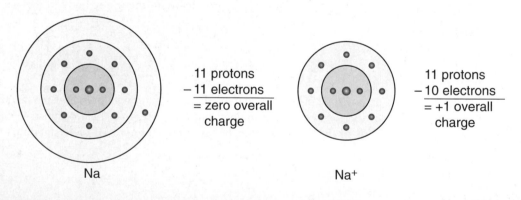

Figure 1-2. Positive Ion Formation
The electron is removed from its path around the nucleus, causing the number of protons to outnumber surrounding electrons.

Molecules and Bonding

A **molecule** is any structure comprised of 2 or more atoms bonded together. These atoms can be the same, as in a molecule of nitrogen or iodine, or they can be different, as when a sodium ion combines with a potassium ion to form potassium chloride.

Within a bond, at least one electron is shared by each of the two atoms. The degree of sharing of this electron classifies the bond as either covalent or ionic. In **covalent bonds**, each atom participating in the formation of a bond provides an electron, and the resulting pair of electrons is nearly equally shared between the two atoms. This occurs in the same or similar patoms, more specifically when two atoms identified as nonmetals bond.

Ionic bonds occur when two charged ions interact. In this bond, at least one electron is completely donated from one atom to another. Ionic bonds almost always occur when a metal and a nonmetal bond together. The most common example of an ionic bond is common table salt, sodium chloride. The sodium atom donates its extra electron to the chlorine atom, forming positively and negatively charged ions, respectively. Because opposites attract, these two ions bind tightly together in an ionic bond.

ACIDS, BASES, AND pH SCALE

From household cleaners to orange juice, almost all daily items can be classified as acids or bases. Most foods and beverages are moderately acidic. Blood, by contrast, is normally slightly basic.

Acids and Bases

The most common way to classify acids and bases is by measuring how they affect the hydrogen ion concentration, designated as $[H^+]$, in water when they dissociate into their component cations and anions. Chemicals that increase the $[H^+]$ are called **acids** (e.g., vinegar, orange and other citrus juices, and the hydrochloric acid in our stomachs). Chemicals that decrease the $[H^+]$ in water when they dissociate are referred to as **bases** (e.g., soap, baking soda [sodium bicarbonate], and bleach). The relative strength of each of these chemicals to increase or decrease the $[H^+]$ in water can be shown with the pH scale.

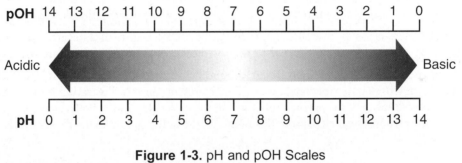

Figure 1-3. pH and pOH Scales
pH + pOH = 14 for aqueous solutions at 298 K.

The **pH scale** is a logarithmic scale ranging from 0 to 14 that is centered around the $[H^+]$ in pure water. Pure water has a pH of 7, which is neutral—neither acidic nor basic. Solutions with increasingly greater $[H^+]$ are increasingly acidic and have progressively *lower* pH, down to the acidic extreme of 0. Solutions with progressively lower $[H^+]$ are increasingly alkaline (basic) and have increasingly *higher* pH, up to an alkaline extreme of 14.

Table 1-1. Hydrogen Ion Concentration and pH

$[H^+]$	pH	Solution
High	Low, <7	Acidic
Low	High, >7	Basic

For biological purposes, the primary focus of acidity and alkalinity is how it relates to blood pH. Blood has a normal pH range of 7.35–7.45. A pH that deviates far outside this range can be lethal. If a person has blood pH <7.35, the person is said to be acidotic or have **acidosis**. When pH >7.45, the person has **alkalosis** or is alkalotic.

Acid-Base Balance and Buffers

Because the body requires a very narrow pH range in which to function optimally, deviations outside this range can have far-reaching effects. Here, the focus is on understanding the most important and often confusing buffer system and chemical reaction in the body: the bicarbonate buffer system. A buffer system, or **buffer**, minimizes the impact on a system's pH from the onslaught of an acid or a base. Buffers are reactions in a dynamic equilibrium that can neutralize bases and acids without meaningfully affecting the pH.

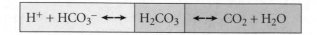

$$H^+ + HCO_3^- \longleftrightarrow \quad H_2CO_3 \quad \longleftrightarrow CO_2 + H_2O$$

Figure 1-4. Acid-Base Buffer Reaction

Central to this reaction is carbonic acid, H_2CO_3. You should be very familiar with this chemical if you have ever had any kind of carbonated beverage or soda. What happens to soda as soon as you pour it into a glass? It almost immediately starts to bubble and foam up, sometimes over the edge of the glass. Sometimes, even before pouring, you can see bubbles forming on the inside of the bottle. This reaction is the side shaded in **blue**, going from the **green** box and moving right. It is spontaneous in that direction and forms the respiratory side of this buffer system.

In the yellow shaded area, you have what often is referred to as the renal component of the reaction. It illustrates an alternative option for breaking down the carbonic acid in the **green** section. It could be broken down into a hydrogen ion and a bicarbonate ion. Carbon dioxide (CO_2) is most commonly transported in the bloodstream as the bicarbonate ion (HCO_3^-). Bubbles of CO_2 do not effervesce in a person's blood.

Keep in mind the following during further analysis of these reactions: Both the **blue** and yellow shaded sides can move left to right through the arrow, or right to left, depending on the needs of the body. Furthermore, you will seldom see this reaction with the intermediate, carbonic acid, present. Yet this illustration hopefully shows why this reaction is possible; it is simply a rearrangement of atoms in the molecules. In the body, enzymes catalyze reactions without stopping at the carbonic acid step. From this point on, the only reaction that will be referred to is the bicarbonate buffer system.

$$HCO_3^- + H^+ \longrightarrow CO_2 + H_2O$$

Figure 1-5. The Bicarbonate Buffer System

This reaction is always happening regardless of whether any species are added or removed on either side of the double-headed arrow. This is what is known as dynamic equilibrium and is illustrated with a double-headed arrow separating the reactants (left side) from the products (right side).

A principle in chemistry dictates in which direction an equilibrium reaction, such as a buffer reaction, will go based on adding or removing chemical species from either side of the arrow. If this system is stressed, by, say, adding H^+ to the system, the reaction would go to the right to eliminate the newly introduced and excess H^+. The reaction would similarly move from left to right if CO_2 is removed from the system; the reaction would move to replace it to maintain equilibrium.

Because this reaction can move in both directions (indicated by the double-headed arrow), if excess CO_2 is added to the system, the reaction will move to the left to relieve the stress. Finally, if it were somehow possible to remove HCO_3^- from the system, the reaction would proceed in the direction that replenishes it (i.e., the left), as shown in Figure 1-5. You can play the equilibrium game by adding or removing any of the species—but *only* these 4 species. Let's take this into the world of the paramedics, shall we?

Acid-Base Disorders

The maintenance of acid-base balance is crucial for survival. The body is relatively adroit at compensating for variations in pH by employing the acid-base buffer reaction discussed previously.

Table 1-2. Acid-Base Disturbances

Condition	Causes	Symptoms
Respiratory acidosis	• Hypoventilation • Cardiac/respiratory arrest • Asphyxiation • Head injury	• Slow/no breathing • Flushed skin • Headache
Respiratory alkalosis	• Fever • Excessive BVM (bag-valve-mask) ventilation • Anxiety	• Carpal-pedal spasms • Tingling lips and face • Dizziness
Metabolic acidosis	• Diabetic ketoacidosis • Lactic acidosis • Aspirin overdose	• Kussmaul respirations • Flushed skin • Shortness of breath
Metabolic alkalosis	• Excessive vomiting • Antacid overdoses • Eating disorders	• Slow breathing • Altered mental status • Vomiting

Respiratory acidosis is a decrease in blood pH that primarily has a respiratory component. The human body has a necessarily efficient way of removing CO_2 from the body so that this does not happen, but let's take a moment to understand what happens if that fails. Looking at the reaction in Figure 1-5, where might respirations come into play? With the CO_2, of course. Now, in which direction would the reaction need to proceed to relieve the stress of excess CO_2? To the left, exactly! When the body's CO_2 level increases, the reaction proceeds to the left to relieve the stress, which has the unfortunate outcome of increasing the $[H^+]$ and decreasing the body's pH, a process called acidosis. Therefore, this condition results from a systemic increase in CO_2 level.

A variety of causes underlie this condition; however, broadly, it always results from decreased respiratory efficiency or hypoventilation. Any condition that causes CO_2 retention can cause respiratory acidosis, including cardiac or respiratory arrest, airway obstruction, asphyxia, or a head injury. As respiratory acidosis progresses, more problems can be seen. To compensate for the acidosis, potassium ions are released from cells, which frequently results in cardiac dysrhythmias. Calcium ions are also released from muscles and cause a decreasing level of consciousness and delayed nerve signal transit, resulting in sluggish pupils and delayed responses to painful stimuli.

Respiratory alkalosis is an increase in pH, or a decrease in $[H^+]$, with a primarily respiratory component. If you're thinking that since acidosis is caused by a retention of CO_2, then alkalosis must be caused by an increase in exhalation of CO_2, you would be correct. An increase in respiratory rate does, indeed, lead to respiratory alkalosis and a resultant decrease in CO_2 in the blood. Looking at the reaction again, if CO_2 is removed from the system, the reaction will work to replace it, thus stripping the body of its hydrogen ion. A decrease in $[H^+]$ results in a higher or more basic pH, the hallmark of alkalosis.

Common causes of respiratory alkalosis are fever, anxiety, and excessive artificial ventilation. As alkalosis progresses, hydrogen ions leave the cells in an attempt to replenish what has been lost from the high respiratory rate. To compensate for this, calcium ions move into the cells, resulting in a state of hypocalcemia, which is responsible for the symptoms that can be seen in many alkalotic patients, including carpal-pedal spasms, tingling in the lips and face, and dizziness.

Pro-Tip

Monitoring end-tidal CO_2, written as $EtCO_2$, will provide an immediate and ongoing assessment of patients experiencing pH problems.

- The patient with **respiratory alkalosis** will have a decreased $EtCO_2$ value because much of it has been exhaled out of the body.
- The patient with **respiratory acidosis** will initially have a high $EtCO_2$ due to hypoventilation but after a few good ventilations, this value should assume normal levels.

Metabolic acidosis is a type of acidosis that results primarily from a metabolic disorder or ingestion and typically does not contain a respiratory component; that is, metabolic acidosis does not need hypoventilation to occur. In this case, the ingestion of a poison or an intentional overdose, or the body's usual production of acids through normal processes, overwhelms the body's ability to remove the acids that are present. Refer back to the reaction in bicarbonate buffer system (Figure 1-5); the body's primary means of relieving a stress of excess acid is to have that reaction proceed to the right, producing more CO_2. The person will then breathe faster and more deeply to try and exhale the CO_2 being produced.

Diabetic ketoacidosis (DKA) heads our list of common causes of metabolic acidosis. DKA occurs in patients who do not take any or enough insulin, which causes cells to shift to using fatty acids for fuel in lieu of glucose. A more detailed treatment of this condition can be found in the diabetic emergencies section of chapter 5. Lactic acidosis, the presumed cause of death in the movie *A Few Good Men*, occurs when the cells are not getting enough oxygen (O_2) and shift to anaerobic respiration, which leaves behind a lot of acids. Aspirin overdoses also cause metabolic acidosis because this is a direct ingestion of an acid: salicylic acid. Signs of metabolic acidosis include Kussmaul respirations (deep, rapid respirations), hot flushed skin, and bounding pulses.

Metabolic alkalosis is perhaps the rarest of acid-base disturbances and occurs when the system loses an excessive amount of acid. Look at the reaction in Figure 1-5 again. You can see that if acid is removed from the system, the reaction will proceed to the left in an attempt to replenish it. It will do this by intentionally retaining CO_2 and thus reducing respirations.

The most likely cause of this in the emergency setting is prolonged vomiting. The elimination of acid in this manner is the fastest way to cause the necessary reduction in circulating hydrogen ions. Excessive intake of acid-neutralizing medication, such as over-the-counter antacids, also could account for metabolic alkalosis.

Pro-Tip

$EtCO_2$ monitoring in metabolic acidosis or alkalosis also can provide valuable insight into a patient's status. The patient with Kussmaul respirations in metabolic acidosis will have a low $EtCO_2$ that continues to decrease slowly across time. $EtCO_2$ will continue to drop as the body attempts to remove more hydrogen ions from solution. Metabolic alkalosis will have a higher than expected $EtCO_2$, thus forcing more hydrogen ions back into solution. More information on $EtCO_2$ is in chapter 3.

CELLULAR STRUCTURE AND FUNCTION

The human body contains approximately 37 trillion cells. These cells create tissues from which organs form. Each cell serves a purpose, communicating and carrying out the reactions that make life possible. Interestingly, bacterial cells outnumber the eukaryotic cells in our bodies about 10 to 1. But the sheer number of cells from which the human body is created is not nearly as impressive as the numerous functions these cells can perform, from conduction of impulses through the nervous system, which allows for memory and learning, to the simultaneous contraction of cardiac myocytes, which pump blood through the entire human body.

The first major distinction that can be made between living organisms is whether they are composed of prokaryotic or eukaryotic cells. Eukaryotic organisms can be either unicellular or multicellular. **Eukaryotic cells** contain a true nucleus enclosed in a membrane; prokaryotic cells do not contain a nucleus. The major organelles are identified in the eukaryotic cell.

Each cell has a **cell membrane** enclosing a semifluid cytosol in which the **organelles** are suspended. In eukaryotic cells, most organelles are membrane bound, which allows for the compartmentalization of functions. Membranes of eukaryotic cells consist of a phospholipid bilayer. This membrane is unique because its surfaces are hydrophilic, electrostatically interacting with aqueous environments inside and outside the cell; its inner portion, on the other hand, is hydrophobic, which helps provide a highly selective barrier between the interior of the cell and the external environment. The **cytosol** diffuses molecules throughout the cell. Within the **nucleus**, genetic material is encoded in **deoxyribonucleic acid (DNA)**, which is organized into **chromosomes**. Eukaryotic cells reproduce by **mitosis**, which results in the formation of 2 identical daughter cells.

The **nucleus** is the control center of the cell, containing all the genetic material necessary for replicating the cell. The nucleus is surrounded by a nuclear membrane or envelope, a double membrane that maintains a nuclear environment separate and distinct from the cytoplasm. Nuclear pores in the nuclear membrane allow for the selective, two-way exchange of material between the cytoplasm and the nucleus.

The genetic material (DNA) contains coding regions called **genes**. Linear DNA is wound around organizing proteins called **histones**, which are then further wound into linear strands called **chromosomes**. The location of DNA in the nucleus allows for the compartmentalization of DNA transcription separate from ribonucleic acid (RNA) translation. Finally, in a subsection of the nucleus known as the nucleolus, ribosomal RNA (rRNA) is synthesized. The nucleolus actually takes up approximately 25% of the volume of the entire nucleus and often can be identified as a darker spot in the nucleus.

Mitochondria often are called *the power plants of the cell*, in reference to their important metabolic functions. The mitochondrion consists of two layers: the outer and inner membranes. The **outer membrane** serves as a barrier between the cytosol and the inner environment of the mitochondrion. The inner membrane, which is thrown into numerous infoldings called **cristae**, contains the molecules and enzymes necessary for the electron transport chain. The cristae are highly convoluted structures that increase the surface area available for electron transport chain enzymes. The space between the inner and outer membranes is called the **intermembrane space**; the space inside the inner membrane is called the mitochondrial **matrix**. The pumping of protons from the mitochondrial matrix to the intermembrane space establishes the proton-motive force; ultimately, these protons flow through *ATP synthase* to generate adenosine triphosphate (ATP) during oxidative phosphorylation.

Mitochondria are different from other parts of the cell because they are semiautonomous. They contain some of their own genes and replicate independently of the nucleus via binary fission. As such, they are paradigmatic examples of cytoplasmic or extranuclear inheritance—the transmission of genetic material is independent of the nucleus. Mitochondria are thought to have evolved from an anaerobic prokaryote that engulfed an aerobic prokaryote, thus establishing a symbiotic relationship.

In addition to keeping the cell alive by providing energy, the mitochondria also are capable of killing the cell by releasing enzymes from the electron transport chain. This release kick-starts a process known as **apoptosis**, or programmed cell death.

Lysosomes are membrane-bound structures containing hydrolytic enzymes that are capable of breaking down many different substrates, including substances ingested by endocytosis and cellular waste products. The lysosomal membrane sequesters these enzymes to prevent damage to the cell. However, release of these enzymes can occur in a process known as **autolysis**. Like mitochondria, when lysosomes release their hydrolytic enzymes, apoptosis occurs. In this case, the released enzymes directly lead to the degradation of cellular components.

The **endoplasmic reticulum** (ER) comprises a series of interconnected membranes that are actually contiguous with the nuclear envelope. The double membrane of the endoplasmic reticulum is folded into numerous invaginations, creating complex structures with a central lumen. The two varieties of ER are smooth and rough.

- The **rough ER** (RER) is studded with ribosomes, which permit the translation of proteins destined for secretion directly into its lumen.
- **Smooth ER** (SER) lacks ribosomes and is used primarily for lipid synthesis (such as phospholipids in the cell membrane) and the detoxification of certain drugs and poisons. The SER also transports proteins from the RER to the Golgi apparatus.

Pro-Tip

Liver cells (hepatocytes) contain a large amount of SER because they are heavily involved in detoxification. SER increases in alcoholics as well. Because the SER also is involved in lipid (fat) synthesis, alcoholics develop fatty livers.

The **Golgi apparatus** consists of stacked membrane-bound sacs. Materials from the ER are transferred to the Golgi apparatus in vesicles. Once in the Golgi apparatus, these cellular products may be modified by the addition of various groups, including carbohydrates, phosphates, and sulfates. The Golgi apparatus also may modify cellular products by introducing signal sequences, which direct the delivery of the product to a specific cellular location. After modification and sorting in the Golgi apparatus, cellular products are repackaged in vesicles, which are subsequently transferred to the correct cellular location. If the product is destined for secretion, then the secretory vesicle merges with the cell membrane, and its contents are released via **exocytosis**.

One of the primary functions of **peroxisomes** is the breakdown of very long chain fatty acids via beta-oxidation. Peroxisomes contain hydrogen peroxide, participate in the synthesis of phospholipids, and contain some of the enzymes involved in the pentose phosphate pathway.

The **cytoskeleton** provides structure to the cell and helps maintain the cell's shape. In addition, the cytoskeleton provides a conduit for transporting materials around the cell. The three components of the cytoskeleton are microfilaments, microtubules, and intermediate filaments.

Microfilaments are composed of solid polymerized rods of **actin**. The actin filaments are organized into bundles and networks and resist both compression and fracture, providing protection for the cell. Actin filaments also can use ATP to generate force for movement by interacting with **myosin**, such as in muscle contraction.

Microfilaments also play a role in cytokinesis, or the division of materials between daughter cells. During mitosis, the cleavage furrow is formed from microfilaments, which organize as a ring at the site of division between the two new daughter cells. As the actin filaments within this ring contract, the ring becomes smaller, eventually pinching off the connection between the two daughter cells.

Unlike microfilaments, **microtubules** are hollow polymers of **tubulin** proteins. Microtubules radiate throughout a cell, providing the primary pathways along which motor proteins such as **kinesin** and **dynein** carry vesicles.

Cilia and flagella are motile structures composed of microtubules. **Cilia** are projections from a cell that are primarily involved in the movement of materials along the surface of the cell; for example, cilia line the respiratory tract and are involved in the movement of mucus. **Flagella** are structures involved in the movement of the cell itself, such as the movement of sperm cells through the reproductive tract. Cilia and flagella share the same structure: they are composed of 9 pairs of microtubules forming an outer ring, with 2 microtubules in the center. This **9 + 2 structure** is seen only in eukaryotic organelles of motility. Bacterial flagella have a different structure with a different chemical composition, which will be discussed later in this chapter.

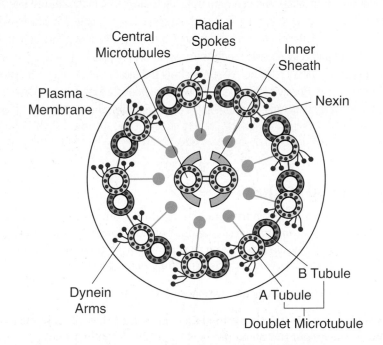

Figure 1-6. Cilium and Flagellum Structure
Microtubules are organized into a ring of 9 doublets with 2 central microtubules.

Centrioles are found in a region of the cell called the **centrosome**. They are the organizing centers for microtubules and are structured as 9 triplets of microtubules with a hollow center. During mitosis, the centrioles migrate to opposite poles of the dividing cell and organize the mitotic spindle. The microtubules emanating from the centrioles attach to the chromosomes via complexes called **kinetochores** and can exert force on the sister chromatids, pulling them apart.

The diverse group of **filamentous (intermediate) proteins** includes keratin, desmin, vimentin, and lamins. Many intermediate filaments are involved in cell-cell adhesion or the maintenance of the overall integrity of the cytoskeleton. Intermediate filaments can withstand a tremendous amount of tension, making the cell structure more rigid. In addition, intermediate filaments help anchor other organelles, including the nucleus. The identity of the intermediate filament proteins within a cell is specific to the cell and tissue type.

SHOCK

For a person to be healthy and sustain life, several things must happen without fail. First, O_2 must be able to enter the alveoli from the atmosphere, in a process called **ventilation**. Once in the alveoli, O_2 must be able to enter the blood vessels at the same time CO_2 is removed without interference, in a process called **respiration**. These two processes must happen in parallel, with the body taking in macronutrients (food) and having the ability to break down food into usable pieces through the process of digestion. These pieces then must be absorbed in the intestines and into the bloodstream and travel in the blood plasma to the destination tissues, with O_2 riding attached to hemoglobin. **Perfusion** is O_2 and nutrients getting to the destination cells and tissues. As long as all these processes continue uninterrupted, there should be no problems. However, if any of these processes is disrupted, hypoperfusion can occur and result in death if not recognized and reversed in a timely manner.

Pro-Tip

You may hear ventilation, respiration, and perfusion used interchangeably. In the strictest interpretation, they are not. **Ventilation** is the act of moving air in and out of the lungs. It does not address whether gas exchange occurs in the alveoli. **Respiration** is gas exchange across the alveoli-capillary border. **Perfusion** is the exchange of gases, nutrients, and waste products across the capillary wall into and out of the cell. From these definitions, "respiratory rate" or "respirations" are technically misnomers; "ventilatory rate" or "ventilations" is more correct. However, these terms have been around a long time, and rather than be pedantic, the terms *respiratory rate* and *respirations* will be used to describe the number of ventilations a patient takes in 1 minute.

Anatomy and Physiology of Shock

To maintain all the requirements for a fully functioning body, among other things, the body needs a functioning pump, a properly sized container, and an appropriate amount of fluid for the pump to move throughout the container. **Shock** can be thought of as any deviation from normal in any of these three requirements. Shock, and its severity, centers around blood pressure, so let's start by explaining blood pressure.

Blood pressure is dependent on peripheral vascular resistance and cardiac output.

Peripheral vascular resistance is the resistance of blood flow through all the vessels of the body, excluding those in the lungs. **Cardiac output** is the amount of blood pumped out of the heart in 1 minute; it is the product of stroke volume and heart rate.

- Stroke volume is the amount of blood ejected from the left ventricle of the heart with each beat or contraction.
- Heart rate is the number of beats in 1 minute.

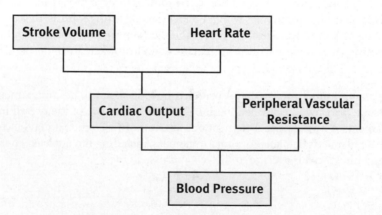

Figure 1-7. Blood Pressure Cascade

Pump

The heart must be able to adequately pump blood around the body, and, most importantly, it must have adequate strength to get blood up to the brain against gravity. By itself, pure muscle strength of the heart is not enough. There must be enough blood returning to the heart from the body to fill and stretch the chambers of the heart, which is called the **preload**. As blood flows into the heart chambers, the chambers stretch, thereby increasing the contraction strength of the heart. Finally, outflow of blood must not be obstructed. This **afterload**, or pressure against which the heart must pump, needs to be lower than the force of the heart's contraction to overcome it. In the cases of myocardial damage, such as from a heart attack or cardiac contusion from trauma, the contractile strength of the heart is diminished, which will eventually lead to shock.

Container

The vasculature (collection of blood vessels) must be of appropriate size for the amount of fluid contained within it. Under normal circumstances this is typically not an issue, but during severe blood loss or dehydration, the container as it is normally may be too large for the volume of blood remaining. In times of crisis, the autonomic nervous system is responsible for shutting down nonessential capillary beds, such as those found in the skin, and constricting the venous and arterial side of the vasculature. This effectively shrinks the overall size of the container to better match the volume within. Taken a step further, this measure will maintain blood pressure at least in the short term until fluid or blood can be replaced. In some instances, the vessels of the container may suddenly dilate, or get larger, resulting in the current fluid volume being too small, which can occur in cases of spinal trauma.

Fluid

The blood has several responsibilities in the prevention of hypoperfusion. There must be an adequate number of red blood cells with hemoglobin capable of carrying O_2. In cases of hemorrhage, insufficient red blood cells may be remaining to carry adequate O_2 to the tissues. In this situation, the best efforts of fluid resuscitation and oxygenation will ultimately prove futile. In the case of anemia, there is insufficient hemoglobin to hold O_2, potentially resulting in shock as well. Finally, the blood must be able to get to the end organ to deliver its O_2 and nutrients. If the container remains constrained for too long, between starvation of the cells from a lack of nutrients and a buildup of waste products, cellular death and—eventually—organ death are inevitable.

Types of Shock

A variety of things can affect the pump, the container, or the fluid. Although they will all produce similar symptoms, their causes, and consequently the optimal treatment, are different. The types of shock you will encounter as a paramedic will be presented first, which is followed by a discussion of the progression and stages of shock. Finally, the end of this chapter addresses the assessment and treatment of shock in broad and general terms. In later chapters, these same causes of shock will be presented, including a discussion of more specific treatments. Here, the phrase *treat for shock* will be defined.

Cardiogenic shock, as the name implies, starts in the heart. This happens when the heart is no longer strong enough to move the blood around the body and through the lungs. It often results from a heart attack, or the cumulative damage from a series of heart attacks. This topic is covered in much greater detail in chapter 5.

Hypovolemic and hemorrhagic shock are forms of shock that are similar but not exactly the same. **Hypovolemic shock** is exactly that; it is shock that results from a low circulating volume. It can be caused by excessive vomiting and diarrhea, poor fluid intake, or extravasation from burns. **Hemorrhagic shock** is a specific form of hypovolemic shock that occurs because of blood loss. The blood loss can be external or internal from trauma or can be from cumulative blood loss from gastrointestinal bleeding or something similar. Hemorrhagic shock carries with it the extra burden during resuscitation of replacing red blood cells. With hypovolemic shock, aggressive fluid administration often is sufficient.

Obstructive shock refers to a variety of disorders that hamper preload or elevate afterload to the point where cardiac function is disrupted. Some examples include pulmonary embolism (PE), pneumothorax, and blood return from the inferior vena cava.

Distributive shock is the collective name for several different causes of shock that all have displacement of fluid as a common thread. In each, fluid is somehow shifted from the vessels to other locations within the body. Septic shock, anaphylactic shock, neurogenic shock, and psychogenic shock are all forms of distributive shock.

Septic shock is caused by bacterial toxins infiltrating the bloodstream from a local infection or a systemic infection. The body's reaction to this infection is to initiate a widespread inflammatory response, which causes systemic vasodilation and increased capillary permeability. In addition to being too small of a volume for the now dilated container, fluid leaks from the capillaries into the interstitial space (the potential space between the cells and outside the vasculature), further worsening hypovolemia.

Although our immune system is truly a marvel, occasionally, it short-circuits and wildly overreacts to an otherwise innocuous invader, such as bee venom or egg proteins. When this happens, it starts a complicated cascade of events that can eventually, and sometimes rapidly, lead to death. This is known as **anaphylactic shock**. During the progression of anaphylaxis, capillaries once again become leaky, and the vasculature dilates, leading to a state of profound hypotension. As if that were not enough, unlike in septic shock, this also happens in the airways, the lips, and the tongue, leading to difficulty breathing and asphyxiation.

Neurogenic shock results from an insult to the spinal cord. Sometimes it is caused by an infection, but most often, trauma is the cause. In addition to paralysis, which may be a patient's complaint, the astute paramedic will be far more wary of systemic, uncontrolled dilation of *all* blood vessels inferior to the injury. Once again, the container is too large for the fluid within (though, thankfully, the capillaries are not leaky), and profound hypotension ensues. In addition, the area affected by the vasodilation will not be sweating like the area superior to it. Because the blood vessels nearest the skin of the affected area also are dilated, the skin also will appear flushed, whereas the remainder of the body will be white or gray.

Psychogenic shock is not mentioned in many texts; however, it is worth noting here. Psychogenic shock is the "see-blood-and-faint" variety of shock, and, yes, it is real. In cases where a person becomes scared or otherwise overwhelmed, such as from negative news, blood vessels dilate, if only transiently, resulting in a container too big for the fluid. Often, the person passes out briefly; once supine, the patient regains consciousness as the nervous system recovers and regains control.

Progression of Shock

Whatever the cause of the shock, all forms will progress through 3 distinct phases, culminating in certain death if not recognized early and treated with definitive steps.

During **compensated shock**, the body's main concern is the preservation of a blood pressure, specifically the mean arterial pressure (MAP). To maintain brain, kidney, and coronary artery perfusion, the MAP must be >60 mmHg. The MAP can be calculated based on the following equation, where DBP is the diastolic blood pressure and SBP is the systolic blood pressure.

$$\text{MAP} = \frac{2(\text{Diastolic}) + \text{Systolic}}{3}$$

Using this equation, the MAP for a person whose blood pressure is 106/70 can be calculated: [2(70) + 106]/3 = 82.

Consider a person who is losing blood over a period of time. As the person first starts to lose blood, the blood vessels begin to constrict, shrinking the container around the diminishing volume of circulating fluid. **Baroreceptors**, specialized areas within blood vessels extremely sensitive to otherwise imperceptible changes in blood pressure, signal this drop to the brain, and the autonomic nervous system responds by constricting blood vessels. The heart rate also accelerates during this phase and is one of the earliest findings in any shock. Remember the relationship of heart rate and blood pressure; as the heart rate increases, so does cardiac output and, therefore, blood pressure. Sweating and pale skin become apparent as the bleeding continues.

In **decompensated shock**, the patient's bleeding continues. The volume of loss has begun to outstrip the body's ability to recover on its own. The heart rate has increased to the point where it cannot go any higher, approaching 140–150 beats per minute in the adult. The capillary sphincters to all nonessential areas are closed, and the patient's skin is now systemically mottled or pale and ashen. Capillaries are now beginning to shut down blood flow to essential areas, including the entire digestive tract and kidneys in a last-ditch effort to maintain the person's blood pressure and MAP to the heart, lungs, and brain. The hallmark of this stage is a measurably low blood pressure because the body's self-protection mechanism has been overwhelmed. External support for the patient is now necessary and should include aggressive fluid replacement before the patient progresses into the final stage of shock.

Irreversible shock is the point at which end organ failure and cellular death have begun and will, ultimately, be unrecoverable. Kidney failure and death have begun; even if the shock is adequately treated at this stage, death is frequently unavoidable. Extended periods of hypotension lead to this stage.

Assessment and Treatment

This section addresses global assessment and treatment of the person in shock. More specific treatments are addressed in later chapters. Be on the lookout for "Practical Point," designed to help you link cognitive knowledge from this book with practical knowledge essential for the psychomotor exam portion of the NRPE.

Patient Assessment

Scene Size-Up

Sizing up the scene begins with any dispatch information you are given and any additional information you are provided during the response. This part of the assessment gives you an opportunity to anticipate and request additional resources, such as police, fire, or additional ambulances. When arriving on the scene, evaluate your safety as you walk up to and enter the patient's location. While you are looking for clues to your patient's condition, be aware of any potential weapons in the vicinity of the patient. Now that you have encountered your patient, will you and your partner alone be able to carry the patient? This is another opportunity to request additional support. Finally, consider any obstructions for accessing the patient or egressing from the scene; the way you came in may not be how you exit. Hazards here could be as insidious as a welcome mat becoming a tripping hazard or as obvious as loose stair treads.

Pro-Tip
Scene size-up should be continuous and ongoing. Previously safe scenes can change in a heartbeat. Anytime you feel uneasy, leave, call the police, and ensure crew safety once again before returning.

Practical Point
Once you take deliberate actions to mitigate perceived or actual threats to your safety, it will garner you 3 out of 3 possible points on the scene safety portion of both Oral Exam stations.

General Impression

The first step is to form a general impression of your patient. This is a simple thought that will frame your thinking about the severity of the patient's condition. It might sound like the following: "A 58-year-old female is seated on her couch in no apparent distress" or "This is a 28-year-old male lying unresponsive on a bed with vomit on the pillow and agonal respirations."

ABCDE

More than just the first 5 letters of the alphabet, ABCDE guides you to what will kill your patient first: Airway, Breathing, Circulation and Consider C-Spine, Disability, and Expose.

- **Airway:** Assess the airway for patency and immediately relieve any obstructions.

- **Breathing**: Check breathing for any increased work of breathing, respiratory rate, and breath sounds. Even if you do not get a respiratory rate immediately, you can note if the respirations are fast or slow or follow an altered pattern from normal. In the patient with shock, respirations should be normal or slightly elevated. Breath sounds of crackles or rales could indicate cardiogenic shock, but further investigation is necessary. Wheezes and stridor might be present in anaphylactic shock as the upper and lower airways swell.

- **Circulation and Consider C-Spine**: A quick check of the pulse, even if a rate is not immediately obtained, can tell you a lot—fast or slow, weak or strong, regular or irregular. During the pulse check, you can assess the patient's skin; here you can notice if the skin is cool or hot to the touch, sweaty, or clammy. The person in shock will have pale skin, plus weak and rapid peripheral pulses as they try to compensate to maintain blood pressure and MAP. Consider the need for cervical spine stabilization at this point.

- **Disability**: This is the neurological assessment and can include any or all of the Glasgow Coma Scale (GCS), any of a variety of stroke scoring techniques, or simply AVPU (alert, voice, pain, unresponsive). Note also the degree of orientation, which should include the patient's orientation to person, place, and time. The AVPU scale helps you determine the shock patient's level of responsiveness. Note the initial level and reassess constantly in the critical patient.

- **Expose**: Here you will expose the patient as needed for assessment and treatment purposes. Many times, this is not required. For the patient in shock, keeping the patient warm is of paramount importance, so undressing the patient is essentially contraindicated except in the cases of external hemorrhage and perhaps cases of neurogenic shock to visualize the injury and other symptoms. If the patient needs to be undressed, ensure that steps are taken to maintain the patient's modesty and temperature during treatment and transport.

After the life threats are addressed, you will need to assess SAMPLE and OPPQRST as you would for any patient. More information on this can be found in the patient assessment chapter.

Treatment

With shock, the same treatment can generally be used regardless of the cause or source. Needless to say, maintaining a patent airway, maintaining an adequate breathing rate and quality, and treating cardiac arrest take priority over all sequential treatment, especially for patients in shock. For a patient in shock, you may need to initiate an advanced airway if the patient is unable to maintain it on their own. At the very least, administer O_2 via a non-rebreathing mask or BVM if breathing quality is inadequate.

As already seen, circulation in shock can be highly compromised, for a variety of reasons. It should go without saying that if a patient is pulseless, high-quality cardiopulmonary respiration (CPR) should be initiated early and continued until a measurable return of spontaneous circulation occurs, and treatment should be continued along cardiac arrest algorithms (see the Cardiology, Cardiac Emergencies, and Resuscitation chapter). Because shock often is a lengthy progression, you will likely encounter patients who still have a pulse, though often weak and "thready," so maintaining and improving pulse quality and rate should be the primary goal once you are confident you have secured an airway. Starting a large-bore (≥18 gauge) intravenous line with a liter of a crystalloid solution is a great first step. Even if the patient is not currently hypotensive, the progression of shock will eventually lead to hypotension, so it is better to be ahead of the curve. The crystalloid solution could be normal saline solution (NSS) or Ringer's lactate and should be administered as a bolus of 20 mL/kg in approximately 500 mL increments. Fluid resuscitation should be titrated to the patient's needs; however, aim for the following perfusion goals:

- Return of radial pulses
- Maintenance of SBP >80 mmHg
- MAP >60 mmHg

These goals should be achieved without pulmonary edema or jugular vein distension.

In addition to O_2 and intravenous fluid therapy, proper patient positioning and core body temperature maintenance are essential steps to be taken for any shock patient. Keep the patient supine. While Trendelenburg positioning was once recommended, it no longer is as it exacerbates too many other problems.

Keeping the patient warm during transport will help the body put energy into addressing the problem rather than shivering to generate heat. Layer on a few blankets and keep the back of the ambulance hotter than you may otherwise prefer. In addition, administer warm fluids whenever possible so the body does not have to work to raise the temperature of that fluid. Avoid localized heat sources such as heat packs and pads because they have the potential to cause more vasodilation and actually worsen hypotension.

Pro-Tip

Intravenous fluid kept at room temperature is not "warmed" because it is still about 30° less than body temperature. Warmed fluid should be at approximately 100°F. If the ambulance does not have a warmer, some paramedics will wrap the intravenous line a few times around a hot pack and then wrap the coil and pack in a towel or blanket. This technique might not produce a meaningful change in the temperature of the fluid, but it can't hurt!

Practical Point

The bleeding and shock station is an optional basic life support (BLS) skill station that may be encountered during the psychomotor skills portion of the NRPE. During voice treatment of a simulated injury on a patient, you will need to identify the BLS. Only treat for shock.

BLS includes the following:
- Provide high-flow O_2.
- Elevate the patient's legs.
- Cover the patient with blankets to maintain body temperature.
- Rapidly transport the patient to a trauma facility.

The first and last bullet points also are critical failure points! There is no benefit in this station to mentioning intravenous fluid resuscitation.

REVIEW QUESTIONS

Select the ONE best answer.

1. A chemical bond formed when an electron is completely donated from 1 atom to another is called a/an:

    A. Covalent bond.

    B. Ionic bond.

    C. Shared bond.

    D. Strong bond.

2. Use the pH information for the following common substances to answer questions 2 and 3.

    • Vinegar: pH = 2.9

    • Ammonia: pH = 10.6

    • Milk: pH = 6.7

    • Urine: pH = 6.0

    • Blood: pH = 7.4

    Which of the following pairs of substances are considered basic according to the indicated pH?

    A. Ammonia and blood

    B. Urine and vinegar

    C. Blood and milk

    D. Blood and urine

3. Which of the following is more acidic than ammonia?

    A. Blood

    B. Urine

    C. Vinegar

    D. All of the above

4. Use the following buffer equilibrium reaction for questions 4 and 5.

    $$HCO_3^- + H^+ \Leftrightarrow CO_2 + H_2O$$

    A patient who is apneic will retain CO_2. This will most likely result in what condition?

    A. Metabolic acidosis

    B. Metabolic alkalosis

    C. Respiratory acidosis

    D. Respiratory alkalosis

5. A 58-year-old female patient with a multiple-day history of eating without taking insulin has fast and deep respirations. This patient is breathing like this because she is in _____ acidosis because acids are building up in the bloodstream from _____.

   A. metabolic; ketoacid production from fat metabolism
   B. metabolic; poor CO_2 exchange at the alveolar level
   C. respiratory; ketoacid production from fat metabolism
   D. respiratory; poor CO_2 exchange at the alveolar level

6. The organelle responsible for >80% of the cell's ATP production is the:

   A. Golgi apparatus.
   B. Mitochondrion.
   C. RER.
   D. SER.

7. Your 40-year-old patient has the following vital signs: HR: 140; BP: 82/48; RR: 30. She is pale, is lethargic, and responds only to painful stimuli. What kind of shock is she most likely experiencing?

   A. Compensated shock
   B. Decompensated shock
   C. Hypovolemic shock
   D. Irreversible shock

8. Your assessment reveals the following about your patient: HR: 123; RR: 24; BP: 104/66. The patient has had a 4-day history of bloody diarrhea and is now weak and passes out when standing for too long. The ECG reveals a normal complex, but it is tachycardic with no ectopic beats. You have established intravenous access with a saline lock. What is the most appropriate next step?

   A. Nothing; the patient is compensating well
   B. Administer 2–5 mcg/kg/min dopamine
   C. Administer 2 L isotonic crystalloid
   D. Administer at least 500 mL isotonic crystalloid

9. Cardiogenic shock results from pump failure. Which of these medications will be most helpful in restoring an appropriate blood pressure to the patient in cardiogenic shock?

   A. Dopamine
   B. Nitroglycerine
   C. Labetalol
   D. Epinephrine

ANSWERS AND EXPLANATIONS

1. **The correct answer is (B).** When an atom loses or donates an electron to another atom, an ion is formed. The bond that forms between 2 ions is called an ionic bond. Covalent bonds (A) form between 2 atoms where the electrons in the bond are shared nearly equally. Shared (C) and strong bonds (D) do not exist.

2. **The correct answer is (A).** A pH >7 is considered basic; the only 2 substances listed that are basic are blood and ammonia. Everything else is acidic.

3. **The correct answer is (D).** All the listed materials are more acidic than ammonia because ammonia has the highest pH listed and therefore is the most basic. The most acidic substance listed is vinegar.

4. **The correct answer is (C).** An increase in CO_2, as a result of decreased respiratory rate or depth, will cause the buffer reaction to progress to the left as written to relieve the stress on the body of excess CO_2. This will then result in an increased $[H^+]$ caused by poor respiratory status and is known as respiratory acidosis. Respiratory alkalosis (D) is caused when the patient exhales too much CO_2, which might happen during hyperventilation. Exhaling too much CO_2 causes the reaction to progress to the right, leading to a reduction of $[H^+]$. Metabolic acidosis (A) is caused by a buildup of $[H^+]$ in the bloodstream as a result of metabolic processes, such as diabetic ketoacidosis. Metabolic alkalosis (B) generally occurs during times of protracted vomiting.

5. **The correct answer is (A).** During times of sugar (food) consumption coupled with an inadequate insulin regimen, the cells will shift to fat metabolism, resulting in a buildup of metabolic acids in the body. The only way the body can mitigate this acid buildup is to breathe faster and eliminate CO_2. This will cause the reaction to progress to the right faster, eliminating the acids and generating more CO_2. CO_2 is eliminated from the body by breathing faster, known as Kussmaul respirations. Water also is produced in excess during these times and is eliminated, with symptoms that include excessive urination and dehydration. Poor CO_2 exchange at the alveolar level could lead to respiratory acidosis.

6. **The correct answer is (B).** The mitochondria are the powerhouses of the cell. They produce much of the ATP along the folds of the inner membrane. SER (D) is responsible for detoxification and transport. RER (C) is responsible for protein synthesis. The Golgi apparatus (A) packages cellular product for exocytosis.

7. **The correct answer is (B).** From the scant details given in the question stem, it is impossible to determine the cause of the shock, so hypovolemic shock (C) is incorrect because there are many reasons for a person to have these vital signs without actually being hypovolemic. Based on the blood pressure of 82/48, the patient is no longer able to compensate for the fluid loss or shift. Therefore, the patient is in decompensated shock. Whether it is irreversible (D) will depend on many factors once the patient's vital signs are corrected in the hospital. A patient in compensated shock (A) will still be maintaining a normal blood pressure.

8. **The correct answer is (D).** The patient is compensating at this point but could benefit from some fluid expansion; 500 mL is an appropriate starting point. Reassessment after the bolus would indicate whether more fluid is needed. The pressor options of dopamine (B) are not yet appropriate because the hypovolemia needs to be first addressed with fluid. Two liters of fluid (C) may be required overall; however, delivering that volume all at once is seldom appropriate, especially in compensated hypovolemic shock.

9. **The correct answer is (A).** Dopamine is the medication of choice for cardiogenic shock. Its positive inotropic effects and minimal effects on peripheral circulation increase the blood pressure in a more desirable way than does epinephrine (D). Labetalol (C) would lower the blood pressure through peripheral vasodilation. Nitroglycerine (B) would lower the blood pressure as well.

Pharmacology 2

Learning Objectives

❑ Describe medication regulation in the United States and the schedule system.

❑ Differentiate between pharmacodynamics and pharmacokinetics.

❑ Explain how to initiate an intravenous line.

❑ Identify indications for initiating an intravenous line.

Understanding pharmacology is paramount to the paramedic's success. Dozens of medications are available that could improve a patient's condition long before arriving at the hospital.

MEDICATION REGULATION

In the 20th century, major laws affecting medication regulation in the United States were passed.

Table 2-1. Major U.S. Laws Regulating Medications

Year	Title of Regulation	Description
1906	Pure Food and Drug Act	Prohibited altering or mislabeling medications
1909	Opium Exclusion Act	Prohibited the importation of opium
1914	Harrison Narcotic Act	Regulated and taxed the manufacture and sale of opiates and cocaine products
1938	Food, Drug, and Cosmetic Act	Gave authority to the U.S. Food and Drug Administration to oversee the safety of food, drugs, and cosmetics
1970	Comprehensive Drug Abuse Prevention and Control Act	Classified potentially abused medications into one of 5 schedules, which included security, record keeping, and dispensing requirements

The Comprehensive Drug Abuse Prevention and Control Act led to the scheduling system that classifies all medications with a potential for abuse, shown in the following table.

Table 2-2. Schedule System for Controlled Substances

Schedule	Medication Example	Description
I	Marijuana, LSD (lysergic acid diethylamide), heroin	No medical purpose; great potential for psychological and physical addiction
II	Oxycodone, methamphetamines, meperidine, fentanyl, morphine	Drugs with a high potential for abuse but less than Schedule I. Continued use could lead to psychological and physical addiction. Contain <15 mg hydrocodone per dosage unit.
III	Ketamine, steroids, acetamino-phen with codeine	Drugs with moderate to low potential for psychological and physical addiction, less than Schedule II. Drugs have <90 mg codeine per dosage unit.
IV	Alprazolam, lorazepam, diazepam, zolpidem	Potential for abuse and any type of addiction
V	Narcotic cough medications, pregabalin	Lowest risk for abuse or addiction; generally for antidiarrheal, antitussive, or analgesic purposes

Sources, Forms, and Names

Medications are derived from multiple different sources beyond synthetic preparation in a laboratory. Medications such as atropine, digoxin, and morphine come from plant sources. Heparin and insulin are most commonly produced in and collected from animals. Many antibiotics are produced from microorganisms such as bacteria and molds. Minerals are essential to our diet and can be mined from the earth. Regardless of the source, however, by the time they reach the consumer, they have been put under rigorous quality control measures to ensure what the label says is what the patient gets.

Medications also can be delivered to the patient in a multitude of forms, which are as follows:

- **Tablet:** powder compressed into a solid to be swallowed
- **Capsule:** powder or gel surrounded with a gelatin shell
- **Suspension:** water-insoluble powder suspended in a thick sugary liquid that separates on standing; shaking is required to achieve the desired dose
- **Solution:** medication dissolved in another liquid, usually water
- **Metered dose inhaler:** liquid or finely powdered solid in a pressurized canister for inhalation
- **Topical:** applied to skin for treatment or moisturization of skin
- **Transdermal/transcutaneous:** medication applied to and absorbed through the skin for absorption into the bloodstream; often comes as a patch, such as a nicotine patch
- **Suppository:** medication contained within a greasy/waxy substance that melts in the body to deliver the medication; often inserted into rectum

Medications can be referred to by any of 3 names. Depending on the medication being requested, the typical person may use either the generic or trade name but never the chemical name.

- **Brand or Trade Name.** Name given to the medication by the manufacturer and approved by the Food and Drug Administration (e.g., Amidate).
- **Generic Name.** Name approved by the US Adopted Names Council and the World Health Organization to minimize medication name duplication. The original developer of a drug frequently suggests this name (e.g., etomidate).
- **Chemical Name.** Long name used by organic chemists to systematically name a structure. For example, the chemical name for etomidate is: ethyl 3-[(1R)-1-phenylethyl]imidazole-5 caboxylate.

Medication Terms

The following terms are used to describe medications:

- **Indications.** Why a drug is given—the symptoms it is used to treat.

- **Contraindications.** Reasons to not give a medication. There may be relative contraindications when a medication should be avoided in favor of another medication but may be given in extreme or emergent circumstances. Absolute contraindications are reasons the drug should never be given at any time, regardless of the circumstance.

- **Adverse Reactions or Side Effects.** These are nontherapeutic effects that a medication has on the body. They are not desired and often can be severe enough for a person to stop taking the medication. Side effects range from annoying or bothersome to dangerous or life threatening. A patient may experience none, one, or all of a drug's listed side effects.

- **Idiosyncratic Effects.** Specific unexpected, nontherapeutic reactions of a patient to a medication. Although side effects are typically predictable and listed on the label, idiosyncratic effects (also called untoward effects) may be unique to one patient or so rare as to have been left off the list of possible side effects.

- **Interactions.** When patients take more than one medication, care must be taken to avoid medication interactions. For example, a medication used to treat Condition A may potentiate (increase) the effects of a second drug used to treat Condition B, potentially to the point of toxicity. Alternatively, Medication X (or Food X) can inhibit or negate the effects of Medication Y. A classic example of this is grapefruit juice enhancing the absorption of certain statin medications that are used to treat high cholesterol, which, in turn, has caused patients to experience more side effects.

PHYSIOLOGY OF PHARMACOLOGY

Pharmacology is the study of medications and their effects on the body. This section addresses the pharmacodynamics and the pharmacokinetics of medications.

Pharmacodynamics

Pharmacodynamics is the process that a drug performs to alter processes in the body to bring about a desired effect. It also includes the overall response of the body to a medication. Here, the discussion focuses on the ways a drug impacts the body as well as other responses to the medication.

The surfaces of the cells within the human body bear many chemical receptors. These receptors bind to chemicals that are produced within the body (**endogenous chemicals**) which allow the body to respond naturally to changes in blood sodium, danger, anxiety, etc. Norepinephrine, dopamine, and acetylcholine are examples of endogenous chemicals. Modern medicine stimulates or inhibits the same cell receptors to induce desired therapeutic effects. These synthetic agents are called **exogenous chemicals** because they originate outside the body. They are more commonly known as *medications*.

Agonist medications bind to these receptor sites and not only act like the endogenous chemical that would naturally stimulate that receptor but also initiate a more magnified cellular response than the endogenous chemical would produce.

Antagonists produce the opposite effect on the receptor (think *anti-agonist*); they can work by competitive inhibition or noncompetitive inhibition.

- In **competitive inhibition**, the medication blocks the effects of the endogenous chemical by binding to the same receptor. How firmly the medication sticks to the receptor depends on the relative concentrations of antagonist versus agonist. If that receptor's agonist is increased, it can overpower and replace the antagonist. Inhibition of the site continues until either concentration of the antagonist falls or concentration of the agonist increases and pushes out the antagonist.

- **Noncompetitive inhibition** can occur in 2 ways (both of which are irreversible):
  - The medication can bind to a site on the receptor at a location other than the active site, which is the location on the receptor to which the endogenous chemical would bind. This type of binding changes the shape of the area on the receptor to which the agonist chemical would attach, because it can no longer bind, i.e., it can no longer exert its agonist effects.
  - The antagonist binds irreversibly to the receptor site. This type of binding is not influenced by the amount of agonist present; it will still exert its inhibitory effects (think *irreversible competitive inhibition*, which is a better description).

Table 2-3. Receptors and Effects of Stimulation

Receptor	Agonistic Effect	Agonistic Medications	Antagonistic Medications
Alpha-1	Vasoconstriction of arteries and veins	Pseudoephedrine, phenylephrine	Phentolamine, prazosin, terazosin
Alpha-2	Inhibits norepinephrine release, inhibits insulin release, stimulates glucagon secretion, and inhibits lipolysis	Clonidine, methamphetamine	Risperidone, olanzapine, aripiprazole
Beta-1	Increases heart rate (positive chronotropy), increases cardiac contractility (positive inotrope), increases myocardial conduction (positive dromotropy), and increases renin production to retain urine	Dobutamine	Atenolol, metoprolol, esmolol, acebutolol
Beta-2	Smooth muscle relaxant that causes bronchodilation and stimulates glycogenolysis and insulin secretion	Albuterol, terbutaline, isoproterenol, formoterol	Propranolol, carvedilol, labetalol, nadolol
Nicotinic	Allows acetylcholine to stimulate muscle contraction at the neuromuscular junction	Nicotine, varenicline, acetylcholine	Bupropion, pancuronium, vecuronium, succinylcholine
Muscarinic-2	Located in the heart, stimulation of these slow the heart down after stimulation by the sympathetic nervous system; completely antagonizes beta-1 receptors	Muscarine, pilocarpine	Atropine, hydroxyzine, ipratropium
Dopaminergic	Found throughout the body in 4 different subtypes; cardiac receptors increase myocardial contractility and output without increasing myocardial O_2 demand while maintaining renal and mesenteric artery dilation	Dopamine, phencyclidine (PCP)	Haloperidol, metoclopramide, melatonin

Medications also exert their therapeutic effects in ways other than targeting the cell receptors. Antibiotics and antifungals are designed to attack certain features of a bacterium or fungus, respectively, which human cells do not possess, such as peptidoglycan on gram-positive bacteria. Chelating agents bind to heavy metals, such as lead, in the blood, which help remove the poison from the body. Electrolytes, such as sodium, magnesium, or calcium, increase the concentration of that electrolyte in the body, which can allow it to function better in all the ways that electrolytes affect the cells of the body.

Responses to Medication

Side effects and idiosyncratic effects were discussed earlier in this chapter, both of which are undesired reactions to a medication beyond the medication's desired therapeutic effect. The **therapeutic effect** is the desired effect of the medication on the body—why it is given in the first place. All medications have a **therapeutic index**, also called the therapeutic window, which is the range of concentrations in the body between the minimum amount of drug needed to generate a therapeutic response and the amount that is toxic or lethal. Some drugs have a wide therapeutic index, such as diphenhydramine, which are difficult to overdose; others have a narrow therapeutic index, such as atropine, making overdose easier to achieve. The minimum concentration in the blood needed to generate a therapeutic response is called the **threshold**. The **potency** of a medication is based on how much of the medication is needed to achieve the threshold. For example, the potency of fentanyl is about 100 times that of morphine sulfate, which is to say that a patient can receive 0.1 mg (100 mcg) of fentanyl and have the same pain relief as from 10 mg morphine.

Efficacy is the ability of a medication to carry out the effects it was designed to do. In most cases and with continued use, efficacy tends to decrease as time progresses. This decline in efficacy indicates that the patient is building a **tolerance** to a medication, which means that the patient requires ever-increasing doses to achieve the same therapeutic effect. Tolerance is caused by the body actually reducing the number of receptors for a given chemical through a process known as downregulation or increasing the ability to metabolize the medication faster to nontherapeutic forms. **Cross-tolerance** can be developed when a person develops tolerance for an entire class of medications.

Through tolerance, patients can develop a dependence and thus abuse certain medications or classes of medications. The phenomenon of needing more and more medication to achieve the same effect is at least partially responsible for the problems of abuse and dependence, but in many cases, the euphoric or stimulant effects of medications can result in both psychological dependence and physical dependence.

Factors Affecting Medication Responses

The first and perhaps most obvious factor impacting how a medication affects an individual is weight. Weight-based dosing is common in the prehospital setting for dopamine and other pressor medications and analgesics because the size of a person dictates circulating volume and, therefore, the concentration of the medication in the bloodstream. Delivering a dose based on weight answers this need to ensure the drug concentration—and therefore therapeutic threshold—is achieved. This is particularly true of medications that stimulate or inhibit receptors. When calculating a weight-based dose, remember to use the patient's weight in kilograms, not pounds.

The age of a patient plays a big role in how medications are absorbed in the body. Alterations in the fluid and fat percentages can change how much medication is needed. Metabolism at the extremes of ages also changes how much of a medication is available at any time and can slow elimination of a medication. Finally, paradoxical reactions also are more common at the extremes of ages; for example, particularly young people tend to get excited or agitated when sedatives are administered.

Hypothermia has the effect of slowing metabolism. Therefore, medications are metabolized more slowly, meaning that medications that are typically repeated will need to be repeated less frequently. Also, because cellular metabolism is slower, the effect of the medication once it arrives at the site of action is slower to occur. Hyperthermia has the effect of accelerating metabolism, so, theoretically, the metabolism of a medication will be faster and the effect will be shorter in duration.

Pregnancy causes a host of changes in the mother that determine how medications affect the body.

- Circulating blood volume increases along with cardiac output.
- Hematocrit decreases because the circulating volume expands faster than the extra red cells can be produced.
- Patients who are pregnant often are tachypneic because of both the reduced hematocrit and the reduced ability of the lungs to expand as the fetus grows larger in the later months of pregnancy.
- Gastrointestinal motility decreases, whereas urinary output increases, which alters elimination patterns for medications.

Pharmacokinetics

Pharmacokinetics is the action of the body on a medication, specifically how a medication is absorbed, distributed, biotransformed, and eliminated. The onset of effect, and peak concentrations of the medication, are determined by how the medication is absorbed and distributed throughout the body. The duration of the medication's effect is largely impacted by how much the body needs to do to the medication through biotransformation and how long it takes for the medication to be eliminated from the body. Some medications are not administered in the form that ultimately exerts the effect; in these cases, the medication needs to be biotransformed by the body's existing enzymes before it can exert its therapeutic effect. The route of administration has the greatest impact on absorption, so selecting the best route of medication administration in the emergent situation is of paramount importance.

Before administering any medication, the paramedic has a responsibility of ensuring that several items have been thoroughly verified. These are referred to as the **7 Rights of Medication Administration**. Some texts and tests will refer to only 5 or 6 "rights," often omitting the last 1 or 2 items. Remembering and verifying all 7 rights, however, is essential for the safe, appropriate administration of medication to patients.

Table 2-4. Seven Rights of Medication Administration

Right	Description
1. Right patient	It is essential for an emergency medical technician (EMT) preparing to administer a medication to ensure it is, in fact, that person's prescribed medication. The paramedic, however, selects the medication supply on the ambulance. In most cases, only a single patient is with a paramedic at any one given time, so this really becomes an issue only during mass casualty incidents.
2. Right medication	In selecting the medication from the bag or cabinet, ensure that the correct one is chosen. This may seem intuitive, but medication errors happen frequently, especially if the medication is similar in name to others in the cabinet. Verify that the medication is clear, not discolored.
3. Right time	This applies to medication that you will either repeat after a certain amount of time has passed or initiate after a patient may take the same medication at home. Nitroglycerine (NTG) is an example of a medication that the paramedic would need to verify is the right time to administer. It also may be the right time only after contacting online medical command for permission to administer the drug.
4. Right route	Many medications come in various forms designed for administration along different routes. If the ambulance is out of D50, for example, Insta-Glucose cannot be substituted because the former is designed for intravenous administration, but the latter is for oral dosing.
5. Right dose	Verifying the right dose is essential for the paramedic. Many medications are available in different concentrations. Morphine can be supplied in 2 mg, 4 mg, or 10 mg prefilled syringes, each with only 10 mL of fluid. Take the extra second to verify the concentration and administer the correct dose.
6. Right documentation	Every time a medication is given, it must be properly documented in the run sheet after the call, and the paramedic must report it to medical control and the nurses and physicians receiving the patient in the emergency department. Failure to do this could lead to accidental overdoses or dangerous medication interactions.
7. Right expiration date	Many texts leave this important piece out. Before administering any medication, verify that the drug has not expired. Using expired medications can open up the paramedic and the service to liability and negligence lawsuits.

Routes of Administration

There are numerous routes of medication administration. In this section, they are broadly categorized as enteral, invasive parenteral, and noninvasive parenteral.

Enteral

Enteral routes of administration use the digestive tract for absorption. Medications absorbed through the gut (stomach and intestines) are subject to first-pass metabolism. When a medication is absorbed through the digestive tract, it first enters hepatic circulation. During this first pass through the liver, a predictable amount of the medication is metabolized to a nontherapeutic form, which results in only a fraction of the medication available to the body for its therapeutic purpose. The amount of drug available for therapeutic effect is known as its **bioavailability**. Typically, medications administered sublingually or rectally, although still considered enteral routes, avoid first-pass metabolism.

Oral. Oral medications are the most commonly prescribed medications for patients to use at home. In the prehospital world, very few medications are administered via this route because oral administration typically has the slowest administration to onset of action time. Many oral medications are subject to first-pass metabolism, which protracts the time to bioavailability and the onset of therapeutic effect. To administer anything via the oral route, the patient must be conscious, able to protect their own airway, and able to swallow. Ideally, the paramedic should also be confident that unconsciousness is not imminent. Baby aspirin, activated charcoal, and Insta-Glucose are given this way.

Sublingual. Some medications can be placed under the tongue and allowed to dissolve. The medication is then absorbed through the mucous membrane into the bloodstream, where it can then reach its target organ. Follow these directions:

1. Wear gloves and ensure that the patient does not have any allergies to the medication about to be received.
2. Obtain medical direction for administration of the medication through either standing or online orders.
3. Verify the 7 rights of medication administration.
4. Ask the patient to lift their tongue to the roof of the mouth while keeping the mouth open wide. Demonstration goes a long way to success with this.
5. Deposit the tablet under the tongue or deliver one spray to that area.
6. Advise the patient that this may taste unusual and may even burn. Also advise the patient not to chew or swallow the tablet.
7. Monitor the patient and document the administration.

Buccal. This is the space between the gum and the cheek, typically on the lower jaw. In the prehospital realm, paramedics can deliver glucose gel this way, although the patient usually swallows it. Follow these directions:

1. Wear gloves and ensure that the patient does not have any allergies to the medication about to be received.
2. Obtain medical direction for administration of the medication either through standing or online orders.
3. Verify the 7 rights of medication administration.
4. Deposit the medication between the cheek and the gum. Some paramedics find it helpful to place the medication on a tongue depressor first and then place the tongue depressor between the cheek and the gum.
5. Advise the patient to try not to chew or swallow the medication.
6. Monitor the patient and document the administration.

Orogastric and Nasogastric Tubes. Paramedics do not commonly use these routes for medication administration; however, it is possible that one will be inserted during patient contact. These routes are ideal for administering activated charcoal, particularly in the patient who is obtunded. After confirming gastric placement as indicated later in this book (chapter 3), draw up the appropriate amount of medication into a syringe and administer it through the tube. Flush the tube with 30–60 mL of warmed saline or sterile water into the tube to ensure the medication has entered the stomach. Close and clamp the tube.

Rectal. The rectum is a highly vascular area where absorption can occur rapidly. Antiemetic and antipyretic medications often are administered via suppositories when a patient is vomiting to ensure that the patient gets a full dose. In the field, paramedics use this route to give sedatives, particularly diazepam, for patients who are seizing, especially in the pediatric population. Follow these directions:

1. Wear gloves and ensure that the patient does not have any allergies to the medication about to be received.

2. Instruct the patient to relax and not bear down.

3. If using a suppository, lubricate it with a water-soluble gel and insert it into the rectum about 1 to 1.5 inches beyond the anal sphincter.

4. For medications that are liquid, draw them up into a syringe in the appropriate dose.

5. Attach a large-bore intravenous catheter to the end of the syringe.

6. Insert the catheter into the rectum about 1 to 1.5 inches beyond the anal sphincter and slowly depress the plunger, observing for any leakage of the fluid out. If this happens, insert the catheter deeper and continue.

7. Monitor the patient's condition and document the administration.

Parenteral, Invasive

The following routes of administration are via the parenteral route, which means outside the digestive tract. Some are used frequently in emergency medical services (EMS), whereas others are rarely used and are indicated as such.

Intradermal. This is rarely used by a paramedic and is most commonly used to administer purified protein derivative testing for tuberculosis (TB). In this procedure, a small amount of liquid medication is delivered in between the layers of the skin to form a wheal, a raised area with a pool of medication resembling a mosquito bite. The needle is typically a 25–27 gauge needle, and the volume of medication does not exceed 0.5 mL. The rate of absorption is extremely slow because of the lack of superficial vasculature in the areas used for injection, so this method does not lend itself well to the emergent administration of medications.

Subcutaneous. This method of medication administration is used in prehospital applications and has a relatively slow rate of absorption. Use a small 24–26 gauge needle and a fluid volume of <1 mL and follow these directions:

1. Wear gloves and ensure that the patient does not have any allergies to the medication about to be received.

2. Obtain medical direction for administration of the medication through either standing or online orders.

3. Verify the 7 rights of medication administration and collect the needed equipment to perform the skill: an alcohol swab and a 1–3 mL syringe with a 24–26 gauge needle to draw up the medication.

4. Subcutaneous injections often are given in the upper arm, buttocks, anterior thigh, or abdomen. Cleanse the selected spot with alcohol, starting in the center of the injection spot and clean from the inside out in a tight spiral.

5. Pinch the skin around the cleansed area, advise the patient of the stick and possible discomfort in the area and insert the needle at approximately a 45° angle.

6. Inject the medication and remove the needle. You may rub the area after the injection to not only distribute the medication but also ease localized pain from the injection.

7. Immediately dispose of the needle in a sharps container without recapping.

8. Monitor the patient's condition and document the administration.

Intramuscular. This technique is highly similar to subcutaneous injections; however, the muscle can handle up to 5 mL of fluid at a time. Absorption rates are about the same for both subcutaneous and intramuscular injections. The deltoid muscle of the lateral shoulder, the vastus lateralis muscle of the lateral upper leg, the rectus femoris muscle of the anterior thigh, and the lateral superior area of the gluteus maximus muscle are ideal locations for intramuscular injections. It is important to stay in the lateral superior area of the gluteus maximus to avoid the even remote possibility of hitting the sciatic nerve in the medial areas of the buttocks. Follow these directions:

1. Wear gloves and ensure that the patient does not have any allergies to the medication about to be received.

2. Obtain medical direction for administration of the medication through either standing or online orders.

3. Verify the 7 rights of medication administration and collect the needed equipment to perform the skill: an alcohol swab and 1–5 mL syringe with a 20–24 gauge needle to draw up the medication. The needle should be at least 1 inch long to ensure entrance into the muscle and not remain in the subcutaneous space.

4. Cleanse the selected spot with alcohol, starting in the center of the injection spot and cleaning from the inside out in a tight spiral.

5. Stretch the skin around the cleansed area to further minimize the amount of subcutaneous area between the skin and the muscle, advise the patient of the stick and possible discomfort in the area, and insert the needle at a 90° angle.

6. Aspirate (pull back on the needle plunger) and check for blood. If blood is present, abandon the site, discard the needle and syringe immediately into a sharps container, and prepare another syringe of medication. Blood means you may have inadvertently entered a blood vessel, which is not desirable in this method.

7. If you do not get anything back with aspiration, inject the medication and remove the needle. You may rub the area after the injection to not only distribute the medication but also ease localized pain from the injection, although this is not necessary.

8. Immediately dispose of the needle in a sharps container without recapping.

9. Monitor the patient's condition and document the administration.

Intravenous Bolus. When it comes to emergency medication administration, intravenous administration is the granddaddy of all methods. The intravenous route is the fastest of all routes at the paramedic's disposal and is the most likely method for administering medications. Bolus means a single dose given all at once, versus intravenous piggyback or drip (discussed next), which is slower and given during an extended time frame. Follow these directions:

1. Wear gloves and ensure that the patient does not have any allergies to the medication about to be received.

2. Obtain medical direction for administration of the medication through either standing or online orders.

3. Verify the 7 rights of medication administration and collect the needed equipment to perform the skill: an alcohol swab and a 3–10 mL syringe with an 18–24 gauge needle to draw up the medication only. Most intravenous line medication ports no longer require needles to draw up the medication.

4. Verify that the established intravenous line is still patent by flushing it with approximately 10 mL of saline. Abandon the site if the line will no longer flush or you see bruising or infiltration around the intravenous site in the patient's arm.

5. Cleanse the selected medication administration port with alcohol and attach the syringe to the medication port.

6. Pinch the tubing between the selected medication port and the bag to prevent the medication from flowing backward away from the patient and into the bag.

7. Inject the medication and disconnect the syringe from the medication port. Release the pinch on the tubing and allow the line to flow.

8. Dispose of the syringe in a sharps container immediately without recapping.

9. Monitor the patient and document the administration.

Intravenous Piggyback. Occasionally, paramedics will be required to give a medication infusion that is a small dose of medication given for a period of time, usually to maintain therapeutic levels of a drug in the bloodstream. The medication is injected into a bag of intravenous solution that is then connected—piggybacked—to a maintenance line of normal saline solution or lactated Ringer solution instead of directly into the vein. Paramedics may initiate only one or two such piggybacked lines, but they may be required to monitor many more during complex interfacility transports. It is highly recommended to use a mechanical pump for administering these medications so that the precise amount of medication is delivered; under- or overdosing patients with these medications can have disastrous effects on a patient's condition.

Intraosseous. This route has absorption rates nearly identical to that of intravenous administration. Initiation of intraosseous lines is discussed later in this chapter. Any medication that can be given intravenously can be given intraosseously. Fluid does not typically flow well through an intraosseous line and may require a pressure infusion, which can be achieved by taking a blood pressure cuff and inflating it until the desired drip rate is achieved.

Occasionally, the pressure may need to be increased as fluid drains from the bag. Pressure infusion bags are available and achieve the same result. Follow these directions:

1. Wear gloves and ensure that the patient does not have any allergies to the medication about to be received.

2. Obtain medical direction for administration of the medication through either standing or online orders.

3. Verify the 7 rights of medication administration and collect the needed equipment to perform the skill: an alcohol swab and a 3–10 mL syringe with an 18–24 gauge needle to draw up the medication. Most intravenous line medication ports no longer require needles to draw up the medication.

4. Verify that the established intraosseous line is still patent by flushing it with approximately 10 mL of saline. Abandon the site if the line will no longer flush or you see bruising or infiltration around the intraosseous site.

5. Cleanse the selected medication administration port with alcohol and attach the syringe to the medication port.

6. Pinch the tubing between the selected medication port and the bag to prevent the medication from flowing backward away from the patient and into the bag.

7. Inject the medication and disconnect the syringe from the medication port. Release the pinch on the tubing and allow the line to flow.

8. Dispose of the syringe in a sharps container immediately without recapping.

9. Monitor the patient's condition and document the administration.

Parenteral, Noninvasive

The following routes of medication administration are still parenteral but are noninvasive.

Transdermal. With this route, medications are absorbed into the bloodstream after passing through the skin. The medication must be fat soluble and small enough to pass through the skin. This route acts similarly to an intravenous piggyback, where the medication is delivered slowly across time and at the same rate. Follow these directions:

1. Wear gloves and ensure that the patient does not have any allergies to the medication about to be received.

2. Obtain medical direction for administration of the medication through either standing or online orders.

3. Verify the 7 rights of medication administration.

4. Cleanse the selected spot with alcohol, starting in the center of the administration site and cleaning from the inside out in a tight spiral. Dry the area thoroughly.

5. If the medication is a cream in a tube, apply the appropriate amount to the application paper and apply to the skin. If it is a premedicated patch, peel the patch from the backing and then apply to the skin.

6. Monitor the patient's condition and document the medication administration.

Inhalation. The inhalation route has several methods of delivery; in chapter 4, information about O_2 delivery devices is given. Patients will have metered dose inhalers (MDIs) for beta-agonists such as albuterol and other medications that exert their effects when breathed into the bronchial tree. Paramedics and EMTs can help their patients administer inhaled beta-agonists from MDIs. Follow these directions:

1. Wear gloves and obtain medical direction for administration of the medication through either standing or online orders. Because it is the patient's MDI, you already know that the patient does not have an allergy to the medication.

2. Verify the 7 rights of medication administration, paying particular attention to whether the patient has taken any medication recently within the prescriber's window, usually within the past 5–10 minutes.

3. Shake the canister and have the patient exhale completely.

4. Have the patient put their lips around the opening of the canister. As the patient begins to inhale, have the patient squeeze the plunger. If the patient uses a spacer, have the patient continue to use it.

5. Direct the patient to hold their breath as long as is comfortable before exhaling.

6. After a couple of breaths, repeat the process until the prescribed dose is completely given. That is, if the prescription says to take 2 puffs every 5 minutes, you can administer a second puff right away. Remember, it is only one squeeze of the canister per breath.

7. Monitor the patient's condition and document the administration.

Inhaled medication also may be given via nebulizer, as follows:

1. Wear gloves and ensure that the patient does not have any allergies to the medication about to be received.

2. Obtain medical direction for administration of the medication through either standing or online orders.

3. Verify the 7 rights of medication administration and collect the needed equipment to perform the skill: a nebulizer kit and an inhaled bronchodilator.

4. Add the medication to the chamber of the nebulizer without the O_2 connected to it.

5. Assemble the nebulizer.

6. Connect the O_2 tubing and start the flow of O_2 at between 6 and 10 L per minute to produce a fine mist.

7. Have the patient securely hold the mouthpiece in their mouth.

8. Coach the patient to take deep breaths and hold their breath as long as comfortable before exhaling each time to give the medication a chance to work. Tap the sides of the chamber occasionally to knock down condensate on the sides of the chamber. Continue until no fluid remains in the chamber of the nebulizer and no mist is produced.

9. Monitor the patient throughout administration and watch for side effects. Advise the patient on the possible feeling of jitters during the treatment.

Pro-Tip

If the patient is unable to hold the mouthpiece in the mouth or is unable to hold the nebulizer by hand, you can remove the bag from the mask of a non-rebreather and insert the chamber of the nebulizer into the hole where the bag came out. Just ensure that the chamber remains upright so that the medication can be nebulized and does not spill. In other words, this route of administration cannot be done in a patient who must remain supine.

Intranasal. Some studies suggest that absorption of a medication through the mucous membranes of the nasal lining is faster than giving a medication intramuscularly because of highly vascularized tissue. This method is available only for certain medications, including midazolam, fentanyl, naloxone, glucagon, ketorolac and flumazenil. Follow these directions:

1. Wear gloves and ensure that the patient does not have any allergies to the medication about to be received.

2. Obtain medical direction for administration of the medication through either standing or online orders.

3. Verify the 7 rights of medication administration.

4. Draw up the appropriate dose of the medication in a syringe, generally 2–2.5 times the usual intravenous dose of the medication.

5. Attach the mucosal atomization device to the syringe.

6. Spray half the volume into each nostril.

7. Immediately discard the syringe and mucosal atomization device into the sharps container.

8. Monitor the patient's condition and document the administration.

Endotracheal. In the absence of any other route of administration, certain medications may be administered through a properly placed endotracheal tube (ETT) and into the bronchial tree. The only medications approved for this are lidocaine, epinephrine, atropine, and naloxone, which can be remembered with the mnemonic LEAN. ETT administration is the last resort if an intravenous or an intraosseous route cannot be established. Follow these directions:

1. Wear gloves and ensure that the patient does not have any allergies to the medication about to be received.

2. Obtain medical direction for administration of the medication through either standing or online orders.

3. Verify the 7 rights of medication administration.

4. Deliver the medication, usually double the intravenous dose, into the ETT and ventilate the patient briskly to deliver the medication out of the tube and into the bronchial tree.

How Medications Are Supplied

Medication packaging varies depending on the stability of the medication and the method in which it will be given to a patient. The types of medication packages are ampules, vials, and prefilled syringes.

Ampules are sealed glass containers that contain a sterile solution of medication and typically contain a single dose of medication. Epinephrine 1:1,000 dilution often comes packaged this way. To extract the medication, follow these steps:

1. Flick the ampule with your finger to get all the fluid into the bottom section.
2. Grip the ampule by the top between your thumb and forefinger on your dominant hand and the bottom in the fist of your other hand and break the top off at the narrowed neck.
3. Insert a filter needle into the bottom portion and draw up the medication. It is important to use a filter needle whenever possible in case some small glass shards fall into the medication. Immediately discard the ampule in the sharps container.
4. With the needle pointed upward, tap the barrel of the syringe to get air in the fluid to bubble up to the top. Expel the air from the syringe, remove the needle, and place the needle into the sharps container.
5. The syringe is now ready to attach to an intravenous medication port. Alternatively, you can attach another needle for administration via the intramuscular or subcutaneous route.

Vials are more common than ampules and are easier to use. Vials are glass or plastic bottles with a rubber stopper that is covered with a plastic breakaway cap. They may contain single or multiple doses of a medication. Many medications come in a ready-to-use solution; however, some may need to be reconstituted. To reconstitute a medication, press the top of the vial down; the center stopper that separates the liquid from the solid pellet in the bottom will dislodge, allowing the liquid and solid to mix. Shake until completely dissolved and use promptly. Follow these steps to withdraw the medication from the vial:

1. Remove the cover and wipe the rubber stopper with an alcohol swab.
2. Draw up air into a syringe with a needle attached equal to or slightly more than the volume of fluid you will need from the vial for the dose.
3. Insert the needle through the center of the stopper (the edges are much thicker) and inject the air into the vial.
4. Invert the vial. With the tip of the needle below the level of the liquid, allow the pressure of the air that was just injected to force the liquid into the syringe. Draw up the remaining fluid to slightly more than what you would need for the dose.
5. Remove the needle from the vial and then from the syringe (unless being used as an intramuscular or subcutaneous injection) and discard immediately. The syringe is now ready to be connected to a medication port on the intravenous line.

Prefilled syringes are ready-to-use syringes that come with a set amount of medication already in a needleless system. Simply screw the plunger piece into the barrel containing the fluid, connect to the medication port on an intravenous line, and deliver the appropriate amount to the patient. Remember, not all the medication in a prefilled syringe may be needed as a single bolus, so be sure to know the dose before connecting.

Distribution of Medication

The second component of pharmacokinetics is the distribution of medication after it has been absorbed into the bloodstream. There are several methods of medication distribution to get the drug into the cells where it will exert its effects. Although medications that attach to receptors do not need to enter the cell, necessarily, they often do need to leave the bloodstream to get to the receptors.

Small molecules that are nonionic, or uncharged, and molecules that are lipophilic, which means fat loving or fat soluble (and therefore hydrophobic or water hating), can pass through cells with relative ease and can easily cross cell membranes to do so.

Larger molecules and molecules that are **hydrophilic**, which means water loving (and therefore fat hating) have a harder time crossing the cellular barrier. Once inside, the molecule can move about freely; it is just crossing the membrane that presents the issue. These types of molecules need help, which can happen in several ways. **Pinocytosis** is where the cell buds small vesicles to bring it inside. The second way is through **facilitated diffusion**, where proteins that stretch from side to side in the membrane provide a pathway for the molecule to enter. Finally, **active transport** requires the use of cellular energy to move the molecule across the membrane.

Some molecules bind to proteins found in the bloodstream; these are called plasma proteins. This phenomenon effectively removes the medication molecules from circulation so that they are no longer available to exert their effects, thus requiring higher doses of the medication. This is a reversible process; therefore, as the plasma concentration of non-protein-bound medication drops, the medication that is bound to the protein can fall off, which can lead to a longer duration of effect for the medication. This also can cause an accidental overdose of a medication when, if a medication with a higher affinity for a protein comes along, the second medication knocks the first off its protein, causing a sudden increase in concentration of the first medication.

Finally, fat stores in the body can be a place where lipophilic medications are stored and removed from circulation. Fat stores can lessen the amount of medication that is available to exert a therapeutic effect.

Biotransformation

Most of the medications prescribed require some form of metabolism once in the body, a process called **biotransformation**. From this process, either active or inactive metabolites are formed. Active metabolites can be the active form of a drug, which is the one that actually exerts its effects on the body. Active metabolites also are an active form if they are harmful to the body. Active just means it is actually doing something in the body. Inactive metabolites are exactly that: inactive—essentially waste. Finally, biotransformation also may play a role in converting a substance to another metabolite that is easier for the body to eliminate.

The sites of biotransformation are as follows:

- The cytochrome P-450 system in the liver is the site of most biotransformation.
- Medications taken orally often are biotransformed by bacteria in the gut.
- The kidneys, skin, and lungs also have the ability to biotransform medications, typically for elimination.

Medication Elimination

Medications that are absorbed after being taken orally most often are removed from the body by the kidneys. Some oral medications never even see the bloodstream and are eliminated in their original form in solid waste. Medication gets removed from the body in one of 2 ways.

- **Zero-order elimination** is not dependent on the concentration of the medication or chemical. Regardless of the amount in the blood, it will continuously be removed at a steady rate until it is completely gone.
- **First-order elimination** is wholly dependent on the plasma concentration and has a half-life associated with the medication.
- In this case, *half-life* refers to the amount of time it takes for the peak plasma concentration to be reduced by half. Once it has been reduced by half, it will take the same amount of time to eliminate half of the remaining amount of medication, and so on. During each half-life time period, half of the amount is eliminated. So if the peak plasma concentration of a medication is 20 mcg/mL and its half-life is 60 minutes, what is the concentration after 4 hours? As shown, after 4 (60-minute) periods (or 4 half-lives), 1.25 mcg/mL remain.

Table 2-5. Half-Life Calculations

Number of Half-Lives Passed	Time (hours)	Medication Concentration (mcg/mL)
Initial	0	20
Half-life 1	1	10
Half-life 2	2	5
Half-life 3	3	2.5
Half-life 4	4	1.25

INTRAVENOUS THERAPY

One of the most common procedures a paramedic will perform is the initiation of intravenous therapy. Frequently, establishing an intravenous line is done primarily as a route of access for medication administration. Other times, it will provide fluid resuscitation for the patient who is at risk of developing shock.

Fluids

The body is in a very delicate state of balance. Although it has many compensatory mechanisms to maintain that state of balance, an important mechanism the body has to work through is the salt balance. If sodium and potassium ions exchange places for too long, death can result. Potassium needs to stay inside the cells, and sodium needs to remain outside the cells. Water follows sodium, so if the body does a poor job at removing excess sodium, fluid overload can result, putting an excess workload on the heart.

When fluid is administered, some stays in the vasculature, some moves into the intercellular fluid, and some moves into the cells, all based on where these ions, or solutes, are located. **Solute** is that which is dissolved and can refer to sugars or salts. A **solvent** is the item, frequently water, into which something dissolves. The body has an overall solute concentration within the cells of approximately 0.9%, which is about 9 g of solute in about 1,000 mL of fluid.

Most fluids that are administered are **isotonic**, which means that they have approximately the same solute concentration as the plasma and intercellular fluid. These fluids include 0.9% saline solution, referred to as normal saline solution (NSS). NSS is the most commonly used prehospital fluid because it is designed to be harmonious with the body's natural salt balance. Lactated Ringer solution also is isotonic, resulting in no net movement of water into or out of the cells.

Paramedics rarely use 5% dextrose in water (D5W) anymore, but it is a unique solution. It is classified as an isotonic solution in the bag; however, shortly after this fluid is administered, the dextrose (a sugar) is metabolized, leaving only water behind. Because pure water is free of any solutes, it is now hypotonic to the surroundings, such as cells. Because a higher solute concentration is in the cell, the water will move into the cell by osmosis in an attempt to bring both solutions—the blood and the intracellular space—closer to equal in solute concentration. If too much of this solution is given during an extended period of time, excess water could move into the cell and cause the cell to rupture.

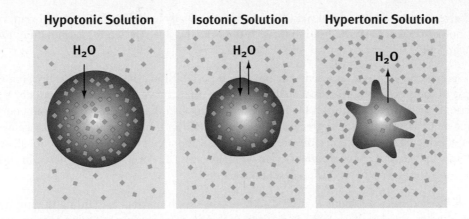

Figure 2-1. Osmosis
Water moves from areas of low-solute (high-water) concentration to high-solute (low-water) concentration.

Fluids also can be classified as crystalloids or colloids. **Crystalloid solutions** are made by mixing water and crystals of something; in the case of NSS, the crystals that go into it are sodium chloride. Other dissolved crystals include sugars to make D5W. **Colloids**, on the other hand, are solutions of proteins. Paramedics do not carry colloid solutions because they need to be reliably refrigerated. Colloid solutions are given because these proteins are too large to move out of the vasculature and have a similar effect of being a hypertonic solution. Egg whites are an example of a colloid solution; medical colloids include albumin and heparin, among others.

Establishing an Intravenous Line

Before even preparing to break skin, select the intravenous solution. Most prehospital providers prefer to go with the saline lock and flush, unless the patient is dehydrated, in shock, or bleeding and a fluid bolus is needed. The saline lock and flush provides the necessary access for potential medication administration without being cumbersome or making extrication more difficult, such as an intravenous line and bag can. To establish an intravenous fluid drip, NSS most common, although lactated Ringer solution is the optimal choice in trauma. When selecting the fluid, ensure that the fluid is clear and not expired.

Equally important is choosing which administration set to use. Generally speaking, administration sets come in microdrip or macrodrip setups. The microdrip setup forms smaller droplets than the macrodrip setup, thus allowing finer control of fluid administration, which is essential in fluid-overloaded patients. The microdrip setup also is the administration set of choice for most medication infusion drips. The microdrip takes 60 drops (gtt) to make 1 mL, which is written 60 gtt/mL. The macrodrip administration set is used in all other situations, especially when large volumes of fluids may need to be given, such as in cases of bleeding, dehydration, and burns. Macrodrips typically can deliver 10 gtt/mL or 15 gtt/mL and are occasionally used for medication infusions.

Once it has been determined that the patient needs an intravenous line and the fluid has been chosen and prepped, where should the line be established? Begin with the straightest, biggest vein you can find using the largest bore intravenous line possible. The vein will be spongy or springy when palpated, which will enhance the chances of success. From a patient's perspective, the least painful spot in which to start an intravenous line is the anterior forearm; the dorsum of the hand and antecubital area can be the most painful, though they usually harbor the finest veins. The anterior wrist just proximal to the palm of the hand should be avoided despite tempting veins because this is the most sensitive area of the arm. Paramedics also can use the external jugular (EJ) vein as an intravenous insertion site on either side of the neck, but this location is preferable only in patients who are unconscious or in extremely dire circumstances.

Some guiding principles for intravenous establishment include starting distally and working proximally to minimize the chances of proximal missed intravenous site infiltrate, or bleeding into the soft tissue surrounding them, when the intravenous line is run. Next, pull traction on the selected site to anchor the vein in place, which can be done by either pulling the skin of the hand distally and over the first knuckle or stretching the skin away from the vein.

To cannulate the vein found on the lateral wrist, flex the wrist medially to anchor it. For the EJ vein, when a cervical spine injury is not suspected, push the head to the side opposite the side selected for cannulation; this will provide most of the anchoring.

Select the intravenous catheter that represents the purpose for establishing the intravenous line. For example, if the primary purpose of the access is to provide a medication route, then a 20-gauge catheter should be sufficient. If the line could potentially be used to administer blood or blood products in the hospital, it is recommended to start with an 18-gauge line or larger. Finally, for aggressive fluid resuscitation in trauma and burns, a 16-gauge or larger line should be initiated. Of course, all these options are determined by the size of the optimal vein; not all veins will accept what the patient really needs. Perhaps a patient's vein will take only a 22- or 24-gauge catheter. In such cases, establishing a patent intravenous line of any size is first and foremost.

At this point, all the necessary decisions that need to be made have been made regarding the intravenous site, the fluid type, and catheter size. Now it is time to actually perform the procedure. Nothing is more important when performing any procedure than gathering all the equipment you could possibly need, which includes preparing for success as well as failure. Some intravenous start kits come complete with everything needed for either case in one neat little package, but this equipment should be on a mental checklist. Have the following items within arm's reach before inserting the needle through the skin:

- The intravenous catheter, appropriately sized for the patient's needs and vein size
- The intravenous administration set with fluid completely run through or a primed saline lock
- Tape, at least three strips torn into 3–4-inch lengths and the roll nearby
- Alcohol, chlorhexidine, or iodine skin prep wipes
- Several gauze pads
- Tourniquet

When all the supplies are present, insert the catheter. The following steps will guide successful placement:

1. Place the tourniquet on the upper arm tight enough to occlude the veins but not hamper arterial blood flow. Although it should go without saying, if using the EJ vein, do not put a tourniquet around the neck. As noted earlier, tape for securing the line (or gauze if the site needs to be abandoned) should be torn and within arm's reach.

2. Next, palpate the vein that is suitable for the purpose. Ensure you know the relative pathway of the vein.

3. Cleanse the site, starting from the point you anticipate inserting the catheter and working outward in a circular motion. Allow to air dry or dry with a sterile gauze pad. Do not palpate the vein in this area again without cleansing the area again.

4. Pull traction on the skin surrounding the vein but not directly proximal to the needle insertion point to minimize the risk of accidental needle stick.

5. With the bevel of the needle up, insert the needle through the skin at an angle low to the skin. The most painful part is getting the needle through the skin, not so much into the vein or manipulating the catheter. Some texts recommend starting at a 45° angle and then dropping down once blood shows up in the flash chamber; however, starting and remaining low places the needle more in parallel with the vein, reducing the risk of going through the backside of the vein before blood is even visible, especially with smaller gauge catheters.

6. When blood is visible in the flash chamber, advance the needle and catheter a little further into the vein, paying particular attention to avoid going through the other side of the vein. This step is crucial because it helps ensure that the catheter, which sits just behind the bevel of the needle, is fully within the lumen of the vein.

7. Advance the catheter off the needle and into the vein until resistance is reached (possibly against a valve) or the hub is in contact with the skin.

8. Place a finger or thumb over where the tip of the catheter should lie to prevent backflow of blood from the catheter. This may require considerable pressure, especially with the EJ vein.

9. Withdraw the needle and immediately place it into a puncture-proof sharps container to reduce the risk of accidental needle-stick (needed even when a protected-tip IV needle is used).

10. Quickly connect the saline lock or administration set to the hub and tighten the locking piece.

11. Remove the tourniquet while still continuing to hold the catheter.

12. Secure the catheter with tape or a commercial device, such as a Tegaderm, being sure to completely cover the entry point into the skin to help keep that area clean.

13. If using a saline lock, flush it with 3–10 mL of saline to prevent blood from clotting the catheter. If using an administration set and an intravenous bag, roll the roller clamp all the way up to flush the line, then adjust it back down to achieve the desired flow rate.

14. Check for signs of infiltration and bruising around the catheter site. If you find any, it is suggested to avoid using the site and remove the catheter.

Pro-Tip

If you know a vein cannot be anchored, i.e., it rolls around under the skin, it may help to start alongside the vein and redirect the needle into the vein from the side (rather than from the top). Because the vein rolls, the needle will push the vein until it cannot roll any further and invariably enter the lumen of the vein. You also can use this technique if you know needle insertion will be painful for the patient. This technique will allow you to enter the skin faster without puncturing the vein right away. Because this is the most painful part of the procedure, take your time to cannulate the vein.

Complications

Although starting an intravenous line is perhaps the most routine, innocuous procedure that paramedics perform, it is not free of complications—some of which are potentially lethal—that need to be weighed when contemplating the potential benefit of starting the line.

Catheter shear occurs when a needle is partially removed from the catheter and then intentionally or accidentally reinserted such that the needle punctures the side of the plastic catheter. This may cut off a small piece of catheter capable of becoming a lethal embolus. The moral of this story is, never reinsert a needle into the catheter after it has been partially or wholly removed.

Infiltration is localized swelling or bruising that typically results from perforation of the vein, by either going through the other side of the vein or penetrating the vein more than once. Infiltration may not produce bruising and may be seen only when you flush the catheter and the fluid flows into the interstitial spaces. Infiltration is not usually a major problem, but it may cause some ugly bruising and discomfort. If the vein is not properly occluded when a catheter is removed for a long enough period of time, a hematoma also may result.

Occlusion can happen when flow through the catheter is not fast enough and blood clots at the tip of the catheter. If it is too difficult to flush the catheter, it is best not to continue to try and inadvertently embolize the clot. Occlusion also may be seen when the catheter rests too close to or against a valve in the vein. This situation often can be resolved by applying pressure to the intravenous bag or withdrawing the catheter slightly and securing it again once the flow is reestablished. Finally, the catheter may be occluded when an intravenous line is inserted into or near a joint and the patient bends that joint.

Although it is possible to tell the difference between a vein and **tendon**, **ligament**, and **nerve** structures simply by palpating, occasionally the sight or feel for the vein is lost and one of these structures is hit. If one of these structures is hit with the needle, remove the needle and catheter and try again elsewhere, after profusely apologizing to the patient.

Occasionally, particularly in the area of the antecubital fossa where the vein and artery are very close, an artery rather the vein can be punctured. After **arterial puncture**, it is possible for the line to flow normally in these cases; however, sometimes the blood pressure is high enough that blood starts pulsing up the line. If an artery is struck, abandon the site and apply direct pressure to the site for at least 5 minutes; a longer period of direct pressure is required for patients who are anticoagulated.

Occasionally, even bags without leaks become contaminated, yet still appear clear. This contamination is then injected into the patient, causing **pyrogenic reactions** and generating a high fever usually within 30 minutes of the initiation of the intravenous line. Such reactions will then rapidly progress to what is essentially septic shock with hypotension, tachycardia, and an altered mental status with an extremely high fever. Stop the infusion and remove that intravenous line. Establish another line and treat the patient for the resulting shock, in addition to what the patient had beforehand that initially necessitated the intravenous line.

Thrombophlebitis is inflammation of the vein that was catheterized and is strongly related to poor aseptic technique. Irritating medications or infusions also can be a cause. If redness develops at the insertion site or the patient complains of pain and itching along the route of the vein, stop any infusion and discontinue the intravenous line. Warm compresses will help reduce the pain.

An **air embolus** results from the introduction of large amounts of air directly into the vein. Properly flushing an intravenous line prior to initiation will prevent this issue.

Vasovagal reactions are essentially syncopal episodes that result from the sight of blood or just the sheer anxiety of needing an intravenous line in the first place. Often it's nothing to worry about in the long run; however, you may have to help the patient regain consciousness by lying them flat and administering O_2. The goal is to have the intravenous line started before they come to.

Intraosseous Therapy

If you are unable to start an intravenous line or if the patient is in cardiac arrest, initiating an intraosseous line is a suitable alternative. Although this has been done for decades in children, it became an option for adults only within the last decade. Intraosseous lines are quick to establish and provide for administration-to-clinical-effect times for all medications that are similar to those for intravenous administration. The needle is driven through the outer compact bone and into the highly vascular marrow. The intraosseous line should not be started in cases of tibial fracture or if there are burns or a skin infection, such as cellulitis, overlying the site of entry.

An intraosseous line can be started in any patient who would otherwise get an intravenous shot and is in a critical, life-threatening situation. Contraindications to initiating an intraosseous administration include the following:

- Osteoporosis
- Osteogenesis imperfecta, a genetic condition in which bone does not form properly
- Fracture in the same extremity into which the intraosseous needle would be placed
- Previous attempts in the same bone
- Infection or burn over the insertion site

The sites for intraosseous initiation are vastly different from those for intravenous administration. Prehospital intraosseous insertions can happen in the proximal humerus or the proximal medial tibia. To locate the proper site on the proximal humerus, have the patient hold their arm at the level of the navel, with the elbow bent at a 90° angle. Place two fingers on the anterior humeral head. As the patient abducts their forearm, a notch in the humeral head can be felt. This is the location for the intraosseous needle. For the anterior medial tibia, find the tibial tuberosity just distal to the kneecap. Move approximately two finger widths inferiorly and slightly medial to the flat part of the tibial shaft. This is the location for the tibial intraosseous needle.

Essentially, two adult intraosseous devices are on the market. The EZ-IO device is basically a driver resembling a drill that uses the needle as a drill bit. The second device is a spring-loaded bone injection gun that uses the same principles as the spring-loaded center punch to launch the needle into the bone. Familiarize yourself with the manufacturer's directions before using these products.

Once it is determined that an intraosseous line will be initiated, gather all equipment necessary and have it within arm's reach. Set up the infusion bag and the administration the same as for an intravenous line. Use an alcohol, chlorhexidine, or iodine swab to cleanse and prepare the area. Select the needle based on the site chosen and the patient's weight. Prepare a syringe of saline connected to a saline lock primed with fluid. As with the intravenous line, cut tape prior to the procedure. Finally, have a commercial device recommended by the manufacturer to secure and stabilize the intraosseous needle once the procedure is complete.

For the following procedure, the proximal tibia and an EZ-IO driver will be used.

1. Cleanse the site, starting at the point you anticipate inserting the needle and working outward in a circular motion. Allow to air dry or dry with a sterile gauze pad. Do not palpate the vein in this area again without cleansing the area again.

2. Attach the needle to the driver.

3. Insert the needle at a 90° angle to and through the skin directly against the bone without activating the driver. Once against the bone, turn on the driver by squeezing fully on the trigger and applying very gentle pressure, letting the spinning needle do the work.

4. Suddenly, there will be a drop in resistance as the needle breaks through the hard outer bone and into the cavernous marrow. As soon as this is felt, stop drilling by releasing the trigger.

5. Remove the driver from the needle. It is acceptable if the plastic hub of the needle is not against the skin when the drop in resistance is felt.

6. Remove the stylet by unscrewing the top half of the needle's hub and pulling it out of the needle while holding the bottom half in place. The needle should stand on its own if properly placed.

7. Attach the saline lock and syringe unit.

8. Draw back on the syringe plunger and attempt to aspirate marrow contents and blood. This may not always happen.

9. Inject 10 mL and observe the area around the tibia for infiltration or bleeding.

10. Disconnect the syringe and connect the administration set to the saline lock. The bag may need to be pressurized with a pressure infuser bladder or a manual blood pressure cuff so that the fluid can flow through the marrow. This is normal and does not indicate a problem unless there is infiltration into surrounding tissues.

11. Secure with a commercial stabilizing device from the manufacturer, or similar to any impaled object, with bulky dressings around the needle and a lot of tape or roller gauze.

Complications to intraosseous therapy are much less likely than with intravenous therapy. Aside from pain being reported only during the infusion, and rarely during the actual insertion, the biggest complication of intraosseous insertion is infiltration. If the site is infiltrating and the infusion is not stopped, compartment syndrome can occur, leading to necrosis (death) of muscle and tissues surrounding the bone. Particularly in small or fragile bones, such as those found in osteogenesis imperfecta or osteoporosis, fracture is a possibility. An extremely rare complication is osteomyelitis, which is inflammation of the bone and muscle surrounding it caused by infection. To prevent osteomyelitis, avoid any area of skin that appears red or inflamed near or over the insertion site.

REVIEW QUESTIONS

Select the ONE best answer.

1. The paramedic withholds NTG from a patient whose SBP is <100 mmHg. In the context of NTG administration, SBP <100 mmHg is an example of a/an:

    A. Contraindication.

    B. Indication.

    C. Side effect.

    D. Idiosyncratic effect.

2. All of the following are parenteral routes of medication administration EXCEPT:

    A. Intravenous.

    B. Subcutaneous.

    C. Rectal.

    D. Transdermal.

3. Medications that undergo first-pass metabolism require a higher dose to maintain therapeutic levels. Medications subject to first-pass metabolism are given via the _____ route.

    A. inhalation

    B. intravenous

    C. oral

    D. sublingual

4. Use the following picture to answer questions 4 and 5.

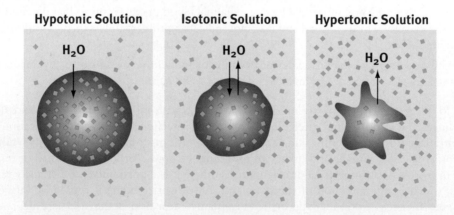

    Which of the following solutions could be an example for the type of solution represented in the third image?

    A. 0.9% saline solution

    B. Dextrose 5% in 0.225% normal saline

    C. Dextrose 5% in water

    D. Dextrose 50% in water

5. In the diagram, the arrows represent the movement of water across the cell membrane. Why would water move into the cell in solution 1?

    A. More solute is inside the cell than outside.

    B. More solute is outside the cell than inside.

    C. More water is inside the cell than outside.

    D. More water is outside the cell than inside.

6. Which of the following poses the most immediate and life-threatening complication from intravenous line placement?

    A. Catheter shear

    B. Pyrogenic reaction

    C. Thrombophlebitis

    D. Vasovagal reaction

7. You are starting an intraosseous line on an unresponsive 4-year-old patient who is in cardiac arrest. You had a sudden decrease in resistance while inserting the needle into the bone; however, you were unable to aspirate any bone marrow or blood with a syringe. What should be your next most appropriate step?

    A. Abandon the site and initiate a 2nd intraosseous line on the other leg.

    B. Connect intravenous tubing from the intravenous bag and run to gravity.

    C. Flush the needle with saline and observe for infiltrate.

    D. Pull back on the needle slightly and aspirate a 2nd time.

ANSWERS AND EXPLANATIONS

1. **The correct answer is (A).** Contraindications are reasons to not give a medication. For NTG, contraindications include recent use of phosphodiesterase-5 inhibitors (sildenafil, among others) and a systolic blood pressure <100 mmHg. Indication (B) is a reason the medication would be administered. Side effects (C) are expected actions of a particular medication that are not therapeutic. For example, for NTG, a side effect could be a headache. Idiosyncratic effects (D) are unexpected effects of a medication that occur in only 1 patient. They can range from severe and life threatening to a nuisance.

2. **The correct answer is (C).** Parenteral medication administration routes include all those that do not use any portion of the digestive tract. Rectal administration of a drug is considered an enteral medication because the rectum is still part of the digestive tract.

3. **The correct answer is (C).** Medications subjected to first-pass metabolism in the liver are those that are absorbed through the digestive tract in either the stomach or the intestines. These routes include oral administration, administration via orogastric or nasogastric tubes, and those medications that are occasionally administered through gastrointestinal tract ostomies (PEG-, G-, and J-tubes). Medications absorbed rectally and sublingually (D) are able to avoid the first-pass effect despite being administered via the oral route and directly enter systemic circulation. Inhalation (A) and intravenous routes (B) are parenteral routes and avoid first-pass metabolism.

4. **The correct answer is (D).** Image number 3 represents a hypertonic solution. The only medications that paramedics can administer that are hypertonic to the cells are D50 and mannitol. Hypertonic solutions will draw fluid out of the cell, which is indicated in the image. Normal saline (A) is isotonic to the cells, meaning there is no net movement of water in or out of the cell. Dextrose 5% in D5 in 0.225% normal saline (B), informally called D5 in 1/4 NSS, is also hypotonic for the same reason. D5 (C) is isotonic in the bag and hypotonic shortly after administration.

5. **The correct answer is (A).** Water will move in a direction of lower solute concentration to an area of higher solute concentration, which is the definition of osmosis. Since the diagram indicates more solute inside the cell than out, the water will move into the cell because that is the area of higher solute concentration.

6. **The correct answer is (A).** Catheter shear can embolize a piece of plastic from the catheter if the needle is removed, in whole or part, from the catheter and reinserted. This piece can block an artery in the lung and cause an almost immediate decline in patient status. Pyrogenic reactions (B), thrombophlebitis (C), and vasovagal reactions (D) are serious complications, but they are rarely life threatening.

7. **The correct answer is (C).** In the event you are unable to aspirate blood or bone marrow after a sudden decrease in resistance, this does not necessarily mean that the needle is misplaced. If the needle still stands freely, the needle has likely entered the bone. The remaining options are not the best choice and should be considered only if the site infiltrates.

Patient Assessment   3

Learning Objectives

❑ Explain and prioritize the facets of a patient assessment.

❑ Conduct an orderly and comprehensive patient assessment on a medical or trauma patient.

❑ Apply patient assessment skills to the psychomotor exam.

Far and away the most important skill a paramedic can possess is the ability to conduct a thorough, accurate patient assessment. As with any skill, it can be developed and refined to flow naturally for both the patient and the paramedic. Throughout their careers, paramedics need to constantly work on the skills of taking a patient history, relating the patient's answers with the physical exam findings, and ensuring that nothing is missed. Using those findings to identify a likely cause for the patient's complaint—in other words, creating the working diagnosis—is where the astute and talented paramedic can flourish. This chapter will help prepare you for both the cognitive exam and the psychomotor exam. Later chapters will address specific assessment points within the focus of those chapters.

This chapter primarily follows the approach to patient assessment of the trauma assessment skill sheet from the National Registry of Emergency Medical Technicians' paramedic psychomotor exam. As of this printing, these sheets are available at no cost online: **nremt.org/rwd/public/document/paramedic**

In addition, the cognitive exam tests these skills and knowledge extensively and relates them to trauma and medical situations. The chapter describes what needs to be done with the patient during that exam (what questions should or could be asked) and how to remember these steps both during the high-stress exam and on the job, when working as a paramedic. Discussion includes a detailed look at history taking and the important assessment points for any medical exam. In addition, this chapter describes what evaluators will be looking for under each heading of the Integrated Out-of-Hospital (IOOH) scenario in box features called Look at the IOOH. Point values are indicated, where applicable.

Look at IOOH: General Format

The IOOH grading sheet is a series of five areas graded on a 0–3 scale. Though the test maker does not publish what point score is needed to pass, generally a score of 2 or higher in each section is required. In all the sections, the points awarded for a 2- or 3-quality score differ essentially only in finesse and nuance. These are the IOOH sections:

- Leadership and Scene Management
- Patient Assessment
- Patient Management
- Interpersonal Relations
- Integration (Field Impression and Transport Decision)

SCENE SIZE-UP

From all perspectives, the Scene Size-Up is the most important phase of any call the paramedic makes. Failing to perform an adequate scene size-up may cause important details to be missed, which may put the paramedic and other responders in unnecessary danger or miss the scope of the problem at hand.

Body Substance Isolation (BSI) and Scene Safety: 2 Points

Scene safety is the part of the psychomotor exam where all testing candidates demonstrate their best "jazz hands." However, it is also something that should not be taken lightly. On the trauma assessment, undertaking BSI and indicating that the scene is safe for EMS to proceed is worth a quick and easy 2 points.

In the psychomotor exam, you receive credit for either donning appropriate BSI for the anticipated call type or stating that you are wearing it. Note that when any BSI component that is actually worn becomes unusable (e.g., a glove rips), it should be replaced as soon as possible, and replacement time counts against total time in the scenario. Simply stating that one would be wearing BSI appropriate for the scenario is enough to be awarded the point.

BSI includes all forms of protection the paramedic may elect to use to remain safe from a patient's bodily fluids, including blood, amniotic fluid, saliva, and semen.

Table 3-1. BSI Precautions

Type	Protection Offered	When to Don
Gloves	Essential protection for the hands	Every call involving a patient
Eye protection	Splatter protection for the eyes	During situations where splashing of bodily fluids is likely (e.g., childbirth, arterial bleeds)
HEPA or N95 mask	Protection from inhaled hazards including pathogens or particulate matter	When respiratory precautions are needed (e.g., patient with suspected respiratory infection, building collapse)
Specialized PPE (e.g., turnout gear, steel-toed boots, helmets)	Protection from scene-specific hazards	When protection from scene-specific hazards is crucial (e.g., fire scenes, motor vehicle collisions, weather-related causes)

Before every patient contact, it is important to change gloves and replace any piece of equipment that may have become contaminated. Doing so helps prevent the spread of disease from one patient to another. Replacement of protective gear is especially important on the scenes of multiple-casualty incidents, where the paramedic moves between patients in rapid succession. Hand hygiene after removing gloves and before seeing the next patient is also highly recommended. While handwashing with soap and water is the best prevention, alcohol-based sanitizers are a suitable substitute when the hands are not visibly soiled.

Scene safety is of paramount concern to the paramedic and all responding personnel, because everyone should be able to go home safely after each and every call. Ensuring scene safety means taking steps to avoid entering a potentially volatile or dangerous scene. Frequently, the best way to do this is to have police secure the scene, confirm that there is no one in the location with a weapon, and ensure that access to any weapon in the house is minimal.

But scene safety is not limited to entry into a house or other location where weapons may be present. Other examples include

- Not entering swift water such as a river without proper training and securing lines.
- Securing any animals on the scene; depending on the region where the paramedic is working, this could mean anything from domestic pets to farm animals.
- Waiting to access a vehicle until it can be properly checked by the fire department.

Maintenance of scene safety is an ongoing process. A scene that initially appears safe may suddenly become insecure; for instance, a violent person might return to the scene in a rage, or a spark could ignite gasoline at a motor vehicle crash. The best course of action always involves preserving the personal safety of the paramedic and the rest of the team. When a scene becomes unsafe and raises the paramedic's concerns about personal well-being, it is not abandonment of the patient to retreat until the scene can be made safe again. Looking out for the potential hazards of a scene is known as situational awareness, and each team leader should possess it.

Mechanism of Injury/Nature of Illness (MOI/NOI): 1 Point

In the trauma assessment station, the exam candidate must distinguish and explicitly identify the patient's probable mechanism of injury. The candidate can ask the room proctor outright, and the proctor will state the mechanism of injury. Because this is a trauma station, the nature of illness is less likely to play a role in the situation, but it is not out of the realm of possibility. For instance, a patient with injuries from a fall could have fallen after a medical event such as syncope or seizure, so keep such possibilities in mind.

Number of Patients: 1 Point

Ask specifically about the number of patients in the scenario. In a real call, the presence of multiple patients in the room would be inherently obvious, and examiners would be unlikely to present a scenario with multiple patients. However, the evaluators here want to know that the provider candidate is always aware of the possibility of multiple patients on a scene (e.g., carbon monoxide poisoning).

Requests Additional Assistance: 1 Point

The exam includes this line to ensure that the candidate is always thinking about an exit strategy: How will the paramedic remove the patient from the location? What resources are needed to make that happen? Consider the needs of the scenario posed. For example:

- If the scenario involves multiple patients or the patient's needs are beyond the capacity of one ambulance crew, the paramedic should request additional EMS units.
- In fire or technical rescue operations, the paramedic should request the assistance of the fire department.
- If the scenario involves unruly mobs of people, have police on scene to assist in crowd control.

Considers Stabilization of the Spine: 1 Point

Stabilization of the spine is included in the Scene Size-Up because it should always be an early consideration for the paramedic. Like the ABCs (airway, breathing, circulation), cervical spine precautions—and by extension, motion restriction precautions for the entire spine—should be considered early and often. This very important step is conducted in relation to the trauma assessment station. In some testing stations, observing this step will simply involve the paramedic stating, "I would apply a cervical collar due to the suspected mechanism of injury stated." Some testing centers will have the assistant in the room actually apply the collar to the simulated patient.

Why These 6 Points Are Important

The candidate can earn a maximum of 6 points in the Scene Size-Up section of the trauma assessment. Given that 42 points are available in this station, 6 points may seem trivial; however, Scene Size-Up includes three items that will fail the candidate if they are missed. Be sure to perform these essential steps:

- Mention scene safety.
- Take (or verbalize) BSI.
- Assess the spine and provide spinal motion restriction when indicated.

Failure to perform any of these steps will result in failure regardless of the remainder of the candidate's performance on the assessment. For a suggested way to navigate this section of the trauma assessment station, see the Pro-Tip.

Look at IOOH: Leadership and Scene Management

In order to achieve the 3-point maximum in this section for the IOOH, candidates must demonstrate that they have assessed the scene and taken deliberate control of it. Scene management depends on the needs presented in the scenario, but here are a few examples of how this requirement might be met:

- Controlling crowd presence with police
- Having the homeowner secure animals in the house
- Removing throw rugs or other tripping obstacles

In some cases, appropriate scene management may mean identifying a situation that involves waiting for other agencies, such as the fire department to secure a vehicle. The provider candidate should also elicit suggestions from other team members.

PRIMARY SURVEY/RESUSCITATION

The trauma assessment scoring rubric from the National Registry of EMTs includes a section called Primary Survey; this set of steps is also known as the primary assessment. In patients who do not require immediate ABC interventions, the primary assessment should generally take less than a minute to complete. The Primary Survey section of the exam includes elements that are not intuitive and are often missed. This part of the chapter discusses all the elements of the primary assessment in the order in which they appear on the rubric. Once again, point values are indicated.

Verbalizes a General Impression of the Patient: 1 Point

To earn this point, the provider candidate must state out loud to the proctor an overarching first impression of the patient. For example, suppose the scenario presents a middle-aged fall victim who is sitting against the wall holding one arm and appearing to be in pain. To verbalize a general impression of this patient, the provider candidate might simply say, "I see an approximately 35-year-old female seated on the ground, holding her arm in apparent pain and distress. She appears to be conscious and alert to her surroundings." That's it. No big deal. But verbalizing a general impression of the patient for the exam feels very unnatural and requires practice to remember, because a paramedic would not typically speak in this ritualized way on an actual scene with an actual patient.

The verbalized general impression must include certain components to receive exam credit:

- **Approximate Estimated Age of the Patient.** While a paramedic will later get the exact age during collection of demographics, this estimate will help guide priority of the patient later in the section.
- **Presumed Sex of the Patient.** This can also be modified later with input from the patient.
- **A "Doorway Assessment" of the Patient's Level of Consciousness.** This spot assessment includes only what is observable and may be limited to the AVPU scale. It is not possible to make a judgment of the patient's level of orientation at this time, nor would it be appropriate to guess.

Determines Responsiveness/Level of Consciousness: 1 Point

This point can be earned in either of two ways. Most commonly, the point is awarded as a result of the statement made in the general impression. The verbalized general impression includes the "doorway assessment," which should satisfy the requirement of determining the level of responsiveness. Alternatively, the point can be awarded when the patient answers the candidate's opening question. For example, if the candidate asks "What seems to be the problem today?" and the patient responds immediately, it is apparent that the patient is alert.

It is worth the momentary pause in the scenario to turn to the proctor and state the findings clearly to ensure the proctor knows you are explicitly aware of the patient's mental status. Additionally, although there is no specific place to be rewarded for assessing the patient's orientation to person, place, time, and event, you should consider whether it is needed in every situation as the assessment dictates.

Pro-Tip

You will begin the trauma assessment station in the room with the patient—essentially on scene with the patient. Before even approaching the patient, mentally tick off a script that will ensure you get **all 8 points** available in the Scene Size-Up. At the conclusion of the vignette presented by the room proctor, state all of the following as appropriate for the scenario presented, pausing at the end of each sentence for an answer or response from the proctor.

"BSI taken. Scene is safe. What is the mechanism of injury or nature of illness? How many patients? At this time I (will/will not) request additional help from (police/fire/additional EMS). I am considering stabilization of the spine and will apply that if my assessment reveals it is indicated. I see an approximately 35-year-old female, seated on the ground, holding her arm in apparent pain and distress. She appears to be conscious and alert to her surroundings."

Determines Chief Complaint/Apparent Life Threats: 1 Point

This is perhaps the easiest point on the entire rubric. Earning it is as simple as asking the patient "What seems to be the problem today?" or some similar opening question. Determining the chief complaint is necessary to guide the remainder of the exam, particularly the focused physical exam later in the encounter, and it establishes the focus of the reassessments.

The remainder of the primary assessment is, in essence, an evaluation of ABC-related threats to life. If the patient in the scenario responds to your opening question with any kind of spoken answer, you can accurately report to the proctor that the patient has an airway, is breathing, and has a pulse sufficient to support brain function. The remainder of the section requires more diligence on the part of the paramedic candidate for full credit, but there is no reason to miss this "gimme."

Airway: 2 Points

Evaluating any patient for a patent airway is second in importance only to scene safety. Without a patent airway, the patient will certainly not survive. The points in this section of the psychomotor exam are awarded for the following:

- Noting an open airway in a talking patient, or opening the airway and assessing with "look, listen, and feel" for breathing in an unresponsive patient
- In an unresponsive patient, providing an airway adjunct of the paramedic's choice that is appropriate for the patient's condition

Though it seems obvious that a patient who is talking does not need an airway adjunct, taking a moment to *state this to the proctor* is always a good idea. (See the Airway, Respirations, Ventilation, and Respiratory Emergencies chapter for more on these topics.)

Breathing: 4 Points

Once an airway is established in the patient, breathing should be assessed for rate and quality. During the primary assessment, breathing can simply be assessed as present or absent. No actual respiratory rate needs to be counted at this time. If the patient is breathing, move on to rapidly assess the quality of those respirations. If instead the patient is not breathing, stop further assessment beyond the ABCs until ventilations can be provided using a bag-valve-mask device or other positive-pressure ventilation system. (Note: According to the most recent CPR protocols from the American Heart Association, the pulse should be checked early and often, and compressions should be started even if the inability to ventilate is identified. Unfortunately, these steps may seem out of sync with each other or even in opposition, but really they are performed in parallel rather than sequentially.)

When assessing for adequate ventilation, the paramedic is looking for the following:

- **Reasonable Rate.** The rate should be within the range of generally acceptable limits, not too fast or too slow. The paramedic is looking for clinically significant hyperventilation or the absence of agonal respirations.
- **Adequate Depth.** Depth should be adequate to produce visible chest rise and fall.
- **No Accessory Muscle Use or Retractions.** The patient should be free from accessory muscle use and retractions. Any elevated work of breathing should be noted.
- **No Interference with the Act of Breathing.** There should not be any chest wall injuries, and chest wall excursion should be unhindered and equal. If an injury is found or indicated, it should be managed immediately.

The final topic in this section is initiation of appropriate oxygen therapy. This topic has recently become somewhat controversial because of the word *appropriate*. Without explicit explanation, instructors and candidates alike are left to wonder what constitutes "appropriate oxygen therapy" from the evaluator's point of view. Theoretically, for a person who is breathing adequately, with an appropriate rate and rhythm and without any presumed chest or head injury, the oxygen present in room air should be appropriate. However, some people insist that providing high-flow oxygen (10 L/minute or more) is the candidate's safest route in all patient situations and cannot ever be marked incorrect. Despite mounting evidence in research literature against the routine use of high-flow oxygen, the National Registry had provided little guidance on this topic at press time. The best recommendation for NRP exam candidates, therefore, is to do what is, in fact, appropriate for patient care.

Circulation: 4 Points

Assuming that assessment of the patient has not identified the need for compressions thus far, the next step is evaluation of circulation. As in the breathing assessment, it is not necessary to determine an actual rate at this point. It is sufficient to determine the presence or absence of a pulse at any of the usual pulse points—but most likely radial or carotid. A radial or carotid pulse ensures, temporarily at least, that the patient has adequate blood circulation to perfuse the brain and vital organs.

When assessing the pulse rate, also evaluate its quality (though this is not a specific point in the rubric). It could be thready and weak or bounding and full. Also take note of any irregularities. The pulse should have a regular beat to it. If not, is the irregularity regular or irregular? A *regularly* irregular pulse could indicate a heart block or geminal pattern such as bigeminy or trigeminy, while an *irregularly* irregular pattern could indicate atrial fibrillation or something more serious. Further evaluation is warranted. (See the Cardiology, Cardiac Emergencies, and Resuscitation chapter for more on these topics.)

As part of this section, a rapid body sweep for major bleeding should be performed. Assessing for and controlling major hemorrhage at this point is necessary to minimize the effects of blood loss. Waiting until the secondary assessment to perform this step and address the findings could be too late.

When checking for a pulse, verbally state that you are simultaneously checking the skin color, temperature, and texture—qualities that are ordinarily easy to observe in a real patient. Linking the pulse evaluation with this second evaluation ensures that it is incorporated into the assessment of the simulated patient. Skin color, temperature, and texture are often difficult to simulate in an otherwise healthy individual.

Finally, evaluate whether the patient is in shock. By now, the paramedic candidate should have enough information to do so. Recall that the first minute or so of the encounter (if done in rubric order) was spent assessing respiratory rate and effort, circulatory rate and quality, and skin color and temperature. When taken together, do the resulting assessments present the picture of a patient in shock? If yes, initiate shock management, which includes the following four components:

- Initiation of oxygen, if not already done
- Proper positioning of the patient
- Careful handling of the patient
- Maintaining the core temperature of the patient

Mentioning these items, rather than enacting them, is all that is needed.

Identifies Priority Patients/Makes Transport Decision Based upon Calculated GCS: 1 Point

The priority and transport decision is another crucial but often overlooked topic on the trauma assessment rubric. It is also related to a critical failure point. This point is awarded, and the critical failure is avoided, if the paramedic candidate identifies the patient as a priority patient (the scenarios are often designed to be a critical or potentially critical patient) and states that immediate transportation is warranted. Both statements must be made within the first 10 minutes of the scenario's start time. Although this topic appears on the rubric after the evaluation of the ABCs, it can be highlighted at any time the paramedic recognizes a threat to life that would warrant rapid transport. For example, if the paramedic finds inadequate breathing that must be managed with a bag-valve-mask device, it is not necessary to wait until the circulatory assessment is completed to state the need for rapid transport.

Look at IOOH: Integration (Field Impression and Transport Decision)

Unlike the trauma assessment station, where the need for priority and transport is decided in the middle of the experience, in the IOOH, the Field Impression and Transport Decision box is at the end of the scenario. This section of IOOH has 3 distinct areas of focus:
- First and foremost, the provider should provide appropriate management.
- The provider must identify at least one working diagnosis, and preferably more than one. The list of possible diagnoses that the paramedic is actively treating or is considering treating, known as the *differential diagnosis*, should also be appropriately prioritized.
- The provider should identify other transport options that would be appropriate for the patient. Transport options are usually based on transport time to the hospitals available in the scenario, and they can also include a more distant hospital that has specialized treatment for the situation. For example, the candidate might opt for a trauma center over a tertiary care facility even if the trauma center is slightly farther, or might opt for aeromedical transport for a stroke patient, and so on.

Recognizing and treating the primary issue and transporting to an appropriate facility are all that is needed for a score of 2. The major difference between 2 points versus 3 points (the maximum for this section) is the prioritized differential diagnosis.

HISTORY TAKING

In the trauma assessment portion of the psychomotor exam, the history taking section is worth only 2 points: 1 point for assessing or directing the assessment of baseline vital signs, and 1 point for making an attempt to obtain a SAMPLE history. This section explores these important aspects of history taking in the context of both medical patients and trauma patients. It also highlights the OPPQRST mnemonic for patient questioning and the vital signs assessment. Finally, this section collects other pieces of patient assessment that do not neatly fall into a mnemonic, such as presenting an organized way to recall them when you enter the testing rooms for any portion of the psycho-motor or cognitive exams.

SAMPLE History

The SAMPLE questions have a long history in the prehospital provider's repertoire for questioning patients. This mnemonic stands for:

- Signs and symptoms
- Allergies
- Medications
- Past medical history
- Last oral intake
- Events prior

Signs and Symptoms

Signs are manifestations the paramedic can visually observe on or around the patient—for example, vomiting, abnormalities of the body (including skin changes or facial droop), or severe respiratory distress. Symptoms are subjective manifestations the patient complains of that are not outwardly observable. In this part of the patient assessment, the paramedic should confirm with the patient that the observed signs are new and ask the patient about as many symptoms as possible or appropriate to the complaint. You should elicit information about symptoms from the patient with open-ended questioning techniques whenever possible, but it may be necessary to ask specifically about some or all of them. Symptoms that are universal and apply across medical and trauma situations include chest pains or discomfort, shortness of breath, nausea, vomiting, diarrhea and other gastrointestinal dysfunction, dizziness, weakness, headache, loss of consciousness or syncope, hunger, and thirst. These cover a wide breadth of problems, can help rule in or rule out various medical problems, and point to possible areas of occult trauma.

Allergies

The paramedic should inquire about any allergies the patient may have, specifically allergies to both prescription and over-the-counter medications. Also inquire about seasonal and environmental allergies as well as food allergies. Should the patient's condition deteriorate, this information can be helpful to the providers caring for the patient.

Medications

On every call, the paramedic should ask the patient about medications taken on a regular basis. These include but are not limited to prescription and over-the-counter medications; also ask about natural remedies, homeopathic medications, vitamins, and other supplements the patient may be using. Try to find out what the patient is using these medications or remedies to treat.

Past Medical History

Paramedics should make a concerted effort to know the patient's medical history. While it is often possible to puzzle this out from the medications the patient takes, that may not give the full picture. The patient may have a condition that is not treated with medication or one that is no longer an active issue, but these need to be known. For example, a patient with a history of cancer may not take medication for it now and may be in total remission, but knowing that cancer is a part of the patient's history could be important to evaluating the patient in the hospital.

Last Oral Intake

Ask what was the last thing the patient took orally. It is not always food; the last oral intake could have been a mouthful of medications or an excess of alcohol that led to EMS being called. Asking about the patient's last oral intake may also remind the paramedic of the possibility of ingested poisons, overdoses, possible food allergies, or contaminated food or drink being at the root of the patient's current problem. Knowing what the patient last consumed is also helpful if the patient requires emergency surgery upon arrival at the hospital.

Events Prior

Events prior information includes everything about the situation leading up to why EMS was called in the first place, regardless of complaint. Answers to these questions often lead directly into the evaluation of the history of the present illness (HPI). The OPPQRST mnemonic (or OPPQRST, depending on the source) helps structure an investigation of the HPI. OPPQRST lends itself best to pain assessment, but portions can apply to all situations. While the list of questions that follows is not necessarily exhaustive, it should be sufficient for the success of any candidate in the various psychomotor exam stations (including oral stations and IOOH).

Table 3-2. OPPQRST

Letter meaning	Suggested question(s)
Onset	What were you doing when this started?
Provocation	What makes this pain worse?
Palliation	What makes this pain better? What have you done to make this pain better?
Quality	How would you describe this pain? (Sharp, dull, achy, tearing, pressured, squeezing, etc.)
Radiation	Does this pain go anywhere else, or does it remain localized? Where else does it move?
Severity	On a scale of 1 to 10, with 10 being the worst pain you have ever felt and 1 being no pain at all, rate this pain.
Time	How long have you been experiencing this pain? Does this pain come and go or remain constant? Has it been getting worse or staying about the same?

Additional Questions

SAMPLE and OPPQRST are useful mnemonics, but some questions do not neatly fit into them. Consider asking the patient these questions as well:

- Has this happened before?
- How long ago did this last happen?
- What was done for you the last time you experienced similar symptoms?
- Have you sought treatment for this issue before?

Generally, if it seems like a question could generate valuable information about the situation at hand, go ahead and ask it. Patients will seldom volunteer information to any medical provider, so it is the paramedic's responsibility to work to pull out that information in a caring and supportive way whenever possible. More information about the assessment of specific complaints is available in the following chapters.

Vital Signs

Obtaining vital signs during an assessment should be an obvious step. Vital signs should be obtained from every patient, unless something prevents it (e.g., patient is violent and will not allow; situation is tense and easily exacerbated). Yet another mnemonic represents the vital signs that should be obtained during every patient encounter, and especially during the psychomotor exam testing stations: B-PRESS. This abbreviation stands for:

- **B**lood pressure
- **P**ulse
- **R**espiratory rate
- **E**yes (pupils)
- **S**kin (color temperature and texture)
- **S**ounds (breath sounds)

Besides B-PRESS, the paramedic should also obtain a pulse oximetry reading on every patient. This measurement is essential to evaluating the patient's end-organ perfusion.

Certain patient populations require additional monitoring of observable vital signs, such as temperature and end-tidal carbon dioxide ($ETCO_2$) monitoring. The patient's temperature can be taken using a tympanic, temporal, or oral thermometer, depending on what is available at local services. Use caution in the tympanic and temporal models in cold environments; these are superficial areas of measurement, so they are prone to false low-temperature readings in and shortly after removal from the cold environment. $ETCO_2$ monitoring should be used in cases of respiratory distress, suspected sepsis, cardiac arrest, and acidosis. Temperature and $ETCO_2$ monitoring and the patients they should be used on are described in more detail in later chapters.

SECONDARY ASSESSMENT (PHYSICAL EXAM)

The trauma assessment rubric refers to this part of the patient encounter as the Secondary Assessment; however, many texts refer to it as the physical exam. This chapter largely uses the term *physical exam*, with the understanding that in life-threatening emergencies, it may be less thorough than in more routine situations and thus "secondary" to ongoing primary assessment and management. In order to ensure that nothing is missed, always perform the physical exam from head to toe on an adult. Some younger pediatric patients may benefit from having it performed toe to head; this topic is discussed later in the book.

During all components of the exam, the paramedic should look for any finding that is out of the ordinary. **Inspect** all areas systematically for DCAP-BTLS. **Auscultate** areas that house hollow organs, e.g., lung sounds in the chest and the bowel sounds in the abdomen. **Palpate** all areas firmly as appropriate for obvious injuries.

Table 3-3. DCAP-BTLS

Deformities	Burns
Contusions	Tenderness
Abrasions	Lacerations
Punctures	Swelling

A fourth assessment modality, called **percussion**, is most commonly used on the abdomen and chest. Despite its usefulness, percussion is rarely performed in the field. This is not only because it takes a lot of practice to hear the differences that percussion tests for, but also because effective percussion requires silence to hear the sound produced when the provider taps. Silence is rarely available in an emergency field setting, making percussion much better suited to an office or hospital setting.

Percussion is used over solid organs such as the liver or over the lung fields of the chest. It is performed by placing the fingers of the nondominant hand over the area to be percussed and tapping the first knuckle of the middle finger with the tip of the middle finger (or tips of the middle and index fingers) of the dominant hand to create a sound. This sound is described as unremarkable, dull, or hyperresonant. Unremarkable percussive findings are reasonably normal; dull percussive sounds could indicate fluid, blood, or other consolidation; hyperresonance under percussion could indicate a buildup of air under pressure, such as in tension pneumothorax.

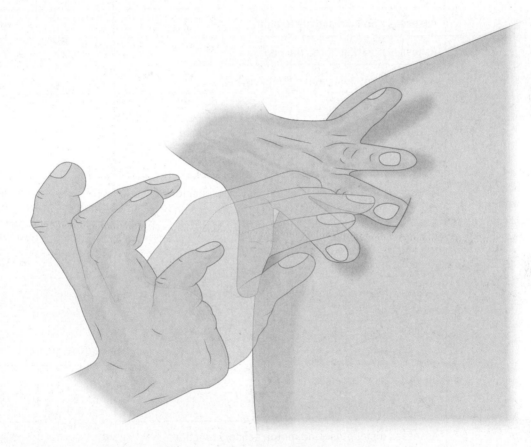

Figure 3-1. Percussion

When an area of the patient's body requires all four modalities for assessment, the paramedic should generally follow IPPA order: inspect, palpate, percuss, auscultate. This is true for the anterior and posterior thorax. For the abdomen, however, *always* auscultate before palpating; the assessment order for the abdomen is IAPP: inspect, auscultate, percuss, palpate. Think of the assessment order of the abdominal exam as progressing from least invasive (inspection) to most invasive (deep palpation).

In the psychomotor exam, 18 points are available for the physical exam component of the trauma assessment—which highlights the importance of the physical exam in the trauma assessment. The following table outlines the order in which the physical exam should be performed in most circumstances (from head to toe) and records how many points each assessment component is worth in the trauma assessment. The table also indicates which components are commonly a part of the medical physical assessment and where in the trauma assessment rubric the assessment component can be found (Body Region column). Not all assessment components in a body region are specifically evaluated there; however, they are important to the physical exam.

Table 3-4. Secondary Assessment/Physical Exam

Body Region	Assessment Components	Trauma	Medical
Head	Inspects mouth, nose, and facial area	1	Yes
	Palpates areas of the face		
	Inspects and palpates scalp/skull and ears	1	
	Assesses pupils' reactivity to light	1	Yes
Neck	Assesses position of the trachea	1	Yes
	Assesses for jugular vein distension	1	Yes
	Palpates cervical spine	1	
Chest	Inspects chest	1	
	Auscultates chest	1	Yes
	Palpates chest, including for equality of expansion, crepitus, and flail segments	1	Yes
Abdomen and pelvis	Inspects and palpates abdomen	1	Yes
	Auscultates abdomen		Yes
	Assesses pelvis using lateral and anterior/posterior compression	1	
	Assesses genitalia/perineum as needed (Verbalized during psychomotor exam)	1	Yes
Lower extremities	Inspects each extremity	2 (1 point per leg)	
	Palpates each entire extremity		
	Assesses distal pulse and motor/sensory function		Yes
	Assesses for pitting or nonpitting pedal edema		Yes
Upper extremities	Inspects each extremity	2 (1 point per arm)	
	Palpates each extremity		
	Assesses distal pulse and motor/sensory function		Yes
Posterior chest, lumbar area, and buttocks	Inspects and palpates posterior chest	1	
	Inspects and palpates lumbar area and buttocks	1	
	Total point value	18	

The full credit of 3 points is awarded to candidates who complete the entire patient assessment—history and physical exam—in an organized and efficient way. The exam candidate must also integrate the findings into the assessment process. In other words, when you are in there, the questions in the history should flow logically and lead to other, patient-specific questions. Using early findings to inform your later questions and assessment steps will indicate to the proctor that you know not only what to ask, but also what the answers mean in relation to the patient's condition. Maintaining situational awareness is another component of the patient assessment, meaning that you should be aware of time on scene, any obstacles to maneuvering the patient to the stretcher, and possible alterations to scene safety (though this is unlikely). In this scenario, the patient can improve or deteriorate regardless of your treatment, so be aware of this possibility as well.

Manages Secondary Injuries and Wounds Appropriately: 1 Point

This is an assessment station, so emphasis is placed on the assessment. This station requires only "voice treatment" of any wounds or injuries found during the assessment. Simply stating the treatment—for instance, "I would have my partner splint the ankle fracture I found"—would count as appropriate treatment. Be careful, however, not to overtreat the injuries found, as doing too much for the patient can be as harmful to your score as doing too little.

Reassesses Patient: 1 Point

Indicate what would be reassessed in this patient and how often. For most patients encountered in this station, it would be appropriate and expected to reassess the chief complaint and the efficacy of treatments performed every 5 minutes until arrival at the hospital (or landing zone, if a flight is the most appropriate transport for the patient).

Look at IOOH: Patient Management

The difference between a score of 2 and 3 in the Patient Management section of the IOOH is based on anticipation and collaboration with your partner in the room. To achieve 3 points, you will need to anticipate the patient's possible further needs and intervene rapidly after confirming interventions with your partner; proceeding in this way demonstrates teamwork, which is crucial in medicine, as well as your proactiveness in caring for your patient. For example, suppose an intubated patient in the scenario begins to decompensate. A score of 3 would go to the paramedic who verifies that the tube is still in place and that ventilations remain as easy as they were at the outset, and who does so with the assistance of the partner, whom the candidate directs to evaluate these areas. Conversely, a paramedic who did not ask the partner if there was a change in ventilatory resistance, and only listened to lung sounds instead, would possibly receive a 2.

Look at IOOH: Interpersonal Relations

Simply interacting with and responding appropriately to the patient, crew, and bystanders while engaging in closed-loop communication is only enough to get the candidate a score of 2. Therapeutic communication and demonstration of empathy are integral to the top score. To achieve a score of 3 in this section of the IOOH, the candidate must go above and beyond the fundamentals by encouraging feedback from the team about the scene, patient, and treatment while also demonstrating leadership, responsibility, and decision-making.

SUMMARY

The information in this chapter is a lot to bring into a room during the psychomotor exam, or even onto a call. In the high-pressure situation of testing, it is easy to omit certain important criteria during the evaluation. While you are not permitted to bring anything into the psychomotor testing stations with you, you can write down anything you want to for a couple of minutes before the scenario is read. The figure illustrates a suggested way to write down memory aids once you arrive in the room and before your time starts. Essential patient demographics are noted at the top of the page. It includes all of the mnemonics discussed here, as well as this artist's rendition of the human body.

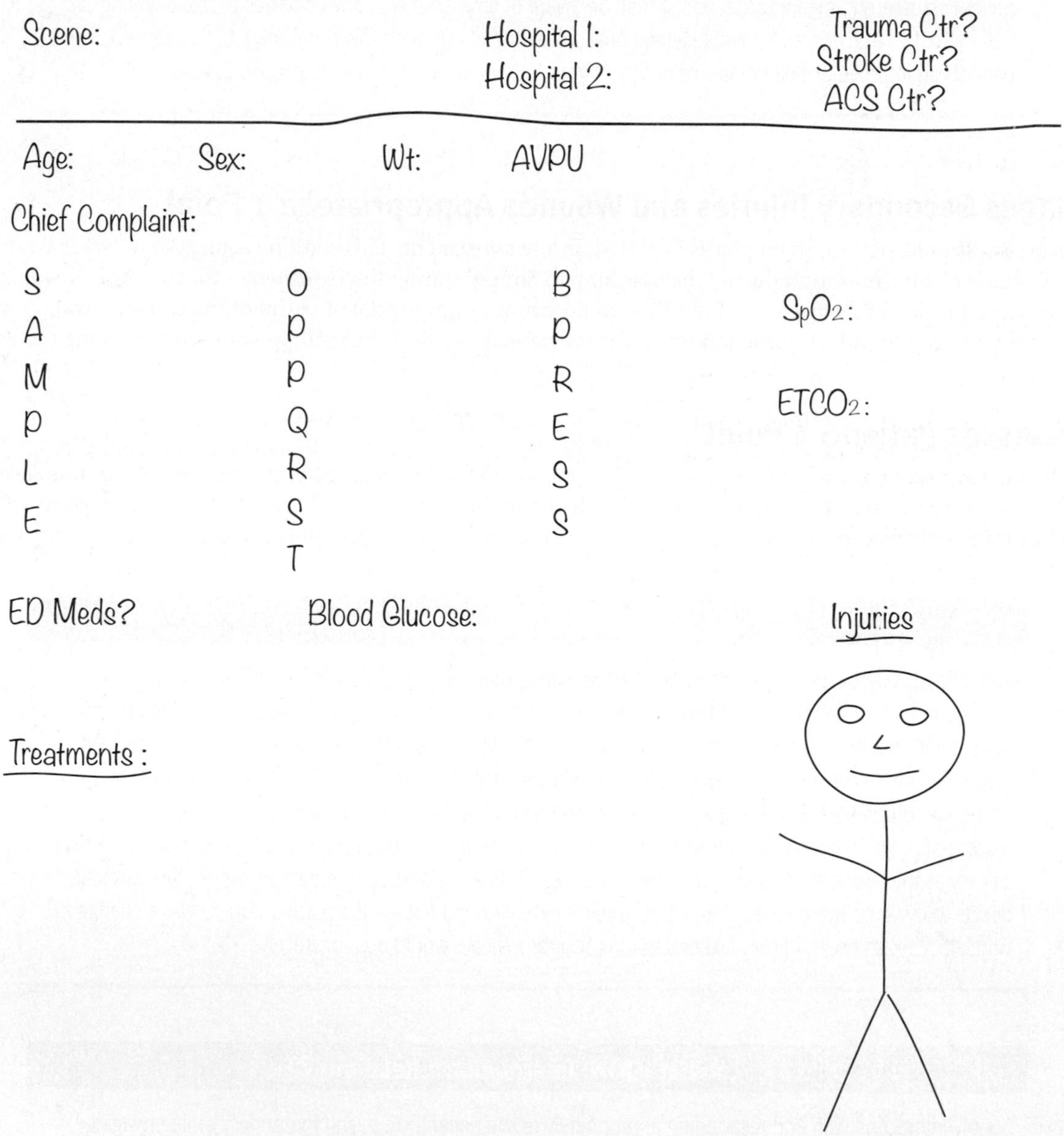

Scene:

Hospital 1:
Hospital 2:

Trauma Ctr?
Stroke Ctr?
ACS Ctr?

Age: Sex: Wt: AVPU

Chief Complaint:

S	O	B
A	P	P
M	P	R
P	Q	E
L	R	S
E	S	S
	T	

SpO_2:

$ETCO_2$:

ED Meds?   Blood Glucose:

Injuries

Treatments :

Figure 3-2. Suggested Write-Up of Memory Aids in the Exam Room

REVIEW QUESTIONS

Select the ONE best answer.

1. During which part of the patient assessment would it be MOST appropriate to determine the patient's level of consciousness?

    A. Scene Size-Up

    B. Primary Assessment

    C. Focused Physical Exam

    D. Secondary Assessment

2. Your patient describes her pain to you as a 5 out of 10. What question did you MOST likely just ask her?

    A. Quality

    B. Radiation

    C. Severity

    D. Type

3. You are on the scene with a 54-year-old male who was the restrained driver in a motor vehicle crash. He is complaining of chest and abdominal pain that he believes is from the seat belt. Which of these should you do SECOND during your assessment of the chest?

    A. Auscultation

    B. Inspection

    C. Palpation

    D. Percussion

4. You are on the scene with a 54-year-old male who was the restrained driver in a motor vehicle crash. He is complaining of chest and abdominal pain that he believes is from the seat belt. Which of these should you do SECOND during your assessment of the abdomen?

    A. Auscultation

    B. Inspection

    C. Palpation

    D. Percussion

5. Which of the following is NOT typically a part of the Primary Assessment?

    A. Checking for a pulse

    B. Assessing skin color, temperature, and texture

    C. Listening to breath sounds

    D. Providing ventilatory assistance

6. Your patient is complaining of respiratory distress and has these basic vital signs: HR: 118; BP: 180/100; RR: 40. Which of the following could provide you the most helpful information about this patient?

    A. End-tidal carbon dioxide
    B. Pulse oximetry
    C. Skin color, temperature, and texture
    D. Temperature

7. A secondary exam should be performed:

    A. On every patient.
    B. Only after the primary exam is completed.
    C. Only once on the ambulance during transport.
    D. When immediate life threats are treated.

8. You are assessing a patient with altered mental status and who is not able to verbalize a complaint; this patient was found sleeping on a park bench and is only making incomprehensible sounds. He is an older adult, is protecting his own airway, and has unremarkable rate and depth of respirations. Radial pulses are present and unremarkable in rate and quality. Your primary assessment reveals no immediate life threats. Which of the following is the most reasonable list of top three possible diagnoses in the differential?

    A. Alcohol intoxication, dementia, diabetic problem
    B. Heat cramps, stroke, diabetic problem
    C. Sepsis, heat exhaustion, alcohol intoxication
    D. Stroke, sepsis, head injury

ANSWERS AND EXPLANATIONS

1. **The correct answer is (B).** Level of consciousness is first assessed during the primary assessment and reassessed in greater detail during history taking. None of the other answers is accurate.

2. **The correct answer is (C).** The question would be, "On a scale of 1 to 10, with 10 being the worst pain you've ever had, rank this pain." This question is typically asked during "Severity" from the OPPQRST mnemonic. The question stem reflects an answer the patient might give to this question.

3. **The correct answer is (C).** The second maneuver you should do when assessing the chest is palpation. This is done after inspection (B) and typically before auscultation (A) and percussion (D), if percussion is done at all by a paramedic. Auscultation is completed second only during the abdominal exam.

4. **The correct answer is (A).** The second maneuver you should do when assessing the abdomen is auscultation. This is done after inspection (B) and typically before palpation (C) and percussion (D), if percussion is done at all by a paramedic. Auscultation is completed second only during the abdominal exam, because palpation done first can alter what would be heard.

5. **The correct answer is (C).** Listening to breath sounds, while important, is typically conducted during the secondary assessment, or physical exam. All of the other answer choices are completed during the primary assessment. Ventilatory assistance (D) is provided during the primary assessment because any problem with the ABCs found during the primary assessment is corrected immediately.

6. **The correct answer is (A).** End-tidal carbon dioxide monitoring would be able to help the paramedic differentiate between possible causes of respiratory distress, specifically asthma/COPD (which would show a shark fin waveform), hyperglycemia/acidosis/sepsis (peak $ETCO_2$ level would be lower than expected), or CHF (peak $ETCO_2$ level would be normal or slightly elevated with a normal waveform). None of the other answer choices can directly rule in or rule out any specific condition. Pulse oximetry (B) values could be similar in both CHF and COPD.

7. **The correct answer is (D).** A secondary exam, or physical exam, is performed only after all the life threats have been remedied. In severe situations, treating the ABCs may be all the paramedic has time for. Therefore, the secondary exam may not be completed on every patient (A). While technically it is done after the primary assessment is completed (B), the more accurate answer is that it is done once the life threats are remedied. There is nothing stating that the secondary assessment can only be carried out in the ambulance (C).

8. **The correct answer is (A).** Based on the limited information on the patient available in the question stem, the key is to select the option with three possible diagnoses that are likely to cause a notable derangement in mental status without appreciably affecting the vital signs. Since both respiratory rate and quality and pulse rate and quality are described as unremarkable, it is reasonable to conclude that they are within normal expected limits. Only answer choice (A) offers conditions that could present with a marked decline in mentation but maintain normal vital signs. Heat cramps (B) would not affect mentation. Sepsis (C) and (D) would likely present with tachycardia and a weak or thready pulse.

Airway, Respirations, Ventilation, and Respiratory Emergencies

4

Learning Objectives

❏ Describe the structures and functions of the airways and the respiratory system.

❏ Explain the physiological regulation of breathing.

❏ Describe and demonstrate techniques for placing basic, advanced, and alternative airways.

❏ Differentiate, assess, and treat respiratory emergencies associated with the upper and lower airways.

Supporting breathing efforts and maintaining an open airway are the most important life-saving treatments that a paramedic will ever perform. They are the bread and butter of the profession. When it comes to airway and breathing problems, the paramedic should be proactive and aggressive in treating the patient. Quick action when faced with a patient with a critical respiratory condition will go a long way in not only preventing the patient from getting worse but also shortening the hospital stay for the patient. In this chapter, the anatomy and physiology of the respiratory system will be reviewed, and intricacies of airway management will be discussed. Medical knowledge will be linked with the practical examination whenever possible. Finally, the assessment, management, and treatment of patients with respiratory issues will be presented.

ANATOMY AND PHYSIOLOGY OF THE RESPIRATORY SYSTEM

The respiratory system includes all the structures relating to the passage of air from the atmosphere to the lungs and associated structures responsible for the actions of breathing, including muscles and nerves. To begin our discussion of the airway, the pathway of air will be followed as it enters the system from the atmosphere during inhalation.

Structures of Breathing

Upper Airway

The upper airway includes the structures superior to and inclusive of the larynx. While air can enter the body by mouth, it primarily enters the nose during quiet breathing at rest. Air passes through the nostrils and enters the nasopharynx. This area is lined with mucous membranes where the air is warmed and humidified, helping protect the body from heat loss and hypothermia. This area also is lined with tiny hairs called cilia. These hairs trap foreign particles, such as bacteria and dust, so that they do not make it to the lungs, helping prevent infection. The turbinates also are located within the nasopharynx and create turbulent flow of air, which helps warm the air and increases the mucosal surface air that further aids in warming and humidification.

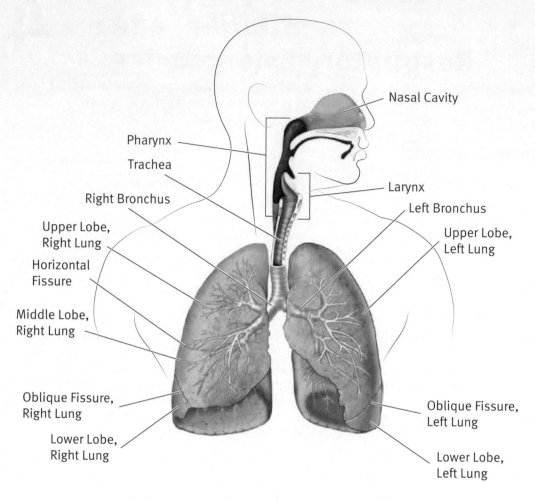

Figure 4-1. Anatomy of the Respiratory System

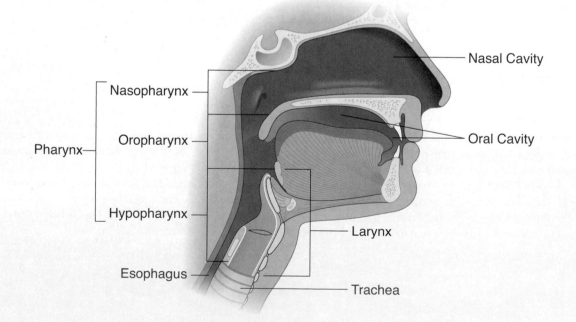

Figure 4-2. Upper Airway Structures

If the patient is breathing through their mouth, air passes between the tongue and the palates. Forming the anterior portion of the roof of the mouth is the hard palate, with the soft palate forming the posterior portion. The focus of many jokes, the uvula marks the division between the mouth and the oropharynx and actually has a purpose: It prevents food from passing upward into the nasopharynx. At the back of the mouth, the oropharynx and the naso-pharynx merge into the pharynx, a muscular tube that helps guide food into the esophagus. Humidification, warming, and filtration of air entering the mouth are less efficient because there is less surface area and no cilia until beyond the oropharynx. Finally, a poorly defined area that represents the most inferior portion of the pharynx is the hypopharynx. Here, the trachea and the epiglottis are anterior, and the esophagus is posterior.

Lower Airway

The lower airway is defined as everything inferior to the larynx, so our journey to the lungs resumes there. The larynx is a rather complicated structure that houses the vocal cords.

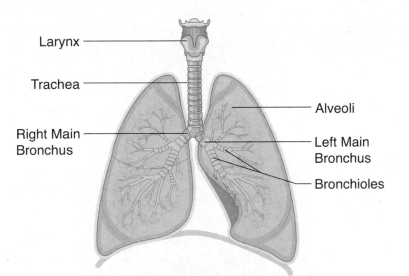

Figure 4-3. Lower Airway Structures

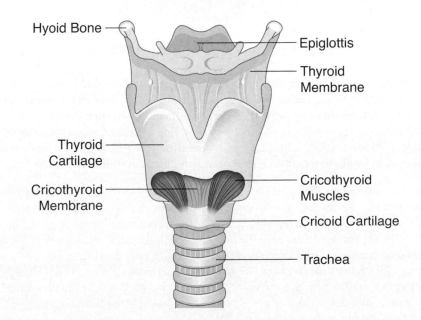

Figure 4-4. Larynx, Anterior View

The superior border to the larynx is essentially the epiglottis and the hyoid bone. The hyoid bone is the point of attachment of the tongue and the epiglottis. Anteriorly, the thyroid cartilage provides protection and is the anatomical reference point on the anterior neck, commonly known as the Adam's apple. The Adam's apple is typically more apparent in men than women. Posteriorly, the larynx is bordered by esophageal muscle. The inferior border of the larynx is marked by the cricoid cartilage. The cricoid cartilage is the only complete ring of cartilage in the trachea; all the others are C-shaped and open posteriorly to allow for easier transit of food through and contraction of the esophagus. The cricothyroid membrane is the midline groove palpable between the cricoid and thyroid cartilages on the anterior of the larynx. This is the site for surgical and nonsurgical airway placement, which will be discussed later in this chapter.

The narrowest part of the airway is the space between the vocal cords called the glottis or the glottic opening. A vocal cord forms each of the lateral sides of the glottic opening. The epiglottis is the superior border, and the inferior border consists of the cuneiform and corniculate cartilages, which, incidentally, are the superior division between the esophagus and the trachea. The epiglottis is a leaf-shaped flap of cartilage that is responsible for covering the glottic opening during swallowing so food does not enter the trachea. It is attached to the tongue, the thyroid cartilage, and the hyoid bone with three different ligaments; these attachments allow for the head tilt, chin lift, and jaw thrust maneuvers to effectively open the airway. The space that exists between the epiglottis and the tongue is called the vallecula and is important for certain intubation attempts, which will be learned later.

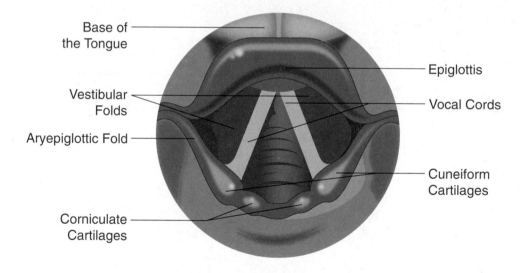

Figure 4-5. Glottic Opening, Superior View

Continuing past the larynx, air enters the trachea, also known as the windpipe. This hollow tube of C-shaped cartilage rings leads from the larynx to the carina, where it bifurcates (divides) into the 2 main bronchi. The cartilage rings are necessary to support the shape of the trachea; without them, the trachea would collapse with each inhalation. The right bronchus is shorter and lies in more of a straight line with the trachea than the left bronchus, which makes a sharper angle with the trachea. Thus, an endotracheal tube (ETT) is likely to enter the right bronchus, resulting in right main-stem intubation and decreased or absent breath sounds over the left lung fields.

The main-stem bronchi continue to divide into bronchioles of decreasing diameter until they reach the biological cul-de-sacs known as alveoli. The trachea, the bronchi, and the bronchioles are lined with sticky mucus secreting goblet cells and cilia that work together to trap and remove potential pathogens and dust from the lungs. The superficial layer of mucus called the gel layer rides atop the lower, watery layer called the sol layer. The contaminants stick to the gel layer of mucus, whereas the cilia sweep back and forth with each breath, continuously moving the mucus up and out of the lungs through a process called the mucociliary escalator system. Unknowingly, humans swallow much of the mucus that our bodies produce each day, which is removed from the lungs or drained from the nose. Beta-2 adrenergic receptors also are present in the linings of the trachea, the bronchi, and the bronchioles. When stimulated, these receptors signal the smooth muscle in these tubes to relax, causing the tubes to dilate, which allows in more air for easier breathing.

Our trip through the airways comes to an end at the alveoli. These microscopic sacs resemble grape bunches and are the primary site of gas exchange. They are surrounded by a web of capillaries and are only one cell layer thick. The capillary delivers CO_2 waste from the cells to the alveoli, which diffuses down the concentration gradient into the alveolus. Concurrently, oxygen will move into the capillaries.

Clinical Correlate

Mucociliary Escalator

In smokers, paralysis of the cilia leads to the inability of the lungs to clear debris from the lungs. This failure of the mucociliary escalator leads to congestion and, eventually, bronchitis. It contributes to the breathing problems of long-time smokers.

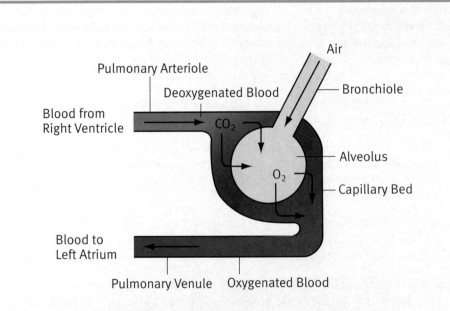

Figure 4-6. Gas Exchange in the Alveolus

Two types of cells make up each alveolus. The 1st type, appropriately named type I pneumocytes, is basically empty, which allows for faster gas exchange. Type I pneumocytes lack any organelles that would allow them to reproduce or conduct cellular respiration (chapter 1). The 2nd type, not surprisingly called type II pneumocytes, is tasked with making new type I cells and producing surfactant. Surfactant is a slippery, soap-like substance that reduces surface tension, keeps the alveoli open, and allows the tissues of the lungs to slide past each other. Without the surfactant, breathing would be at the very least painful and at worst impossible. Smoking, infections, and trauma can destroy type II cells, causing the alveoli to collapse, effectively killing them. This process is called atelectasis.

Alveoli

Healthy adult lungs can hold about 6 L of air and contain five distinct lobes: two in the left lung and three in the right lung. The lungs are covered by a tough membrane called the visceral pleura, and the inner chest wall is lined with a parietal pleura. In between these membranes is more surfactant, allowing the lungs to slide along the inside of the chest wall nearly frictionlessly.

Pro-Tip

You can remember which lung has only two lobes because the heart takes up the space of the third lobe and lies on the left of the chest. Therefore, the left lung has only two lobes.

PHYSIOLOGY OF BREATHING

The act of breathing requires several systems to work together. The musculoskeletal system must be intact and functioning, and nothing can inhibit the transfer of O_2 from the atmosphere to the blood or inhibit CO_2 wastes from reaching the lungs and being exhaled. In this section, the physiology behind how people breathe is presented.

Ventilation

Ventilation is the process of moving air into and out of the lungs and should always be among the highest priorities in the treatment plan for any patient. Ventilation can be divided into two phases: inhalation and exhalation. Inhalation is the act of moving air into the lungs and is regarded as the active phase of ventilation because the body must use energy to make muscles contract. The primary muscle of breathing is the diaphragm, a large sheet of muscle that separates the abdominal cavity from the thoracic, or chest, cavity containing the lungs. When this muscle contracts, it descends into the abdominal cavity, displaces abdominal organs, and creates negative pressure in the thoracic cavity, specifically the lungs. It is negative pressure because it is less than the surroundings. Atmospheric air then rushes into the lungs to quickly equalize the pressures. The intercostal muscles located between the ribs also are considered the primary muscles of ventilation and help generate this negative pressure. When they contract, the ribs are lifted anteriorly and superiorly, further increasing the thoracic cavity volume to allow for more air to rush in.

Except in special cases, everything diffuses along the concentration gradient. The chemical in question will diffuse across a permeable membrane from an area of higher concentration to an area of lower concentration.

The concentration of gases is measured as the partial pressure of that gas; that is, the portion of the total pressure caused by that specific gas. **Henry's Law** states that as the partial pressure of a particular gas present over a liquid decreases, so does the amount of that gas dissolved in the liquid. If that partial pressure of a gas present over a liquid increases, the amount of gas dissolved in a liquid will also increase. This law is at work in the lungs.

In the lungs, O_2 has a higher partial pressure in the alveolus than in the capillary, so O_2 will move into the capillary according to Henry's Law. The opposite is true for CO_2 in the alveolar capillaries. Because the partial pressure of CO_2 in the alveolus is less than that in the capillary, CO_2 will preferentially diffuse out of the capillary and into the alveolus.

To help understand this, think about opening a brand new bottle of soda. When you twist the cap, you hear the rush of gas from the bottle and you immediately see bubbles form inside the liquid that percolate up to the top. This process will continue in an effort to reestablish the balance of partial pressures of CO_2 in both the liquid and the space above the liquid. If you tightly seal the container again, this bubbling stops when the partial pressure of CO_2 in the soda equals the partial pressure of CO_2 in the space above the liquid.

You may have noticed that you do not breathe in the same amount of air each time. Sometimes, you may take a really big breath after a few minutes of quiet breathing. You may yawn, taking in even more air than usual. There are terms for this varying volume of air that the lungs can hold. First, during normal inhalation, the **tidal volume** is the tide of air in and out or, more formally, the volume of air moved in or out during a single breath. The tidal volume can be broken down further into the alveolar volume and the dead space volume. The **alveolar volume** is the amount of air that actually reaches the alveoli. The **dead space volume** is the amount of air in each breath that fills the portion of the lungs not involved with gas exchange. **Physiologic dead space** is the normal dead space plus the dead space resulting from atelectasis of any etiology.

With normal breathing tidal volume as a baseline, the volume of air a person can inhale with the deepest breath possible is called the **inspiratory reserve volume**. The amount of air a person can forcibly exhale after a normal exhalation is called the **expiratory reserve volume**. The **inspiratory capacity** is the total volume that can be inhaled, whereas the **functional residual capacity** is the expiratory reserve volume combined with the residual volume. The **vital capacity** is the sum of three volumes: the expiratory reserve capacity, the tidal volume, and the inspiratory reserve capacity. Even after forcing out as much air from the lungs as possible, air is still left in the lungs. This remaining air is called the **residual volume**. Residual volume plus the vital capacity gives the total lung volume.

Finally, when it comes to lung volumes and capacity, it often is more helpful to talk about these volumes during the span of 1 minute, rather than breath to breath as discussed previously. **Minute volume** is the amount of air that is

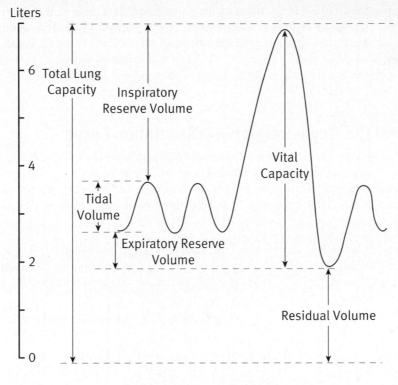

Figure 4-7. Lung Volumes

moved through the lungs in 1 minute and can be calculated by multiplying the respiratory rate by the tidal volume. The alveolar minute volume is the tidal volume minus the dead space volume multiplied by the respiratory rate.

Unlike inhalation, exhalation in the healthy person is passive; it does not require the body to spend energy to expel the air from the lungs. As the muscles of inhalation discussed earlier relax, the pressure within the thoracic cavity increases, until it exceeds that of the atmosphere. At that point, air leaves the lungs without much effort. This becomes an active process in people with asthma or chronic obstructive pulmonary disease (COPD), as will be seen later in this chapter.

Regulation of Ventilation

Have you ever noticed that you cannot hold your breath for more than about 30 seconds to a minute? Or that you cannot keep your breath exhaled without being forced to take what ends up being a deeper breath than usual? Breathing is regulated primarily through chemical control and neural control, with chemical control being the most sensitive and complex. Chemoreceptors located throughout the body monitor all the body's metabolic processes; the chemoreceptors concerned with respiration are located in the carotid arteries, the aortic arch, and the central chemoreceptor.

The aortic and carotid chemoreceptors monitor the partial pressure of carbon dioxide ($PaCO_2$) dissolved in arterial blood to help it determine when to breathe. The central chemoreceptors are located near the respiratory centers in the brain and monitor the pH of cerebrospinal fluid (CSF). When the pH of CSF decreases, that is, CSF becomes more acidic, the central chemoreceptors send a signal to increase the rate and depth of breathing. These centers are not only important in driving respirations but also integral to holding the body's pH and acid-base balance within a narrow range.

Under normal circumstances, breathing is regulated primarily by these methods: $PaCO_2$ monitoring by the chemo-receptors in the carotid arteries and the aortic arch and by the pH in CSF. However, some patients, particularly those with COPD, live with an increased CO_2 level and more acidic CSF because they have difficulty removing CO_2 from the blood. Consequently, changes in CO_2 level are not enough to drive respiration, so the chemoreceptors in the aortic arch and the carotid arteries begin to stimulate breathing based on a drop in the partial pressure of oxygen (PaO_2) levels in the blood. This is called the hypoxic drive and is a fail-safe for the body to continue breathing under extreme circumstances. It is believed that giving patients with end-stage COPD excess O_2 could override this hypoxic drive and cause them to stop breathing altogether. The medical community has no consensus for this, so the best practice in these patients is to not deny O_2 to them if they need it and to be prepared to support their breathing as it becomes necessary.

Oxygenation and the Oxyhemoglobin Dissociation Curve

Ventilation is the act of moving air into the lungs. **Oxygenation** is specifically the loading of O_2 onto the hemoglobin, the O_2-carrying molecule in red blood cells. Oxygenation cannot occur without ventilation; however, ventilation can occur without oxygenation actually taking place. This can happen whenever the amount of O_2 is not found in adequate concentrations in the inhaled air, such as at high altitudes or in confined spaces where another gas has displaced the O_2.

Monitoring pulse oximetry is the best way to assess the oxygenation and perfusion status of a patient. As with any device, the history and clinical presentation of the patient should trump any number from any monitoring device. Pulse oximeters can give a false reading in certain situations, so consider if any of the following situations are playing a role in the oximeter reading:

- Nail polish may give a false high or low reading depending on color or prevent the machine from giving a reading at all.
- Cold extremity/poor perfusion: If the location of the sensor—typically a finger, a toe, or an earlobe—is cold, blood may be shunted away from that area, resulting in a false low reading. Raynaud disease, wherein otherwise healthy people have cyanotic fingers in cool weather, is another example of poor perfusion.
- Low hemoglobin: This condition may be deceptive because the readout will likely indicate normal oximetry. Remember, this is the percentage of red blood cells that are carrying O_2. For example, if normally 400 red blood cells pass by the sensor in a second, and 396 of them are carrying O_2, the oximetry is 99%. The oximetry is the same if 200 red blood cells pass by a sensor and 198 of them are carrying O_2. In the latter example, however, the person may still have a reduced carrying capacity requiring O_2.
- Bright ambient light: If ambient light enters the sensor, it could give a false reading.
- Carbon monoxide (CO) poisoning: CO binds with hemoglobin on the order of 250 times more strongly than O_2. A patient experiencing CO poisoning will have a pulse oximetry reading of 100%, even though CO is replacing O_2 on the hemoglobin. A device is available that can distinguish between hemoglobin loaded with O_2 and hemoglobin loaded with CO; however, this is not a necessary value to get because exposure to CO warrants high–flow O_2 under all circumstances.

The oxyhemoglobin dissociation curve illustrates the relationship between the partial pressure of the O_2 dissolved in arterial blood and the saturation of the hemoglobin molecules with O_2: SpO_2 if measured through pulse oximetry, and SaO_2 if measured from an arterial blood gas (ABG) draw. Because paramedics typically do not have ABG results, only the SpO_2 is referenced; however, paramedics should be aware that both exist. The Hb-O_2 dissociation curve shows the oxyhemoglobin dissociation curve, and, under normal conditions, the PaO_2 is about 105 mmHg when the SpO_2 reads 98%. There is a steep drop-off of the partial pressure of O_2 dissolved in the plasma when the SpO_2 is <80%. When the blood reaches the tissues, dissolved O_2 is taken up by the cells, first causing the PaO_2 to drop. As this occurs, O_2 bound to the hemoglobin detaches and dissolves in the plasma. In this way, O_2 supply often far exceeds demand.

Several factors affect how tightly O_2 is held to the hemoglobin. Several factors cause the curve to shift right, meaning that O_2 is released more readily from the hemoglobin. These factors are increased CO_2 levels in the blood, acidosis, higher concentrations of 2,3-diphosphoglycerate (an intermediate of glucose metabolism), exercise, and increased temperature. This actually works in our favor because the area where O_2 would need to be released—in the capillary bed of the receiving tissues—is an area that will be higher in CO_2 concentration, higher in 2,3-diphosphoglycerate, and more acidic. Naturally, when the curve shifts to the left, O_2 binds more tightly to the hemoglobin in alkalosis or areas rich in O_2 or in areas devoid of CO_2. This area would include the pulmonary capillaries where CO_2 is being actively removed from the blood.

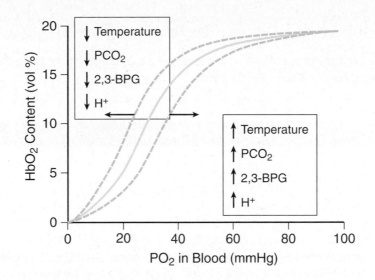

Figure 4-8. Shifts in Hb-O_2 Dissociation Curve
The oxyhemoglobin dissociation curve with left and right shifts.

Pro-Tip

Oxyhemoglobin curve mnemonic: CADET, face RIGHT! **C**O_2, **a**cidosis, 2,3-**d**iphosphoglycerate, **e**xercise, **t**emperature moves the curve to the **right**. These are the conditions under which O_2 is bound less tightly to the hemoglobin. Fortunately, they also are conditions common to tissues where O_2 should be offloaded from the hemoglobin.

Respiration

Respiration is another term related to gas movement. **Respiration** is the process of exchanging O_2 and CO_2. The key here is the exchange of gases, which makes respiration different from oxygenation. The distinct forms of respiration are external respiration and internal respiration. **External respiration** is the exchange of gases at the alveolar level in the lungs. **Internal respiration** is where the cells of the tissues receive O_2 and expel their waste CO_2 into the bloodstream for removal. Internal respiration also is more frequently called cellular respiration. The cell uses O_2 during aerobic metabolism within the mitochondria of the cell during the complete oxidation of glucose to CO_2. Refer to chapter 1 for more information on cellular metabolism.

Table 4-1. Summary of O_2 Transport-Related Terminology

Ventilation	Process of Moving Air into and out of the Lung
Oxygenation	Loading of O_2 onto the hemoglobin
Perfusion	Circulation at the cellular level, including the delivery of O_2 and nutrients and the removal of wastes
Respiration	Exchange of O_2 and CO_2 between blood and the alveoli (external respiration) or cells (internal respiration)

Pro-Tip

You can associate the word *external* with meaning external to the body to help you remember that this occurs in the lungs, and atmospheric air is external to the body.

Clinical Correlate

Geriatric Corner

Many changes take place in the respiratory system as a person ages.

- The lungs become less elastic, and the portions of the ribs that are made of cartilage in youth ossify and become bone in adults age 65 and older. Combined with an overall weakening of the respiratory muscles, these lead to a reduction in vital capacity and an increase in residual volume.
- The PaO_2 dissolved in the lungs declines from 90 mmHg at 30 years old to about 75 mmHg at 80 years old, which is caused in large part by changes in the distribution of pulmonary blood flow.
- Older adults are more likely to live with hypoxemia and hypercarbia (high blood CO_2) because of decreasing sensitivity to minute changes in ABGs and pH in the central nervous system.
- The presence of kyphosis, a hump-shaped curvature of the spine, results in a decreased ability to perform ventilations in the older adult patient, reducing inspiratory volume.
- Weakened muscles of respiration, decreased inspiratory volume, and changes in blood flow all lead to defense mechanisms in the lungs declining, which leads to more frequent and longer lasting infections.

AIRWAY MANAGEMENT AND SUCTIONING

Getting O_2 to the lungs is the single most important thing that the paramedic can ensure happens in every patient encountered. This section will discuss obstructions to the airway and how to relieve them and will conclude by discussing the airway adjuncts available to the paramedic, including BLS airways through surgical airways.

Airway Obstruction

Assessing airway patency in a person who is talking is about as easy an assessment a paramedic will ever make. If the person is talking, then the airway is patent. Check. But if the person is unresponsive, ensuring that the person has an adequate airway is a greater challenge. When assessing the airway, listen for stridor. This upper airway sound is sometimes the only clue to a narrowed airway passage. The following are common causes of airway obstruction.

- **Tongue.** In the person who is unresponsive, the tongue is the most common obstruction to the airway. In this group of patients, the muscles relax, and the tongue falls back against the posterior wall of the pharynx, effectively shutting off the airway.
- **Foreign Body Aspiration.** Choking often is associated with alcohol consumption, loss of a gag reflex in those with a stroke, and laughing or talking with food in the mouth.
- **Laryngeal Spasm, Edema, and Injury.** Laryngeal spasm occurs when the vocal cords close off the airway, which can happen from intubation attempts or can be a diver's reflex. Edema is swelling and results from a fluid shift in the larynx that closes or nearly closes off the airway. Allergic reaction, trauma, or inhaling hot air or steam are common causes of laryngeal edema.

Patient Positioning and Manual Airway Maneuver

Any patient who has a GCS reading <8 or who is unresponsive should be immediately placed in a supine position if not found that way. This allows paramedics to quickly assess airway patency, breathing effort, and circulatory status with minimal difficulty. Sometimes simple repositioning of the head is all that is needed to relieve the obstruction and restore spontaneous breathing.

Head Tilt/Chin Lift

Indications: A patient who is unresponsive does not show any signs of trauma.

Contraindications: Patients suspected of having a cervical spine injury.

Procedure:

1. While at the patient's side, place the hand nearest the head on the forehead.
2. Place two fingers on the mandible, staying clear of the soft tissue under the chin.
3. Simultaneously apply pressure to the patient's forehead while lifting up on the mandible.

Jaw Thrust

Indications: A patient who is unresponsive and suspected of having a cervical spine injury.

Contraindications: None in unresponsive trauma. Otherwise, the head tilt/chin lift maneuver is preferred. This maneuver can be painful if performed on a person who is conscious.

Procedure:

1. Position yourself superior to a supine patient's head.
2. Place your thumbs on the cheekbones of the patient and the tips of your first two fingers posterior to the angle of the jaw.
3. Pull the jaw upward (anteriorly) using your thumbs on the cheeks for leverage. This position is difficult to maintain for long periods of time, so be sure to have a plan for inserting an airway adjunct.

Suctioning

When repositioning alone fails to open an occluded airway, suctioning may be needed to remove debris in the airway. The suction unit must be capable of generating 300 mmHg of vacuum force; have rigid-suction catheters, soft-suction catheters, and large-bore noncollapsible tubing to connect the catheter with the suction unit; and include an unbreakable, disposable collection vessel to go along with a supply of water for rinsing the catheters after each suctioning run. The rigid-suction catheters, or Yankauer catheters, are ideal for suctioning the mouth of vomit and blood and are easy to control. The soft-suction catheters, or French catheters, are best suited for suctioning out the lumen of an ETT or a naso-pharyngeal airway.

Indications: The airway has excessive blood, vomit, or secretions that pose an aspiration threat.

Contraindications: None.

Procedure, no advanced airway:

1. Select a rigid-suction (Yankauer) catheter.
2. Measure from the corner of the mouth to the earlobe. This is the maximum depth of insertion.
3. Open the mouth using the cross finger technique.
4. Kink the tubing or leave the catheter port open to ensure no suctioning on the way into the mouth. Insert the catheter to the depth measured in step 2.
5. Unkink the tubing or cover the catheter port to initiate suctioning when the premeasured depth is reached.
6. Suction on the way out of the mouth for a period of not longer than 15 seconds in the adult, 10 seconds in the child, or 5 seconds in the infant.
7. Dip the suction catheter into water to rinse. This prevents blood from clotting in the catheter.

Procedure, ETT in place:

1. Select a soft-suction (French) catheter.
2. Observe sterile technique. Measure from the end of the ETT to the earlobe to the suprasternal notch. This is the maximum depth of insertion.
3. Lubricate the tip of the catheter.
4. Preoxygenate the patient.
5. Kink the tubing or leave the catheter port open to ensure no suctioning on the way into the mouth. Insert the catheter to the depth measured in step 2.
6. Unkink the tubing or cover the catheter port to initiate suctioning when the premeasured depth is reached.
7. Suction only while slowly withdrawing the catheter from the ETT for a period of not longer than 15 seconds in the adult, 10 seconds in the child, or 5 seconds in the infant.
8. Dip the suction catheter into water to rinse. This prevents blood from clotting in the catheter.
9. Ventilate or direct the ventilation of the patient.

BASIC AIRWAY ADJUNCTS

Although no adjunct can take the place of manual head positioning, adjuncts can help maintain an airway in patients who are unresponsive. They are designed to hold the tongue off the posterior wall of the pharynx.

Oropharyngeal Airway

Indications: The patient is unresponsive, breathing or not, without gag reflex.

Contraindications: A gag reflex is present.

Procedure:

1. Measure the airway from the corner of the mouth to the earlobe.
2. Open the mouth with the cross finger technique.
3. Insert the airway upside down until the distal tip reaches the soft palate.
4. Rotate the airway 180° with gentle pressure so that it slips under the tongue. The flange should rest against the lips.

Nasopharyngeal Airway

Indications: Patients who are unresponsive and patients with an altered mental status who have an intact gag reflex and cannot tolerate an oropharyngeal airway.

Contraindications: Facial or head trauma; a basal skull fracture is suspected or possible.

Procedure:

1. Measure the nasopharyngeal airway from the tip of the nose to the earlobe.
2. Lubricate the tip with water-based lubricant.
3. Select the larger nostril and apply gentle pressure posteriorly. A common error here is to aim the device superiorly, when the nasal passage is almost directly posterior to the nostril.
4. Advance the airway until the flange rests against the nose. If resistance is encountered, do not force it. Remove it and attempt the other nostril.

Pro-Tip
Oropharyngeal airways can be left in patients who have been intubated as a bite block. In the event the patient regains consciousness, seizes, or for some other reason experiences trismus (clenching of the jaw), this will prevent them from biting and crimping the ETT.

ADVANCED AIRWAY MANAGEMENT AND ADJUNCTS

It is worth repeating: Conduct BLS before advanced life support (ALS). This means that an advanced airway adjunct should be attempted only when any of the following conditions are met:

- After attempting and failing to establish a patent airway using any previously discussed method.
- Prolonged airway management is required.
- Continued bleeding into the airway, excessive secretions, or vomiting require nearly continuous suctioning.
- Laryngeal fracture.

Before deciding to move to an advanced airway, evaluate the patient and anticipate and prepare for a difficult airway. If assessment reveals it will be difficult to successfully intubate the patient or current ventilation efforts are successful with minimal difficulty, sometimes it may be best to stay with what is working, rather than risk a bad outcome for the patient. A good mnemonic to assess for a difficult airway is LEMON, as follows:

- **L, Look Externally.** Look for things that may pose a problem, such as loose teeth or dentures. Short thick necks or severe overbite are clues that intubation may be difficult.
- **E, Evaluate 3-3-2.** The 3-3-2 rule is a quick way to assess for a difficult airway. The first 3 indicates the distance of mouth opening; it should be at least 3 of your fingers wide, or about 5 cm. The second 3 indicates that the distance between the chin and the trachea should also be 3 fingers wide. Finally, the 2 is the finger width distance between the soft tissue under the chin to the top of the thyroid cartilage.
- **M, Mallampati.** This scoring system evaluates the mouth opening by how much of the oropharynx is visible when the patient opens their mouth as wide as possible.
- **O, Obstructions.** Any other potential problem in the mouth that could inhibit intubation.
- **N, Neck Mobility.** Ideally, the patient should at least be able to attain the sniffing position with some recommendations suggesting getting the external auditory meatus even with or anterior to the suprasternal notch.

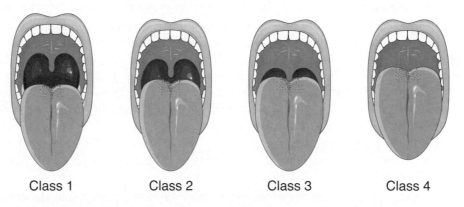

Class 1   Class 2   Class 3   Class 4

Figure 4-9. Mallampati Classification System

Orotracheal Intubation with Direct Laryngoscopy

The crowning achievement of any paramedic is walking into the emergency department with a successful intubation. Nothing feels better than when the resident or attending looks into the mouth and declares, "Yup! It's in!" That sense of accomplishment can last the rest of the tour at least. To be successful at this, prepare for the procedure completely before making an attempt. Set out all the necessary equipment, including laryngoscope blades, the stylet, the water-based lubricant, the ETT, a 10 mL syringe, and suction. Put on gloves; because blood or bodily fluid splashing is possible, wearing a surgical mask with a face shield also is recommended.

Indications:

- Prolonged ventilation expected (i.e., cardiac arrest, head injury)
- Absence of a gag reflex
- Anticipated airway compromise in respiratory failure, anaphylaxis, or airway burns
- A last resort for administering certain medications

Contraindications:

- Oral trauma
- Oral pathologies such as cancer, angioedema, and poor oral opening
- Inability to visualize glottic structures

Procedure:

1. Preoxygenate the patient for 2–3 minutes prior to the intubation attempt. This helps elevate the PaO_2 so that the patient can tolerate a minute or so without ventilation and oxygenation.

2. Select and set out desired equipment, which includes the laryngoscope blade type and size, the ETT, the stylet if using one, a syringe for inflating the cuff later in the procedure, and the water-based lubricant. Check all the equipment to make sure it is functioning. Ensure the cuff on the tube holds air and that the light on the laryngoscope blade is bright to see into the dark recesses of the pharynx. If using a stylet, ensure that it does not protrude beyond the end of the tube.

3. Position the head into the sniffing position.

4. Insert the blade, displacing the tongue to the patient's left. Insert the Miller (straight) blade all the way into the pharynx and lift straight up while controlling the epiglottis. If using a Macintosh (curved) blade, insert the blade by sliding it down the curve of the tongue and into the vallecula; lifting up on a curved blade will pull the tongue up directly and the epiglottis up indirectly because both are attached to the hyoid bone. This will reveal the rest of the glottic structures.

5. Elevate the mandible with the laryngoscope. Remember, it is a lift of the laryngoscope along the axis of the handle, not a ratcheting movement using the upper teeth as a fulcrum.

6. Insert the ETT to the proper depth. Consider adding some sterile water-based lubricant to the tip of the tube prior to insertion. Anything that will help ensure success on the first try should always be employed.

7. Inflate the cuff and immediately disconnect the syringe. Leaving the syringe attached will allow the cuff to deflate.

8. Connect a BVM to the ETT and have another rescuer ventilate the patient while listening to lung sounds over both lung fields and the epigastrium. Breath sounds over the epigastrium likely indicate intubation of the esophagus and a failed attempt. Breath sounds should be heard equally over both lung fields. If, during auscultation, lung sounds are heard over the right lung fields only and diminished or absent sounds over the left, the tube was likely inserted too deeply and has entered the right main-stem bronchus. To alleviate this, pull back on the tube 1 cm at a time and listen again over both lung fields. Stop once breath sounds have returned to the left side.

9. Secure the ETT using a commercial device or tape. Note the depth of insertion at either the teeth or lips as the reference point in centimeters. Any deviation from this number found later in the transport could indicate a displaced tube.

10. Confirm tube placement by at least one additional method. Waveform capnography shows the amount of CO_2 exhaled after each ventilation and is the ideal method for confirming tube placement. Colorimetric capnography is an alternative to waveform. Litmus paper placed at the end of the tube will turn from purple to yellow and back again several times during ventilations. Another option could be an esophageal detection device, which is a device placed on the end of the tube that will not inflate if placed in the esophagus.

Other methods of intubation exist and are frequently taught during paramedic classes. Because none of these methods or techniques have been tested, only their indications and contraindications will be discussed. A step-by-step procedural outline, as done with other procedures that have been tested, is not included here.

Nasotracheal intubation, where the ETT is inserted through the nostril, is an alternative to orotracheal intubation when it would be extremely difficult for oral intubation. The patient must be breathing to perform this skill, unlike orotracheal intubation. Indications for this procedure include trismus, intractable seizures, mandibular fractures or wiring, or any oral pathology that would inhibit oral intubation. This technique is contraindicated in patients who have facial trauma, who are not breathing, or who have anatomic abnormalities such as a deviated septum or a history of cocaine abuse. Nasal trauma and bleeding are the most common problems associated with this procedure.

Digital intubation involves the rescuer inserting their fingers into the patient's mouth and feeling for the epiglottis. Next, direct the ETT over the fingers along the middle finger and into the glottic opening. This should be attempted only in extreme circumstances, such as when a laryngoscope has malfunctioned or is not available, the patient is in an extremely confined space, or when other techniques have failed. When performing this skill, ensure that the patient is either deeply unconscious or apneic. If the patient seizes or goes into trismus, the patient may bite down hard enough to actually cut off the fingers. Using a bite block in these situations is highly recommended. A misplaced ETT is the most common complication of this procedure. Because of the availability of alternative airway devices, such as the Combitube or King LT, among others, digital intubation is rarely performed and not typically recommended.

Other less commonly used intubation methods also exist in certain systems. Local protocols will indicate whether other alternate forms of intubation are available. First, a lighted stylet that illuminates the trachea internally and is visible through the skin externally when correct placement is achieved may be an intubation option. A 2nd option may be retrograde intubation, which involves inserting a large-bore intravenous catheter into the cricothyroid membrane in a cephalic direction and threading a guide wire through it until it is visible in the pharynx. The guide wire is then pulled out through the mouth, and an ETT is placed over it and slid directly into the trachea blindly. This very complex procedure should be performed only under the strictest of sterile techniques.

Alternative Airway Devices

While direct laryngoscopy is still currently the preferred method of securing an airway, other devices can be used in the event that orotracheal intubation is not possible or proves extremely difficult. In many cases, these devices and procedures should be used before attempting alternative intubation techniques, such as those discussed previously in this chapter because placement of and successful ventilation with these techniques is often quicker than digital, nasal, or retrograde intubation will be.

Multilumen Airways

The Combitube is a preformed dual lumen plastic tube that is blindly inserted into a patient's mouth and can be used for ventilation regardless of whether it is inserted into the esophagus or the trachea. This tube is expected to enter the esophagus but occasionally will enter the trachea, so, essentially, it cannot be misplaced.

Indications: The patient is older than 16 years old and has a height of 5 feet 7 inches (4 feet 5 inches for the Combitube SA); an ETT cannot be placed for any reason.

Contraindications: Esophageal trauma, alcoholism (esophageal varices)

Procedure:

1. Wear gloves. A surgical mask with a face shield is recommended.
2. Preoxygenate the patient prior to attempt.
3. Test both cuffs to ensure that they hold air. Lubricate the distal tip of the Combitube.
4. Position the patient supine and in the neutral or sniffing position.
5. Open the mouth with the tongue/jaw lift maneuver.
6. Insert the device midline into the patient's mouth and advance it until the patient's teeth rest between the 2 black reference marks on the device.
7. Inflate the pharyngeal cuff to the proper volume (100 mL) and remove the syringe.
8. Inflate the distal cuff with the proper volume (15 mL) and remove the syringe.
9. Ventilate the patient through the longest tube first. This tube is marked with the number 1 and is usually blue. Listen over the lung fields and the epigastrium and watch for chest rise during ventilation.
10. If there is no chest rise or breath sounds, ventilate over port number 2, the shorter tube, and listen again. If ventilation is successful with this tube, the tube accidentally went into the trachea.
11. Secure the device with tape or a commercial tube holder.

Supraglottic Airways

Laryngeal Mask Airway

The laryngeal mask airway (LMA) is designed to wedge itself into the hypopharynx and cover the entire glottic opening. Ventilation is then directed into the trachea after the cuff is inflated, sealing off the entire hypopharynx. Insertion for these types of airways is blind, similar to the Combitube. LMAs come in a variety of sizes and are not limited based on height, like the Combitube. A drawback for these devices, compared with the Combitube or the ETT, is that they do not completely prevent vomiting or aspiration.

Indications: An alternative to BLS airway when an ETT cannot be placed

Contraindications: Morbid obesity because the seal for these patients is not as tight as for others; patients with COPD may require higher airway pressures, which is not accomplished well with the LMA.

Procedure:

1. Wear gloves. A surgical mask with a face shield is recommended.
2. Preoxygenate the patient prior to attempt.
3. Inflate the cuff to ensure that it holds air. Lubricate the entire cuff of the LMA.
4. Position the patient supine and in the neutral or sniffing position.
5. Open the mouth with the tongue/jaw lift maneuver.
6. Insert the device midline into the patient's mouth and advance it until resistance is met.
7. Inflate the cuff with the proper volume for the size of LMA used and remove the syringe.
8. Ventilate the patient. Listen over the lung fields and the epigastrium and watch for chest rise during ventilation.
9. Secure the device with tape or a commercial tube holder.

King LT

The King LT is very similar to the Combitube, except that it is only a single lumen and must be inserted into the esophagus to work. Similar to the Combitube, it has a distal cuff that seals the esophagus and a pharyngeal cuff that seals the oropharynx; however, it has only one tube for ventilation. Unlike the Combitube, it comes in a variety of sizes and can be used in children as small as 12 kg.

Indications: Inability to place an ETT for any reason

Contraindications: Esophageal trauma, alcoholism (esophageal varices)

Procedure:

1. Wear gloves. A surgical mask with a face shield is recommended.
2. Preoxygenate the patient prior to attempt.
3. Test both cuffs to ensure that they hold air. Lubricate the distal tip of the King LT.
4. Position the patient supine and in the neutral or sniffing position.
5. Open the mouth with the tongue/jaw lift maneuver.
6. Insert the device into the corner of the patient's mouth and advance it while gently rotating it until the blue line faces the patient's chin and the connector is at or near the patient's teeth.
7. Inflate both cuffs to the proper volume and remove the syringe.
8. Ventilate the patient. Listen over the lung fields and the epigastrium and watch for chest rise during ventilation.
9. Secure the device with tape or a commercial tube holder.

Cricothyrotomy

The cricothyrotomy is not common in or out of the hospital, accounting for less than 1% of all cases of airway management. Whether accomplished through transtracheal needle insertion or open surgical intervention, the cricothyrotomy is a life-or-death last resort for establishing airway patency. It is used only in patients who cannot be ventilated or intubated successfully and cannot maintain an oxygen saturation above 90% via any other method. Even then, the paramedic must ensure that local protocols allow this procedure to be performed; in many cases, online medical control needs to be contacted first to verify permission. Complications may arise using either technique. These include incorrect placement, mediastinal or esophageal tears, aspiration, damage to the adjacent thyroid, and subcutaneous emphysema.

The following sections describe the indications, contraindications, and procedures for both needle cricothyrotomy and surgical cricothyrotomy.

Needle Cricothyrotomy

The needle cricothyrotomy has the advantage of speed. This procedure is much quicker to implement than a surgical airway. It also carries significantly less risk of bleeding. An important disadvantage, however, is that needle cricothyrotomy is not considered a definitive airway because it does not place a cuffed tube inferior to the vocal cords.

Indications: Inability to ventilate by any other method; severe facial trauma and severe oral bleeding, upper airway edema

Contraindications:

- Complete obstruction superior to the needle insertion point (prevents effective exhalation, leading to hypercarbia, and increases the risk for barotrauma to the lungs); be prepared to treat pneumothorax if overinflation of the lungs occurs from high-pressure ventilations.
- Inability to identify landmarks for intervention

Procedure:

1. Wear gloves. A surgical mask with a face shield is recommended.
2. Ideally, preoxygenate the patient prior to attempt.
3. Position the patient supine and in the neutral or sniffing position. Palpate the cricothyroid membrane and cleanse the area, preferably with iodine-containing solution.
4. Insert a 16-or 14-gauge intravenous catheter into the cricothyroid membrane at a 45° angle toward the feet. Remove the needle, leaving the catheter in place. Discard the needle in a sharps container. Attach a syringe to the catheter and aspirate to confirm placement. If the catheter is in the tracheal lumen, the syringe plunger will be easily removed. The plunger creates a vacuum and will feel as if it is being pulled back down if the catheter is still in the soft tissue surrounding the trachea.
5. Connect the transtracheal jet insufflator to the catheter hub. Press the O_2 delivery valve on the insufflator for 1 second or enough to see the chest rise. Release the button for at least 4 seconds to allow for adequate exhalation.
6. Listen over the lung fields and the epigastrium and watch for chest rise during ventilation.
7. Secure the catheter with tape and gauze as if it were an impaled object.
8. Closely monitor pulse oximetry.

Surgical Cricothyrotomy

Service medical directors are increasingly authorizing the paramedics in their service to perform the surgical crico-thyrotomy. In a patient who cannot otherwise be ventilated, surgical cricothyrotomy is a valuable option to establish airway patency. This method of cricothyrotomy provides enhanced airway control compared with needle cricothyrotomy, because it places a cuffed tube inferior to the vocal cords, similar to that of an intubation. There are several techniques for performing the surgical cricothyrotomy. (For instance, some services may prefer the technique that employs a bougie.) Here we will focus only on the standard technique.

Indications: Inability to ventilate by any other method; severe facial trauma and severe oral bleeding, upper airway edema

Contraindications: Inability to identify landmarks for intervention

Procedure:

1. Wear gloves. A surgical mask and face shield are recommended.
2. Ideally, preoxygenate the patient prior to attempt.
3. Collect the necessary equipment: suction, BVM, scalpel #10 or #11, size 6 ETT (with one half-size up and down), and antiseptic (preferably iodine solution). Dilator and tracheal hook are recommended but not essential in the emergency situation.
4. Position the patient supine and in the neutral or sniffing position. Identify the landmarks of the thyroid and cricoid cartilage and the cricothyroid membrane in between. Cleanse the area.
5. Stabilize the trachea with the thumb and middle finger of the nondominant hand, leaving the index finger free to repalpate the cricothyroid membrane as needed.
6. Using the scalpel, make a vertical incision over the membrane, approximately 3.5 cm long.
7. Re-identify the membrane inside the incision with the index finger. Blunt dissect the area as needed to clear the soft tissue. Ignore the blood for now, as tube insertion generally has a tamponading effect.
8. Make a 1 cm transverse (horizontal) incision through the membrane. Aim caudally with the scalpel and make as low an incision as possible.
9. Insert the tracheal hook, transversely rotate it 90 degrees toward the head, and lift the trachea upward and superiorly.
10. Insert the dilator to expand the opening. This can also be accomplished with a finger. (Note that this is the point at which a bougie would be inserted caudally, if available.)
11. Insert a tracheostomy tube or ETT (usually a 6) into the ostomy caudally and inflate the cuff. Ventilate using a BVM. Cut the ETT to eliminate excess tube length as needed. Secure the tube.
12. Listen over the lung fields and the epigastrium and watch for chest rise during ventilation.
13. Closely monitor pulse oximetry and $EtCO_2$.

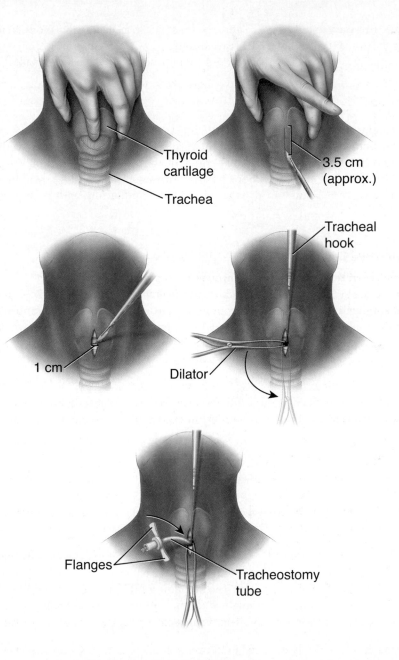

Figure 4-10. Emergency Surgical Thyroidotomy

Special Patient Populations: Stomas and Tracheostomy Tubes

Some patients have a stoma or a tracheostomy tube and are in need of O_2 or ventilatory assistance. Many of these patients need to be suctioned frequently and will sometimes have a sudden onset of severe respiratory distress until they are suctioned. Simply inserting a soft-suction catheter until resistance is felt but no more than 12 cm and suctioning only on the way out as described previously should clear up most respiratory issues. The patient will cough as the suction catheter is inserted, so use caution in case of airborne mucus.

Any ventilation that is necessary for this patient population must be performed through the stoma or the tracheostomy tube. If the patient has only a stoma, using a pediatric mask attached to an adult BVM should work to get an adequate seal for ventilation through the stoma. Tracheostomy tubes are manufactured with the same size connector as ETTs, which means the BVM can be connected directly to it. Then ventilate as usual.

Occasionally, it may be necessary to insert an ETT through the stoma to facilitate ventilations. In this case, take a tube that just fits the lumen of the stoma (usually a size 6 ETT; avoid going below size 5). Insert it 1–2 cm beyond the cuff and inflate the cuff. Ventilate normally. Cut the ETT so that only 3–4 cm protrudes from the neck to make it a little less unwieldy.

O$_2$ Delivery

After ensuring a patent airway, preferably by ensuring the patient can talk to you, evaluate and treat any breathing problems. Before exploring the variety of respiratory emergencies, this section reviews all the O$_2$ administration methods that are available to the paramedic in the field. In addition, ventilatory support methods, including BVM techniques and continuous positive airway pressure (CPAP) will be presented. Finally, the section will conclude with a discussion on special patient populations who may present a challenge with breathing problems.

O$_2$ Therapy and Delivery Devices

Designed for low concentrations of O$_2$, **nasal cannulas** are typically used to deliver O$_2$ to a breathing patient at a flow of 1–6 L per minute (LPM), providing a fraction of inspired oxygen (FiO$_2$) of 24% to 45%. Remember, each liter per minute of supplemental O$_2$ delivers 3% more O$_2$ to the patient over the atmospheric concentration of 21%, so the equation to estimate FiO$_2$ is FiO$_2$ = 21 + (3 * liter flow). This can be used when a patient is unable to tolerate a non-rebreathing or simple face mask or does not require high concentrations of O$_2$ to maintain adequate perfusion. It also is highly recommended that the patient be placed on nasal cannula O$_2$ at 6 LPM during intubation attempts.

Simple face masks fit over the patient's mouth and nose and are used to deliver moderate levels of O$_2$, typically 6–10 LPM. The mask allows atmospheric air to mix with O$_2$ and will deliver between 35% and 60% FiO$_2$.

The **non-rebreathing mask** is used to deliver high concentrations of O$_2$ to a spontaneously and adequately breathing patient. At liter flows between 10 and 15 LPM, the non-rebreathing face mask can reliably deliver a FiO$_2$ of 90% to 100%. Use of this mask is indicated in any patient who requires high concentrations of O$_2$, such as a person in shock or hypoxia. This mask has a bag—the O$_2$ reservoir—attached to it which should be filled prior to placing it on the patient. The liter flow should be increased to the point that when the patient takes a breath, the bag does not deflate. This will help ensure that the patient is getting the maximal flow of O$_2$ with each breath.

The **Venturi mask** is not typically initiated by the paramedic; however, it may be used during interfacility transfers, where the sending provider wants to strictly control FiO$_2$ for the patient. This mask is designed to mix pure O$_2$ and atmospheric O$_2$ to obtain specific concentrations. The liter flow for this device is either 3 LPM or 6 LPM, depending on the desired concentration. It should be maintained for the duration of patient contact unless the patient's condition deteriorates and higher concentrations or an alternate delivery device (i.e., BVM) is warranted.

The **tracheostomy mask** is specifically designed to fit over a stoma or a tracheostomy tube and may not be available in the emergency setting. A tracheostomy mask may be improvised using a simple face mask or a non-rebreather mask to cover the stoma.

O$_2$ humidifiers are designed to add moisture to the O$_2$ being delivered to the patient. O$_2$ delivered to a patient from a concentrator or a sealed bottle or cylinder is completely devoid of any moisture or humidity. Delivering dry O$_2$ to a patient for extended periods can dehydrate the patient and the mucous membranes, which becomes an issue with long transport times, such as those on interfacility transfers, but not during a typical emergency where patient contact time is limited.

Ventilatory Support

As mentioned earlier in this chapter, normal ventilation is accomplished by creating negative pressure in the chest when the diaphragm contracts and descends into the abdominal cavity and the intercostal muscles contract and the rib cage raises anteriorly and superiorly to increase the volume of the thoracic cavity. This is important to the circulatory system as well. During the creation of negative pressure, not only is air drawn in but also blood is pulled up from the extremities and head, returning it in greater quantity to the heart. When artificial ventilation methods must be employed, however, the enhanced venous return is not only lost but also actually reduced because of the now positive pressures used to push air into the lungs. Finally, because positive pressures are used, the air that is squeezed into the chest enters the lungs; occasionally, if too much force is provided to deliver the breath, air will enter the stomach, a condition known as gastric insufflation or gastric distension.

As a patient's breathing worsens, before the patient stops breathing altogether, the paramedic should begin assisting the patient's existing respiration using a BVM device. This is a very difficult skill and requires the paramedic's full concentration. Losing concentration while assisting ventilations will inadvertently make the patient's breathing and their already high anxiety worse.

Indications: Inadequate breathing based on fast rate or shallow depth

Contraindications: Patient's increased anxiety when hands and the BVM are on the face

Procedure:

1. Connect the BVM to an O_2 source and explain the procedure to the patient.
2. Place the mask over the patient's mouth and nose.
3. Observe the patient closely and squeeze the bag each time the patient initiates a breath. This will get easier as the squeezes get more in sync with the patient's natural breathing rhythm. The patient will drive the exhalations. Do not try to force air in while the patient is trying to exhale. This will serve only to further worsen the patient's apprehension.
4. Slowly increase the volume delivered with each breath, which will do the most in attempting to control the breathing.

Artificial Ventilation

Multiple ways can be used to deliver a breath to a patient who has stopped breathing; however, the most effective way is with two rescuers using a BVM. Mouth to mask with supplemental O_2, as is taught in most CPR classes, is second. Once a patient has stopped breathing, or is in respiratory arrest, paramedics need to breathe for them entirely. This is arguably the most important skill any prehospital provider can master at any level. There are no contraindications to this skill; even when there is massive facial trauma, still attempt to establish a seal with the mask to the face to deliver ventilations.

Procedure:

1. Kneel superior to a patient's head (assuming the patient is on the floor) and hyperextend the neck. If trauma is suspected, perform the modified jaw thrust maneuver instead and maintain the head in a neutral in-line position.
2. Place the mask of the BVM over the patient's mouth and nose and use both hands to simultaneously press the mask to the face with both thumbs and forefingers while pulling the patient's jaw into the mask with the remaining fingers of both hands. Take care not to press on the patient's eyes or the soft tissue under the jaw during this procedure. Establishing a seal and successfully ventilating may be difficult in patients with BONES: beard, obese, no teeth, elderly, snores.
3. Connect the reservoir to O_2 set to at least 15 LPM or higher. Connect the BVM to the mask if not already done. While holding the mask securely to the face, have a second rescuer squeeze the bag with both hands enough to have visible chest rise. Squeezing the bag should be done slowly over 1–2 seconds to help minimize the chances of gastric distension. Repeat this 10–12 times per minute or give one breath every 5–6 seconds for the adult and 3–5 seconds for the infant and child. Ventilating faster than this will not be of any more benefit to the patient. If there are limited rescuers, use just one hand to secure the mask to the face using the E-C technique: the thumb and index finger form a C, and the other three fingers form a capital letter E under the jaw bone.
4. Observe for changes in pulse oximetry readings and document those. Also observe for any developing gastric distension.

Practical Point

Although it may seem easy, ventilating a patient with a BVM is decidedly an underrated skill. This is a critical skill to practice and ensure that you are ventilating at the correct rate (10–12 per minute for an adult) and at the appropriate depth. Examiners pay particular attention to this skill.

Continuous Positive Airway Pressure (CPAP)

CPAP is essentially the same as the assisted ventilations described previously; however, it is controlled by a machine and does not require the provider to hold the mask to the face of the patient. It uses straps that fasten to the mask and wrap around the head. It has been shown to decrease the morbidity and mortality of patients with severe respiratory distress who, prior to the use of CPAP, would have been intubated. CPAP provides continuous pressure into the lungs and opens collapsed alveoli while preventing further atelectasis. It is not uncommon for patients who are found with respiratory rates in the 40s and oximetry readings <80% to dramatically improve with CPAP application to having a slowed respiratory rate and pulse oximetry reading approaching 100%.

Indications: Patients in severe respiratory distress caused by congestive heart failure (CHF), exacerbation of COPD, or asthma; patients also need to be breathing spontaneously and able to exhale forcefully enough to stop the flow.

Contraindications: Respiratory arrest, bradypnea, chest trauma, altered mental status and unable to follow verbal commands, excessive facial hair or facial deformities such that the mask does not have a tight, complete seal

Procedure:

1. Connect the circuit (mask and tubing) to the CPAP device. Connect to the O_2 source.

2. With O_2 flowing and the CPAP unit turned on, place the mask on the patient's face, covering the mouth and nose.

3. Have the patient breathe normally. Connect the strapping system to one side of the mask first. Wrap the straps around the head and connect to the posts on the other side of the mask. Adjust for a tight, secure fit and check that it is comfortable for the patient.

4. Set the positive end expiratory pressure (PEEP) to 5 cm H_2O to start and titrate to achieve improvement in respiratory status. Do not increase PEEP beyond more than 15 cm H_2O.

5. Continuously monitor the patient for decline in their status. Although CPAP often results in rapid improvement of the patient, it does not treat the underlying cause of why the patient began with respiratory distress in the first place; it treats only a symptom, and it also can be overpowered by a relentless disease process.

Gastric Distension

Any time artificial ventilation is used in the absence of an ETT, it is very likely that air enters the stomach in addition to the lungs, resulting in gastric distension. This presents the very real possibility of projectile vomiting as the stomach suddenly and spontaneously decompresses, further complicating the airway and respiratory problem at hand, not to mention creating a nightmare of a cleanup. Furthermore, as the stomach expands and pressure within it builds, it will become increasingly more difficult to ventilate the patient because the lungs can no longer expand into the abdominal cavity as they normally would.

Minimize the development of gastric distension by positioning the airway correctly and hyperextending the neck, delivering breaths slowly over 1–2 seconds, and allowing full exhalation before delivering the next breath. Even observing these suggestions will likely result in some distension. To relieve it, the paramedic can insert a nasogastric tube or an orogastric tube if protocols allow. The nasogastric tube is contraindicated in patients with facial fractures because the tube can enter the cranium through a fractured basal skull. The orogastric tube should be used only in the cases of facial fractures and in patients who are unresponsive and do not have a gag reflex. Because the orogastric tube is used only during these conditions, it is nearly always inserted after ETT placement and cannot be placed if any other advanced airway device is used. (It can be used with a Combitube if it was placed in the esophagus and the patient is being ventilated through blue tube number 1.)

Nasogastric tube placement procedure:

1. Explain the procedure to the patient while donning gloves and a face shield.
2. Whenever possible, use a topical anesthetic spray to suppress the gag reflex and make the whole procedure a little more comfortable for the patient.
3. Measure the tube for depth of insertion from the tip of the nose to the earlobe to the xiphoid process.
4. Lubricate the tube with a water-based lubricant and insert it into the larger nostril. While advancing the catheter, have the patient swallow if possible to help guide the tube into the esophagus. Advance it to premeasured depth.
5. Inject approximately 50 mL of air and listen over the epigastrium for the sounds.
6. Apply suction to the tube.
7. Secure the tube to the tip of the nose and cheek.

Orogastric tube placement procedure:

1. Position the patient's head in a neutral position.
2. Measure the tube for depth of insertion from the corner of the mouth to the earlobe to the xiphoid process.
3. Lubricate the tube with a water-based lubricant and insert it along the midline into the oropharynx. Advance it to premeasured depth.
4. Inject approximately 50 mL of air and listen over the epigastrium for the sounds.
5. If intubated, listen over the lung fields while ventilating to confirm that the ETT is still in place.
6. Apply suction to the tube.
7. Secure the tube to the cheek.

RESPIRATORY EMERGENCIES

Respiratory emergencies are one of the most common reasons for a person to call an ambulance. The reasons can range from a foreign body airway obstruction to a severe asthma attack. Respiratory emergencies can affect patients of any age or medical history. The paramedic needs to be prepared for managing a wide variety of respiratory distress calls.

Pathophysiology of Breathing

Breathing can fail in a multitude of ways, such as a closed airway or obstructions in the alveoli, among other things. Hypoxia or hypoxemia is a state of low O_2 levels in the blood that ultimately results in tissue and organ death if the condition is not quickly treated and reversed. Some tissues are more sensitive to hypoxic conditions than others. For example, the brain can tolerate a decline in blood O_2 levels only for a few minutes; after 10 minutes without O_2, irreversible brain damage occurs.

Respiratory success is dependent on several things to maintain health: ventilation, oxygenation and respiration, and perfusion. If any of these fail, the patient will be short of breath. The various derangements in each of these will be presented in order.

Many factors can affect ventilation in a patient, and these can be further divided into intrinsic and extrinsic factors. Intrinsic factors that affect ventilation include anything caused by the body's processes, such as anaphylaxis, infection, and the tongue in cases of unconsciousness while supine. These conditions all affect ventilation by hindering the ability of air to reach the alveoli. Other factors within the body but outside the respiratory system also can affect ventilation. Central nervous system disturbances that affect the neuromuscular control of breathing can prevent breathing altogether or cause abnormal breathing patterns that reduce alveolar ventilation. Extrinsic factors that can impact ventilation are those that occur outside the body. Trauma to the chest will impair the ability of a patient to expand the chest, thus reducing alveolar ventilation. Trauma to the trachea may cause the trachea to collapse during inhalation, preventing the inspiration of any air.

If ventilation can be performed without deficit, look at the issue of oxygenation and respiration. Because impairment to oxygenation also likely affects the transposition of CO_2 from the blood into the alveolus, if one is affected, both are likely similarly hindered. As with ventilation, impairments to respiration come in both extrinsic and intrinsic flavors. An extrinsic factor affecting respiration is, for example, if the patient is in an environment where the concentration of O_2 in the environment has been reduced or eliminated, oxygenation cannot happen. This can happen at high altitudes, where the pressure of O_2 is the leading problem, or in places where other gases have displaced O_2, such as a silo or a closed garage with a running car. CO is of particular concern because it will not only displace the O_2 in the environment but also cross the membrane and bind to hemoglobin more strongly than O_2.

Internal factors also can reduce respiration. Any condition that reduces the available surface area for O_2 to enter the blood and CO_2 to leave it is an example of such internal factors. Pneumonia, COPD, and pulmonary edema all affect gas exchange in the alveoli, by either reducing the number of alveoli available for respiration or filling them with fluid. Such a process is called intrapulmonary shunting because blood entering the lungs to be oxygenated goes to nonfunctional alveoli and just continues back to the heart without O_2—similar to walking into a room and forgetting what you went in there for and simply returning to where you started. Intrapulmonary shunting can be seen as decreased pulse oximetry. Pneumothorax (also known as a collapsed lung), pulmonary contusion, cardiac tamponade, and CHF also inhibit gas exchange as a result of circulatory problems. Finally, as seen earlier, the acid-base balance can impact respiration.

Assessment

Any patient with a respiratory complaint must be assessed carefully because so many different factors go into successful breathing. The **respiratory rate**, the number of times a person breathes in one minute, is the easiest portion of the breathing assessment to ascertain. Immediately evaluate any person found breathing outside these ranges for respiratory problems because alveolar ventilation and tidal and minute volumes can start to be affected. It's essential to know the normal respiratory rates for adults, children, and infants. Assessing the remainder of the history and physical examination is more involved.

Table 4-2. Normal Respiratory Rates

Age Range	Respiratory Rate Range
Adult	12–20
Child	15–30
Infant	25–50

The specific signs and symptoms and how they relate to each respiratory problem will be discussed later in this chapter. For now, the focus is on some generalities that should be assessed in every patient, but especially in the patient who is respiratory compromised. When entering where the patient is, use all of your senses to evaluate their condition. Some questions patients should be asked and the associated physical examination findings to be looked are as follows:

- **General Information.** In what position was the patient found? Is the patient tripoding? A patient in severe respiratory distress will not be lying down because it will worsen breathing. Assuming a tripod position—hands on the knees and back straight—will put the airways in line and allow for the least inspiratory resistance. As with every patient, remember to get a complete SAMPLE history, paying particular attention to the events leading up to the incident.

- **Head and Skin.** Are the nostrils flaring? Is there pursed lip breathing? Patients will flare their nostrils to create more space for air to enter with inhalation. When they exhale, they exhale almost exclusively through their mouth and purse their lips as if blowing out candles on a cake. This creates about 2 cm H_2O of PEEP and helps keep the alveoli open. Assess the pupils for equality and reaction. This may indicate a neurological problem that could be the source of the patient's respiratory problem. Remember that not all respiratory problems originate in the lungs. Check the skin for color, temperature, and texture. Findings of pale and sweaty or clammy skin could indicate shock, whereas flushed skin could be a clue for a fever, and hives indicate an allergic reaction.

- **Neck.** Is the patient using accessory muscles to breathe? Accessory muscles are most visible in the neck, and they stand out when in use. They are used to help elevate the rib cage. Is there jugular vein distension (JVD)? Is the trachea midline? JVD indicates increased intrathoracic pressure, commonly from CHF or pneumothorax, whereas a trachea that is displaced from the midline is a late finding in a pneumothorax.

- **Chest.**
  - Are retractions present? Retractions form as a result of a combination of extremely high negative pressure in the thoracic cavity in an attempt to draw air in and a blockage, whether internal or external, in the airways. The following are locations for retractions: intercostal retractions (between the ribs), supraclavicular retractions (to the right and left of the neck), suprasternal retractions (above the sternal notch), and subcostal retractions (under the rib cage in the area of the epigastrium). Retractions indicate severe airway compromise.

  - Are the rise and fall of the chest adequate? Equal? Unequal rise and fall of the chest indicates that the lung underneath is not getting ventilated with each breath. It often signals a pneumothorax. Paradoxical motion is the movement of a segment of the rib cage in the opposite direction of the rest of the ribs; on inhalation, a rib segment moves inward; on exhalation, the segment moves outward. This motion occurs in a flail segment and indicates chest trauma and broken ribs.

  - Is there a regular rhythm to breathing? The rhythm of breathing should be regular; in slowly and out slowly, and the whole process should take about 3–5 seconds to complete. The following table illustrates irregular breathing patterns that a patient may exhibit.

  - Are there any adventitious breath sounds? Listen to the breath sounds of every patient. This can be done on either the anterior or posterior chest, but the bell of the stethoscope should always be placed directly against the skin for the best transmission of the clearest sound. More on breath sounds a little later.

- **Abdomen.** Is it distended and hard? Although not much is going on in the abdomen that would be a clue to a problem in a patient with respiratory issues, if it is hard and distended, it could impact how much air can easily get into the lungs. This can happen after a big meal or after overzealous BVM ventilations.

- **Lower Extremities.** Is bilateral pitting edema present? Edema is simply swelling, and it is said to be pitting if a fingerprint remains after pressing into it. Also assess how far up the leg this edema travels. Is edema in only one of the lower extremities? This could indicate a clot in one of the veins of the leg, called **deep vein thrombosis (DVT)**. A piece of that clot could then break off and travel to the lungs, where it gets caught and blocks off blood flow to a section of lung. This results in sudden chest pain and shortness of breath.

- **Upper Extremities.** Is clubbing present on the fingers? Clubbing indicates chronic hypoxia.

Table 4-3. Abnormal Respiratory Patterns

Type	Description	Pattern
Cheyne-Stokes respirations	Periodic breathing with cycles of increasing rate and depth of breathing followed by gradual decrease in depth and rate of breathing in between periods of apnea that can last up to 60 seconds	
Kussmaul respirations	Continuous, deep sighing breaths with a rapid rate; usually >40 when the body is responding to metabolic acidosis	
Biot's (ataxic) respirations	Irregular rate, rhythm, and depth with intermittent apnea	
Apneustic respirations	An ominous sign of a brain-stem injury, prolonged inhalation followed by short ineffective exhalation	
Agonal respirations	An ineffective form of breathing that is characterized by slow gasping breaths often seen in pulseless patients	
Central neurologic hyperventilation	Essentially the same as Kussmaul respirations but from a different cause—brain injury and increased intracranial pressure (ICP), resulting in respiratory alkalosis	

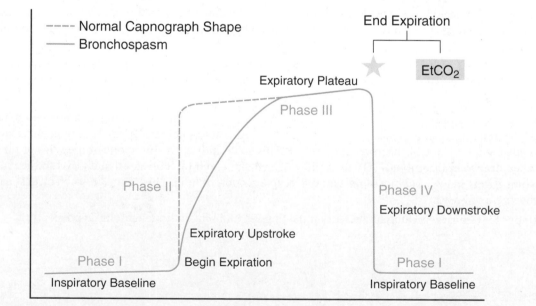

Figure 4-11. End-Tidal CO_2 Waveform Morphologies and Phases

Breath Sounds

Listening to lung sounds is an essential piece of the assessment puzzle in the patient with respiratory issues. It helps discern among the various pathologies that will be learned, which provides clues to the treatment that needs to be administered. When listening to breath sounds, it is important to listen on the same level, side to side, not up and down, first one lung and then the other. Look for equality of sound between the lungs at the same location, as well as the sound itself. Different volumes of sound in one lung versus the other lung at the same level could indicate that the diminished side is collapsing or filled with fluid, which indicates that air movement is not happening in that particular area. Remember to listen to all lung fields. This means listening to the following: listen to the apices by placing the stethoscope on the patient's back just superior to the shoulder blade on each side; listen to the middle lung fields by listening between the shoulder blades and the spine on each side; listen to the lower lung fields by placing the stethoscope on the midaxillary line at about the level of the fifth rib. As a new paramedic, listen to as many "normal" lungs as possible so that it will be easier to differentiate subtle differences in lungs with adventitious breath sounds. Adventitious breath sounds are simply abnormal in some way. There are several lung sounds with which to be familiar.

Wheezing is a breath sound that is higher in pitch than normal and is associated with a narrowing of the bronchioles. The bronchioles could themselves be constricted, swollen, or lined with thick mucus, thus creating a whistling sound, particularly on exhalation. The exhalation phase is prolonged in patients with bronchoconstriction and presenting with wheezing, which is indicated in an I/E ratio (inspiratory/expiratory ratio) that might be, for example, 1:4 instead of normal breathing, which has an I/E ratio closer to 1:2. Another way to think about this is that air has little trouble getting into the lungs but lots of trouble getting out. Unlike normal exhalation, wheezing exhalation is active; it requires energy expenditure and contracting intercostal and diaphragm muscles.

Rales or Crackles. Providers at all levels of medicine use these interchangeably, although the more commonly used term is crackles, which indicates thin fluid in the lower airways. Such sounds are heard in patients with pulmonary edema, where pressure in the pulmonary arterioles is high enough to force plasma to leak out into lung tissue. When the patient takes a breath into the affected alveoli, it sounds like bubbling, predominantly on inhalation. This sound does not clear with repeated deep breathing and does not typically clear with coughing. Patients who seldom take deep breaths, who are now asked to do so for a breath sound assessment, may have sounds similar to crackles on the initial inhalation. In this case, it is merely unused, collapsed alveoli popping open, and it is heard less and less on sequential deep breaths.

Rhonchi. Patients who have a buildup of mucus in the lower airways, such as smokers or those with pneumonia, have sounds called *rhonchi* (singular *rhonchus*). Rhonchi are snapping sounds, not bubbly sounds, because they are caused by the movement of thick mucus rather than the thinner plasma. Rhonchi may clear temporarily with a cough as the mucus gets moved out of the lower airways, if the patient can cough forcefully enough. In patients with pneumonia, rhonchi tend to be localized, only over the lobe(s) that have the infection. Lung sounds can otherwise be clear.

Stridor is a very high-pitched sound generated by the upper airway in inspiration and often expiration. This often ominous sound can be heard in a person with nearly complete closure of the upper airway. Stridor can occur in patients with a foreign body airway obstruction, anaphylaxis, croup, epiglottitis, or inhalation burns.

Pleural friction rub is the least common sound heard during a lung sounds assessment. As a result of an infection that gets into the pleural space, the friction rub occurs when the space between the pleura dries out and the inflamed pleura rub against each other. This becomes painful for the patient and causes the patient to self splint so that the area moves less. The patient does this by breathing more shallowly and not allowing full inflation of the lung underlying the area of inflammation.

End Tidal CO_2

A tool to help us evaluate patients' respiratory status is the measurement of their $EtCO_2$. It is measured as a patient exhales and can be done either with a colorimetric detector or as capnography that produces an actual numerical value and waveform on a monitor. Normal $EtCO_2$ values range between 35 and 45 mmHg. Using a colorimetric detector is typically good only for a few breaths—until the litmus paper gets saturated with CO_2 and no longer changes color from purple (unsaturated) to yellow (saturated).

Waveform capnography is useful in cardiac arrest as well as respiratory distress. In cardiac arrest, a sudden jump in $EtCO_2$ values could signal the return of spontaneous circulation. In a person with respiratory distress, high values indicate retention of CO_2 and possibly acidosis as the body attempts to shift the reaction from chapter 1 to make more CO_2. Low values could indicate hyperventilation or alkalosis. High values could indicate hypoventilation and CO_2 retention or metabolic alkalosis.

The shape of the waveform can help us as well. Normally, it is more of a boxy shape represented as the dotted line. The expiratory upstroke, phase II, begins abruptly from the inspiratory baseline (phase I) and represents the start of the exhalation phase. Next, the flat part is the plateau phase, or phase III, which represents the ongoing exhalation and essentially consists entirely of alveolar gases. The $EtCO_2$ value is read at the end of expiration, just prior to the expiratory downstroke.

Finally, the expiratory downstroke, phase IV, represents the start of the next inhalation and a return to the baseline of atmospheric conditions. In cases of bronchospasm, as found in asthma and exacerbation of COPD, the waveform takes on the appearance of a shark's dorsal fin. Following the solid line, the upslope is no longer abrupt, and there is an overall loss of the plateau phase. This provides a graphical representation of the difficulty a patient is having initiating their own exhalation. The distance from the start of the shark fin to the expiratory downstroke also tends to be longer and achieves a higher $EtCO_2$ number in the patient with bronchospasm, illustrating the prolonged expiratory phase.

CONDITIONS WITH A COMPLAINT OF SHORTNESS OF BREATH

Many conditions will lead to a chief complaint from a patient of shortness of breath. This section will discuss those that are primarily caused by a problem with the respiratory system. Starting the discussion as done for the anatomy, the progression will be problems affecting the upper airway, followed by those affecting the lower airways and pulmonary circulation. Alternate causes of shortness of breath, such as diabetic ketoacidosis, myocardial infarction, and pulmonary contusion, among others, will be discussed in later chapters. With that in mind, when faced with a breathing complaint in the field, do not just focus on the respiratory issue. There may be a more insidious problem, such as diabetes or an aspirin overdose, at the root of the respiratory problem. As for all patients, always rule out other potential causes for the signs and symptoms found.

Upper Airway Pathologies

Foreign Body Airway Obstruction

Many everyday objects can cause a foreign body airway obstruction (FBAO), from toys and other small items within a child's reach to a shrimp served at a fancy restaurant. The patient will be coughing if there is any air movement whatsoever; this is known as a partial FBAO because the patient can still exchange air in the lungs, albeit poorly. The patient may also have stridor during inhalation. In partial FBAO, the patient will do a better job of relieving the obstruction on their own, through forceful coughing, without any intervention from a paramedic. As the responder, remain close to the patient if the obstruction moves, becoming a complete FBAO, and be prepared to help should the patient lose consciousness due to the obstruction. Anticipation of patient need is key in such a case.

In a complete FBAO, the obstructing object completely covers the entire trachea, typically at the glottic opening, totally preventing air exchange. The patient with a complete FBAO often will show the universal sign of choking, which is two hands holding the neck. If the patient is able to respond to the question, "Are you choking?" with a verbal response, continue to encourage the person to cough. If the person is able to answer only with a head nod, then actively try to squeeze the obstruction out of the trachea. This can be accomplished with abdominal thrusts known as the **Heimlich maneuver**. The rescuer wraps their arms around the patient's waist at the level of the navel from behind and squeezes forcefully inward and upward until the object is expelled or the patient becomes unconscious.

Unless this occurs as just described, the paramedics often will arrive on scene long after the patient has lost consciousness from a lack of O_2, finding the patient unresponsive on the floor. With the patient supine, immediately begin 30 chest compressions as if doing CPR (15 in the infant or child). Next, open the airway using the head tilt/chin lift maneuver and remove any object you see, with either your fingers or suction. Attempt to ventilate at this point regardless of whether you actually removed anything or not because the obstruction may have moved enough to allow air to pass. If breaths are delivered, continue the assessment as if this patient was found unresponsive, including pulse check and CPR. If breaths fail to go into the lungs, continue chest compressions, alternating with airway checks and ventilation attempts. At any point during this process, prepare to use the Magill forceps, which are curved tweezers specially designed to be used along with direct laryngoscopy to reach in and remove a FBAO in any patient.

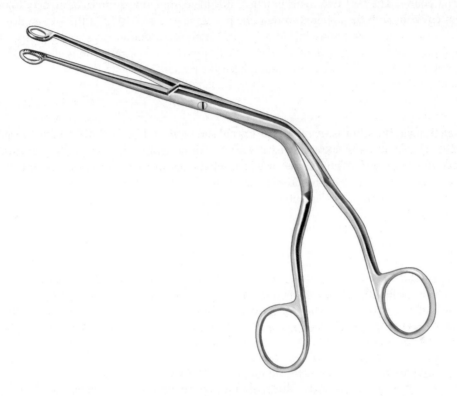

Figure 4-12. Magill Forceps

Swelling

Upper airway burns, anaphylaxis, croup, and Magill forceps are all possible causes for stridor and respiratory distress related to an upper airway problem. In most of these cases, getting a good history of the present illness from the patient or caregiver will help differentiate the likely reason and guide effective treatment. Aside from stridor, a complaint of difficulty breathing and, in most cases, an observable increase in the work of breathing, figure out which of these is the primary culprit and treat accordingly.

Croup

Croup is most commonly found in children between 6 months and 3 years old, although it can affect a person of any age. It is caused by swelling of the upper airways and is most commonly caused by a viral infection. It is often preceded by cold- or flu-like symptoms until the airway begins to swell. Croup's hallmark sign is a barking seal-like cough that is unmistakable. The treatment for these children often is as simple as a change in environment; if the child is in a warm environment, having the child breathe cold air, such as outside during winter months or from a freezer, may help. If the child is already in a cool, dry environment, bringing the child into a steamy bathroom where a hot shower is running often can result in profound improvement. Although it is typically more scary because of the sounds the child is making, it is rarely life threatening, so manipulation of the airway with oral adjuncts or intubation is rarely needed. If the stridor persists after a change in environment, and the pulse oximetry is falling or remains low after blow-by O_2 therapy, racemic epinephrine is the medication of choice. To administer racemic epinephrine, dilute 0.25–0.75 mL of a 2.25% solution in 2.0 mL normal saline and administer via a nebulizer for 5 minutes.

Epiglottitis

Epiglottitis is a severe and often life-threatening emergency characterized by swelling of the epiglottis caused by infection with the flu virus. In children, the epiglottis can swell to the point it completely closes off the airway. Adults, with larger airway diameters, rarely progress to that point; however, both populations present the same way. The typical presentation of a patient with epiglottitis includes sitting bolt upright to allow for the straightest pathway of air into the lungs. Because of a profoundly sore throat, these patients often will be drooling to avoid swallowing, and their voice will be hoarse. The best treatment practices include eliminating sources of anxiety for the patient and providing a calm environment. Be prepared to treat the patient aggressively should the airway close off but do not manipulate the airway in any way—this includes tongue depressors, oral airways, and attempts at intubation— because the likelihood of causing more damage than actually remedying the situation is greater. Blow-by O_2 should be provided as long as it does not create more agitation for the patient.

Anaphylaxis

Anaphylaxis is swelling of the soft tissues of the mouth and throat, including the lips, tongue, hypopharynx, larynx, and vocal cords, as a result of a systemic release of histamine from exposure to any number of allergens. Interventions that involve manipulation of the airway should be performed only with extreme caution and should not include oral or nasal airways; any intubation attempt should be performed only by the most experienced provider available, if at all, and with a smaller tube than anticipated. Much more on assessment and treatment of this condition is in chapter 5.

Airway Burns

Airway burns are caused when superheated air or steam is inhaled and can occur even in the absence of fire. For example, a person can sustain airway burns when the oven is first opened and the air that first comes out is inhaled. The treating paramedic should be prepared for intubation and cricothyrotomy because the swelling will continue until the burning process is complete, which may not be for hours after the initial exposure. More discussion on this topic can be found in chapter 7.

In summary, any severe upper airway problem should be treated with caution and preparations should be made to treat a difficult airway. Manipulation of the airway should not be performed prophylactically because it may precipitate worsening of the current condition and, in some cases, actually cause the airway to close.

Lung Tissue and Lower Airway Pathologies

Asthma

Asthma is a condition that affects millions of people in the United States and results in hundreds of thousands of hospital stays each year. Asthma is a collective term for a trio of lower airway issues that combine to cause dyspnea. First, there is bronchospasm, where the muscles in the bronchioles constrict, causing difficulty in exhaling air. The air becomes trapped in the alveoli, requiring increased pressure to exhale. This prolongs the exhalation time and causes normally passive exhalation to become an active process where muscle use is required. Second, increased mucus production further clogs already constricted airways. Finally, swelling in the lower air passages from infection or irritation can further worsen the breathing ability of the asthmatic. Any or all these issues may occur in varying degrees at all times during the life of an asthmatic and can worsen during an attack or exacerbation of the disease.

The patient with an exacerbation of asthma will be wheezing if there is sufficient air movement in the lower airways. The patient also may have diminished or absent breath sounds anywhere in the lungs if the airways are so tight that they are not allowing any movement. The patient may have had exposure to a trigger—such as smoke, animal dander, or mold—that precipitated this attack. The patient often will be found in a tripod position trying to expand the lungs as much as possible and frequently will have taken multiple extra doses from an MDI or even a home nebulizer with little improvement. Inhaled beta-agonists treat only the bronchoconstriction piece of the asthma triad and do little to address edema or secretions.

The paramedic has many treatment options available for asthma and status asthmaticus. The following therapies should be attempted in the order listed.

1. Inhaled, nebulized beta-agonist such as albuterol. The usual dose is 2.5 mg in 3 mL saline nebulized with a flow of at least 8 LPM O_2. The dose may be repeated as often as necessary during transport.

2. Ipratropium bromide often is given concurrently with albuterol. The usual dose is 500 mcg (0.5 mg) inhaled.

3. CPAP is recommended if the albuterol and ipratropium combination does not improve the patient's status.

4. Epinephrine 0.3 mg IM for adults or 0.15 mg IM for children can help relieve status asthmaticus.

5. Corticosteroids such as methylprednisolone can be given to address the airway edema that may be happening. The dose for methylprednisolone is 125 mg intravenously.

6. Magnesium sulfate, which is a strong smooth muscle relaxant, can be administered when all previous options have failed to bring about relief. Magnesium sulfate is usually administered slowly over several minutes with a max dose of 2 g.

Chronic Obstructive Pulmonary Disease (COPD)

COPD is a name given to emphysema and chronic bronchitis. Patients with COPD often have a significant history of smoking and a barrel-shaped chest caused by the chronic collapse of alveoli and the trapping of CO_2 in the bullae. People are able to live normally with COPD and tend to live in a constant state of shortness of breath. They will call the ambulance when the shortness of breath gets worse and when they can no longer control it with their rescue inhalers or daily medication regimen. A good question to ask these patients is, "What made it worse today to call the ambulance?" Patients with COPD may indicate that they have had a change in the amount or color of sputum, indicating that they may have a new onset of pneumonia.

The patient with COPD will present differently depending on what caused the exacerbation. If the overall condition worsens, the patient will likely present much like someone diagnosed with asthma (e.g., wheezing and tightness in the chest). A patient with COPD who is developing pneumonia may present with wheezing and rhonchi as lung sounds; they also may have a fever and a change in the color of sputum. Remember, patients with pneumonia who do not have COPD will have a fever, a productive cough, and dehydration as well. Patients with COPD and pneumonia tend to be more difficult to manage and to get pneumonia more often. This is because patients with COPD have increased mucus and secretions in the lungs and decreased ability to expel those secretions.

Treatment will be determined largely by identifying what is causing the exacerbation. Beta-agonists will help with bronchial constriction, and steroids will help with the bronchial edema as in asthma. Patients also may benefit from magnesium sulfate, as in asthma. CPAP benefits these patients because the PEEP keeps the lower airways open. However, the higher volume of air and the continuous pressure has the potential to cause barotrauma, especially in the delicate lungs of the patient with COPD. Despite the assertion that giving O_2 will cause overdependence, the idea of "eliminating the hypoxic drive" is not accurate. If the patient needs oxygen, do not withhold it. An oxygen-assisted patient who stops breathing probably would have done so anyway; in addition, this complication can be managed.

Pulmonary Edema and Congestive Heart Failure (CHF)

Generically, fluid building up within the lung tissues and alveoli, and eventually out into the bronchioles, is referred to as **pulmonary edema**. CHF is just one of many causes of the pulmonary edema. It is caused by dysfunction in either the right or left ventricle of the heart, resulting in the poor movement of blood through the lungs. As the pressure in the capillaries builds and the blood stagnates, the capillaries become leaky, causing plasma and sometimes red blood cells to seep into the lung tissues. If this continues long enough, eventually the level of the fluid rises from the bases to the apices of the lungs, causing a person to expel foamy sputum from the mouth that is blood streaked or tinged.

Other causes of pulmonary edema include the inhalation of toxic gases, high-altitude pulmonary edema (HAPE), and drowning. These are noncardiogenic and do not result from high pressure; they are a generalized increase in the permeability of the capillaries. Each of these noncardiogenic causes of pulmonary edema results in an irritation to the alveoli, which in turn causes the capillaries to swell and eventually leak, similar to the way an abrasion on the skin oozes plasma and blood.

Patients with pulmonary edema will present with crackles in the dependent lung fields; in a person who can sit upright or stand, crackles would start in the bases and move superiorly until eventually filling the entire lung. Patients with noncardiogenic causes of pulmonary edema will have symptoms consistent with the specific cause. Patients with HAPE will have a history of recent mountain climbing with extended time at the higher altitude. Patients with toxic gas exposure may be among a group of patients with similar complaints or work with gases that could cause irritation, such as chlorine at a pool or ammonia at food processing plants. Pulmonary edema is a late finding in patients who are drowning, and the patient may have been treated and delivered to the emergency department long before the edema occurs. Treatment largely depends on the cause but centers on removing the patient from the environment and providing high-flow O_2. CPAP is recommended to help increase intrapulmonary pressures and push the fluid back into the circulation. This also will help keep open alveoli that have collapsed and provide additional surface area for the exchange of gases.

Patients with CHF will have additional signs to look for in the physical examination, in addition to crackles in the lungs and information to gather (if possible) during the interrogation. The shortness of breath will have increased during the course of several days. The patient may no longer be able to sleep lying flat, using pillows to prop up or sleeping in a semi-seated position in a recliner. The patient may complain of associated chest pain. The patient often will be pale and very diaphoretic. Because of the failure of the pump to move blood around the body, JVD and swelling in the dependent areas of the body—feet, ankles, and lower extremities if the patient can sit or stand and the sacrum or hip area if the patient is bedridden—are common findings. The patient also typically has high blood pressure and tachycardia.

The treatment of a patient with pulmonary edema from CHF is one of the more intensive treatments that paramedics can complete. Delivering high-concentration O_2 is the first priority. CPAP will be the best treatment for these patients as long as they can tolerate the mask. Next is the administration of large quantities of nitrates in the form of NTG. Before the CPAP mask is placed, administer 1 tablet of 0.4 mg NTG sublingually at once, depending on the patient's blood pressure. Once the CPAP mask has been applied to the patient, removing it to administer additional doses of NTG can be difficult and is not recommended. Instead, if permitted in local protocols, apply a 1-inch strip of NTG paste to the patient's chest or arm. Morphine sulfate is a great medication because it will not only treat any existing chest pain, thus making the patient more comfortable, but also act as a mild vasodilator, lessening the preload on the heart. Finally, furosemide is a potassium-wasting loop diuretic that is used to help the patient eliminate any excess fluid. Furosemide use is rapidly decreasing in paramedic treatments and is being eliminated in many systems. Higher doses of nitrates are far more helpful than furosemide in treating the patient with CHF.

Pneumothorax

Pneumothorax in the nontrauma patient is caused when a weakened area of the lung, called a bleb, ruptures. The bleb can be pathological (i.e., congenital) or caused by COPD. The rupture could be caused by any event that increases pressure inside the chest, including a sneeze or a cough or positive pressure ventilation. Air then leaks out of the lung from this ruptured bleb into the intrapleural space and collects there. After a certain amount of time, the lung will be crushed by the building pressure in that space, and difficulty in breathing will begin as the surface area for gas exchange is reduced.

These patients will have shortness of breath and decreased or absent lung sounds over one or more lung fields on the same side of the chest or back. As intrathoracic pressure builds, the mediastinum will shift toward the unaffected side. This shift will minimize the pumping ability of the heart, which is seen as JVD, and it will cause the trachea to deviate from the midline toward the unaffected side late in the process. These patients also may have a ventilation-perfusion mismatch; despite giving high-flow O_2, their pulse oximetry readings do not increase above a certain number, which is expected. The affected side also becomes hyperresonant to percussion, that is, it will sound hollow.

Treatment beyond O_2 includes a procedure called needle thoracostomy. During this procedure, an over-the-needle catheter is inserted into the chest through the second intercostal space—the midclavicular line—just above the third rib on the affected side. There will be a rush of air when the needle is removed as the pressure is released, which will allow the lung to slowly reinflate. If this is the cause of the difficulty breathing, the patient will improve rapidly after the needle insertion.

Pleural Effusion

Fluid collecting in the intrapleural space is a **pleural effusion** that often is caused by trauma, cancer, or infection. As with a pneumothorax, as pressure builds up, the lung begins to collapse, and respiratory distress begins. The position of the patient will affect the location and distribution of the fluid. Lung sounds may be difficult to hear over the effused area. Definitive treatment for this effusion is a thoracentesis, which can be done only at a hospital. The paramedic should provide supportive care, including O_2 if needed, and transport the patient in the position of maximal comfort, which is usually sitting up.

Pulmonary Embolism

PE is most commonly caused when a piece of a clot that formed in the deep veins of the leg (DVT) travels through the right side of the heart and lodges in the lung somewhere. Large clots will block off a larger percentage of the lung, resulting in a large area of the lung that is ultimately well ventilated but completely lacking in circulation. DVT can form in people who are bedridden for long periods of time, people on birth control pills for any reason, or people who have a clotting disorder. Other sources of an embolism include fat embolism from a broken bone, air embolism from a laceration to a large vein or an incompletely flushed intravenous line where a large amount of air is injected, or amniotic fluid during pregnancy.

A patient with a PE often will complain of a sudden onset of chest pain with a sudden onset of shortness of breath. The patient will be tachypneic, trying to compensate for the area of lung that is no longer exchanging gases. There often is a marked ventilation perfusion mismatch because it will appear that the patient is moving air appropriately, and lung sounds over all lung fields will be clear; however, the pulse oximetry readings will be low, and the patient will have extensive cyanosis. A large enough embolus, such as a **saddle embolus,** could result in almost immediate cardiac arrest, which is typically not survivable. A saddle embolus is a clot that forms across where the pulmonary artery bifurcates into the left and right pulmonary arteries. Patients in cardiac arrest from such a large embolus will present with cape cyanosis, which is deep, irreversible cyanosis of the head, neck, chest, and back despite otherwise effective CPR and rescue breathing with 100% O_2.

Clinical Correlate

Geriatric Corner

When it comes to pneumonia, geriatric patients are at increased risk of both infection and hospitalization. Aside from simply age, adults age 65 and older are at increased risk for pneumonia because they tend to have more underlying health problems, which increase the pneumonia risk. People who have vascular disease or COPD and those receiving cancer therapy are more vulnerable to any infectious disease, including pneumonia. In addition, bed confinement or any condition that limits the ability to take deep breaths exacerbates the risk. Older adults often have several of these associated risks, resulting in a longer, more severe illness than a younger adult might experience. Furthermore, older adults typically lack the telltale pneumonia symptoms of fever, chills, and a productive cough; instead, they may simply become suddenly confused.

Older adults also tend to be more at risk of a PE because of decreasing mobility and the resulting venous stasis it causes. Assume that any patient who presents with *shortness of breath and tachycardia alone* (with no other complaint or symptom) has a pulmonary embolus until proven otherwise. In a patient who presents this way, look for a swollen leg that is cooler than its counterpart, indicative of DVT. After ensuring an airway and adequate ventilation, provide supplemental O_2 and transport the patient carefully; rough handling could cause more of the clot to break free and worsen the patient's condition.

REVIEW QUESTIONS

Select the ONE best answer.

1. Use the following information to answer questions 1 and 2.

   I. Trachea

   II. Oropharynx

   III. Bronchioles

   IV. Bronchi

   V. Cricoid cartilage

   Place these 5 structures in order according to the way inhaled air would encounter them.

   A. V, II, I, IV, and III

   B. V, II, I, III, and IV

   C. II, V, I, III, and IV

   D. II, V, I, IV, and III

2. Which of the structures listed above is/are part of the upper airway?

   A. II only

   B. V only

   C. II and V only

   D. I, II and V only

3. Which of the following is true about the lung volumes of a person with COPD?

   A. Residual volume increases.

   B. Tidal volume increases.

   C. Expiratory reserve volume increases.

   D. Total lung volume increases.

4. A patient who twisted their ankle while running is found to be tachypneic during your assessment. Possible reason(s) for this include:

   A. Increased pH of the CSF.

   B. Increased pH of the blood.

   C. Increased pCO_2 of the blood.

   D. Increased FiO_2 of the atmosphere.

5. Consider the following scenario for questions 5 and 6:

    A 42-year-old female patient is complaining of a sudden onset of dizziness that started while at rest and is constant but not worsening with a change in position. She has been on bed rest for the past 2 weeks after an infection to her incision for a total knee replacement. Her vital signs are HR: 108; RR: 24; SpO_2: 91% (on 15 LPM O_2 via mask); BP: 132/88. Her lung sounds are clear in all fields and equal bilaterally. Her skin color and temperature are unremarkable. She has not passed out, and her blood sugar is within normal limits.

    This patient is most likely having a problem with:

    A. Ventilation.
    B. External respiration.
    C. Internal respiration.
    D. Perfusion.

6. Based on the assessment information given, select the most likely condition this patient is experiencing.

    A. Pulmonary edema
    B. Pulmonary stenosis
    C. Pulmonary embolism
    D. Pulmonary contusion

7. In which of the following patients would the use of a nasopharyngeal airway be most appropriate?

    A. A 7-month-old female found apneic in a crib
    B. A 17-year-old female struck in the face with a batted softball during a game
    C. An awake, combative, 27-year-old male who consumed half a bottle of bourbon
    D. An 86-year-old male responsive only to painful stimuli with hyperglycemia

8. You are doing an interfacility transport of a patient who was intubated prior to your arrival at the sending facility. The chest x-ray from the previous facility confirmed proper placement before you departed. During transport, the patient's pulse oximetry begins to drop, and the $EtCO_2$ waveform is slightly lower than earlier. The patient still has a pulse. Of the following, which should you do first?

    A. Using a laryngoscope, check that the tube is still in the trachea.
    B. Suction the ETT with a soft-suction catheter.
    C. Perform a bilateral needle thoracostomy.
    D. Remove the ETT and attempt to reintubate.

9. The ETT of the patient in the previous question is confirmed as still being in the trachea. It has been suctioned, all equipment is functioning properly, and O_2 is flowing at 15 LPM. However, the pulse oximetry is continuing to drop, and the $EtCO_2$ is starting to increase. It is notably harder to ventilate the patient, and the left side of the chest is not rising as it was earlier in the transport. What should you do next?

    A. Perform a bilateral needle thoracostomy.
    B. Perform a needle thoracostomy on the left anterior chest.
    C. Perform a needle thoracostomy on the right anterior chest.
    D. Pull the ETT back 1 cm at a time to relieve bronchial intubation.

10. Which of the following sets of signs and symptoms would you expect to find to help confirm your diagnosis from question number 9?

    A. Decreased breath sounds on the left side, trachea deviated to the left side, and JVD
    B. Decreased breath sounds on the left side, trachea deviated to the right side, and JVD
    C. Decreased breath sounds on the right side, trachea deviated to the right side, and JVD
    D. Decreased breath sounds on the right side, trachea deviated to the left side, and JVD

11. For a 55-year-old male patient in status asthmaticus on 10 LPM O_2 via a nebulizer who has already received 2 nebulized albuterol treatments and 500 mcg of ipratropium bromide, which of the following would be the next best treatment option?

    A. 2 g of magnesium sulfate intravenously
    B. 0.3 mg of 1:1,000 epinephrine intramuscularly
    C. Continuous positive airway pressure (CPAP)
    D. 125 mg of methylprednisolone

12. You have arrived at the home of a 3-year-old female who is in respiratory distress. She is seated in a tripod position and drooling, stating she is unable to swallow. Her mother indicates that she has recently been sick with a strep throat infection. You suspect your patient has:

    A. Anaphylaxis.
    B. Croup.
    C. Epiglottitis.
    D. Laryngitis.

13. Which of the following is the best indication for the paramedic to perform a needle or surgical cricothyrotomy?

    A. Anaphylaxis
    B. Facial Trauma
    C. Superior airway burns
    D. Unable to ventilate or intubate.

ANSWERS AND EXPLANATIONS

1. **The correct answer is (D).** The order would be oropharynx, cricoid cartilage, trachea, bronchi, and bronchioles.

2. **The correct answer is (A).** The lower airway is defined as all structures inferior to the larynx. Therefore, the cricoid cartilage, trachea, bronchi, and bronchioles are all considered part of the lower airway. The oropharynx is the posterior portion of the mouth, is superior to the larynx, and therefore the only structure listed that is part of the upper airway.

3. **The correct answer is (A).** In a person with COPD, atelectasis and the retention of CO_2 result in an increase in the residual volume in the lungs, which is the amount of air left in the lungs after a forceful exhalation. All the other volumes will remain the same or decrease as the residual volume takes up an increasing amount of the total available lung volume.

4. **The correct answer is (C).** An increase in CO_2 concentration in the blood is more likely to make a person breathe faster. When pH increases, the solution becomes more basic and the concentration of hydrogen ions decreases. Remember the equation:

$$HCO_3^- + H^+ \Leftrightarrow CO_2 + H_2O$$

According to this equation, if $[H^+]$ decreases, the reaction will proceed to the left to create more. This means that the patient will breathe less frequently to retain some CO_2. An increase in acidity—and, therefore, a decrease in pH—is 1 of the primary stimuli prompting a person to take a breath. This makes (A) and (B) incorrect. Increased FiO_2 of the atmosphere means that a person is getting more O_2 with each breath and is more likely to cause their breathing to slow down, if there is any change at all, making (D) incorrect.

5. **The correct answer is (B).** External respiration is the ability to load O_2 into the bloodstream at the alveolar level. This is most likely causing her low O_2 saturation and dizziness. In this case, the patient is ventilating well, as indicated by the clear and equal lung sounds, making (A) incorrect. Perfusion (D) and internal respiration (C) have to do with the delivery of blood to the tissues and the offloading of O_2 to those tissues, respectively. Problems with each of these are ruled out because her skin color and temperature are unremarkable, and she is not showing signs of hypoperfusion (shock).

6. **The correct answer is (C).** This patient is most likely experiencing a new PE. Because of her lengthy bed rest from her total knee replacement and resulting infection, it is possible for a clot to develop in the deep veins of the leg (DVT). If a piece of this clot breaks free, it could travel to and become lodged in the lungs. This condition is called a PE. Pulmonary edema (A) would have adventitious breath sounds. Pulmonary stenosis (B) is a narrowing of the pulmonary artery and is not typically a sudden onset. There is no indication of chest trauma that would suggest a pulmonary contusion (D).

7. **The correct answer is (D).** This patient is the most appropriate patient to receive a nasopharyngeal airway because he may still have a gag reflex, ruling out the use of oropharyngeal airway, and has not sustained any trauma to his head or face but may have difficulty maintaining his own airway. (A) should receive an oropharyngeal airway or be intubated because she is apneic. The patient in (B) may have sustained facial and head trauma, increasing the likelihood that the basal skull also is fractured; here is it best to avoid. The patient in (C) should not receive the nasopharyngeal airway because he is awake at this point, although he may become a candidate later.

8. **The correct answer is (A).** Whenever a previously successfully intubated patient has a decline in pulse oximetry, EtCO$_2$, or both, immediately check the DOPE mnemonic: displacement, obstruction, pneumothorax, and equipment. Of the choices given, checking to see if the tube is still in the trachea is the best option. Suctioning (B) and thoracostomy (C) are considered only after correct placement is confirmed. Reintubation (D) should be done only as a last resort.

9. **The correct answer is (B).** The presented symptoms likely indicate a left-sided pneumothorax. Once other noninvasive problems have been ruled out, needle thoracostomy is the best option. This patient needs only a left thoracostomy, making (A) and (C) incorrect. (D) would be most appropriate if the lung sounds and chest rise were diminished on the right side; a right main-stem intubation is much more likely than a left main-stem intubation.

10. **The correct answer is (B).** During a pneumothorax, breath sounds will be diminished on the side of the collapsing lung, and the trachea deviates to the unaffected side. Tracheal deviation is a late sign and indicates a significant buildup of pressure. JVD will become more pronounced as venous return to the heart becomes inhibited.

11. **The correct answer is (C).** The best option here would be to initiate CPAP. Answer choices (A), (B), and (D) are all reasonable options and should be attempted after CPAP is initiated.

12. **The correct answer is (C).** This is a classic presentation of epiglottitis with tripod positioning and drooling. *Streptococcus pyogenes* also is one of the more common causes of epiglottitis and strep throat. Anaphylaxis (A) is a possibility if the patient is still on penicillin; however, the patient should be able to swallow. Croup (B) is almost always accompanied with the "barking seal" cough. Laryngitis (D) is possible but does not usually prevent a person from swallowing.

13. **The correct answer is (D).** Though the remaining answers may lead to the need to perform a cricothyrotomy, the best answer here is the scenario of "can't ventilate, can't intubate." Without any further description, each of those could be capable of being ventilated or even intubated.

Cardiology, Cardiac Emergencies, and Resuscitation

5

Learning Objectives

❏ Describe cardiovascular anatomy and physiology.

❏ Identify normal and abnormal electrical cardiac rhythms.

❏ Interpret 12-lead ECGs (electrocardiograms).

❏ Differentiate, assess, and treat cardiac emergencies.

In most systems, cardiac-related emergencies make up a significant portion of a paramedic's call volume, especially when you consider all the ailments that can result from a failing cardiovascular system. Each year, new treatments are added and some are taken away from the repertoire of assessment and treatment possibilities for the patient with a cardiac condition.

This chapter will focus on all things cardiac, from anatomy to electrophysiology.

CARDIOVASCULAR ANATOMY AND PHYSIOLOGY

The human heart is a muscular structure about the size of a fist and consists of four separate chambers. It is uniquely designed to pump blood throughout our bodies. The entire heart is encapsulated by the **pericardium**, a tough fibrous sac that protects the heart from other structures of the chest and contains lubricating fluid to reduce friction generated by the moving heart. There are three layers to the muscular walls of the heart.

- The **epicardium** is the outermost layer of the heart and protects the muscle from friction generated when it beats.

- The **myocardium** is the actual contractile muscle of the heart. All the myocytes (muscle cells) are able to not only contract and conduct electrical impulses efficiently through them to neighboring myocytes but also generate their own electrical impulse in the absence of a coordinated, propagated impulse that normally occurs and initiates the contraction of the heart.

- The final layer of the heart is the **endocardium**, which is the layer that lines the inside of the heart and protects muscle tissue from the friction of the blood traveling through it.

The cardiac muscle tissue needs all these levels of protection to function properly because any outside irritation could generate an electrical and mechanical impulse and start a new beat when the heart is not ready to beat.

Despite being surrounded by and, in fact, bathed in blood, the heart derives none of its O_2 supply from the blood within its chambers; it has its own vasculature and is entirely supplied by the coronary arteries. Two coronary artery sinuses originate in the root of the aorta and flow along the surface of the heart.

- The **right coronary artery** (RCA) follows the AV sulcus between the right atrium and the right ventricle, and the branches from the RCA service the right atrium and ventricle and part of the left ventricle and septum. The RCA services the AV node in approximately 85% of the population.

- The **left main coronary artery** (LMCA) comes off the aorta and travels about 10–25 mm and branches into the left anterior descending (LAD) and the left circumflex (LCx) arteries. These heavily branched arteries deliver blood to the left atrium; the left ventricle's lateral, posterior, and anterior walls; and most of the septum. The LCx provides most of the blood for the lateral wall and the posterior wall. A branch of the LCx services the AV node in those people whose AV node does not get its blood supply from the RCA.

This extensive network of branches, called **collateral circulation**, creates multiple routes of flow for oxygenated blood to reach the cells. It develops across time to ensure continuous blood flow to the heart.

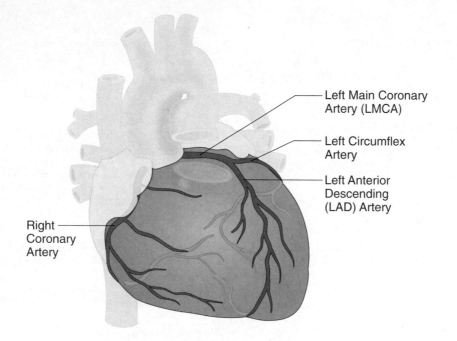

Figure 5-1. Arterial Supply to the Heart

As with any capillary system, the capillaries empty into venules and eventually veins that go around the heart in a groove called the **coronary sulcus**. They empty into the **coronary sinus** before making their way back into the right atrium directly.

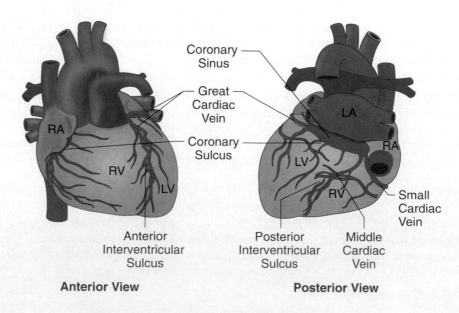

Figure 5-2. Venous Drainage of the Heart

Blood Flow through Heart and Cardiac Structure

To make a complete circuit from systemic circulation back to systemic circulation, a blood cell must go through the heart twice. The heart is actually two pumps within the same organ, each with a distinct purpose. The right side of the heart is responsible for the pulmonary circuit and getting O_2 from the lungs, whereas the left side is responsible for the systemic circuit and getting blood to every cell of the body. Each blood cell begins its journey through the heart at the vena cava.

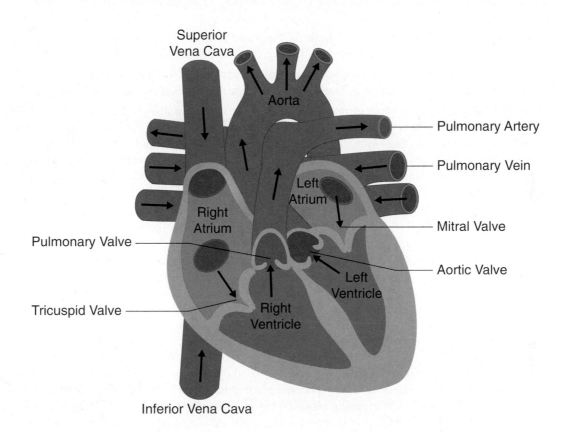

Figure 5-3. Bloodflow through the Heart

1. The **vena cavae** are the collecting veins where all the blood drains as it completes its circuit through the body. They are named according to their relative position to the heart: the superior vena cava drains the head and upper limbs, and the inferior vena cava drains the lower extremities, abdomen, and pelvis. Both empty into the right atrium.

2. The **right atrium** is the initial holding area for blood and is the site of the sinoatrial (SA) node. (The SA node will be discussed in more detail later when the electrical system is discussed.) The atria contract together under normal circumstances. The right atrium sends blood through the tricuspid valve and into the right ventricle.

3. The **tricuspid valve** is composed of three leaflets that are designed to prevent the backflow of blood during ventricular contraction into the atrium and make up the physical barrier between the right atrium and right ventricle. During atrial systole, or contraction, the leaflets are pushed open. As the atria relax, the valve leaflets swing shut again. The leaflets of the valve are prevented from inverting, or prolapsing, because they are attached to chordae tendineae. These "heartstrings" are attached at the other end to the wall of the right ventricle to specialized muscles called papillary muscles.

4. After the **right ventricle** squeezes out its blood, it relaxes and refills. The motion of relaxing draws in blood from the right atrium down the pressure gradient. When the atria beat, they kick a little extra blood into the ventricles than would otherwise be able to fit. This is called the atrial kick, and it has the effect of stretching the ventricles just a fraction more, helping maintain cardiac output. The blood is now in a

second, larger chamber called the right ventricle. This chamber is more muscular than the previous one because it is responsible for moving blood through all the lung capillaries.

5. Next the blood is squeezed out through the **pulmonary semilunar valve**, sometimes called the pulmonic valve. This valve is shaped like a half moon, hence its name. This valve deposits the blood into the pulmonary artery.

6. The **pulmonary artery** is the only artery in the body that carries deoxygenated blood. It eventually bifurcates into the left and right pulmonary artery and down into capillaries within the lung tissue itself.

7. The **pulmonary vein** returns blood only from the lungs and is the only vein to carry oxygenated blood. This vein also completes the pulmonary circulation as blood is delivered to the left atrium.

8. Now back at the left side of the heart, blood enters the **left atrium**, which is the holding chamber for the left ventricle. As this atrium contracts, blood within it is shuttled through the bicuspid or mitral valve.

9. The **mitral valve** is the gatekeeper of the left ventricle. It lets blood in during diastole and when the atrium contracts. Diastole is the phase where the heart is at rest, relaxing from the previous systole, and the chambers are refilling. The mitral valve, like its counterpart the tricuspid valve, is prevented from inverting with chordae tendineae attached to papillary muscles. However, because of the high pressures exerted by the left ventricle during systole, the mitral valve has a greater tendency to prolapse, which is why it is more common to hear of mitral valve prolapse than tricuspid valve prolapse. The left ventricular papillary muscles also are more prone to rupture than those in the right ventricle because of the higher pressures needed to keep this valve closed, especially in patients with chronic or uncontrolled high blood pressure.

10. The **left ventricle** needs fanfare, because a lot happens here. First, it is the most muscular of all the chambers by a wide margin because it needs to move blood throughout the entire body, including the head, which is typically against gravity. The atrial kick here is important because it stretches the large muscular walls of the ventricle, which allows it to pump more forcefully. This is referred to as the **Frank-Starling principle**, which is a property of cardiac muscle: As it gets stretched more, it contracts with greater force. The initial total pressure coming into the ventricle is known as the preload; think of it as the load placed on the heart before contraction. Now the left ventricle is ready to contract. It is stretched as far as it can, even after the atrium kicked in what it has to offer, so it squeezes most of the blood out into the aorta; yet some remains in it for the next cycle. This is called the ejection fraction, or how much of the blood is ejected as a percentage of the total volume of the ventricle, which is normally between 55% and 70% at rest in a healthy heart. The amount of blood that makes it out of the ventricle is known as the stroke volume and ranges from 60 mL to 100 mL. Finally, when the stroke volume is multiplied by the number of times the heart beats in 1 minute, or the heart rate, the resulting product is cardiac output. Cardiac output is measured in liters per minute and is typically between 5 and 6 LPM.

11. The **aortic semilunar valve** is the final way station in the cardiac cycle. It is positioned between the left ventricle and the aorta and systemic circulation beyond. The left ventricle must pump against a back pressure, called the afterload, which is caused by the collective pressures in the systemic arteries. Overcoming the afterload, the blood go on to deliver its O_2 to whatever organ lies at the end of its journey, only to return to the place it all started again—the vena cava.

Blood Vessels

Blood vessels have basically the same structure, whether in an artery or a vein. Three distinct layers of tissue in the walls of the blood vessel surround the lumen: the tunica adventitia, the tunica media, and the tunica intima. The **tunica intima** is the innermost layer and provides a smooth surface for blood to slide against. The **tunica media** is the middle layer, which is thickest in arteries and is composed of smooth muscle. The tunica media is responsible for the dilation and constriction of arteries and veins. The **tunica adventitia** is the outermost layer and is composed of a fibrous connective tissue that holds the vessels together against the high pulsing pressures.

Pro-Tip

To remember the layers, the tunica intima is intimate with blood and the tunica media is the medium layer. Therefore, the tunica adventitia is the outside layer.

The arteries are the most sensitive to nervous system signals because they have the most smooth muscle. Therefore, they are instrumental in regulating blood pressure. Blood pressure is based on the total systemic vascular resistance and the cardiac output. The veins are thinner because much of the pressure produced by the pulse is dissipated in the capillary bed. Some of the fluid that was present on the arteriole side of the capillary got squeezed out and will return to the heart as lymph.

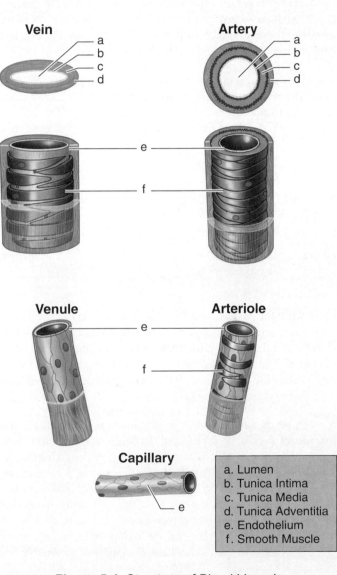

Figure 5-4. Structure of Blood Vessels

ELECTRICAL CONDUCTION SYSTEM

The heart is special in that it is the only organ to completely generate its own electrical impulse, conduct it through the entire muscle, and operate entirely free innervation. Four properties contribute to this unique ability of the heart.

- The myocytes possess **automaticity**, which is the ability for any cell in the heart to initiate an electrical impulse.
- **Excitability** refers to a cell's responsiveness to that electrical impulse simply by being in contact with the cell next to it; this does not happen in skeletal or smooth muscle.
- **Conductivity** is the ability of each cell to pass along the electrical impulse.
- **Contractility** is common to all muscle types in the body.

The SA node is the pacemaker of the heart and is an area in the right atrium that normally sets the rate of the heart. However, any area that sets the heart rate is called the pacemaker site. For now, the focus will be on the normal electrical pathways of the heart and what passage of the electrical impulse through these pathways means for both the mechanical action of the heart and the appearance on the electrocardiogram (ECG). To fully understand all of this, a discussion on cellular polarity, depolarization, and repolarization is needed.

When muscle cells are relaxed, an electrical potential is established across the muscle cell membrane. Muscles actively pump out positively charged sodium ions into the intercellular space, which leaves the inside of the cell negatively charged relative to the outside. This establishes an electric gradient across the cell membrane of approximately −90 millivolts (mV), indicating that the inside of the cell is negatively charged. Once this is established, the cell is said to be polarized.

Pro-Tip

Potential here means "difference in electrical charge," which also is known as voltage. It does not mean "possible"—although without electrical potential, muscle contractions would not be possible.

When the cell receives the signal from the nervous system, or in this case the electrical conduction system of the heart, this polarized muscle cell depolarizes. When this happens, the permeability of the muscle cell membrane changes, and Na^+ ions rush into the cell along with some calcium ions, effectively reducing the electrical gradient to 0 mV. In muscle cells, a depolarized cell is contracted. Therefore, when it is said that, for example, "the ventricles are depolarized" or "a part of the ECG refers to the depolarization of the ventricles," this means that the ventricles are contracted or contracting at that time.

Once a cell has depolarized, it cannot do anything more until it has repolarized. Repolarization can begin only when the stimulus to the cell to contract or depolarize is removed. To begin repolarization chemically, the sodium and calcium channels that allowed those ions into the cell during depolarization close, shutting off the flow of these ions into the cell. Meanwhile, the potassium channels simultaneously open, allowing potassium to flow out of the cell, which allows for a rapid reestablishment of the electrical gradient needed for depolarization to occur. However, potassium is not the correct ion that is needed on the outside of the cell. Next, the potassium channels close, and specialized pumps aptly named the sodium-potassium pump in the cellular membrane work to move 3 Na^+ ions out of the cell and 2 K^+ ions back into the cell. At the end of this process, Na^+ ions are back outside the cell, and K^+ ions are now back inside the cell where they belong, and the polarity of the cell has been reestablished at −90 mV. The cell is now ready to depolarize once again.

One point already mentioned is worth repeating: While the cell is depolarized, it cannot respond to further electrical stimulus. This condition is referred to as the refractory period. In the heart, there is an absolute refractory period and a relative refractory period. During the **absolute refractory period**, no amount of external stimulus will cause another contraction. During the **relative refractory period**, cells that have fully repolarized can and will depolarize if the stimulus is strong enough, whereas the others that have not yet completed repolarization will remain unaffected. Stimulus during the relative refractory period can cause electrical rhythm disturbances that could prove to be lethal, such as ventricular fibrillation.

With the chemical basis of depolarization and repolarization in mind, along with what these processes mean for the heart mechanically, we now turn to how all of these apply to the creation of a normal ECG. When the SA node discharges, the electrical impulse travels down the internodal pathways and pauses briefly at the atrioventricular (AV) node near the AV junction. As the impulse travels through the internodal pathways, the atria are caused to depolarize and contract. On the ECG, this event is represented as the 1st upward deflection or the P wave.

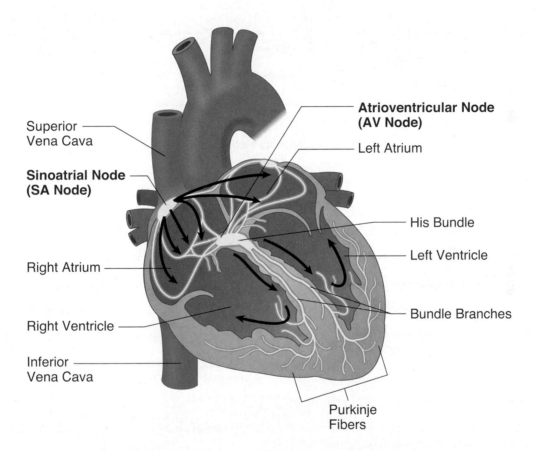

Figure 5-5. Cardiac Conduction System

The AV node then "collects" the charge transmitted through the internodal pathways and delays transmitting it for approximately 0.12 seconds, which gives the atria time to empty into the ventricles. This pause is represented on the ECG as the PR interval (PRI). When the AV node discharges, the electrical charge travels through the bundle of His. The bundle subsequently divides into the right and left bundle branches, which travel down the septum and divide further into the Purkinje fibers. The Purkinje fibers divide countless times, and each branch will ultimately innervate only a single cardiac muscle cell. This system is efficient enough to deliver the charge to every cell in the ventricles in about 0.08 seconds, allowing the large ventricles to depolarize and contract simultaneously and uniformly. This event is represented on the ECG as an upright spike called the QRS complex. The final notable part of the ECG is a hump immediately after the QRS complex, which is the repolarization of the ventricles and is referred to as the T wave.

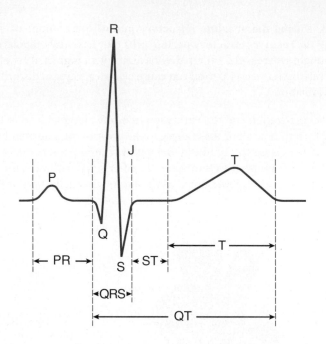

Figure 5-6. Normal Pattern of ECG

P wave: atrial depolarization

QRS complex: ventricular depolarization (40–100 msec)

R wave: first upward deflection after the P wave

S wave: first downward deflection after an R wave

T wave: ventricular repolarization

PR interval: start of the P wave to start of the QRS complex (120–200 msec); mostly due to conduction delay in the AV node

QT interval: start of the QRS complex to the end of the T wave; represents duration of the action potential (see Figure 5-6)

ST segment: ventricles are depolarized during this segment; roughly corresponds to the plateau phase of the action potential

J point: end of the S wave; represents isoelectric point

Note: Height of waves is directly related to (a) mass of tissue, (b) rate of change in potential, and (c) orientation of the lead to the direction of current flow.

The SA node, as the pacemaker of the heart, has an intrinsic rhythm of approximately 60–100 beats per minute. This means that, under normal circumstances, at rest, the SA node will discharge 60–100 times per minute, sending its electrical charge through the normal pathway and generating what is known as a normal sinus rhythm (NSR). If the SA node fails, the rest of the heart serves as a fail-safe pacemaker, capable of taking over and maintaining the heartbeat, though usually at a slower rate. The AV node is the first fail-safe and will take over the pacemaker activities if needed at a rate of 40–60 beats per minute. In the event that both the SA and AV nodes fail, the ventricles and the Purkinje fibers will take over at their intrinsic rate of 20–40 beats per minute. This rhythm can be generated from anywhere within the ventricles and often is referred to as a ventricular escape rhythm because, by its mere presence, a person escapes death.

Nervous System Control of Heart

The heart is under complete control of the autonomic nervous system, meaning that its activities are completely regulated outside of conscious direction. The autonomic nervous system has 2 branches that are always working in opposition to each other.

- The **parasympathetic nervous system** exerts its control on the heart through the vagus nerve. It has a slowing effect on the heart and has as its neurotransmitter acetylcholine, which acts directly on the SA node. Parasympathetic stimulation unopposed by sympathetic nervous input may result in profound bradycardia.
- The **sympathetic nervous system** is responsible for speeding up the heart and increasing its contractility, conduction, and thus the cardiac output.

Cardiac Monitoring

One of the most common procedures a paramedic will perform is placing a patient on the cardiac monitor. This is done alike for patients with and without a cardiac condition. Although it is rather simple to accomplish, accuracy is important to be able to get the best views of the heart that cardiac monitoring can afford, especially in cases of heart attack. Cardiac monitoring will allow you to observe the electrical activity of the heart from a variety of different views and allow you to determine the rhythm that the patient's heart is displaying. It also can allow you to figure out not only if but also where a patient is having a heart attack or other ischemic problem. This section explains everything about cardiac monitoring, including how to apply it to your patient and what the paper can tell you about your patient's rhythm. The section concludes by delving even deeper into the normal ECG, expounding on what has been learned already.

Every patient who requires advanced care beyond the scope of the EMT–Basic will need to be placed on a cardiac monitor for continuous monitoring. This is accomplished through any of the three standard limb leads—lead I, lead II, and lead III—but most commonly lead II. Capturing the limb leads requires the placement of four electrodes on the patient, one on each limb, hence the name. The leads are color coded regardless of the manufacturer and can be placed on the patient in any order; however, they need to be placed in the following specific locations:

- The white lead is placed on the right arm or shoulder.
- The black lead is placed on the left arm or shoulder.
- The red lead is placed on the left hip or anywhere on the lateral surface of the left leg.
- The green lead is placed on the right hip or anywhere on the lateral surface of the right leg.

The leads are placed in these locations to establish Einthoven's triangle. Similar to a battery that has positive and negative ends, or poles, each of the standard limb leads has one of the electrodes designated either positive or negative, which means that leads I, II, and III are the bipolar leads. The green lead is always the ground lead, which means that it helps minimize artifact generated from skeletal muscle activity or patient motion of any kind.

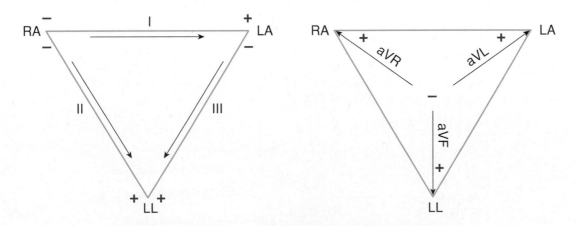

Figure 5-7. Einthoven's Triangle and Limb Lead Polarity
Leads I, II, III (left) and augmented voltage leads (right).

Using just these 3 electrodes, the cardiac monitor is able to generate 3 alternate views of the heart, called the augmented voltage leads. These leads are unipolar leads in that only one of the electrodes on the patient has a true polarity. The second pole is an average of the remaining electrodes. The augmented voltage leads are designated by the letters *aV* followed by the first letter of the electrode that is the positive pole. For example, the lead that has as its positive pole the red lead, near the left foot, is designated as lead aVF; the lead that has as its positive pole the white lead, near the right arm, is designated as lead aVR; finally, the lead that has as its positive pole the black electrode, near the left arm, is designated lead aVL.

Table 5-1. Polarity of Electrodes

Lead	+ Pole	– Pole
I	Black	White
II	Red	White
III	Red	Black
aVL	Black	Average of white and red
aVF	Red	Average of black and white
aVR	White	Average of red and black

The precordial leads are six electrodes that are placed on the anterior and lateral left chest, basically circling around the heart. These 6 leads, combined with the six limb leads, comprise the 12-lead ECG, which is the gold standard in cardiology for determining cardiac events. These leads also are referred to as the V leads because they are all designated with a capital V followed by a subscript number, V_1 to V_6. The precordial leads are all unipolar leads that are positive at the point of electrode placement, and the negative terminal is at a calculated point of reference, which is called Wilson's central terminal. The location and order of placement of these electrodes are specific:

- V_1: 4th intercostal space, immediately to the right of the sternum
- V_2: 4th intercostal space, immediately to the left of the sternum
- V_4: 5th intercostal space, midclavicular line
- V_3: halfway between V_2 and V_4
- V_5: 5th intercostal space, left anterior axillary line
- V_6: 5th intercostal space, left midaxillary line

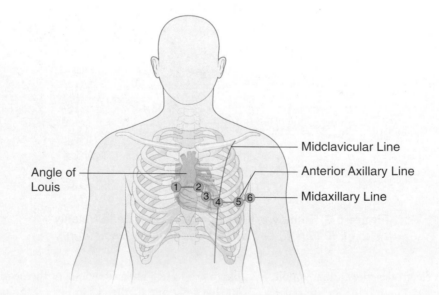

Figure 5-8. Precordial Lead Placement

All of the electrodes pick up small electrical currents traveling through the body, and the monitor converts these signals to the image on the screen and the rhythm strip on the paper. The flat part of the ECG tracing is known as the isoelectric line, and every electrical activity of the heart, whether depolarization or repolarization, can be seen as a deflection from the isoelectric baseline. If the overall direction of the electrical impulse is toward the positive electrode, it will be seen as a positive deflection above the isoelectric line. If the overall direction of the electrical impulse is away from the positive electrode, it will be seen as a negative deflection below the isoelectric line. When the overall electrical impulse is traveling perpendicular to the lead, there may be no discernible deflection at all in that lead, whereas it can be found in others. Finally, there could be a portion of time where the impulse is traveling toward the positive electrode followed immediately by a period of time where it is traveling away or vice versa. In this instance, the deflection is described as biphasic where part of it is above the baseline and another part is below the baseline.

ECG Paper and Appropriate Interval Lengths

ECG paper is designed to help you determine the rate and regularity of the heart's rhythm. The paper moves at 25 mm per second under normal use, which means that horizontally, the paper represents time. The deflections generated by the heart's electrical activity are vertical, which represent voltage, specifically millivolts. Each small box is 1 mm square. Two large boxes represent 1 mV; although this value is adjustable, it defaults to the 1 mV value. The small and large boxes are each necessary in discerning the time component to the ECG. Each large box has 5 small boxes. Each large box represents 0.20 second; therefore, each small box is 0.04 second. It takes 5 large boxes to make up 1 second, and 15 large boxes to make up 3 seconds. At the top of the paper, hash marks represent 3-second intervals, which can help you count the heart rate. Each component to the ECG discussed previously will print out against this paper and, therefore, have normal interval ranges of which the paramedic needs to be aware in determining the rhythm.

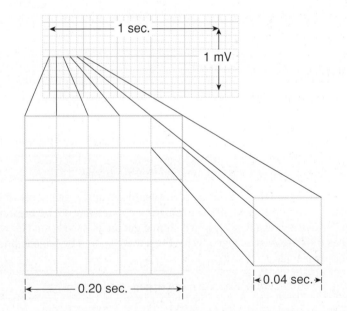

Figure 5-9. ECG Paper and Normal ECG

Table 5-2. ECG Waves and Intervals

P Wave	
Event	Depolarization and contraction of the atria
Shape	Upright, smooth curve
Duration	<0.12 second, or 3 small boxes
Amplitude	<2.5 mm
PRI	
Event	Depolarization of the atria and the delay in the AV node
Duration	0.12–0.20 second; 3–5 small boxes or <1 large box
QRS Complex **Q Wave**	
Event	If present in an otherwise healthy person, it represents the normal left-to-right depolarization of the ventricular septum. Q waves often are more indicative of an old, fully evolved infarction and are then referred to as pathologic Q waves.
Shape	First negative deflection after the P wave; generally pointed
Duration	<0.04 second, or 1 small box
Amplitude	<1/3 the overall height of the succeeding R wave; pathologic Q waves tend to be deeper.
R Wave	
Event	Depolarization and contraction of the ventricles
Shape	First positive deflection after the P wave; generally pointed
Duration	Because the R wave makes up the bulk of the complex, the R wave and, by extension, the entire complex should not be >0.12 second or 3 small boxes.
Amplitude	Could be in excess of 2 large boxes; much more than this could indicate other problems.
S Wave	
Event	Represents the final depolarization of the ventricles and is seen only when the electrical impulse is traveling away from the positive electrode. May not be present in the limb leads. A large S wave is present in V_1, which should get progressively smaller with each successive V lead as the R wave gets larger. By V_6, the R wave should be largest, and almost no S wave should be present.
Shape	First negative deflection after the R wave; generally pointed
Duration	Generally <0.04 second, or 1 small box
Amplitude	Lead dependent; could be in excess of 2 large boxes, although most often it is <1 big box.
J Point	
Event	Point where the QRS complex ends and the ST segment begins; elevation or depression of this point relative to the baseline indicates infarction or ischemia, respectively.

ST Segment	
Event	Begins at the J point and ends with the upslope of the ensuing T wave. This represents a delay between ventricular depolarization and repolarization.
Duration	Typically 0.08–0.12 second, or 2–3 small boxes
T Wave	
Event	Represents ventricular repolarization. From the start of the T wave to its peak represents the absolute refractory period. From the peak to the completion of the T wave represents the relative refractory period.
Shape	Typically upright (positive deflection) and a smooth curve; inverted or negatively deflected T waves also indicate ischemia.
Duration	Typically <0.25 second
Amplitude	Approximately 5 mm; taller, peaked, and more pointed T waves could indicate hyperkalemia.
QT Interval	
Event	Represents a full cycle of ventricular electrical activity; it is measured from the start of the QRS complex to the return to baseline of the T wave.
Duration	Should not be >0.44 second

There are a few ways of calculating heart rate using the rhythm strip:

- **6-Second Strip.** For this method, simply count the number of QRS complexes that appear between the first and third of three sequential hash marks on the top of the strip. Remember, the elapsed time between each hash mark is 3 seconds. Then multiply the number of QRS complexes in that range by 10. This is the only method of the methods presented here that should be used for irregular rhythms.

- **Sequence Method.** This method is a quick way of estimating the rate of a regular rhythm. It is not particularly helpful for irregular rhythms. Find a QRS complex that is on a heavy line—one of the lines that outlines the large boxes. Then recite the following numbers on each successive heavy line until the next QRS complex is reached: 300, 150, 100, 75, 60, 50. Chunking the numbers together in the following way is helpful to remember this because it becomes almost rhythmic, so say to yourself, "300, 150, 100, . . . 75, 60, 50." If the QRS complex falls between two heavy lines, estimate the value, but remember that the lighter lines represent logarithmic values. For example, the light lines between 100 and 75 are not 95, 90, 85, and 80 but really 94, 88, 83 and 79. It is not necessary, nor is it realistically possible, to memorize every light line.

- **1500 Method.** This method is highly accurate; however, it should be used only for regular rhythms, particularly those with rates in excess of 150 beats per minute. Start by counting the number of small boxes between two sequential QRS complexes; this is known as the R-R interval. Then divide that number into 1500. For example, a certain regular rhythm has 8 small boxes between QRS complexes. Doing the math, 1500/8 gives a heart rate of about 187 beats per minute.

DYSRHYTHMIAS

This section addresses the likely rhythms that a patient may generate. Each rhythm is described in the same manner, which will coincide with the process described later of how to differentiate between each rhythm. A picture of each rhythm strip is included to illustrate its typical appearance. The treatment plan for a patient exhibiting the rhythm, whose chief complaint can be attributed to being in that rhythm, then follows.

Sinus and Atrial Rhythms

Sinus and atrial rhythms are generated either within the SA node or from the automaticity of the atrial muscle tissue.

Table 5-3. Sinus Bradycardia

Origination Point: SA Node		Differential Causes
P Wave		• Athletes (not clinically significant)
Shape	Upright	• Increased vagal tone
P rate	<60	• Myocardial infarction (MI)
P wave for every QRS?	Yes	• Increased ICP
QRS complex for every P wave?	Yes	• Hypothermia
PRI		• Beta-blocker and calcium channel blocker overdose
Duration	<0.20 second	• Hypoxemia
QRS Complex		• Sick sinus syndrome
Shape	Normal	• Electrolyte imbalances
Duration	0.08–0.12 second	• Hypothyroidism
R-R Interval		• Idiopathic
Regularity	Regular	
Rate	Normal (60–100 per minute)	

Treatment Options. The treatment for sinus bradycardia is largely dependent on the hemodynamic stability of the patient and the root cause for the bradycardia. If the patient is stable and has not displayed any change in mentation while in this rhythm, aggressive treatment likely is not indicated.

1. For situations thought to be related to increased vagal tone or parasympathetic stimulation, 0.5–1 mg atropine is the first-line treatment of choice. If this fails and the patient remains symptomatic, transcutaneous pacing (TCP) should be considered and initiated. The TCP procedure is discussed later in this chapter.

2. In cases of acute myocardial infarction (AMI), increasing the rate may have a negative effect on the condition of the patient because of the concurrent increase in myocardial O_2 demand. In this case, increasing blood pressure without appreciably increasing the workload of the heart is desirable. This can be accomplished with fluid.

3. For presumed hypoxemia, administer O_2. This is particularly important for pediatric patients.

4. An overdose of any of a variety of drugs can cause symptomatic bradycardia. An effort should be made to determine the drug and administer its antidote; in cases of opiate or calcium channel blocker overdose, administer naloxone or calcium, respectively. If unable to determine the specific drug, treat the patient symptomatically and support the ABCs.

Table 5-4. Sinus Tachycardia

Origination Point: SA Node		Differential Causes
P Wave		• Exercise (not clinically significant)
Shape	Upright	• Fever/hyperthermia
P rate	>100	• Hypoxia (early)
P wave for every QRS?	Yes	• Hypotension/dehydration
QRS complex for every P wave?	Yes	• MI
PRI		• Beta-agonist, caffeine, and cocaine
Duration	<0.20 second	• CHF
QRS Complex		• Anxiety/stress
Shape	Normal	• Hyperthyroidism/thyroid storm
Duration	0.08–0.12 second	• Serotonin syndrome
R-R Interval		
Regularity	Regular	
Rate	>100	

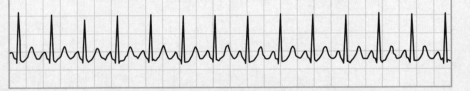

Treatment Options. In many cases, treatment for sinus tachycardia is based on the underlying cause if rhythm-specific treatment is needed. Because tachycardia is the body's natural response to shock, infection, and stress, among other issues, treatment specific to this rhythm often is limited to fluid bolus. If the patient is in this rhythm as a result of CHF, however, fluid would be inappropriate, and O_2 and nitrates would be the best options. See chapter 4 for more information on CHF.

Table 5-5. Sinus Arrhythmia

Origination Point: SA Node		Differential Causes
P Wave		• Normal finding if rate accelerates with inhalation and slows with exhalation.
Shape	Upright; same shape throughout	
P rate	Usually 60–100; could be faster or slower	• If not tied to respiratory rate, it could indicate ischemia of the heart.
P wave for every QRS?	Yes	
QRS complex for every P wave?	Yes	
PRI		
Duration	<0.20 second	
QRS Complex		
Shape	Normal	
Duration	0.08–0.12 second	
R-R Interval		
Regularity	Regularly irregular; could be irregularly irregular	
Rate	Usually 60–100; could be faster or slower	

Treatment Options. The treatment for sinus arrhythmia is limited and should focus on the factors surrounding it. Remember, this is a normal finding in the pediatric population.

Table 5-6. Sinus Arrest and Sick Sinus Syndrome

Origination Point: SA Node		Differential Causes
P Wave		**Sinus Arrest**
Shape	Upright	• Ischemia of SA node
P rate	Usually 60–100; could be faster or slower	• Increased vagal tone
P wave for every QRS?	Yes	• Digitalis use
QRS complex for every P wave?	Yes	• Quinidine use
PRI		• Idiopathic; only significant if it causes hemodynamic instability
Duration	<0.20 second	**Sick Sinus Syndrome**
QRS Complex		• Simply a poorly functioning SA node
Shape	Normal	• May present as alternating bradycardia and tachycardia
Duration	0.08–0.12 second	
R-R Interval		
Regularity	Regular, except during unpredictable arrest where an entire P-QRS-T cycle is dropped.	
Rate	Usually 60–100; could be faster or slower	

Treatment Options. Occasional dropped beats are typically not an issue. If they happen frequently enough, essentially resulting in a marked bradycardia, initiate treatment similar to that for sinus bradycardia.

Table 5-7. Wandering Atrial Pacemaker

Origination Point: SA Node and Atrial Muscle, >3 Foci		Differential Causes
P Wave		• Respiratory failure
Shape	May be upright or inverted; notched, biphasic, or have two humps depending on foci	• COPD
P rate	Usually 60–100; could be faster or slower	• Electrolyte imbalances
P wave for every QRS?	Yes	• Nicotine and caffeine
QRS complex for every P wave?	Yes	• Alcohol
PRI		• Enlarged atria
Duration	Varied but always <0.20 second	• Treated symptomatically
QRS Complex		
Shape	Normal	
Duration	0.08–0.12 second	
R-R Interval		
Regularity	Very slightly irregular	
Rate	Rate dependent upon conduction ratio; rate for 2:1 conduction is 150; rate for 3:1 conduction is 100; rate for 4:1 conduction is 75	

Treatment Options. Treatment usually is not necessary for the wandering atrial pacemaker. However, the treatment of respiratory problems associated with this rhythm, such as respiratory failure and COPD, often relieves this rhythm.

Table 5-8. Multifocal Atrial Tachycardia

Origination Point: Atrial Muscle, Multiple Foci		Differential Causes
P Wave		• Respiratory failure
Shape	May be upright or inverted; notched, biphasic, or have two humps depending on foci	• COPD
		• Digoxin toxicity
P Rate	100–150; could reach 250	• Hypomagnesemia
P wave for every QRS?	Yes	• Hypokalemia
QRS complex for every P wave?	Yes	• Nicotine, alcohol, and caffeine
PRI		
Duration	Varied but always <0.20 second	
QRS Complex		
Shape	Normal	
Duration	0.08–0.12 second	
R-R Interval		
Regularity	Irregularly irregular	
Rate	100–150; could reach 250	

Treatment Options. Treatment is primarily related to the underlying cause. Because it is most commonly associated with COPD and hypoxia, appropriate treatment of the breathing issues is important. Also, if hypomagnesemia is the suspected cause, give 2–4 g magnesium sulfate.

Table 5-9. Atrial Flutter

Origination Point: Atrial Muscle, Single Focus		Differential Causes
P Wave		• MI
Shape	Absent; F waves present; sawtooth baseline	• Atherosclerosis
P rate	200–400 or higher; rate of 300 most common	• Digoxin
P wave for every QRS?	No	• Rheumatic heart disease
QRS complex for every P wave?	Most commonly 2 F waves for every QRS complex (2:1 conduction); 3:1 and 4:1 possible as well	• Alcoholism
PRI		• Thyrotoxicosis (hyperthyroidism)
Duration	Not applicable	• Pulmonary embolus
QRS Complex		• Pneumonia
Shape	Normal	• Pericarditis—infection of the pericardium
Duration	0.08–0.12 second	
R-R Interval		
Regularity	Regular	
Rate	Specific rates based on conduction ratio of F wave to QRS complex: 1:1 Conduction = 300 bpm 2:1 Conduction = 150 bpm 3:1 Conduction = 100 bpm 4:1 Conduction = 75 bpm	

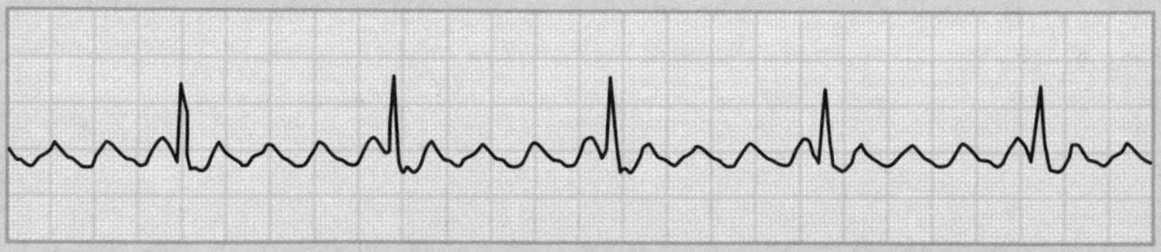

Treatment Options. Not commonly treated in the field, unless the patient is showing signs of altered mental status related to hypotension most likely caused by the rate. The rate pictured here would not warrant emergency treatment interventions; however, if the ratio was 2:1 (instead of the 4:1 pictured here), the ventricular rate would be 150 or higher. Treatment in that case would include electrical cardioversion or medications including diltiazem.

Table 5-10. Atrial Fibrillation

Origination Point: Atrial Muscle, Countless Foci		Differential Causes
P Wave		• Age
Shape	Absent; course to fine fibrillating baseline	• Idiopathic
P rate	Not applicable	• Left atrial enlargement
P wave for every QRS?	Not applicable	**MAD RAT PPP**
QRS complex for every P wave?	Not applicable	• MI
PRI		• Atherosclerosis
Duration	Not applicable	• Digoxin
QRS Complex		• Rheumatic heart disease
Shape	Normal	• Alcoholism
Duration	0.08–0.12 second	• Thyrotoxicosis (hyperthyroidism)
R-R Interval		• Pulmonary embolus
Regularity	Irregularly irregular	• Pneumonia
Rate	Varies anywhere from <60 to >150; hemodynamic stability based mostly on rate	• Pericarditis

Treatment Options. People live their daily lives with their heart in an atrial fibrillation rhythm, so treatment of this rhythm is strongly dependent on its underlying ventricular rate. Atrial fibrillation with a rapid ventricular response, (pulse >150) is associated with decreased blood pressure and altered mental status. This needs to be aggressively treated with fluid first, followed by 0.25 mg/kg diltiazem if the rate remains high after fluid and the patient is still showing signs of hemodynamic instability. Amiodarone is also an option. It is given as a secondary medication to diltiazem at a dose of 150 mg slow over ten minutes. Amiodarone is preferred in AF with RVR in patients with CHF.

Table 5-11. Supraventricular Tachycardia

Origination Point: AV Nodal Reentry Cycle		Differential Causes
P Wave		• Idiopathic
Shape	Not visible; if present, typically buried in T wave of preceding cycle	• Caffeine
P rate	Unable to be discerned	• Nicotine
P wave for every QRS?	Unable to be discerned	• Cocaine
QRS complex for every P wave?	Unable to be discerned	
PRI		
Duration	None	
QRS Complex		
Shape	Normal	
Duration	0.08–0.12 second	
R-R Interval		
Regularity	Regular	
Rate	>150	

Treatment Options. Supraventricular tachycardia (SVT) is a rhythm that is too fast to be able to generate adequate cardiac output for a long period of time. Patients may present initially stable and deteriorate the longer they are in the rhythm. For stable SVT, treatment includes a regimen of 6 mg adenosine followed by a rapid saline flush of at least 10 mL. If that is unsuccessful at converting the rhythm to a sinus rhythm, the dose may be repeated with double the initial dose, 12 mg adenosine, an additional 2 times. If that is unsuccessful, diltiazem can be considered.

Unstable SVT, designated as SVT associated with a change in mentation, chest pain, syncope, or other symptoms related to hemodynamic instability, is treated more aggressively than stable SVT. Unstable SVT is treated with synchronized electrical cardioversion—described later in this chapter—at 100 J initially, with sequential doses of 150 J, 200 J, 300 J, and 360 J if the initial cardioversion is unsuccessful.

Junctional Rhythms and AV Blocks

When the SA node and subsequently the atria fail to maintain the pacemaking duties for the heart, the junction, or the AV node, will take over. These are referred to as junctional rhythms. These 3 rhythms are closely related, varying only in rate. In distinguishing these rhythms apart from each other, pay particular attention to the rate.

AV blocks vary by how well the atria successfully communicate with the AV node and therefore the ventricles. A delay in communication could present as a lengthened PR-interval, greater than 1:1 ration of P waves to QRS complexes, or absolutely no coordination between P waves and QRS complexes.

For example, in first-degree block, there is still a 1:1 ratio of P:QRS, but the PRI is lengthened. In a second-degree Mobitz type I block, the PRI lengthens until one entire QRS complex is omitted; then the process begins anew. In a Mobitz type II block, there is a regular ratio of P:QRS, but it is not 1:1. It can be 2:1, 3:1, or even 3:2; it is similar to banging on a door multiple times until it opens. Finally, in third-degree heart block, there is no communication whatsoever between the SA node and the ventricles, and, therefore, no relationship of P waves to QRS complexes; they each just do their own thing at their own rate.

Table 5-12. Junctional Rhythm

Origination Point: AV Node		Differential Causes
P Wave		• Increased parasympathetic tone
Shape	Typically absent (buried within the QRS); possibly inverted before or after QRS complex	• Digoxin, beta-blocker, or calcium channel overdose
P rate	Unable to be discerned	• Myocardial ischemia or MI
P wave for every QRS?	Unable to be discerned	• Sick sinus syndrome
QRS complex for every P wave?	Unable to be discerned	• Electrolyte imbalances
PRI		• Increasing ICP
Duration	Not applicable	• Idiopathic
QRS Complex		
Shape	Normal, possibly wide	
Duration	0.08–0.12 second	
R-R Interval		
Regularity	Regular	
Rate	40–60, junction's intrinsic rate	

Treatment Options. Treatment is limited to treating the underlying cause and symptoms. The junctional rhythm, with its rate of 40–60, may require treatment for bradycardia. In that case, 0.5–1 mg atropine should be given initially, followed by TCP if the rate and blood pressure do not improve. Administration of 1 g calcium chloride is recommended if calcium channel blocker toxicity or overdose is suspected.

Table 5-13. Accelerated Junctional Rhythm

Origination Point: AV Node		Differential Causes
P Wave		• Increased parasympathetic tone
Shape	Typically absent (buried within the QRS); possibly inverted before or after QRS complex	• Digoxin, beta-blocker, or calcium channel overdose
P rate	Unable to be discerned	• Myocardial ischemia or MI
P wave for every QRS?	Unable to be discerned	• Sick sinus syndrome
QRS complex for every P wave?	Unable to be discerned	• Electrolyte imbalances
PRI		• Idiopathic
Duration	Not applicable	• Recent heart surgery
QRS Complex		
Shape	Normal, possibly wide	
Duration	0.08–0.12 second	
R-R Interval		
Regularity	Regular	
Rate	60–100; faster than the junction's intrinsic rate but <100	

Treatment Options. Treatment is limited to treating the underlying cause and symptoms. Only in the basic junctional rhythm, with its rate of 40–60, would treatment for bradycardia likely be necessary. An accelerated junctional rhythm is likely fast enough to be able to maintain viable cardiac output; therefore, focusing on the rhythm is unnecessary. Fluid for hypotension and 1 g calcium chloride for suspected calcium channel blocker toxicity or overdose are recommended treatments.

Table 5-14. Junctional Tachycardia

Origination Point: AV Node		Differential Causes
P Wave		• Increased parasympathetic tone
Shape	Typically absent (buried within the QRS); possibly inverted before or after QRS complex	• Digoxin, beta-blocker, or calcium channel overdose
P rate	Unable to be discerned	• Myocardial ischemia or MI
P wave for every QRS?	Unable to be discerned	• Sick sinus syndrome
QRS complex for every P wave?	Unable to be discerned	• Electrolyte imbalances
PRI		• Idiopathic
Duration	Not applicable	• Recent heart surgery
QRS Complex		
Shape	Normal, possibly wide	
Duration	0.08–0.12 second	
R-R Interval		
Regularity	Regular	
Rate	>100	

Treatment Options. Junctional tachycardia is likely fast enough to be able to maintain viable cardiac output; therefore, focusing on the rhythm is unnecessary. A fluid bolus of 500–1,000 mL may correct hypotension. Calcium is again recommended.

Table 5-15. First-Degree AV Block

Origination Point: SA Node, AV Nodal Delay		Differential Causes
P Wave		• Idiopathic
Shape	Upright, normal	• Myocardial ischemia or MI
P rate	SA nodal rate	• Calcium channel blocker or beta-blocker overdose
P wave for every QRS?	Yes	• Increased vagal tone
QRS complex for every P wave?	Yes	• Surgery or trauma to the heart
PRI		• Myocarditis
Duration	Prolonged, >0.20 second	• Infections
QRS Complex		• Congenital heart diseases
Shape	Normal	
Duration	0.08–0.12 second	
R-R Interval		
Regularity	Regular	
Rate	>150	

Treatment Options. First-degree AV block is rarely treated in the prehospital environment, unless it is associated with severe bradycardia.

Table 5-16. Second-Degree AV Block, Mobitz Type I, Wenckebach

Origination Point: SA Node, AV Conduction Delay		Differential Causes
P Wave		• Idiopathic
Shape	Upright, normal	• Myocardial ischemia or MI
P rate	SA nodal rate	• Calcium channel blocker or beta-blocker overdose
P wave for every QRS?	Yes	• Increased vagal tone
QRS complex for every P wave?	No	• Surgery or trauma to the heart
PRI		• Myocarditis
Duration	Increasing in sequential cycles until 1 QRS complex is dropped	• Infections
QRS Complex		• Congenital heart diseases
Shape	Normal with 1 missing	
Duration	0.08–0.12 second	
R-R Interval		
Regularity	Regularly irregular	
Rate	60–100	

Treatment Options. Treatment for second-degree AV block, Mobitz type I (Wenckebach), is generally limited to treatment for the bradycardia, which can include atropine and TCP as with earlier bradycardic rhythms. Although this rhythm can result from an active evolving AMI, traditional treatments for AMI, such as morphine and NTG, may not be possible because those medications may be contraindicated in the presence of hypotension. If the patient possibly overdosed on beta-blockers, blood pressure support with pressors and fluid may be indicated in addition to TCP. For calcium channel blocker overdose, calcium also should be considered.

Table 5-17. Second-Degree AV Block, Mobitz Type II

Origination Point: SA Node, AV Conduction Delay		Differential Causes
P Wave		<ul><li>Idiopathic</li><li>Myocardial ischemia or MI</li><li>Calcium channel blocker or beta-blocker overdose</li><li>Increased vagal tone</li><li>Surgery or trauma to the heart</li><li>Myocarditis</li><li>Infections</li><li>Congenital heart diseases</li></ul>
Shape	Upright, normal	
P rate	SA nodal rate	
P wave for every QRS?	Yes	
QRS complex for every P wave?	No	
PRI		
Duration	The P waves that have the QRS complex immediately after it usually have a normal PRI (<0.20 second). The PRI is always constant.	
QRS Complex		
Shape	Normal	
Duration	0.08–0.12 second	
R-R Interval		
Regularity	Regularly irregular	
Rate	<100, dependent on conduction ratio	

Treatment Options. Treatment for second-degree AV block, Mobitz type II, is generally limited to treatment for the bradycardia, which can include atropine and TCP as with earlier bradycardic rhythms. Although this can result from an active evolving AMI, traditional treatments for an AMI, such as morphine and NTG, may not be possible because those medications may be contraindicated in the presence of hypotension. If the patient possibly overdosed on beta-blockers, blood pressure support with pressors and fluid may be indicated in addition to TCP. For calcium channel blocker overdose, calcium also should be considered.

Table 5-18. Third-Degree AV Block

Origination Point: SA Node and Ventricular Tissue, Separately		Differential Causes
P Wave		• Idiopathic
Shape	Upright, normal	• Myocardial ischemia or MI
P rate	60–100	• Calcium channel blocker or beta-blocker overdose
P wave for every QRS?	No	• Increased vagal tone
QRS complex for every P wave?	No	• Surgery or trauma to the heart
PRI		• Myocarditis
Duration	Not applicable	• Infections
QRS Complex		• Congenital heart disease
Shape	Wide, bizarre	
Duration	>0.12 second	
R-R Interval		
Regularity	Regular	
Rate	<60	

Treatment Options. Third-degree heart block, also known as AV dissociation, has no communication from the atria to the ventricles; it is typically treated in the field only if the resultant bradycardia is so severe that the patient is hypotensive and displaying signs of altered mental status. At that point, the best option is TCP because atropine will serve only to accelerate the P rate, leaving the ventricular R rate unchanged.

VENTRICULAR RHYTHMS
Ventricular rhythms are those that originate within the ventricles.

Table 5-19. Idioventricular Rhythm

Origination Point: Ventricular Muscle or Purkinje Fibers		Differential Causes
P Wave		• Idiopathic
Shape	None	• Myocardial ischemia or MI
P rate	Not applicable	• Failure of supraventricular pacemakers
P wave for every QRS?	Not applicable	• Cardiomyopathy
QRS complex for every P wave?	Not applicable	• Drug overdose
PRI		
Duration	None	
QRS Complex		
Shape	Wide, bizarre	
Duration	>0.12 second	
R-R Interval		
Regularity	Regular	
Rate	20–40, intrinsic ventricular rate	

Treatment Options. The idioventricular rhythm, also known as the ventricular escape rhythm, is the heart's last ditch effort to keep the rest of the body alive. Often caused by a massive AMI, mechanical function of the heart may or may not be present; therefore, this rhythm is frequently pulseless. Initiation of CPR as soon as possible is critical to the patient's chances of survival if there is a pulseless electrical activity (PEA). Identifying and treating any reversible causes (H's and T's) in a timely manner also is essential.

Table 5-20. Accelerated Idioventricular Rhythm

Origination Point: Ventricular Muscle or Purkinje Fibers		Differential Causes
P Wave		• Idiopathic
Shape	None	• Myocardial ischemia or MI
P rate	Not applicable	• Failure of supraventricular pacemakers
P wave for every QRS?	Not applicable	• Cardiomyopathy
QRS complex for every P wave?	Not applicable	• Drug overdose
PRI		
Duration	None	
QRS Complex		
Shape	Wide, bizarre	
Duration	>0.12 second	
R-R Interval		
Regularity	Regular	
Rate	40–100	

Treatment Options. The accelerated ventricular rhythm is the heart's last ditch effort to keep the rest of the body alive. Often caused by a massive AMI, mechanical function of the heart may or may not be present; therefore, this rhythm is frequently pulseless. Initiation of CPR as soon as possible is critical to the patient's chances of survival if there is PEA. Identifying and treating any reversible causes (H's and T's) in a timely manner also is essential.

Table 5-21. Ventricular Tachycardia

Origination Point: Ventricular Muscle or Purkinje Fibers		Differential Causes
P Wave		• Idiopathic
Shape	Not visible; if present, typically buried in T wave of preceding cycle or retrograde	• Myocardial ischemia or MI
P rate	Unable to be discerned	• Cocaine overdose
P wave for every QRS?	Unable to be discerned	• Electrolyte imbalances
QRS complex for every P wave?	Unable to be discerned	• R-on-T phenomenon (when a PVC lands on the relative refractory period of the T wave)
PRI		
Duration	None	
QRS Complex		
Shape	Wide, bizarre	
Duration	>0.12 second	
R-R Interval		
Regularity	Regular	
Rate	100–250	

Treatment Options. Ventricular tachycardia (VT) can present with or without pulses. It also can be stable or unstable when pulses are present. Let's look at each case individually.

- **Stable VT with Pulses.** In this case, the patient will have a rather benign chief complaint, such as feeling as if the heart is beating too fast, and perhaps mild chest pain or shortness of breath. The patient will be basically free of dizziness, mental status deficits, syncope, or any other signs of hemodynamic instability. Treating this patient's rhythm should begin with either 150 mg amiodarone given slowly over 10 minutes or 1.5 mg/kg lidocaine while monitoring the patient for changes.

- **Unstable VT with Pulses.** The rhythm is classified as unstable when there are observable or verbalized symptoms of hemodynamic compromise. As previously, these can include syncope, dizziness, altered mental status, or hypotension, among others. Inadequate ventricular filling time caused by the excessive rate is largely responsible for all the symptoms, thus making treatment of the rhythm an urgent priority. Treatment for this begins with electrical synchronized cardioversion at 100–150 J, followed by escalating doses of 200 J, 300 J, and 360 J until the rhythm converts to a more viable rhythm.

- **Pulseless VT.** This is a cardiac arrest situation and is treated as if it were ventricular fibrillation (VF). For this treatment, see the treatment options after the VF description.

Table 5-22. Ventricular Fibrillation

Origination Point: Multiple Foci in Ventricles		Differential Causes
P Wave		• Cardiac arrest
Shape	None	• MI
P rate	Not applicable	
P wave for every QRS?	Not applicable	
QRS complex for every P wave?	Not applicable	
PRI		
Duration	Not applicable	
QRS Complex		
Shape	None	
Duration	Not applicable	
R-R Interval		
Regularity	Not applicable	
Rate	Fibrillation waves	

Treatment Options. VF, along with pulseless VT, is the most treatable of pulseless lethal rhythms. Without prompt recognition and treatment, the patient will not survive either rhythm. Initiation of CPR and rapid delivery of electrical defibrillation provide the best chances of survival from this rhythm. After each defibrillation, CPR should be provided for 2 minutes, during which time, the patient should be administered 1 mg bolus of the 1:10,000 solution of epinephrine intravenously, alternating with either 300 mg amiodarone or 1.5 mg/kg lidocaine. Amiodarone may be repeated once after 10 minutes at half the original dose (150 mg), and lidocaine may be administered again after 5 minutes at half the original dose (0.75 mg/kg) to a maximum dose of 3 mg/kg. Epinephrine can be repeated every 3–5 minutes with no maximum dosage.

Table 5-23. Polymorphic Ventricular Tachycardia (Torsade de Pointes)

Origination Point: Ventricular Muscle or Purkinje Fibers		Differential Causes
P Wave		• Any drug that has a chance of prolonging the QT (quinidine, procainamide, TCA, and many others)
Shape	Not visible; if present, typically buried in T wave of preceding cycle or retrograde	• Hypokalemia
P rate	Unable to be discerned	• Hypomagnesemia
P wave for every QRS?	Unable to be discerned	• Hypocalcemia
QRS complex for every P wave?	Unable to be discerned	• Starvation/anorexia
PRI		• Alcoholism
Duration	None	• Cholinergic overdose
QRS Complex		
Shape	Wide, bizarre, and twisting about an axis	
Duration	>0.12 second, varying	
R-R Interval		
Regularity	Regular	
Rate	>150	

Treatment Options. Polymorphic VT (also known as torsade de pointes) is not treated with the same tools as monomorphic VT because it (a) is refractory to defibrillation and cardioversion, and (b) does not respond to amiodarone or lidocaine. First-line treatment is 1–2 g magnesium sulfate given intravenously, because hypomagnesemia is the most common cause. Any drug or drug combination that has a lengthening effect on the QT interval also can cause the patient to go into polymorphic VT.

Table 5-24. Asystole

Origination Point: No Electrical Activity at All		Differential Causes
P Wave		• Hypothermia
Shape	Absent	• Hypokalemia
P rate	Not applicable	• Hyperkalemia
P wave for every QRS?	Not applicable	• Hypoxia
QRS complex for every P wave?	Not applicable	• Hypovolemia
PRI		• Hypoglycemia
Duration	Not applicable	• Acidosis
QRS Complex		• Trauma
Shape	None	• Cardiac tamponade
Duration	Not applicable	• PE
R-R Interval		• MI
Regularity	None	• Tension pneumothorax
Rate	Not applicable	• Drug overdose or poisoning

Treatment Options. Few people survive asystole because it represents a complete lack of electrical activity in the heart. This should be confirmed in multiple leads (at least 2) to ensure that the electrical activity in the observed lead is not merely traveling exactly perpendicular to the lead or that an electrode did not fall off. Treatment is CPR, epinephrine 1:10,000 every 3–5 minutes, and assessment/treatment of the reversible causes listed earlier. If none of these efforts results in even a transient return of spontaneous circulation, termination of resuscitative efforts is recommended except in patients who are hypothermic and have not been rewarmed.

Artificial Pacing

In situations when medications can no longer increase the heart rate or maintain adequate blood pressure, a patient will receive an implanted artificial pacemaker, which is designed to send small electrical impulses to the heart to generate a beat. The pacemaker consists of a small case that houses the battery and generator of the electrical pulse and one or two wires that connect directly into the myocardium. The pulse generator is about the size of half a deck of cards and is generally housed in the soft tissue of the anterior left shoulder. Two common types are used:

- The **ventricular pacemaker** has a single wire leading from it to the heart and is attached somewhere in the ventricle, usually near the apex of the internal right ventricle. Ventricular pacing produces a rhythm similar to what is shown; however, the exact tracing will vary based on where in the ventricle it is attached. The vertical spike seen just before the wide and bizarre QRS complex is the small electrical current the pacemaker delivers to the myocardium. It is not always visible, and it is not visible in every lead. The spike will likely be upright, but it may be inverted or biphasic.

- The **AV sequential pacemaker** has 2 leads coming from it; in addition to the lead attached to the internal right ventricle like the ventricular pacer above, a second lead connected to the internal right atrium generates an atrial contraction as well. The leads fire sequentially, first the atrial lead followed a short time later by the ventricular lead. This may result in 2 pacer spikes visible on the ECG; the first just prior to what looks like a P wave, and a second following the P wave ahead of the wide QRS complex.

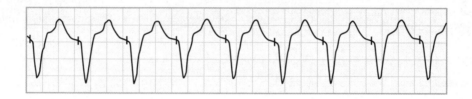

Figure 5-10. Ventricular Artificial Pacemaker Trace

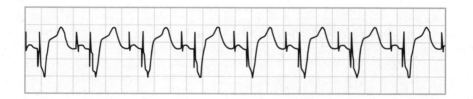

Figure 5-11. AV Sequential Artificial Pacemaker Trace

Ectopic Rhythm Disturbances

Occasionally, within an otherwise normal heart rhythm, a beat occurs earlier than it would have been predicted to happen. This premature beat comes from a place other than the baseline rhythm's pacemaker, and thus looks different from the other complexes in the strip.

- If the beat originates somewhere in the atria, it is called a **premature atrial contraction (PAC)**.
- If the beat comes from the junction, it is called a **premature junctional contraction (PJC)**.
- If the beat comes from somewhere within the ventricles, it is called a **premature ventricular contraction (PVC)**.

PAC and PJCs

PAC and PJC can be caused by various drugs (e.g., caffeine, nicotine, and cocaine), by ischemia, or by an underlying heart problem that has not shown itself in any other way. They are mostly of little cause for concern beyond documenting their presence, and seldom require treatment in the field.

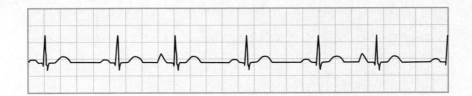

Figure 5-12. Premature Atrial Contraction

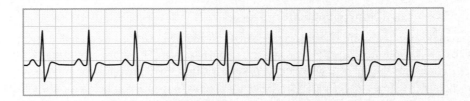

Figure 5-13. Premature Junctional Contraction

PVC

PVC is somewhat more complicated. It can be caused by the same conditions as PAC and PJC, but more often it is caused by ischemia within the ventricular tissue. This ischemia causes the tissue to become irritable and spontaneously depolarize, generating a beat within the entire heart that appears as a wide and bizarre complex among the baseline rhythm on ECG.

PVC may be unifocal, be multifocal, or occur in couplets or runs. Unifocal PVCs originate from a single location or focus in the ventricles and have the same morphology or shape on the ECG. Multifocal PVCs appear on an ECG as premature complexes that originate in the ventricles but have different shapes. The different shapes indicate that the complexes are coming from two or more locations within the ventricles. When two premature ventricular complexes occur back to back without an intrinsic, or baseline, beat between them, they are called couplets. Three or more premature ventricular complexes in a row constitute a run of VT and are the most ominous sign of all.

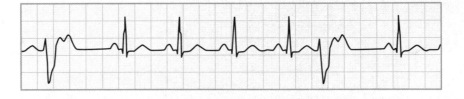

Figure 5-14. Unifocal Premature Ventricular Contractions

PVC also may become frequent enough that its presence creates recognizable patterns with the normal (intrinsic) beats. When PVC alternates with normal beats in a 1:1 ratio, the pattern is called **bigeminy**. If the PVC-to-normal beat ratio drops to 1:2, the rhythm is referred to as **trigeminy**.

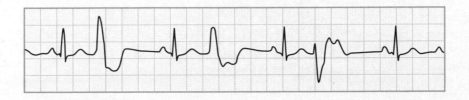

Figure 5-15. Multifocal PVCs in a Bigeminy Pattern

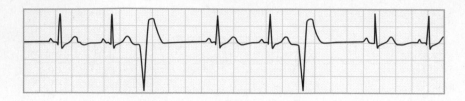

Figure 5-16. Unifocal PVCs in a Trigeminy Pattern

Compensatory Pauses and Noncompensatory Pauses

The ectopic beats all cause the same physiological changes in the myocardium as a regular beat; the potassium is moved out of the cell as sodium rushes in causing the depolarization. Therefore, the same "resetting" physiology must take place in order for the heart to generate its next beat. Since these premature complexes (either PACs, PJCs, or PVCs) happen earlier than a regular beat would have, a distinctive pause can be seen on the ECG tracing. These pauses are described either as compensatory or noncompensatory. Which type of pause, and therefore which type of ectopic beat, can be determined with confidence only in otherwise regular rhythms.

A compensatory pause is one that "compensates" for the presence of the extra beat. That is, the distance from the last normal beat before the ectopic beat to the first normal beat after a single ectopic beat is exactly twice the distance as the overall R-R interval in the rhythm. A compensatory pause indicates that the ectopic beat was a PVC.

A noncompensatory pause is one that fails to fully compensate for the presence of the extra beat. Here, the distance from the last normal beat before the ectopic beat to the first normal beat after a single ectopic beat is less than twice the distance as the overall R-R interval in the rhythm. A noncompensatory pause is seen in both PACs and PJCs.

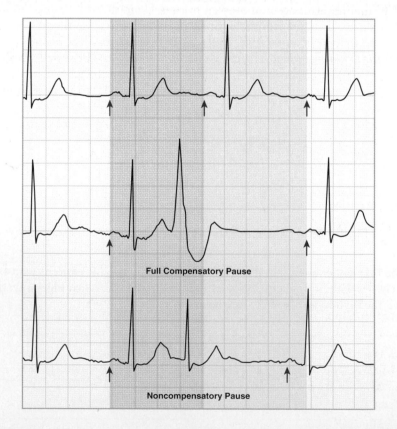

Figure 5-17. Full Compensatory Pause vs. Noncompensatory Pause
Measure a full compensatory pause as follows: 1. Mark off 3 normal cycles (indicated by the arrows). 2. Places the first mark on the P wave of the normal cycle preceding the premature complex. The third mark should fall exactly on the P wave following the premature complex (i.e., the P wave following the compensatory pause).

12-LEAD ECG INTERPRETATION

The 12-lead ECG is the defining method for rhythm interpretation and a determination of what is happening within the heart. It provides a snapshot of the patient's heart rhythm at the time it was taken and combines 12 different views on one page. The leads are always arranged in the same way. Each lead represents a particular area of the heart. Leads I, aVL, V_5, and V_6 look at the left lateral wall of the heart. Leads II, III, and aVF look at the inferior wall. Leads V_1 and V_2 represent the junction and the ventricular septum. Finally, leads V_3 and V_4 look at the anterior wall of the heart.

Lead aVR (colored gray, in the figure) is often referred to as the "forgotten lead." It records the right superior portion of the heart and can provide information about the right ventricular outflow tract and the basal septum. Lead aVR is also reciprocal to leads 2, aVL, V5, and V6. (Reciprocal leads are discussed in more detail later in this section.)

Areas of a 12-Lead ECG			
Lead I High Lateral Wall of LV LCx	aVR	V_1 Septum LAD	V_4 Anterior Wall LV LAD
Lead II Inferior Wall of LV RCA	aVL High Lateral Wall of LV LCx	V_2 Septum LAD	V_5 Low Lateral Wall of LV LCx
Lead III Inferior Wall of LV RCA	aVF Inferior Wall of LV RCA	V_3 Anterior Wall of LV LAD	V_6 Low Lateral Wall of LV LCx

Figure 5-18. 12-Lead ECG
This table shows the arrangement of the leads on an ECG printout. Colors indicate which leads represent the same general area of the heart.

It is important to approach the 12-lead ECG in a systematic way to extract all of the information it can provide, without missing anything. You must determine the underlying rhythm (using the systematic process described previously) and also monitor for a few added phenomena:

- Axis deviation
- Electrical disturbances including bundle branch blocks
- Left ventricular hypertrophy (LVH)
- Infarction or ischemia (presence and location)
- Hyperkalemia

The first 4 steps of the following sequence help to determine the rhythm of the heart, while the last 3 help identify potential underlying cardiac disturbances.

1. **P Waves.** Are they upright and smooth? Are they the same shape? Is there a P wave for every QRS?
2. **PR Interval.** Is it <0.20 second (1 large box)? Is it the same duration in each sequential cycle?
3. **QRS Complex.** Is there a QRS for every P wave? What is the orientation of the lead: upwardly deflected or downwardly deflected? Is it wide (>0.12 second or >3 small blocks) or narrow? How many millimeters high is it from isoelectric line to peak?
4. **R-R Interval.** Is it the same (or regular)? Is it different (or irregular)? What is the rate?
5. **R Wave Progression.** Observing sequentially from V_1 through V_6, does the R wave progress smoothly from inverted in lead V_1 to upright in V_6?
6. **ST Segment and J Point.** Is the segment elevated, isoelectric, or depressed? Does this happen in contiguous leads?
7. **T Wave.** Is the T wave upright or inverted? Is it peaked (or taller than its QRS complex)?

Axis Determination

Every muscle cell, or **myocyte**, emits a small amount of electrical current as it depolarizes. This electrical current has a defined direction of travel associated with it. Any value that has both magnitude and direction associated with it is called a **vector**. If you were able to add together all these tiny vectors (which involves taking into consideration both the magnitude and direction of each), the result is called the resultant vector. In the heart, this resultant vector has a special name, the **axis**. In the normal heart, the position of the axis is down and to the patient's left. If there is damage to the heart or if one side of the heart is much larger than normal, this axis can shift from the normal predicted area. Paramedics can determine if there has been what is called an axis deviation by looking at two leads, lead I and lead aVF, and evaluating the orientation of the QRS complex in each.

Table 5-25. Determining Axis from QRS Direction

Axis	Lead I	aVF
Normal	↑	↑
Left axis deviation	↑	↓
Right axis deviation	↓	↑
Extreme right axis deviation	↓	↓

Arrows represent the direction of QRS from baseline.

Conduction Disturbances

Conduction disturbances can be seen as changes in the overall rhythm of the heart, which we have discussed at length. Here, we will focus on the ECG changes that can be seen in essentially any rhythm. These include chamber size, hypertrophy, and bundle branch block.

Chamber Size

The 12-lead can identify enlarged chambers of the heart. Look for the following hallmark signs on an ECG tracing to identify enlargement of one or more of the heart's chambers.

Right atrial enlargement (RAE) (or *right atrial dilation*) often results from chronic pulmonary disorders. It can be seen as a P wave >2.5 mm in height in lead II and/or >1.5 mm in lead V_1.

Left atrial enlargement (LAE) identified by itself on an ECG is usually associated with mitral valve stenosis. It is often found in association with left ventricular hypertrophy and aortic stenosis. Put more simply, LAE can be seen in patients with left ventricular or left atrial outflow dysfunction. LAE is illustrated on an ECG with the following:

- Notched (or bifid) P wave in lead II
- Peaks of P wave >0.04 second (1 small box) apart in lead II
- P wave duration >0.12 second in lead II
- P wave inverted (negative deflection) in lead V_1
- Inverted negative portion >1 mm deep in lead V_1

The figure compares the shape of P waves seen in RAE, LAE, and conditions in which both atria are enlarged versus normal P wave findings recorded by lead II and lead V_1.

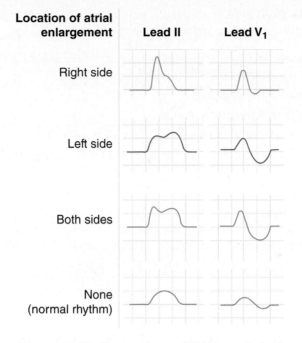

Location of atrial enlargement	Lead II	Lead V$_1$
Right side		
Left side		
Both sides		
None (normal rhythm)		

Figure 5-19. Comparison of P Waves in Left and Right Atrial Enlargement

Hypertrophy

Hypertrophy refers to the enlargement of any organ or tissue as a result of the enlargement of its component cells.

Left ventricular hypertrophy (LVH) can be a normal finding in an athletic heart, but more commonly it occurs when the left ventricle has to contract against high outflow pressures ("high afterload"). These pressures can be caused by systemic hypertension, aortic stenosis, or both. Stenosis is an abnormal narrowing of an opening or passageway of the body.

- Diagnosis requires both ECG and echocardiogram. The ECG can confirm only that the patient's heart meets the voltage criteria for LVH.
- When the patient meets the voltage criteria for LVH, the following are seen on the ECG (wave height and depth are measured in millimeters from baseline to peak or baseline to trough):
  - Most commonly, the **Sokolow-Lyon voltage criteria**: deepest S wave (between leads V$_1$ and V$_2$) + tallest R wave (between leads V$_5$ and V$_6$) >35 mm total
  - R wave in lead I + S wave in lead III >25 mm total
  - R wave in lead aVL >1.1 mV (11 mm when 1 mV is represented by 2 large boxes)
  - R wave in aVF >20 mm
  - S wave in aVR >14 mm
  - R wave in V$_4$, V$_5$, or V$_6$ >26 mm by itself
- Other findings often include left atrial enlargement and left axis deviation.

Right ventricular hypertrophy (RVH) is seen in chronic pulmonary conditions, mitral valve stenosis, pulmonary embolism, primary pulmonary hypertension, and some congenital heart disease such as tetralogy of Fallot.

- RVH is characterized on the ECG when findings include any of the following (wave size is measured in millimeters from baseline to peak or baseline or trough):
  - R wave in V_1 is large (>7 mm in height)
  - R wave in V_1 is larger than S wave (R/S ratio >1)
  - Dominant S wave in lead V_5 or V_6 is larger than 7 mm (R/S ratio <1)
- Other findings often include severe right axis deviation ("+110° or more") and RAE on the ECG.

Bundle Branch Block

After the electrical impulse leaves the bundle of His, it divides into the right and left bundle branches. When there is a lesion (from ischemia or infarction) in the area of the septum that contains the bundles, it can cause the electrical impulse to travel noticeably slower through one bundle versus the other. This condition is referred to as a **bundle branch block**, and it can be evaluated in the QRS complex of lead V_1.

In the lead V_1 tracing, **right bundle branch block (RBBB)** is characterized by an RSR′ (pronounced "R-S-R prime") appearance, often referred to as "rabbit ears," and a widening of the QRS beyond 0.12 seconds. The tracing begins with a positive deflection, which represents the first R, followed by a downward deflection, which constitutes the S. In a normal ECG, this is where the QRS complex ends. In RBBB, however, there is a second, larger positive deflection that is labeled as R′. The slope does not have to descend to or below the baseline to be considered an S wave, and the R waves do not have to be different sizes to establish an RSR′ pattern. The QRS could simply appear notched, and it qualifies. RBBB can be confirmed by the presence of terminal S waves in the lateral wall leads: leads I, aVF, and V_6.

Left bundle branch block (LBBB) can be seen when there is a widening of the QRS beyond 0.12 second and a terminal S wave in lead V_1. Although there is normally a terminal S wave in lead V_1, the key here is a widened complex overall. LBBB can be further confirmed by the presence of terminal R waves in the lateral wall leads: leads I, aVL, V_5, and V_6.

Infarction and Ischemia

Infarction and ischemia have distinct markers that can be seen in the 12-lead ECG as an elevation of the ST segment in a number of contiguous leads. Based on the location of these changes on the ECG (refer to the earlier figure "Areas of a 12-Lead ECG"), it is possible to identify the area of the heart and, by extension, the coronary vessel involved.

In a patient with chest pain, the goal of the 12-lead ECG is to localize the ischemia and infarction. This can be accomplished through systematic evaluation of the ST segment and T wave in each lead on the ECG. While identifying the location or severity of the ischemia and infarction will not change the treatment that the paramedic provides, this information is valuable: It could shorten the time that a patient with an active infarction must wait to receive definitive treatment and, thus, minimize the long-term damage done to the heart. In this way, the paramedic not only plays a key role in treating patients with acute coronary syndrome (ACS) in the prehospital setting, but also impacts length of hospital stay and even quality of life after discharge for these patients.

With this in mind, it is crucial that the paramedic minimize time spent on scene either obtaining a 12-lead ECG or initiating treatment, and instead do as much as possible en route to the hospital, including the 12-lead ECG. This approach supports the American Heart Association's goal of minimizing "door to balloon" time (i.e., the time elapsed between the patient's arrival at the hospital and the inflation of an angioplasty balloon in the blocked arteries). Accomplishing all this time-sensitive work as efficiently as possible will come with practice, rest assured.

The 12-lead ECG can reveal ischemia and infarction (current and prior) in most patients. To identify the presence of these pathologies, look at the Q wave, ST segment, J point, and T wave of every lead. The following sections look at each change as the patient progresses from normal to ischemic, then to evolving injury (or active infarction), and finally to completed infarction (or cellular death).

Q Waves

The first negative deflection after the P wave is the Q wave. The presence of a Q wave is considered pathologic (abnormal) if it is wider than 1 small box (or 0.04 seconds). Q waves also must be deeper than 1/3 the height of the R wave in the lead in which it is found. The presence of a Q wave indicates an old MI that has completed its evolution, typically after several hours or days.

ST Segment and J Point

The ST segment and the J point are the areas to pay the most attention to in a patient with suspected ACS. The J point represents the start of the ST segment; since the ST segment includes the J point, we will refer to this area collectively as the ST segment. Under normal circumstances, the ST segment is isoelectric with the baseline of the ECG, which can be seen in the PR interval (the area between a T wave and the following P wave). During a cardiac event, however, the ST segment can fall below or rise above the isoelectric line.

As an area of the heart begins to be ischemic (that is, to be starved of nutrients and O_2), the ST segment begins to dip below the baseline, a pattern referred to as **ST depression**. As this ischemia progresses to injury, the cells that were ischemic begin to die, or infarct. At this point, the ST segment begins to rise above the isoelectric baseline, a pattern referred to as **ST elevation**.

Pro-Tip

Widespread ST elevation across many or all leads of the ECG is more likely to indicate endocarditis and not massive myocardial infarction. For example, the lateral wall of the heart is typically serviced by the LCx arteries, while the inferior wall is most often serviced by the RCA and sometimes the LAD. Simultaneous occlusion of all these vessels is particularly unlikely.

When the ST segment rises >1 mm above the isoelectric line, it is considered diagnostic for an active, evolving MI. As the infarct worsens in the area, the ST segment will continue to rise, sometimes nearing the height of the R wave (7–10 mm above the baseline). This level of elevation in a QRS complex and its associated ST segment is said to look like the silhouette of a firefighter helmet in profile or the outline of a tombstone. While the ST segment is elevated (indicating the evolution of an active MI), the patient is said to be having an **ST elevation MI (STEMI)**. It is important to know that only approximately 50% of patients with active injury and infarction will have a STEMI. The other 50% will have what is referred to as a **non-STEMI**; these patients have normal ECGs or nondiagnostic changes on the ECG. (Diagnostic versus nondiagnostic changes will be discussed in greater detail later in this section.)

Once the injury to the tissue has reached its maximum through either reperfusion of the area or full-thickness MI, the ST segment will return to baseline, leaving a Q wave as a marker of this trauma.

The following table summarizes the anatomic areas of the heart and associated ECG leads; these locations are color-coded earlier in this chapter in the figure "Areas of a 12-Lead ECG." Once you identify the location of the ST elevation—and the reciprocal ST depression, if present—you can identify the locations of the MI. ST segment elevation must be present in at least 2 of the listed leads to identify the MI.

Table 5-26. Location of MI Based on 12-Lead Presentation

Anatomic Location	Coronary Artery	Leads with ST Changes
Inferior wall	RCA	II, III, aVF
Septal wall	LAD branch	V_1, V_2
Anterior wall	LAD	V_3, V_4
Lateral wall	LCx, possibly LAD	I, aVl, V_5, V_6
Left ventricle	Left main occlusion	aVR, with widespread ST depression

T Wave

The T wave also is an area of dynamic change in the ECG during cardiac ischemia, injury, and infarction. Normally, the T wave is upright and smooth. As ischemia begins, however, the T wave may be inverted in the leads corresponding to the affected area of the heart. T wave inversion is a classic sign of ischemia. Other possible indications of ischemia that may be seen on ECG are hyperacute and broad-based, upright T waves. Hyperacute T waves are larger than normal (exceeding half the height of the QRS in that lead). Broad-based T waves have a less discernible initial ST segment; the T wave almost seems to begin at the J point.

ST segment and T wave changes may be diagnostic or nondiagnostic, as mentioned earlier. These changes are considered diagnostic of an acute myocardial infarction (AMI) when they appear in 2 or more contiguous leads. An isolated finding, such as ST elevation found in 1 lead on the ECG, is nondiagnostic. In leads that represent areas of the heart that are serviced by the same artery, it is possible to have ST changes in >1 area; for example, an occlusion in the LAD could cause ST changes in both the septal and anterior leads. Areas of the heart that are serviced by the same artery, and their corresponding leads, are as follows:

- Inferior wall: leads II, III, and aVF
- Septum: leads V_1 and V_2
- Anterior wall: leads V_3 and V_4
- Lateral wall: leads V_5, V_6, I, and aVL

Hyperkalemia

As noted in the previous section, tall and pointed ("hyperacute") T waves on ECG can indicate ischemia when confined to a particular area of the heart or found in contiguous ECG leads. By contrast, tall, pointed, or sharply peaked T waves *that appear in all leads* could indicate hyperkalemia.

The rule of thumb for identifying hyperkalemia on the ECG is "T wave up, P wave down." However, the ECG of a patient with hyperkalemia may show any of the following changes:

- Flattened P wave
- Widened QRS
- Peaked T wave
- Presence of a U wave; this is a second positive deflection after the QRS complex
- Sinusoidal ECG (a presentation in end-stage hyperkalemia)

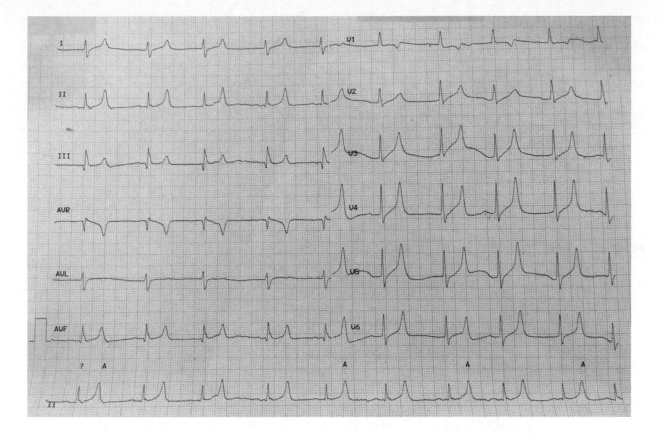

Figure 5-20. Hyperkalemia on the ECG

An example of many possible presentations of hyperkalemia. Note the peaked T waves (taller than the QRS complex) in lead II and pointed T waves in the precordial leads.
© Dr. Michael-Joseph F. Agbayani and Dr. Eddieson Gonzales (Manila, Philippines);
license: https://creativecommons.org/licenses/by/4.0/deed.en

Reciprocal Leads

Finding ST elevation in contiguous leads of a 12-lead ECG is often enough to isolate and diagnose an evolving AMI. Two special cases should nonetheless be noted, in which AMI produces reciprocal changes in the leads opposite the area of the heart where the AMI is occurring.

- When ST elevation is found in the **lateral leads** (V5, V6, I, and aVL), simultaneous ST depression can often be seen in the inferior leads (II, III, and aVF).

- The opposite also is true: When ST elevation is found in the **inferior leads**, ST depression is often seen in 2 or more of the lateral leads.

- If ST elevation is found in inferior or lateral leads, reciprocal changes are not required for a diagnosis of AMI to be made. However, when they are seen, reciprocal changes should be documented.

Unfortunately, paramedics cannot compare old ECGs with the current ECG to look for new onset changes. This means that, until proven otherwise, any deviations from what is considered normal on an ECG should be regarded and treated as acute.

CARDIAC EMERGENCIES:
PATHOPHYSIOLOGY, ASSESSMENT, AND TREATMENT

So far, we have been talking at length about one tool in our assessment arsenal for patients who are suspected of having a cardiac event: the **ECG**. We have not in any meaningful way covered the patient interrogation and physical examination of the cardiac patient. As noted previously, every assessment begins with ensuring scene safety, followed by evaluation and rapid treatment of the ABCs. During the evaluation of the history of present illness, use the OPPQRST and SAMPLE mnemonics to guide questioning. In the following sections, we will cover questions that should be asked that are specific to the cause of the problem that are not obviously addressed elsewhere in SAMPLE or OPPQRST. We will then go into cardiovascular emergencies you will likely encounter in the field, including additional questions for those patient populations. Each cardiovascular emergency section also will cover the treatments recommended for that ailment.

Acute Coronary Syndrome

Pathophysiology

ACS refers to any of a variety of symptoms associated with coronary artery disease (CAD) that results in symptoms of cardiac ischemia, including Prinzmetal angina, stable and unstable angina pectoris, and AMI. Symptoms of ACS can include any of the following: chest pain, pressure, tightness, or general discomfort; shortness of breath; nausea with or without vomiting; dizziness; weakness; or syncope. Patients also may become diaphoretic and pale while experiencing the pain. Each of these has a different pathophysiology; however, the prehospital management for each is highly similar. Paramedics are not required to differentiate between the ultimate cause for the symptoms or diagnose the patient as having one cause of ACS versus another.

Coronary artery spasm is the principal cause of Prinzmetal angina. It causes a sudden onset of chest pain or pressure and often occurs while at rest, usually during sleep. It occurs in a younger population than would be expected to be in the advanced stages of CAD from atherosclerotic plaque buildup. This also is closely associated with cocaine use or smoking. The spasming coronary artery interrupts blood flow to the myocardium, resulting in severe pain.

Stable and unstable anginas differ in their predictability. Stable angina is highly predictable and typically occurs after exertion of some kind. It is caused by advanced CAD and occurs during exercise because of the increased workload placed on the heart at that time. The narrowing of the coronary arteries limits the amount of blood and, therefore, O_2 that can get to areas of the heart, resulting in ischemia. The level of exercise that will cause a bout of chest pain from stable angina does not have to be much; it can simply be walking up a flight of stairs. The amount of exercise varies from patient to patient but is predictable, nonetheless.

Unstable angina is far more serious because it can occur at any time and without warning. Unstable angina indicates a higher degree of obstruction to at least one of the coronary arteries. It also is unpredictable in duration, degree of pain felt, and frequency of occurrences. With unstable angina, exercise and stress are not required to precipitate an event.

The ACS of greatest concern to the paramedic, however, is the AMI or heart attack. This occurs when there is a blockage to coronary blood flow for a long enough period of time that death to the myocardium occurs. This blockage can have several causes.

- **Thrombus.** A clot can form in the already narrowed artery, preventing blood flow to areas beyond.
- **Embolus.** A clot formed elsewhere in the body can travel to the coronary artery.
- **Spasm.** Similar to Prinzmetal angina but for a much longer duration than that typically associated with Prinzmetal angina, a spasm could be severe enough and of long enough duration to cause permanent damage to the heart muscle.

The location, size, and severity of an MI depend on the location of the blockage, as we have seen in the 12-lead discussion. If the full thickness of the cardiac muscle is involved in the infarction, it is called a transmural MI; if the infarction is affecting only the inner layers of muscle, it is called a subendocardial MI. The area surrounding the infarcting area will be ischemic yet still viable. This area can become irritable and therefore the potential source of dysrhythmias. All this information should be thought of as "nice to have" rather than "need to have" because knowing any of it will not change the prehospital management for the most part and should not be evaluated if it means delaying treatment or transport to the nearest appropriate facility.

Assessment of ACS

No patient with ACS will have exactly the same complaints as others with ACS nor will every patient have a single complaint in common. That said, there is a basket of symptoms and examination findings that tend to go hand in hand for patients experiencing ACS. To make sure we approach each of these cases systematically, we will fill in the blanks for SAMPLE and OPPQRST with questions and answers, followed with pertinent head-to-toe physical examination findings.

Symptoms. Chest pain or discomfort and shortness of breath are common complaints associated with ACS. If a patient complains of chest pain or discomfort, you should ask them about shortness of breath. Nausea with or without vomiting may also be present, so be prepared to manage this potential complication. Patients may report dizziness or syncope if cardiac output is impaired as a result of the syndrome.

It is worth noting that up to 25% of people actively experiencing an MI or other ACS do not experience chest pain. This is particularly common among women, adults age 65 and older, patients with a heart transplant, and patients diagnosed with diabetes, so be alert to other subtle, seemingly unrelated complaints and be aware of general or nonspecific complaints. Seemingly unrelated complaints could be upper abdominal (epigastric) pain, back pain, or shoulder pain without identifiable trauma. General or nonspecific complaints could include general malaise, the global feeling of being run down or ill. When an older adult female patient with a history of diabetes complains of "just not feeling well," this may be the subtle, atypical presentation of a heart attack.

Allergies. These are patient specific. Because aspirin and morphine sulfate are an important part of prehospital ACS treatment, make sure to ask specifically about these.

Medications. These are important to evaluate, and the patient's list of medications should be gathered and taken to the hospital with the patient. Common medications for the patient with CAD will include antihypertensives, statins for cholesterol, and calcium channel blockers for heart rhythm. Here, also evaluate if the patient is compliant with their medication regimen. Because the administration of NTG is the hallmark treatment for ACS, be sure to inquire about medications commonly prescribed for erectile dysfunction and primary pulmonary hypertension, including sildenafil, tadalafil, and vardenafil.

Past Medical History. Patients may have a history of a previous heart attack or cardiac-related chest pain, so they may be able to state whether their current situation resembles in any way that of previous episodes. Note all of their history. Also, note if they have any history that could compromise their feeling of chest pain, such as open heart surgeries, especially valve replacements or heart transplants.

Last Oral Intake. Although mostly important to know what may be coming back up if the patient vomits, knowing this could help determine what caused this new problem. For example, heart attacks often occur after a large meal, particularly a meal high in sodium, because the heart will have to work harder to get blood to the gut for digestion. In addition, the systemic parasympathetic stimulation could have a vasoconstrictive effect on the coronary arteries, enhancing the chances of a blockage occurring.

Events Prior. This leads the assessment nicely into OPPQRST. Evaluation of what the patient was doing at the onset of the complaint can help differentiate between stable and unstable angina but not necessarily between angina and an AMI.

Onset. What were you doing when this started? This is of particular concern if the pain started while at rest or while sleeping.

Provocation/Palliation. Does anything make this feeling better or worse? Have you done anything to make it better, such as take a medication or rest? Did the pain start suddenly or come on gradually over time? Patients experiencing

Prinzmetal, stable, or unstable angina may be able to obtain full relief from NTG administration, either on their own or from the paramedics. For those suffering an AMI, NTG may not provide any relief. Because the AMI is not, in most cases, caused by spasms or constriction of the vessels and is more likely the result of a clot, NTG is not able to remove or break up the clot. If they are previous angina sufferers, they may be able to explain that the feeling would normally be able to be made better with NTG, but this time it is not.

Quality. How would you describe the pain? Although open-ended questions should be used whenever possible, a patient may need some guidance with this question. Offering multiple options can help the patient select the best description or help the patient find their own description. If you were trying to make me feel the same pain, what would you do to me to give me that same feeling? ACS pain often is described as a pressure, tightness, or a squeezing sensation and less commonly as a stabbing or tearing pain. Patients also may describe it as someone or something sitting on their chest.

Radiation. Can you show me where the pain is? Does the pain you are having go anywhere? Does it go to the shoulder? Back? Abdomen? Neck or jaw? ACS pain frequently radiates to nearby structures, such as the left shoulder, neck, jaw, back, and abdomen. A patient experiencing radiation of pain should be treated as if there is a cardiac problem until proven otherwise.

Severity. On a scale of 1–10, with 10 being the worst pain you have ever had and 1 being very minor or no pain, what number would you give this feeling? The first time the patient answers this question establishes a baseline for tracking changes in pain as treatments are administered because what is a 10 to a person may be only a 4 for another. A move from an initial answer of 8 to a reassessed answer after some treatment has been given of 6 denotes a potential improvement in patient condition. Serial evaluations of this question help the paramedic decide what is working and perhaps what is not.

Time. When did this begin? Is it constant or intermittent? ACS pain, specifically pain related to an AMI, often will be constant and increasing as the ischemic or infarcting area broadens. If the pain is intermittent and the patient gets relief from NTG, it is likely it is unstable angina or something not cardiac related.

Physical Examination. The patient may present a variety of physical examination findings, but the following are the most common and concerning. The patient may be pale and diaphoretic. Either of these by themselves is cause for concern; both together likely indicates a serious emergency.

Vital Signs. Monitoring the patient's vital signs is paramount as they may change without warning if the condition worsens. The pulse rate could be fast, slow, or normal, and the blood pressure could be high, low, or normal depending on what part of the heart is affected.

Treatment of ACS

The patient with ACS is one of the most critical and time-sensitive patients a paramedic will encounter. A lot of things can and should be done for the patient before arrival at the emergency department; however, none of it should cause a delay in the arrival to the hospital. The following are the treatments that should be attempted and considered for all patients with ACS.

Ensure that the patient is in a place of emotional and physical rest. The best thing a paramedic can do for a patient experiencing ACS would be to keep them calm and mitigate as much anxiety as possible. This will reduce myocardial O_2 demand to a reasonable extent and essentially help patients help themselves.

Monitoring ECG and Obtaining 12-Lead. These are essential to determine the rhythm of the patient and identify the existence of ischemia or infarct. Whenever possible, the 12-lead should be obtained prior to the administration of any medications because they may change the overall baseline rhythm. The prehospital 12-lead has effectively lowered door-to-balloon times for patients experiencing a heart attack. Some systems have even implemented a process where the 12-lead can be continuously transmitted to the hospital receiving the patient so that the emergency physicians and cardiac catheterization team can remain up-to-date on the incoming patient and offer real-time treatment suggestions, should they become applicable.

Oxygen. This formerly was given in high quantities to every patient with a complaint of chest pain; however, in recent years, research has shown that unless a patient is hypoxic with a reliable pulse oximetry reading <94%, supplemental O_2 can actually worsen a patient's prognosis. Because of the prevalence of reperfusion therapies, where the obstruction to the coronary artery is removed and fresh oxygenated blood is able to get to the previously ischemic area of the heart, high levels of O_2 cause reperfusion arrhythmias, occasionally leading to sudden cardiac arrest. Only administer O_2 enough to maintain a pulse oximetry reading at or equal to 95%.

Aspirin. A patient with chest pain of a cardiac origin or symptoms thought to indicate a cardiac problem should be given 162–324 mg chewable baby aspirin as soon as possible. This will help the patient by preventing further platelet aggregation in any clots. Ensure that the patient does not have any history of gastrointestinal bleeding or aspirin allergy before administration. If the patient has taken aspirin within an hour of calling the ambulance it is acceptable to avoid repeating the dosage.

Initiation of Intravenous Access. This is largely preventive in the event that if the patient's condition deteriorates, access has already been established. In addition, if the patient's blood pressure drops after the administration of NTG, the paramedic is ready to quickly administer fluids. Although not necessarily required to happen before NTG is given, it is strongly recommended in case of an adverse event.

Nitroglycerine (NTG). In the case of ACS, 0.4 mg NTG is given sublingually as a spray or a tablet. NTG is a potent smooth muscle relaxant that dilates the coronary arteries with the hope of getting more O_2 to the ischemic areas of the heart. It also reduces myocardial preload because it dilates the venous side of the vasculature. NTG can be repeated every 3–5 minutes up to a total of 3 doses as long as the patient still has pain and the systolic blood pressure (SBP) remains >100. The patient should be advised not to chew or swallow the medication and that it may cause side effects of a burning sensation under the tongue and a headache. NTG should not be administered if the patient has taken any erectile dysfunction medications in the past 24–36 hours. NTG should be withheld in patients who are having an MI that affects the right ventricle. Decreases in preload resulting from NTG administration can be catastrophic if given to a patient with ischemia or infarct extending to the right ventricle. Right-sided involvement is a concern only in patients whose 12-lead ECG shows an inferior MI (ST elevation in leads II, III, and aVF). To assess this crucial piece of information, whenever the 12-lead ECG shows that a patient is having an inferior MI, take the lead V_4 and move it over to the mirror image position on the right side of the patient's chest and rerun the 12-lead. This will give you a lead called V4R. If in V4R, the ST segment is altered—either elevated or depressed—it indicates right-sided involvement of the MI, and NTG should be withheld until medical control is contacted.

Morphine Sulfate. For pain that continues despite NTG administration, 2–4 mg morphine as an intravenous bolus can be administered. Morphine, in addition to providing pain relief, can help the patient relax: As it takes the pain away, the patient slowly stops thinking about their condition. Morphine should be withheld for patients with a SBP <100 and used with caution in patients who are at risk for respiratory compromise. Morphine, like NTG, can have the effect of reducing preload. Therefore, for the same reasons, morphine should be withheld in patients having an MI involving the right side of the heart. Fentanyl citrate can be an alternative to morphine because it has a faster onset and fewer side effects than morphine. If fentanyl is the analgesic of choice, administer 1 mcg/kg slowly over 1–2 minutes intravenously.

Congestive Heart Failure

Pathophysiology

CHF occurs whenever the heart is unable to pump effectively. As a result, blood backs up into the systemic circuit, the pulmonary circuit, or both. Most commonly, the left side of the heart fails before the right side for any of several reasons. First, the left side is more likely to sustain damage from a heart attack than the right side. This damage can then limit the overall function of the heart and reduce its ability to empty the chambers. The heart now has a reduced ability to push blood around the body, which leads to pooling. Second, the left side must consistently push against afterload, which, especially in cases of long-term hypertension, can cause LVH. The thickened walls of the left ventricle have a more difficult time squeezing together, further worsening the heart's ability to eject the blood.

These cases are further impacted by a normally functioning right side of the heart. As the right side continues to function, it efficiently moves blood through the lungs to the poorly functioning left side of the heart. This causes a backup of blood behind the left ventricle into the left atrium and, eventually, the lungs. Slow transit of blood through the lungs combined with increased pressures in the pulmonary capillaries causes those capillaries to become leaky, which allows some of the plasma to enter the alveoli and bronchioles. This is where it gets the term *congestive* because the lungs are now congested with excess fluid, similar to how they can get congested with mucus during an infection.

As the fluid enters the alveoli, it inhibits gas exchange between the alveoli and blood. As more and more alveoli are affected, poor oxygenation will result in hypoxemia. This hypoxemia is then recognized by the body's chemoreceptors, triggering the body to attempt to rectify the problem. Like most sympathetic responses, this actually makes matters worse for the patient with CHF because the body's reaction is to activate the sympathetic nervous system. First, the heart rate will increase in an effort to try and move more blood through the lungs and body. This only worsens the backup of blood into the lungs and the rest of the body. Second, the peripheral arteries constrict in an effort to shunt blood to the vital structures in the chest and abdomen. This serves to further increase the afterload on the left ventricle, further limiting its ability to eject blood. Third, the bronchioles dilate in an effort to allow more air to reach the alveoli. Unfortunately, this serves to further increase the pressure in the lungs, increasing the amount of fluid that escapes the pulmonary capillaries and worsening the hypoxemia. If not addressed quickly, further deterioration can result in cardiac arrest.

Eventually, as the left side continues to fail and pressures build up in the lungs, right-sided heart failure can begin. Left-sided heart failure is the most common reason for right-sided heart failure. As the right side of the heart fails, blood backs up behind the right ventricle that is no longer able to push blood through the lungs and back into systemic circulation. The venous side of the vasculature can hold fluid when it is in excess—but only to a point. Once that point is exceeded, the fluid begins to leak out of the venules of the capillary beds. This is particularly true of those capillary beds in the dependent areas of the body—the legs and feet of patients capable of sitting upright and standing and the sacral and lower back area of those who are bedridden. In something of a surprising twist, right-sided heart failure can actually help left-sided heart failure because as the right side fails, it can no longer push blood into the already failed left side. This reduces left-sided preload and, therefore, the workload of the left side of the heart.

Assessment of CHF

CHF generally results in a syndrome, or several signs and symptoms that generally occur together and relate to the same problem. When we talked about ACS, we said patients may exhibit any of a basket of symptoms. However, in CHF, patients typically present with similar signs and symptoms. As with ACS, we will approach assessment of the patient with CHF systematically and will fill in the blanks for SAMPLE and OPPQRST with questions and answers, followed with pertinent head-to-toe physical examination findings.

Symptoms. Shortness of breath is the most common chief complaint for patients in the throes of CHF. Chest pain or discomfort may or may not be present and often is related more to the workload of the heart exceeding its O_2 supply because of the poor oxygenation status in the lungs than to blockage. That said, keep in mind that it is possible to have a heart attack and CHF concurrently, so chest pain here is worth assessing in the same fashion as previously. Some patients will complain of dizziness or syncope, most likely caused by the overall drop in O_2 in the blood. Nausea, with or without vomiting, is always a possibility with increased sympathetic tone, so be prepared to manage this potential complication.

Allergies. These are patient specific. Morphine sulfate is again a treatment option for patients with CHF because of its mild diuretic properties in addition to analgesia, so ask specifically about morphine allergies.

Medications. These are important to evaluate, and the patient's list of medications should be gathered and taken to the hospital with the patient. Common medications for the patient with CHF will include many of the same as for CAD in addition to diuretics, such as furosemide or bumetanide, and positive inotropes, such as digoxin, to help the heart beat more forcefully. Also evaluate if the patient is compliant with their medication regimen. Because administration of NTG in large quantities is the treatment of choice in patients with CHF, once again ask about medications commonly prescribed for erectile dysfunction and primary pulmonary hypertension, including sildenafil, tadalafil, and vardenafil.

Past Medical History. Patients may have a history of a previous heart attack, which is now causing them to go into CHF. They also may have had episodes of CHF before, so they may be able to state whether their current situation resembles in any way that of previous episodes. They also may be able to tell you what worked best for them in the past.

Last Oral Intake. Although mostly important to know what may be coming back up if the patient vomits, knowing this could help determine what caused this new problem. For example, a recent meal that was high in sodium, which transiently increases blood pressure, may have been enough to "tip the scales" and send the patient into CHF.

Events Prior. This leads the assessment nicely into OPPQRST. Evaluation of what the patient was doing and how the patient was feeling over the hours or days leading up to the call is important.

Onset. What were you doing when this started? This may not yield a specific answer because CHF takes time to develop and worsen to the point that the patient will call for an ambulance. A common answer might be something like "Nothing specific, but I have been getting more and more short of breath over the past few days." At this point, it is worth looking into the progression of the issue. Ask when the patient first noticed a change in breathing and if any factors may have contributed to the respiratory symptoms.

Provocation/Palliation. Does anything make this feeling better or worse? Have you done anything to make it better, such as take a medication or rest? With these questions, patients may indicate symptoms of orthopnea, or difficulty breathing based on position. This might manifest as the inability to sleep lying flat or needing to sleep propped up on multiple pillows. The patient also may reveal sleeping in a recliner rather than a bed.

Quality. How would you describe the pain? This one does not make the most sense to ask in a patient with CHF unless there is associated chest pain or pressure.

Radiation. Can you show me where the pain is? Does the pain you are having go anywhere? Does it go to the shoulder? Back? Abdomen? Neck or jaw? Again, reserve these questions for patients with chest pain associated with the respiratory distress.

Severity. On a scale of 1–10, with 10 being the worst pain you have ever had and 1 being very minor or no pain, what number would you give this feeling? At first look, this may seem to be a question to avoid asking; however, if we reword it slightly to "On a scale of 1–10, with 10 being the shortest of breath you have ever been and 1 being not short of breath at all, how would you rank today's shortness of breath?" Now we can establish a numerical baseline and follow how the treatments are improving the patient's status.

Time. When did this begin? Is it constant or intermittent? This is related to the onset questions noted previously but focuses more on timing.

Physical Examination. The patient will very likely be pale and diaphoretic and cool to the touch because of the shunting of blood away from the skin and the increased sympathetic tone. The patient will likely have JVD when evaluated, with the patient sitting upright or in the semi-Fowler's position with the head raised higher than 45°. Evaluation of lung sounds will reveal rales in the dependent areas, usually the bases, from fluid seeping into the alveoli. Lung sounds also may include wheezing from the interstitial pressure narrowing the bronchioles. Patients with CHF also will have pitting edema in the dependent areas of the body. The edema is said to be pitting when you push your thumb into the edematous tissue and the indent remains for an extended period of time.

Vital Signs. The patient's vital signs in CHF also can be predictable. The heart rate will be elevated, often in the 120–130 range. The patient will be hypertensive, with blood pressure values often exceeding 200/100 on both the systolic blood pressure (SBP) and diastolic blood pressure (DBP) numbers. The patient also will be breathing faster than usual, sometimes in excess of 30 breaths per minute. A decreased pulse oximetry may be present, sometimes so low that the pulse oximeter cannot even pick up a signal.

Treatment of CHF

The primary goal in treating the patient with CHF is to increase oxygenation. This will reduce the patient's work of breathing and, therefore, the anxiety associated with not being able to get enough O_2. Secondarily, the goal should be reducing the blood pressure so that the workload being placed on the heart can be reduced. Both angles of CHF management will be discussed here. Before initiating any of the following, ensure that the patient is at least in a full Fowler's position (seated upright with the legs outstretched). Ideally, although difficult to achieve in an ambulance, the patient should be seated with the legs dangling to aid in venous pooling, limiting the amount that can return to the heart.

Oxygen. In ACS, administration of O_2 was restricted to those with a pulse oximetry <95%. Here, begin treatment with high-flow O_2 via a non-rebreathing mask at 15 LPM. In some patients, this will not improve their pulse oximetry into the desired range of >95%, so CPAP will be needed. Moving to CPAP quickly in the patient with CHF can avert the need for intubation and ventilation, treatment from which the patient may not ever recover.

Monitoring ECG and Obtaining 12-Lead. Continuous cardiac monitoring is essential to determine the rhythm of the patient. It also helps monitor patient improvement. If possible, obtain a 12-lead ECG to rule out ischemia and infarct; however, obtaining a 12-lead ECG should not delay initiation of the CPAP or other treatments that follow here.

Initiation of Intravenous Access. This is largely preventive in the event that the patient's condition deteriorates, access has already been established. In addition, if the patient's blood pressure drops after the administration of NTG, the paramedic is ready to quickly administer fluids. Although not necessarily required to happen before NTG is given, it is strongly recommended in case of an adverse event.

Nitroglycerine. Nitroglycerine is given primarily to reduce myocardial preload and create more venous pooling. In CHF, NTG is given sublingually as a spray or a tablet and is dependent on the blood pressure. Administer one 0.4 mg SL tablet initially, then follow the sliding scale based on the sequential blood pressures in the table.

Table 5-27. NTG Tablets Based on Blood Pressure

Systolic Blood Pressure	Nitroglycerine tablets
100–140 mmHg	1 tablet
141–180 mmHg	2 tablets
>181 mmHg	3 tablets

The patient should be advised not to chew or swallow the medication and that it may cause side effects of a burning sensation under the tongue and a headache. NTG should not be administered if the patient has taken any erectile dysfunction medications in the past 24–36 hours.

If the patient is on CPAP, whenever possible, the seal of the mask of the CPAP should not be broken to administer the NTG. In this situation, if local protocols allow, apply 1 inch of NTG paste to the patient's chest. Some systems may increase the number of inches according to blood pressure as well. Check local protocols.

Morphine Sulfate. Morphine can be given to patients to assist the NTG with reducing preload and increasing venous pooling. A typical CHF dose of morphine is between 2 and 6 mg. Because morphine is not usually used in CHF for its pain-relieving properties, fentanyl citrate is not an ideal alternative because its smooth muscle relaxant properties are not as potent as morphine's. Morphine is falling out of favor for a variety of reasons and may be eliminated from use in CHF in the near future. Check your local protocols.

Beta-adrenergics. Inhaled beta-adrenergic medications should be used with caution in the patient who is wheezing. Frequently, when the patient presents with wheezing and other symptoms consistent with CHF, such as pitting edema, hypertension, and orthopnea, administering albuterol can cause the patient to have what is called flash pulmonary edema, or flash CHF. It gets this name because rales appear, and the patient's work of breathing dramatically increases in a very short period of time. It is recommended that these medications be given only after initiation of the above treatments and on orders from medical control.

Cardiac Tamponade

Pathophysiology

Cardiac tamponade occurs when fluid accumulates between the tough fibrous membrane surrounding the heart, called the pericardial sac, and the heart itself. The fluid can be blood if a coronary aneurysm ruptures or a myocardial rupture occurs after a heart attack; it also can be serous fluid resulting from an infection. Penetrating chest trauma is the most common reason for traumatic tamponade. Blunt chest trauma also can result in tamponade; however, it is more likely to result in myocardial rupture than tamponade. Regardless of the fluid type and cause, it can build up, putting pressure on the heart. If unrecognized, the fluid can build to the point that the heart collapses and is no longer able to expand, preventing the chambers from filling. This can go on until there are no more palpable pulses, at which point in time the patient is essentially in cardiac arrest.

Assessment of Cardiac Tamponade

Symptoms. These are largely dependent on the cause; however, we will ignore trauma as a cause until chapter 7. Slow onset of progressively worsening chest pain is a common symptom. Dizziness or syncope become more likely as the stroke volume, and by extension the blood pressure, drops. Finally, if the cause is an infection, the patient can present with fever.

There are 3 signs and symptoms that when found together strongly signal pericardial tamponade. They are JVD, muffled or distant heart sounds, and low and narrowing pulse pressure. Collectively, these are known as Beck's Triad.

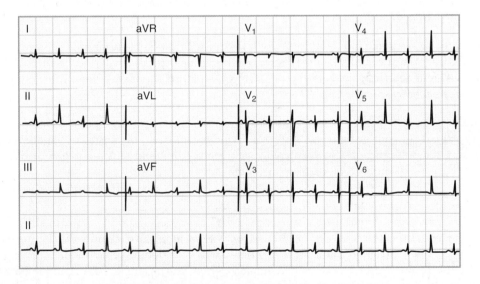

Figure 5-21. Electrical Alternans
The noticeable axis changes found on the ECG of a patient with pericardial tamponade.

Electrical alternans may also be observed. Electrical alternans is a condition that manifests on the ECG running rhythm later in the tamponade. As the fluid builds up, each contraction of the heart causes it to swing around in the fluid that now surrounds it. This causes variations in the size of the QRS complexes throughout each lead.

Allergies and Medications: These are related to the patient's health history and often do not offer any clues that would lead toward a notion of tamponade.

Past Medical History. If the patient has a history of a heart attack, cardiac rupture is a possible cause. The heart attack causes myocardial tissue to die, which over time weakens the structure of the heart. A patient with this and a history of uncontrolled or poorly controlled high blood pressure is at high risk for cardiac rupture.

Last Oral Intake. Important only for documentation purposes. This information likely will not impact any treatment plans.

Events Prior. Evaluate what led up to the patient calling for an ambulance.

Onset. What were you doing when this started? This may not yield a specific answer if the tamponade develops over time. Again, clarify when the patient first noticed the reported symptoms.

Provocation/Palliation. Does anything make this feeling better or worse? Have you done anything to make it better, such as take a medication or rest? With these questions, patients may indicate that chest pain and dizziness get better when they lie down. This can happen because the fluid around the heart spreads out and allows the ventricles to fill more efficiently; also, a lower overall blood pressure is needed when lying down to get blood to the brain.

Quality. How would you describe the pain?

Radiation. Can you show me where the pain is? Does the pain you are having go anywhere? Does it go to the shoulder? Back? Abdomen? Neck or jaw?

Severity. On a scale of 1–10, with 10 being the worst pain you have ever had and 1 being very minor or no pain, what number would you give this feeling? Now we can establish a numerical baseline and follow how the treatments are improving the patient's status. Because chest pain is a very common complaint with this issue, assess or treat as if the patient has ACS. Remember, chest pain is ACS until proven otherwise.

Time. When did this begin? Is it constant or intermittent? This pain is likely to be constant and progressively worsening over time. Dizziness, if present, also would be worsening over time, especially when changing positions (going from lying down to sitting or sitting to standing).

Physical Examination. The skin color and texture of a patient with cardiac tamponade can vary from normal, to cool, to pale and diaphoretic depending on the degree of tamponade that has already occurred. JVD will be present in later stages as venous return to the heart becomes impaired. Heart sounds will be muffled and sound distant compared with normal heart sounds.

Vital Signs. Tachycardia is frequently present as the body raises the heart rate to try and maintain blood pressure. The respiratory rate tends to not be significantly altered. Blood pressure may be normal or hypotensive. As the tamponade progresses, the pulse pressure—the difference between the SBP and DBP—narrows or becomes progressively smaller with each sequential blood pressure measurement.

Treatment of Cardiac Tamponade

Prehospital treatment of tamponade is very limited and focused on supportive measures, including maintaining an airway, providing O_2, and managing pain if present. A fluid bolus of 500 mL Normal saline solution (NSS) may be given to help support blood pressure; however, this should be given with an abundance of caution because too much fluid could precipitate pulmonary edema because of the poor functioning of the heart. Ultimately, the patient needs to receive a procedure called pericardiocentesis. This procedure involves inserting a long needle into the pericardial sac and drawing off the fluid. This is not a procedure typically performed by paramedics because it is extremely dangerous and carries with it many possible side effects. With this in mind, rapid transport to the nearest facility often is the best treatment.

Cardiogenic Shock

Pathophysiology

Cardiogenic shock occurs when >40% of the left ventricular muscle is damaged as a result of a heart attack or a series of heart attacks. This level of damage ultimately prevents the heart from ejecting enough blood to move it around the body and prevents the heart from maintaining a viable blood pressure. It often is lethal to the patient and, therefore, is always a true emergency.

Assessment of Cardiogenic Shock

Symptoms. Shortness of breath and extreme fatigue or general malaise are the most common chief complaints for cardiogenic shock. Chest pain or discomfort also may be a complaint if the developing cardiogenic shock is caused by an ongoing AMI. Some patients will complain of dizziness or syncope related to the hypotension. Nausea, with or without vomiting, is always a possibility with increased sympathetic tone, so be prepared to manage this potential complication.

Allergies. These are patient specific.

Medications. These are patient specific and widely varied depending on the patient's history. Because cardiogenic shock usually follows an MI, the patient will likely be on medications consistent with CAD.

Past Medical History. Patients often have a history of a recent heart attack.

Last Oral Intake. This information will seldom be important to the overall assessment. It may be helpful only if the patient ate recently to help prepare for the potential to vomit.

Events Prior. Evaluation of what the patient was doing and how the patient was feeling over the hours or days leading up to the call is important.

Onset. What were you doing when this started? Patients who suffer from cardiogenic shock typically are not very active, resulting from their diminished cardiac ejection fraction and poorly functioning heart. This answer, therefore, will vary from patient to patient.

Provocation/Palliation. Does anything make this feeling better or worse? Have you done anything to make it better, such as take a medication or rest? With these questions, patients may indicate symptoms of orthopnea. This might manifest as the inability to sleep lying flat or needing to sleep propped up on multiple pillows. This condition can mimic CHF in a variety of ways, including what makes the feeling better or worse.

Quality. How would you describe the pain? Chest pain concurrent with cardiogenic shock is unlikely because the AMI often has already passed.

Radiation. Can you show me where the pain is? Does the pain you are having go anywhere? Does it go to the shoulder? Back? Abdomen? Neck or jaw? Reserve these questions for patients with chest pain associated with the respiratory distress.

Severity. On a scale of 1–10, with 10 being the worst pain you have ever had and 1 being very minor or no pain, what number would you give this feeling? Because pain may not be present, this should be ascertained only if the patient has pain, or it can be adjusted to evaluate respiratory status and severity.

Time. When did this begin? Is it constant or intermittent? The patient may be able to share when this happened. Most likely, the shortness of breath or general malaise felt with cardiogenic shock will be constant and possibly progressively worsening.

Physical Examination. The patient may present with an altered mental status resulting from poor cerebral perfusion from the hypotension. The patient will very likely be pale and diaphoretic and cool to the touch because of peripheral vasoconstriction and increased sympathetic tone as the body tries to correct the blood pressure. The patient may have JVD when evaluated with the patient sitting upright or in the semi-Fowler's position with the head raised higher than 45° because the heart is not able to move blood around the body, leading to venous pooling. Evaluation of lung sounds will reveal rales in the dependent areas, usually the bases, from fluid seeping into the alveoli. Lung sounds also may include wheezing from interstitial pressure narrowing the bronchioles. Depending on how long heart failure has been present, the patient may have dependent pitting edema. If all of this is a relatively sudden onset, the patient may not have peripheral edema.

Vital Signs. Patients with cardiogenic shock will be tachycardic with low blood pressure—the clinical picture of shock. Their respiratory rate could be slow, normal, or fast depending on how well they are compensating. Pulse oximetry will be low, owing to poor blood flow through the lungs and the resulting pulmonary edema.

Treatment of Cardiogenic Shock

Increasing oxygenation and increasing cardiac output are the primary goals for treating the patient with cardiogenic shock. Position the patient according to their mental status in the position. If the patient is able to maintain consciousness in a semi-Fowler's or high Fowler's position, do this because it will help with the pulmonary edema. If the patient cannot maintain consciousness in this position or needs to have an airway adjunct placed, then transport in the supine position.

Oxygen. Begin treatment with high-flow O_2 via a non-rebreathing mask at 15 LPM. CPAP does not improve the patient outcome in cardiogenic shock as it does in CHF, so it is not a treatment option here, despite similar presentations. If the patient's pulse oximetry does not improve with high-flow O_2, consider placing an advanced airway as soon as possible, especially in cases of severe altered mental status or unresponsiveness.

Monitoring ECG and Obtaining 12-Lead ECG. Continuous cardiac monitoring is essential to determine the rhythm of the patient. It also helps monitor patient improvement. If possible, obtain a 12-lead ECG to rule out ischemia and infarct; however, obtaining a 12-lead ECG should not delay other treatments that follow here. Treat any rhythm disturbances appropriately.

Initiation of Intravenous Access. The patient will need intravenous access for medication administration. If the patient does not have JVD when the head of the bed is elevated >45°, it is possible that the patient is hypovolemic in addition to cardiogenic shock. This patient may benefit from a fluid bolus of 200 mL. If, however, the patient does have JVD when the head of the bed is elevated, the patient is likely fluid overloaded and would not benefit from a fluid challenge.

Vasopressors. Depending on the transport time to the hospital, paramedics may need to start a vasopressor that is a positive inotrope and has minimal impact on renal blood flow and myocardial oxygen demand. Dopamine is the preferred choice because it maintains renal blood flow at low doses while increasing myocardial contractility. The dose is typically started at 5 mcg/kg/min and titrated upward to obtain the desired effect of a systolic blood pressure between 90 and 100 mmHg. A dopamine drip is commonly prepared by injecting 400 mg into a 250 mL intravenous bag of normal saline. This yields a 1,600 mcg/mL concentration of dopamine.

Aortic Aneurysm

Pathophysiology

An **aneurysm** is a widening of any blood vessel. The vessel can be anywhere in the body, in this case, specifically the aorta. An aneurysm can form in 3 areas in the aorta: the ascending aorta leading from the aortic valve, the aortic arch, and the descending or abdominal aorta. Because the aorta endures higher pressures during systole than any other vessel in the body, it stands a greater chance of sustaining damage, especially those with untreated or poorly managed hypertension. Degenerative weakening in the middle layer, the tunica media, allows for a ballooning out of the aortic wall. Consequently, the tunica intima is left to bear the brunt of the systolic pressure, which will inevitably cause it to tear under the pressure. This tear will allow blood to get in between the intima and the media, effectively tearing the 2 layers apart. This is referred to as a **dissecting aortic aneurysm**.

Aortic aneurysms are differentiated by their location. When damage to the aorta is localized to the ascending aorta or the aortic arch, it can be called a **thoracic aortic aneurysm**. This aneurysm is concerning because the damage may not be limited to the aorta. The vessels branching off the aorta in this area also could sustain damage. In addition, the dissection could move toward the heart and involve the aortic valve. Because this is the area where the coronary arteries begin, they too could become compromised, therefore altering coronary artery blood flow. In an **abdominal aortic aneurysm** (AAA), the descending portion of the aorta is involved. Although there are many smaller arteries that branch off the descending aorta and service the abdominal viscera and the spinal column, damage to these is less concerning.

Assessment of Aortic Aneurysm

Symptoms. Chest or abdominal pain are the most common symptoms with an aortic aneurysm. Back pain is sometimes the chief complaint.

Allergies. These are patient specific.

Medications. These are patient specific and widely varied depending on the patient's history. Because aortic aneurysms are more common in people with uncontrolled or poorly controlled hypertension, patients often are on several antihypertensive medications.

Past Medical History. Patients may have a documented history of hypertension; however, if they have not been seeing their primary care physician regularly, they may not have had any diagnoses.

Last Oral Intake. This information will seldom be important to the overall assessment. It may be helpful only if the patient ate recently, to help prepare for the potential to vomit.

Events Prior. Evaluation of what the patient was doing and how the patient was feeling over the hours or days leading up to the call is important. This line of questioning is important to help decide between possible causes of the symptoms you are finding.

Onset. What were you doing when this started? Frequently, the pain from the aneurysm starts suddenly and at any time so this can vary widely from person to person.

Provocation/Palliation. Does anything make this feeling better or worse? Have you done anything to make it better, such as take a medication or rest? The AAA causes pain that is excruciating and constant, as long as the dissection is progressing. Many patients will not be able to find a position of comfort that suits them for the duration of the patient contact.

Quality: How would you describe the pain? This pain is frequently described as tearing, shredding, ripping or stabbing pain. It also is most often the worst pain of the patient's life.

Radiation: Can you show me where the pain is? Does the pain you are having go anywhere? Does it go to the shoulder? Back? Abdomen? Neck or jaw? Pain from an AAA that starts in the abdomen frequently radiates around the flank to the back. In a thoracic aortic aneurysm, the pain often is described as straight through to the back. Occasionally, if the dissection travels down into one of the branches of the aorta in the pelvis, pain can be felt in the pelvis or down into the legs. Radiation will be heavily dependent on the location of the original dissection.

Severity: On a scale of 1–10, with 10 being the worst pain you have ever had and 1 being very minor or no pain, what number would you give this feeling? Almost always, it will be the worst pain the patient has ever experienced.

Time. When did this begin? Is it constant or intermittent? The patient may be able to pinpoint the exact starting time of the pain because this tends to start so suddenly.

Physical Examination. In helping differentiate between an AAA and other abdominal ailments, a complete and thorough physical examination is crucial so that important signs are not missed or overlooked. Skin color and temperature often are pale and diaphoretic owing to the increased sympathetic tone and the body's response to severe visceral pain.

In a thoracic aortic aneurysm, blood flow may be disrupted into any of the 3 major branches coming off the aortic arch. If the aortic dissection affects either the brachiocephalic or left subclavian artery, the blood pressure in each arm may be different. This also is true if the aneurysm exists between the 2 arteries, so whenever an aortic aneurysm is suspected, take the blood pressure in both arms. Disruption of blood flow into either the brachiocephalic or the left common carotid artery may cause stroke symptoms, including 1-sided weakness, visual and speech disturbances, or facial droop.

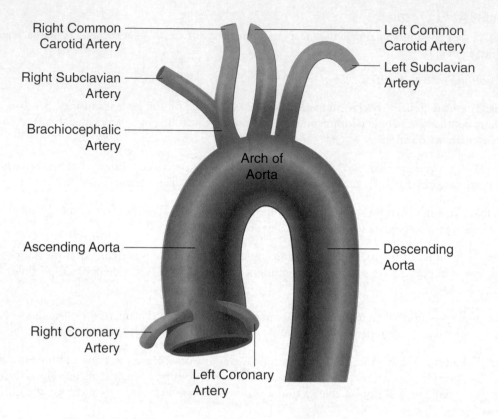

Figure 5-22. Thoracic Aorta and Branches of the Aortic Arch

In an AAA, there may be a palpable pulsating mass near the midline during the abdominal examination. If this is found, gently release the pressure placed over the abdomen and do not palpate that area again. Palpating it only adds to the already high pressure in the area and could accelerate a complete tear of the aortic wall, leading to intra-abdominal bleeding. This bleeding can be so intense that the patient completely exsanguinates (bleeding sufficient to cause death) in minutes. One leg may be cooler than the other. The same leg that is cooler also will likely have a notably weaker or possibly absent pulse; it also may appear mottled or pale compared with the other leg.

Vital Signs. More than likely the patient will be hypertensive. A patient who is hypotensive with any of the above signs, symptoms, or complaints may very well be bleeding out and rapidly approaching death. The patient's heart rate will most likely be normal to tachycardic. The ECG will be unremarkable except in the case of a thoracic aortic aneurysm that is affecting blood flow into the coronary arteries. If this is the case, the ECG may show ischemia or infarct and greatly complicates treatment. The respiratory rate will probably be elevated because of the pain, but breathing will not necessarily be labored. Pulse oximetry will be at the patient's usual baseline.

Treatment of Aortic Aneurysm

The primary goal of prehospital care of an aortic aneurysm is to calm and reassure the patient. Anything that can be done to reduce the patient's anxiety will go a long way in helping the patient reduce their blood pressure. Next is to help manage the patient's pain because this also will help reduce the patient's blood pressure. Paramedics do not frequently carry antihypertensive medications other than NTG, so directly addressing the blood pressure is not likely to happen in a meaningful way in the field. Therefore, rapid, stress-free transport is always indicated for the patient with an aortic aneurysm. Keep lights and siren use to a minimum so as not to alarm or agitate the patient because this will serve only to increase the blood pressure.

Hypertensive Emergencies

Pathophysiology

The full pathophysiology of **hypertension**, and why some people are chronically hypertensive whereas others are not, is poorly understood. The most widely accepted explanation is associated with progressing atherosclerosis, which has the ultimate effect of narrowing the arteries and reducing their elasticity. As this worsens over time, the afterload of the heart increases, which causes the heart to work harder, resulting in systemic hypertension. People walk around on a daily basis with hypertensive blood pressures and generally do not experience any symptoms that would require a hospital visit. It is when their hypertension is uncontrolled during an extended period of time that the symptoms develop and systemic problems arise. Left-sided heart failure and aortic aneurysm, discussed previously, are 2 conditions closely tied to hypertension. Paramedics may encounter a hypertensive blood pressure in a patient that can be associated with stress and anxiety of the situation; however, this is not likely to be life threatening. A sudden onset of hypertension, in very rare instances, can cause a condition known as posterior reversible encephalopathy syndrome (PRES), which can be devastating. The discussion about hypertension will center on this issue.

PRES is at greatest risk of occurring when the blood pressure exceeds 200/130, or, more specifically, whenever the mean arterial pressure (MAP) exceeds 150 mmHg. Recall that MAP is calculated by taking 1/3 the difference of the SBP and adding to that value the DBP:

$$MAP = DBP + [1/3(SBP - DBP)]$$

As the MAP exceeds 150 mmHg, the vessels in the brain begin to become leaky, resulting in cerebral edema, particularly in the occipital and parietal regions. This causes a breakdown of the all-important blood brain barrier and increases ICP. The areas of the brain most affected will determine the type and severity of the symptoms the patient will exhibit.

Patients may present with widely varied symptoms, but headache, dizziness, ringing in the ears (tinnitus), and visual disturbances are most common. These also can be accompanied by nausea and vomiting. Occasionally, global muscle twitching can be seen as a result of neuromuscular irritability, possible progressing to seizures. Sudden onset of confusion also is seen as the encephalopathy worsens.

Treatment of Hypertensive Emergencies

Lowering catastrophically high blood pressure must be done in a highly controlled and gradual fashion. Therefore, prehospital treatment of this issue is largely related to supportive treatment, including maintaining an airway and adequate oxygenation, establishing intravenous access, and monitoring the patient's ECG for the duration of the transport. Paramedics working in areas with transport times >30 minutes or so may need to initiate more definitive treatment related to lowering the blood pressure.

Labetalol is the drug of choice for PRES because it has alpha- and beta-blocking effects. As an alpha blocker, it helps relieve peripheral vasoconstriction, and its beta blocking effects prevent the possibility of rebound tachycardia that may accompany a drop in blood pressure. The beta blockade also will have negative inotropic effects. To administer, mix 250 mg in 250 mL NSS and begin to infuse as an intravenous piggyback at a rate of 2 mg/min, being careful to avoid accidentally giving the patient a large bolus of labetalol. Assess the blood pressure every 2–3 minutes and turn off the infusion when the desired blood pressure is reached.

If labetalol is not available, 0.4 mg NTG sublingually can be used in its place. In this case, multiple doses may need to be given to achieve the desired blood pressure. Ensure that adequate time passes between each administration of NTG so that there is not a large, sudden drop in blood pressure.

Cardiac Arrest

Cardiac arrest can have many etiologies, including massive AMI, severe respiratory distress, drug overdose, and electrolyte imbalance to name a few. Ultimately, in cardiac arrest, the heart is simply not producing a palpable pulse. We saw earlier in the chapter that the resulting rhythm can be the primary cause for pulselessness in the cases of

VF and VT. However, occasionally, the electrical cardiac rhythm looks as if it should be generating a pulse, even a normal pulse. This phenomenon is referred to as PEA. When presented with a patient with PEA, assess the patient for the following reversible causes, often referred to as the H's and T's. In the following list, the H or T that will serve as the memory aid is listed first, then the problem if it is not completely obvious, followed by a description of how the problem can present as cardiac arrest. Finally, each section will address the requisite treatment for the particular cause.

H's

- **Hypoxia.** If the patient does not get enough O_2 for a long enough period of time, the heart will lose the ability to contract forcefully enough to generate a pulse. To treat this, ensure high-flow O_2 at all times and continually monitor pulse oximetry.

- **Hypovolemia.** It is possible for a person to have lost such a large amount of their circulating volume that the heart is beating normally, with an organized electrical rhythm, but will not produce a palpable pulse, even when the patient is supine. This can be caused by profound fluid loss from burns, sepsis, dehydration, or severe bleeding. Treatment for this situation involves aggressive fluid replacement therapy. Fluid boluses of 500–1,000 mL are common during any cardiac arrest situation; however, they are essential if hypovolemia is a suspected contributing cause.

- **H^+ Acidosis.** As we talked about in chapter 1, the body needs to maintain the blood acidity within a fairly narrow pH range: 7.35–7.45. If it deviates outside this range, the cellular enzymes necessary for the metabolism of nutrients and other cellular activities begin to fail as the proteins that make them begin to change shape. Most commonly, the blood becomes more acidic (pH decreases) because of the production of metabolic acids and ketones and/or the inability for the body to reduce CO_2. Treating this involves 1 of 2 options—or both. In the cardiac arrest situation, CO_2 can build up in the blood because the patient is no longer breathing adequately. Here, treatment will focus first on restoring a patent airway and adequate ventilation and oxygenation. This should remedy most of the acidosis in cardiac arrest. If the patient is on dialysis or has a diagnosis of diabetes and has not taken insulin, metabolic acidosis may be playing more of a role than simply inadequate ventilation. In this case, while reestablishing an airway and ventilation remain the priority, 1 mEq/kg sodium bicarbonate may be beneficial in attaining a viable pH.

- **Hyperkalemia/Hypokalemia.** Cardiac arrest can be caused when the potassium levels are either elevated or deficient. Hyperkalemia is possible in patients who are on dialysis, especially if they do not follow their diet or have missed treatments, or in cases of profound cellular damage such as rhabdomyolysis. Rhabdomyolysis should be suspected in patients with a crush injury that has not been relieved for >1 hour, fall victims who have not been able to move for a couple of days, or weight lifters who have overdone the workout. Any of these situations will cause potassium to enter the blood in lethal quantities where it does not belong; as long as potassium remains within the cells, it tends to be relatively harmless. Hypokalemia is much less common and can occur in patients who have consumed excess volumes of water (relative hypokalemia) or more likely overdosed on potassium-wasting diuretics, such as furosemide, or in profound diabetic ketoacidosis. Prehospital providers can moderately treat hyperkalemia only with the administration of 1 g of calcium chloride or calcium gluconate as an intravenous bolus.

- **Hypothermia.** Long-term exposure to cold temperatures can result in slowing of the metabolism and eventually death. Treatment for this is slow, controlled rewarming, including warm intravenous fluids. More on this in later chapters.

- **Hypoglycemia.** As the blood sugar level drops in a patient, consciousness will be lost first as the body reduces its glucose consumption. If it drops far enough, the heart will stop moving but will continue to display a normal electrical rhythm. If the patient has a diagnosis of diabetes, or perhaps intentionally overdosed on insulin, hypoglycemia should be suspected. Check the patient's blood sugar level using a glucometer. If it is found to be <60 mg/dL, administer 25 g of a 50% solution of dextrose (D50). Administering D50 should not be a routine treatment in all cardiac arrest cases; however, it is a first-line treatment in hypoglycemia. **Note:** Officially, hypoglycemia has been eliminated from the list of H's and T's according to the American Heart Association. It is still considered an important assessment point in unresponsive patients. Additionally, glucose is needed for energy (ATP) production and is more efficient in its production than other sources. For these reasons, it is included here.

T's

- **Thrombosis (Cardiac Thrombus).** This is better known as a massive AMI. If the blockage is in the left main coronary artery, this could be sufficient enough to put the patient into sudden cardiac arrest because that would effectively eliminate blood flow to the entire left ventricle and therefore its ability to contract. Because the electrical signal would come from an area unaffected by the blockage, it would continue uninterrupted and unchanged. Treatment is minimal in the prehospital and hospital environments once the patient has gone into cardiac arrest. Unless pulses can be restored, this is likely a lethal event for the patient.

- **Thrombosis (Pulmonary Thrombus).** Also known as a PE, which was discussed at length in chapter 3. If the blockage occurs in a larger pulmonary vessel, profound and irreversible hypoxemia will quickly ensue. This is usually enough to cause catastrophic systemic cellular failure, resulting in patient death. This is irreversible in the field and in many cases in the hospital as well. The best treatment for this situation is aggressive ventilation and oxygenation with intubation and BVM ventilations.

- **Tamponade (Cardiac Tamponade).** Cause and treatment were discussed earlier in the chapter.

- **Tension Pneumothorax.** Cause and treatment were discussed in chapter 3.

- **Toxins (Drug Overdose).** Nearly every drug—street, prescription, or over the counter—in the right concentration can result in an overdose. Even water can be a toxin in the right quantity. Paramedics carry an antidote only for 1 family of medications and can mitigate only the effects of others. Opiate overdoses can quickly and effectively be treated in the field with 0.4–2 mg naloxone. Calcium channel blocker overdoses can be overcome with administration of 1 g calcium chloride or calcium gluconate. Other overdoses, such as aspirin, acetaminophen, benzodiazepines, and beta blockers, need to be treated in the hospital and can be treated only symptomatically in the prehospital environment. Maintenance of the ABCs is of primary concern in overdoses that cannot be definitively treated. This includes CPR, ventilation, establishing an intravenous line, and evaluation of the blood sugar level.

Treatment for VF and pulseless VT was covered earlier in this chapter, but a review of the global treatment options for a patient in cardiac arrest is worthwhile. First and foremost, high-quality CPR must be performed at a rate of 100–120 per minute. The chest should be compressed approximately 5–6 cm. Ensure that the chest fully recoils so that the heart has an opportunity to refill. It is now recommended that the rescuer lift the heel of their hand completely off the sternum to accomplish this; the fingers may remain in contact with the chest.

Compressions should be alternated with ventilations at a ratio of 30 compressions to 2 ventilations until the patient has a definitive airway in place, at which point compressions should be continuous, with a breath administered every 5–6 seconds, or 10–12 per minute. Each ventilation should be delivered slowly over 1 second so that the risk of gastric insufflation is minimized. Adequate time for exhalation of the previous breath should be allowed. After 2 minutes or 5 cycles of CPR, the electrical rhythm may be rechecked and the patient evaluated for a pulse. Stopping compressions for any reason (e.g., patient movement from floor to stretcher) should be kept as short as possible, preferably no more than 10 seconds.

Electrical defibrillation is needed for the patient who presents with VF or pulseless VT. If either of these are the presenting initial rhythm, give 1 defibrillation at 360 J or the manufacturer's recommended dose (often 200 J) as soon as possible if EMS witnessed the arrest or after 2 minutes of CPR if EMS did not witness the arrest. Defibrillations then should happen after 2 minutes or 5 cycles of CPR at about the same time as the pulse/rhythm check described above. Follow each shock immediately with high-quality CPR and ventilations for 2 minutes. Defibrillation is not a treatment option for patients in PEA or asystole.

An intravenous or intraosseous line should be established early in the resuscitation attempt for fluid and medication administration. In most cases, running the intravenous line wide open is recommended.

- The first medication of choice is **1 mg of 1:10,000 epinephrine**.
  - Give epinephrine every 3–5 minutes for the duration of the resuscitation attempt.
  - As per the **2020 AHA updates**, administer epinephrine as early as possible in non-shockable rhythms.
  - Always follow medications with CPR so that they can be moved around the body and reach the central circulation to receive its effects.

- When the patient is in VF or VT, follow the first dose of epinephrine with an appropriate antidysrhythmic medication. Choose between 300 mg amiodarone and 1.5 mg/kg lidocaine as the first-line antidysrhythmic. (Whichever one is chosen, continue for the duration of the resuscitation; i.e., do not alternate medications or use both at any time on a patient.)

- While epinephrine can be continued throughout, the use of amiodarone and lidocaine in the treatment of cardiac arrest is limited.

   - Amiodarone can be given only a second time, approximately 10 minutes after the first dose at 150 mg.

   - After the initial dose of lidocaine, each subsequent dose should be half the previous dose until a maximum of 3 mg/kg has been given. (If the first dose is 1.5 mg/kg, the second dose given about 5 minutes later is 0.75 mg/kg, and the third [and generally accepted final dose] 5 minutes after that would be approximately 0.5 mg/Kg.)

Waveform capnography is the best way to confirm effective CPR and **should be a point of emphasis during and after the resuscitation attempt**. After intubation, or placement of another alternative airway such as a Combitube, monitor the patient's exhaled CO_2.

- If the patient is still metabolizing glucose at a cellular level, CO_2 will still be produced. As long as that CO_2 can make it to the lungs, it will be picked up by the $EtCO_2$ sensor.

- If a sudden spike is noticed in the $EtCO_2$, it is very likely that the patient has had or will have a return of spontaneous circulation (ROSC).

ELECTRICAL THERAPIES

Paramedics can perform different therapies involving direct delivery of electricity to the heart. For each therapy discussed, indications/contraindications, recommended settings or dose, precautions, considerations, and therapeutic process will be described.

Transcutaneous Pacing

TCP is the temporary application of an electrical pacemaker to the chest of a patient. TCP delivers a small electrical current to the heart, stimulating it to beat faster than it already is. It will help the patient reach the hospital in a better overall cardiovascular condition than without this procedure.

Indications. Bradycardic rhythm with hemodynamic compromise, refractory to atropine and fluid administration. If the patient is in a rhythm with associated signs of hemodynamic compromise that does not respond to the initial dose of atropine—typical bradydysrhythmias that do not respond to atropine include high 2nd- and 3rd-degree AV blocks and idioventricular rhythms—then move rapidly to initiate TCP.

Contraindications. Bradydysrhythmias without hemodynamic compromise or pulseless bradycardic rhythms. Aggressive treatment of bradydysrhythmias that are not hemodynamically unstable is not warranted because the patient is maintaining blood pressure and mentation successfully, despite the bradycardic rhythm. Although it may seem that a pulseless bradycardic rhythm is the ultimate description of hemodynamically unstable, pacing a person in this condition often is fruitless. For pulseless bradycardic rhythms, instead of TCP, look to treat underlying problems such as hypoxia or hypovolemia along with providing high-quality CPR.

Recommended Settings or Dose. Eighty pulses per minute, 80 mA to start, titrate milliamps to the minimum needed for electrical and mechanical capture.

Precautions. Wet patients and excessively hairy patients.

- A wet chest area (from perspiration or being in water e.g., shower, pool) should be dried off prior to the initiation of therapy. This step helps prevent arcing of the electricity across the chest and helps the pads adhere more effectively throughout the course of treatment.

- A hairy chest area may make it difficult to get the pads and electrode gel to make a strong contact with the chest (possibly causing electrical burns to the patient's chest or, worse, setting the hair on fire). The following procedure should be done prior to the initiation of therapy. (Shaving also works, though it can take longer.)
  − Firmly apply one set of pads and rip them off (hopefully taking a swath of the patient's hair with them).
  − Next, place a new set of pads in the newly waxed area and proceed as normal.

Considerations. Pain management and/or sedation in patients who are conscious at the start of the procedure or whose consciousness improves with TCP. There is no hiding it; having electricity course through one's chest wall cannot possibly be a pleasant experience under any circumstance. In these cases, consider pain management or sedation but not until after obtaining electrical and mechanical capture. Once capture is obtained, the patient's hemodynamic status should improve by observing better blood pressure and mentation. At that point, the paramedic can address the pain and discomfort caused by the electrical current. This can be accomplished with fentanyl 1 mcg/kg for pain or with 2–5 mg of midazolam. Midazolam is preferred because it not only sedates but also induces amnesia.

Therapeutic Process.

1. Take standard precautions if not already done. The patient should meet criteria described above, including hemodynamic instability and atropine unsuccessful at raising the heart rate. Obtain and document an initial set of vital signs, including an initial cardiac rhythm strip and whenever possible a 12-lead ECG.

2. Place pacing pads on the patient. One pad should be placed inferior to the right clavicle, and the other should be placed on the left anterior axillary line at about the level of the 5th intercostal space. It is important that you explain to the patient and any family members who are present what is about to happen.

3. Attach wires from the pads to the pacing/defibrillation cable of the cardiac monitor.

4. On the monitor, activate the pacer. Different monitor manufacturers accomplish this differently. Be familiar with the one you will use.

5. Set the pacing rate to 80 pulses per minute.

6. Set the pacing current to 80 mA and adjust until there is electrical and mechanical capture. Electrical capture is represented on the running ECG lead when there is a wide and bizarre QRS complex following most if not all pacer spikes. Mechanical capture is verified when a palpable pulse matches the pacer output rate. That is, 80 beats can be counted at any pulse point on the patient.

7. Now that capture has been achieved, this should be the lowest energy that achieves consistent capture. To check this, drop the current slightly until capture is lost.

8. Once it is lost, return it back to the level that capture is consistent. This step helps minimize discomfort for the patient. Obtain a rhythm strip for documentation purposes and transport the patient to the closest facility capable of TCP, transvenous pacing, or pacemaker placement.

9. Consider sedation and pain management.

Synchronized Cardioversion

Synchronized cardioversion is used to interrupt the cardiac cycle of tachydysrhythmias with the delivery of an impulse of electricity. To reset the heart rate at a lower rate while simultaneously minimizing the chances of setting off a lethal dysrhythmia such as VF, this electrical impulse must be delivered at precisely the right moment in the cardiac cycle. If the electricity is delivered on the first half of the T wave, nothing will happen, and the electricity could serve only to hurt the patient. Similarly, if the electricity is delivered on the 2nd half of the T wave, the heart could be sent into VF or VT, either option potentially leading to death. Therefore, the impulse delivery is synchronized with the QRS complex the heart is already generating. The monitor predicts when the next QRS will fall and discharges the electricity only then. This creates a momentary disruption in the entire cardiac cycle, allowing the heart's pacemaker to take over at a presumably slower rate, immediately improving cardiac output.

Indications. Unstable SVT, unstable VT with pulses, and unstable atrial fibrillation (AF) with rapid ventricular response. These rhythms are hemodynamically unstable because they are too fast to support viable cardiac output for an extended period of time. Although more stable versions of the same rhythms can and should be treated with medications, unstable rhythms need to be treated more aggressively with electricity to promptly restore effective cardiac output. An unstable rhythm is characterized by any of the following symptoms: dizziness, syncope, altered mental status, hypotension, or orthostatic hypotension.

Contraindications. Stable SVT, stable VT with pulses, stable AF with rapid ventricular response, and pulseless VT. The stable rhythms are treated with a variety of medications. Pulseless VT is treated with defibrillation and medications.

Recommended Settings or Dose. The settings vary based on rhythm.

- **SVT & Atrial Flutter:** 50–100 J initially, increasing by at least 50 J until monitor maximum is reached.
- **Atrial Fibrillation:** 120–200 J initially, increasing by at least 50 J until monitor maximum is reached.
- **Unstable Ventricular Tachycardia with Pulses:** 100–150 J initially, increasing by at least 50 J until monitor maximum is reached.

Precautions. Electrical shock, postcardioversion cardiac arrest, and wet and/or hairy patients.

- The electrical impulse delivered during cardioversion is much larger than that given during TCP, so the possibility of bystanders or rescuers getting a shock is very real. It is important to "clear" the patient before delivering the shock: announce that the shock is about to be delivered and perform a visual inspection so that no one is in contact with the patient or anything the patient is in contact with (including the stretcher, ETT, or intravenous line).
- After the shock is delivered, reevaluate the patient not just for the resulting rhythm but also to ensure that the patient is not in cardiac arrest (a possible untoward effect of the treatment).
- Patients who are wet or excessively hairy should be handled as described in the TCP section.

Considerations. Pain management and/or sedation in patients who are conscious at the start of the procedure and SYNC button deactivation. In these cases, consider pain management or sedation early in the process but do not delay electrical therapy to provide sedation. One option is to have another paramedic prepare and give the medication as the other prepares the patient for the procedure. This can be accomplished with fentanyl 1 mcg/kg for pain or with 2–5 mg midazolam. Midazolam is preferred because it not only sedates but also induces amnesia. Some machines automatically turn off the SYNC button after the synchronized shock has been delivered, whereas others leave it activated. Therefore, if another synchronized cardioversion is needed, make sure the SYNC button is reactivated. Similarly, if a defibrillation is now needed, ensure that the SYNC button is deactivated.

Therapeutic Process.

1. Take standard precautions if not already done. The patient should meet criteria described above. Obtain and document an initial set of vital signs, including an initial cardiac rhythm strip and whenever possible a 12-lead ECG.
2. Place pacing pads on the patient. One pad should be placed inferior to the right clavicle, and the other should be placed on the left anterior axillary line at about the level of the 5th intercostal space. It is important that you explain to the patient and any family members who are present what is about to happen.
3. Attach wires from the pads to the pacing/defibrillation cable of the cardiac monitor.
4. If time permits, have another paramedic sedate the patient.
5. Turn on the SYNC button. Failure to perform this step will result in defibrillation, not cardioversion, and increase the odds of a negative outcome for the patient.
6. Select your initial setting according to above.
7. Charge the system. During the time that the system is charging, clear all personnel and bystanders from the patient.
8. Announce loudly, "Everyone clear!"

9. Press and hold the SHOCK button until the shock is delivered. Remember the shock must be delivered at a specific time in the cardiac cycle, so the button must be held until that point is predicted by the machine and the shock is delivered.

10. Reassess the patient immediately, focusing on electrical rhythm, the presence of a pulse, and blood pressure if the pulse is present.

11. Still in the same rhythm? Increase the joule level and repeat the process. New rhythm and improved blood pressure? Treat to prevent reentry into the dysrhythmia. Cardiac arrest? Initiate CPR and treat according to appropriate protocol for the resulting rhythm.

Defibrillation

Defibrillation delivers a surge of electricity to a heart that is currently generating disorganized electrical activity in the hopes of reorganizing that activity. The amount of electricity delivered through defibrillation is significantly higher than that used in TCP and cardioversion. This is because in defibrillation, the amount of electricity delivered needs to overcome that which is already present and redirect it, whereas in TCP, just enough electricity needs to be delivered to stimulate a single myocyte to contract, creating a cascade where the rest of the heart contracts.

Indications. VF and pulseless VT. Defibrillation can be used only when the heart is fibrillating and displaying a rhythm of VF. Pulseless VT is treated identically to VF.

Contraindications. Any rhythm with pulses. including AF and SVT; asystole and PEA. A patient with pulses in any rhythm, including VT, should not be defibrillated. AF should not be defibrillated, even though part of the heart is, in fact, fibrillating. SVT can sometimes look like VT if it is conducted aberrantly (through an alternate electrical pathway), but similarly, it should not be defibrillated. In addition, SVT, aberrantly conducted or not, will have pulses. Pulseless VT and VF are shockable cardiac arrest rhythms; asystole and PEA are not. Defibrillation needs the heart to have its own electrical activity to reorganize it into a meaningful rhythm that produces a pulse. Asystole does not have any electrical activity to reorganize. In PEA, the electrical activity is already organized; it is just not producing a palpable pulse for any of a variety of reasons.

Recommended Settings or Dose. Biphasic machines: 200 J to start or the manufacturer's recommended setting for first and successive doses. Monophasic machines: 360 J, all shocks.

Precautions. Electrical shock, SYNC button activated, patients who are wet and/or hairy.

- The electrical impulse delivered during defibrillation is much larger than that given during TCP, so the possibility of bystanders or rescuers getting a shock is very real. It is important to "clear" the patient before delivering the shock: announce that the shock is about to be delivered and perform a visual inspection so that no one is in contact with the patient or anything the patient is in contact with (including the stretcher, ETT, or intravenous line).

- If the defibrillation shock will not deliver (even if the machine is charged and pads are making good contact with the patient's skin), ensure that the SYNC button is not activated. If it is, the machine is waiting to figure out when to deliver the shock. This will never happen because there is no QRS to find in VF.

- Patients who are wet or excessively hairy should be handled as described in the TCP section.

Considerations. Continuity of CPR. Minimize interruptions in CPR during pulse and rhythm checks or intubation attempts. The continuity of high-quality compressions at a rate of at least 100 per minute and approximately 2 inches deep is crucial to the patient having any chance of survival. After the shock is delivered, immediately resume CPR for 2 minutes unless the patient immediately regains and maintains consciousness.

Therapeutic Process.

1. Take standard precautions if not already done. The patient should meet criteria described above.

2. Place pads on the patient. One pad should be placed inferior to the right clavicle, and the other should be placed on the left anterior axillary line at about the level of the 5th intercostal space. It is important that you explain to any family members who are present what is about to happen.

3. Attach wires from the pads to the pacing/defibrillation cable of the cardiac monitor.

4. Ensure the SYNC button is not activated.

5. Select your initial setting according to above.

6. Charge the system. During the time that the system is charging, clear all personnel and bystanders from the patient.

7. Announce loudly, "Everyone clear!"

8. Press the SHOCK button. The machine will discharge the shock immediately.

9. Resume CPR immediately, unless the patient regains consciousness. This is regardless of whether there was a rhythm change.

10. Repeat until the patient regains spontaneous circulation, enters a nonshockable rhythm such as PEA and asystole, or a physician gives orders to terminate the resuscitation effort.

POSTRESUSCITATION CARE

When a patient achieves ROSC, the paramedic's new priority is to prevent a reentry back into cardiac arrest. This is a multistep process that involves stabilizing the heart rate and rhythm, maintaining a viable blood pressure, and maintaining an airway and ventilation if not previously secured.

1. Stabilize the Rhythm

For patients coming out of a cardiac arrest that presented with VF or VT at any time during the resuscitation, the first priority is to prevent recurrence of these rhythms. If not done during the resuscitation, administer a loading dose of amiodarone (1.5 mg/kg) or amiodarone (300 mg). Once this bolus has been administered, initiate an infusion of that same medication. For lidocaine, inject 100 mg into 100 mL NSS to create a 1 mg/mL solution and run the infusion at 1–4 mg/min according to medical control's direction. For amiodarone, run the infusion at 1 mg/min for the first 6 hours after ROSC. If an antidysrhythmic was used during resuscitation prior to ROSC, stay with that medication for postresuscitation care.

2. Stabilize the Heart Rate

Frequently, a patient's heart resumes slowly after conversion from a nonperfusing rhythm and gradually accelerates to a more normal heart rate. If the patient's rhythm is bradycardic, consider a bolus of 0.5–1 mg atropine intravenously, especially if the blood pressure is low. If the atropine does not work, initiate TCP for bradycardia with low blood pressure (symptomatic bradycardia).

3. Stabilize the Blood Pressure

The goal of post-resuscitation care should include maintenance of a blood pressure. The systolic blood pressure (SBP) should be a minimum of 90 mmHg with a MAP of at least 65 mmHg. Ultimately, the BP and overall patient status should return to pre-arrest values.

The first step in stabilizing the blood pressure (as noted) is to administer a fluid bolus of 500 mL of normal saline. This will directly increase preload, which should translate into a higher blood pressure. More than that amount in a short time on an already sick heart could precipitate pulmonary edema and other signs of fluid overload. This is not a case where if some is good, more is better.

If a fluid bolus has not sufficiently increased blood pressure, a vasopressor may be given. The options available to the paramedic are dopamine and epinephrine. For dopamine, inject 400 mg into a 250 mL bag of NSS to create a 1,600 mcg/mL concentration. Run this at 2–5 mcg/kg/min to start and titrate to effect up to 20 mcg/kg/min. The goal of the titration is an SBP of 100 mmHg. Once that value is achieved, turn down the infusion rates and maintain that blood pressure.

Epinephrine may be given to the patient as either a drip or a push, depending on protocols. Prepare an epinephrine drip infusion by injecting 1 mg of a 1 mg/mL concentration into a 100 mL bag of NSS to create a 10 mcg/mL concentration. Run this at 0.1–0.5 mcg/kg/min and titrate to effect.

The push-dose route of epinephrine creates the same concentration of epinephrine as the infusion, but it is faster to prepare and easier to administer. First, expel 9 mL of epinephrine from a 1 mg/10 mL prefilled syringe. Next, replace that volume with 9 mL of saline and mix well; this new mixture contains a 10 mcg/mL concentration of epinephrine. Then administer the new mixture by injecting 1–2 mL as needed to maintain the target SBP and MAP (typically every 1–5 minutes).

Finally, if the blood pressure allows, raise the head of the bed to about 30° to promote cerebral drainage. Once concerns with rate, rhythm, and blood pressure have been addressed, therapeutic hypothermia may be considered and initiated, depending on local protocols. Note that some recent studies do not support the use of therapeutic hypothermia in the prehospital environment for these patients.

4. Stabilize the Airway and Oxygen Saturation

If not already done, secure the airway and maintain the patient's oxygen saturation. Airway may be secured via intubation, supraglottic device, or other method based on local protocols or medical direction. (See the airway chapter for detailed discussion of these procedures.) Carefully maintain the oxygen saturation at 95–99% to minimize the risk of hyperoxia or hypoxemia, and continue to monitor the $ETCO_2$ to guard against hypercarbia, as well.

AHA Updates for CPR and ECC

The 2020 AHA Guidelines for CPR & ECC (available in full at **cpr.heart.org**), largely retain and re-emphasize the AHA's preceding recommendations. This document's key points for paramedics are as follows:

Adult patients:

- Early initiation of CPR continues to be emphasized.
- Early access to defibrillation and initiation of ACLS procedures are still recommended.
- Early administration of epinephrine is still recommended.
- Continuous $ETCO_2$ monitoring and early administration of epinephrine to nonshockable rhythms continue to be emphasized.
- Close attention to blood pressure, oxygenation, and core temperature is needed to enhance likelihood of long-term survival.

Pediatric patients:

- Cuffed endotracheal tubes are suggested.
- Routine use of cricoid pressure is not recommended.
- Administration of epinephrine within 5 minutes is recommended in cardiac arrest, particularly in nonshockable rhythms.
- Titrated fluid resuscitation in combination with epinephrine (vasopressor) is recommended in septic shock.

Withholding Resuscitative Efforts

Withholding CPR means either deciding not to provide it in the first place or ceasing efforts once they have begun. A paramedic may encounter 3 situations that will signal that the patient has already been in cardiac arrest for too long to merit any attempts to even begin.

- **Putrefaction (rot)** and signs inconsistent with life: If the patient has been deceased for so long that putrefaction has begun, nothing can be done. Other signs inconsistent with life may also be present, such as decapitation.
- **Rigor mortis:** Rigor starts to set in approximately 8 hours after death and lasts 12–16 hours. During this time, the body is stiff from all the muscles becoming rigid.
- **Dependent lividity:** Lividity is the pooling of blood in the lowest areas of the body in response to gravity. It starts to be noticeable around 30 minutes after death and continues indefinitely because the heart is no longer pushing the blood around.

While these situations are pretty straightforward and easily observable, deciding when to stop resuscitative efforts after they have been begun—whether by the paramedics, other first responders, or bystanders—can be much more difficult.

There are very few hard and fast rules as to when to stop CPR versus bringing the patient to the hospital. For example, the patient's family may expect you to bring the patient to the hospital; bystanders similarly may view the paramedics and other responders negatively if they appear to just "give up." Next to consider is what to do with the body? It is becoming increasingly common to terminate resuscitations in the field rather than waste prehospital and in-hospital resources on a futile effort. The recommendation is that if **the paramedic believes that continuing resuscitative efforts will only prolong the inevitable**, contact medical control and solicit their input and acceptance. This is particularly true in the following situations:

- ROSC did not occur after all first-line treatments have been completed
- Patient has been in asystole for an extended period with no rhythm changes; no shocks administered
- No bystander CPR provided at any time
- Unwitnessed arrests

REVIEW QUESTIONS

Select the ONE best answer.

1. Which layer of the heart is damaged in a heart attack?

    A. Epicardium

    B. Myocardium

    C. Endocardium

    D. All of the above

2.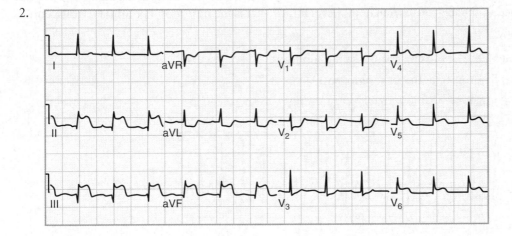

    Your patient presents with chest pain and the above ECG. Which coronary artery most likely is occluded?

    A. LAD

    B. LCx

    C. LMCA

    D. RCA

3. Mitral valve regurgitation means that blood flows backward through the mitral valve. Into which of the following structures does blood flow during mitral valve regurgitation?

    A. Left atrium

    B. Left ventricle

    C. Right atrium

    D. Right ventricle

4. During myocardial contraction, which of the following is true?

    A. Myocytes depolarize, and the cell potential becomes more negative.

    B. Myocytes depolarize, and the cell potential becomes more positive.

    C. Myocytes polarize, and the cell potential becomes more negative.

    D. Myocytes polarize, and the cell potential becomes more positive.

5. You notice an ECG of a patient has a PRI that is consistently 0.20 second long. There is a P wave for every QRS complex, but there is not a QRS complex for every P wave. Which of the following is most likely this patient's rhythm?

    A. First-degree block
    B. Second-degree heart block, Mobitz type I
    C. Second-degree heart block, Mobitz type II
    D. Sinus arrest

6. During a successful intubation attempt of a patient in severe respiratory distress, you notice your patient's heart rhythm is now marked sinus bradycardia at a rate of 34 when it was previously in the high 70s. The pulse oximetry remained in the high 90s throughout the attempt. What is the next most appropriate treatment?

    A. Begin CPR.
    B. Administer a 500 mL bolus of normal saline solution.
    C. Administer 0.5–1 mg atropine intravenously.
    D. Administer 1 mg epinephrine 1:10,000 intravenously.

7.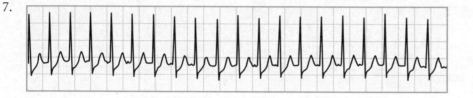

    You arrive at a residence for a 50-year-old female complaining of dizziness after syncope. Her vital signs are HR: 190, BP: 84/36, RR: 24, SpO$_2$: 99%. Her lead II tracing is above. What is the most appropriate treatment?

    A. Performing synchronized cardioversion at 100 J
    B. Performing synchronized cardioversion at 150 J
    C. Administering 6 mg adenosine followed with a 10 mL flush in a large vein
    D. Administering 12 mg adenosine followed with a 10 mL flush in a large vein

8. You have a 66-year-old patient found pulseless and apneic in his home. CPR was initiated by family members and is still continuing to produce a strong carotid pulse. The ECG shows the following rhythm, and you have started a 16-gauge intravenous line in the right EJ. Which medication is the best option for this patient?

    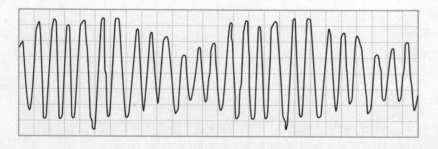

    A. 300 mg amiodarone
    B. 1 g calcium chloride
    C. 1 mg epinephrine 1:10,000
    D. 2 g magnesium sulfate

9. A 12-lead ECG reveals a QRS above the baseline in lead I and below the baseline in lead aVF. It also shows an RSR′ pattern in lead V$_1$. What is the most likely explanation for these findings?

   A. Left axis deviation and left bundle branch block

   B. Left axis deviation and right bundle branch block

   C. Right axis deviation and left bundle branch block

   D. Right axis deviation and right bundle branch block

10. Your patient is in cardiac arrest and the rhythm shows a pulseless 3rd-degree heart block at a rate of 30. All of the following are appropriate treatments for this patient EXCEPT:

    A. Continuous CPR.

    B. Treat the reversible causes (H's and T's).

    C. Pace the patient at a rate of 80 bpm.

    D. Epinephrine 1:10,000, 1 mg IVP every 3–5 minutes.

ANSWERS AND EXPLANATIONS

1. **The correct answer is (B).** The myocardium is the actual muscle layer of the heart, and it is the part of the heart that is damaged during a heart attack. The epicardium (A) and endocardium (C) are fibrous layers that are not generally damaged during a heart attack.

2. **The correct answer is (D).** The ECG shows ST segment elevation in leads II, III, and aVF, which indicates an inferior wall MI. The RCA services the inferior wall of the heart in most of the population.

3. **The correct answer is (A).** The mitral valve is the valve between the left atrium and the left ventricle. During systole, this valve ordinarily prevents backflow of blood from the left ventricle into the left atrium. This is not the case in mitral valve regurgitation.

4. **The correct answer is (B).** When myocytes are polarized just prior to contraction, the resting potential is approximately −90 mV. During contraction, the myocytes depolarize, which means the potential becomes approximately 0 mV. This means that the cell potential has become more positive.

5. **The correct answer is (C).** First-degree heart block (A) would not typically drop a complex after a P wave. Second-degree heart block, Mobitz type I (B) does not have a consistent PR. Sinus arrest (D) would drop the entire complex, including the P wave, not just the QRS complexes.

6. **The correct answer is (C).** Intubation attempts in patients with a pulse often can lead to a bradycardic rhythm because of stimulation of the vagus nerve. Administration of a parasympatholytic such as atropine should be the next step. Fluid (B) will not improve the situation. Epinephrine (D) is a little too aggressive a treatment for this. CPR (A) could be appropriate in a child but not an adult.

7. **The correct answer is (A).** The rhythm is SVT, and the low blood pressure combined with mentation changes illustrated by the syncope and ongoing dizziness indicate that the rhythm is hemodynamically unstable. The initial treatment for this is synchronized cardioversion at 50–100 J. (B) is correct for a wide, complex tachycardia. If the rhythm was stable and not associated with hypotension or mentation changes, then (C) would be correct, followed by (D) if not successful.

8. **The correct answer is (D).** Magnesium sulfate is the definitive treatment for torsade de pointes or polymorphic VT. Treatment with amiodarone (A) and epinephrine (C) are secondary to magnesium because polymorphic VT is refractory to treatments typically used with monomorphic VT. Calcium chloride (B) is a tertiary treatment in cases that may have resulted from hyperkalemia.

9. **The correct answer is (B).** The QRS up in lead I and down in lead aVF indicates a left axis deviation and the RSR′ pattern in lead V_1 indicates a right bundle branch block.

10. **The correct answer is (C).** Although the rhythm is a bradycardic rhythm, because there is no pulse, pacing is not an appropriate treatment. Once pulses return, pacing can then be an option.

Medical Emergencies 6

Learning Objectives

❏ Differentiate, assess, and treat neurological emergencies, including stroke, seizures, and syncope.

❏ Differentiate, assess, and treat various disorders of the endocrine system.

❏ Differentiate, assess, and treat allergic reactions, anaphylaxis, and other derangements of the immune system, including infectious diseases.

❏ Differentiate, assess, and treat poisonings and overdoses from common and uncommon sources of exposure.

❏ Differentiate, assess, and treat various conditions associated with gastrointestinal bleeding, the acute abdomen, and abdominal pain.

❏ Differentiate, assess, and treat various disorders of the genitourinary system, including kidney and bladder problems.

❏ Differentiate, assess, and treat various disorders of the blood, including hemophilia, polycythemia, and sickle cell disease.

❏ Differentiate, assess, and manage behavioral disorders, including depression, suicidal ideation, mania, and bipolar disorders.

❏ Differentiate, assess, and treat environmental emergencies.

This chapter addresses all the medical emergencies a paramedic could encounter that are not cardiac or respiratory in nature, whether they are neurological emergencies or environmental. The discussion includes the pathophysiology, assessment, and treatment of ailments for which a paramedic may be summoned.

NEUROLOGICAL EMERGENCIES

Neurological emergencies include any problem that involves the brain, the spinal cord, or peripheral nerves—including all supporting circulation. This section will discuss such life-threatening problems as stroke and seizures, plus other issues of the central and peripheral nervous system.

Anatomy and Physiology

The nervous system can be divided into the central nervous system (CNS) and the peripheral nervous system (PNS). The CNS consists of the brain and the spinal cord, while the PNS includes all the nerve branches emanating off the spinal cord and those arising directly from the brain itself (called cranial nerves). The PNS connects the CNS with the rest of the body through its vast network of nerves, and those nerves can be somatic or autonomic. Somatic nerves include all the sensory nerves (also called afferent neurons) leading from the body to the brain, and all the motor nerves (also called efferent neurons) that carry signals from the brain to the muscles and glands of the body. The autonomic nervous system regulates the automatic, or involuntary, activities of the body, including heart rate, breathing, digestion, and pupil size, among many others. Finally, the autonomic nervous system can be further divided into the sympathetic and parasympathetic nervous systems.

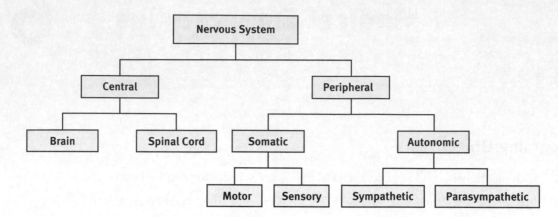

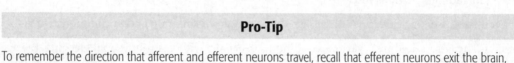

Figure 6-1. Major Divisions of the Nervous System

> ### Pro-Tip
>
> To remember the direction that afferent and efferent neurons travel, recall that efferent neurons exit the brain, and are thus motor nerves.

Brain

The brain is covered with tough and comparatively thick connective tissue called meninges. The 3 layers from the inside (closest to the brain) to the outside (closest to the skull) are the pia mater, the arachnoid mater, and the dura mater. Together, they help protect the brain, anchor it within the skull, and contain within the layers CSF, which further cushions the brain when it moves inside the skull.

The **cerebrum** or cerebral cortex is the biggest part of the brain. Its surface has many folds and bulges, called **sulci** (sulcus, singular) and **gyri** (gyrus, singular), which increase the surface area. It is divided into right and left hemispheres, or halves, and each half receives sensory information from and sends motor direction to the opposite side of the body.

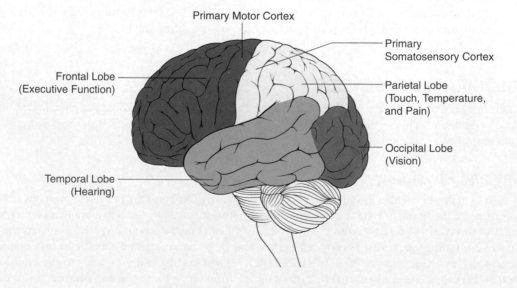

Figure 6-2. Lobes of the Brain

The outer surface of the brain is called the **cerebral cortex** (sometimes called the **neocortex**, a reminder that the cortex is the most recent brain region to evolve). The cerebrum is divided into 2 halves, called **cerebral hemispheres**. The surface of the cortex is divided into 4 lobes: frontal lobe, parietal lobe, occipital lobe, and temporal lobe (identified above as a side view of the left cerebral hemisphere).

The **frontal lobe** is composed of 2 regions: the prefrontal cortex and the motor cortex. The **prefrontal cortex** manages executive function by supervising and directing the operations of other brain regions. This region supervises processes associated with perception, memory, emotion, impulse control, and long-term planning. In memory, for instance, the role of the prefrontal cortex is not to store any memory traces; rather, it reminds the individual of having something to remember at all. To regulate attention and alertness, the prefrontal cortex communicates with the reticular formation in the brainstem, telling an individual either to wake up or relax, depending on the situation.

Damage to the prefrontal cortex impairs its overall supervisory functions. A person with a prefrontal lesion may be more impulsive (generally less in control of behavior) or depressed. It is not unusual, for instance, for someone with a prefrontal lesion to make vulgar and inappropriate sexual remarks or to be apathetic.

Pro-Tip

Because it integrates information from different cortical regions, the prefrontal cortex is a good example of an **association area**, an area that integrates input from diverse brain regions (e.g., multiple inputs may be necessary to solve a complex puzzle or plan for the future). Contrast an association area with a **projection area**, which performs more rudimentary perceptual and motor tasks (e.g., the visual cortex, which receives visual input from the retina, and the motor cortex, which sends out motor commands to the muscles).

The **primary motor cortex** is located on the **precentral gyrus** (just in front of the **central sulcus** that divides the frontal and parietal lobes) and initiates voluntary motor movements by sending neural impulses down the spinal cord toward the muscles. As such, it is considered a projection area in the brain. The neurons in the motor cortex are arranged systematically according to the parts of the body to which they are connected. This organizational pattern can be visualized through the **motor homunculus**. Because certain sets of muscles require finer motor control than others, they take up additional space in the cortex relative to their size in the body.

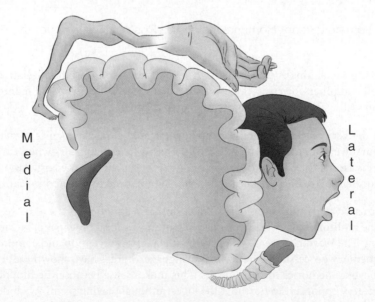

Figure 6-3. Motor Homunculus on the Precentral Gyrus of the Frontal Lobe

A third important part of the frontal lobe is the **Broca area**, which is vitally important for speech production. The Broca area is usually found in only one hemisphere, the so-called dominant hemisphere. For most people—both right- and left-handed—the dominant hemisphere is the left hemisphere.

The **parietal lobe** is located to the rear of the frontal lobe. The **somatosensory cortex** is located on the **postcentral gyrus** (just behind the central sulcus) and is involved in somatosensory information processing. This projection area is the destination for all incoming sensory signals for touch, pressure, temperature, and pain. Despite certain differences, the somatosensory cortex and the motor cortex are very closely related. In fact, they are so interrelated they sometimes are described as a single unit: the sensorimotor cortex. The somatosensory homunculus is shown here.

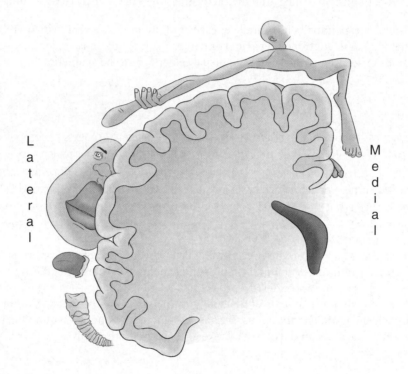

Figure 6-4. Somatosensory Homunculus on the Postcentral Gyrus of the Parietal Lobe

The central region of the parietal lobe is associated with spatial processing and manipulation. This region makes it possible to orient oneself and other objects in three-dimensional space, perform spatial manipulation of objects, and apply spatial orientation skills, such as those required for map reading.

The **occipital lobes**, at the very rear of the brain, contain the **visual cortex**, which is sometimes called the **striate cortex**. Striate means furrowed or striped, which is how the visual cortex appears when examined under a microscope. The visual cortex is one of the best-understood brain regions, owing to the large amount of research that has been done on visual processing. Areas in the occipital lobe also have been implicated in learning and motor control.

The **temporal lobes** are associated with a number of functions. The auditory cortex and Wernicke's area are located in the temporal lobe. The **auditory cortex** is the primary site of most sound processing, including speech, music, and other sound information. The **Wernicke area** is associated with language reception and comprehension. The temporal lobe also functions in memory processing, emotion, and language. Studies have shown that electrical stimulation of the temporal lobes can evoke memories for past events. This makes sense because the hippocampus is located deep inside the temporal lobe. It is important to note that the lobes, although having seemingly independent functions, are not truly independent of one another. Often, a sensory modality may be represented in more than one area.

Cerebral Hemispheres and Laterality

In most cases, each side of the brain communicates with the opposite side of the body. In such cases, the cerebral hemisphere communicates **contralaterally**. For example, the motor neurons on the left side of the brain activate movements on the right side of the body. In other cases (for instance, hearing), the cerebral hemispheres communicate with the same side of the body. In such cases, the hemispheres communicate **ipsilaterally**.

The dominant and nondominant hemispheres can be distinguished. The dominant hemisphere is typically defined as the one more heavily stimulated during language reception and production. In the past, hand dominance was used as a proxy for hemispheric dominance; that is, right-handed individuals were assumed to have left-dominant brains, and left-handed individuals were assumed to have right-dominant brains (because the brain communicates contralaterally with the hand). However, this correlation has not held up under scrutiny; 95% of right-handed individuals are indeed left-brain dominant, but only 18% of left-handed individuals are right-brain dominant.

The **dominant hemisphere** (usually the left) is primarily analytic in function, making it well suited for managing details. For instance, language, logic, and math skills are all located in the dominant hemisphere. Again, language production (the Broca area) and language comprehension (the Wernicke area) are primarily driven by the dominant hemisphere.

The **nondominant hemisphere** (usually the right) is associated with intuition, creativity, music cognition, and spatial processing. The nondominant hemisphere simultaneously processes the pieces of a stimulus and assembles them into a holistic image. The nondominant hemisphere serves a less prominent role in language. It is more sensitive to the emotional tone of spoken language and permits us to recognize others' moods based on visual and auditory cues, which adds to communication. The dominant hemisphere screens incoming language to analyze its content, and the nondominant hemisphere interprets it according to its emotional tone. The roles of the dominant and nondominant hemispheres are summarized only; remember that the left hemisphere is the dominant hemisphere in most individuals, regardless of handedness.

Diencephalon

The **diencephalon** is a region near the center of the cerebral cortex composed of several distinct structures: the thalamus, the hypothalamus, the posterior pituitary gland, and the pineal gland. The basal ganglia and the limbic system are closely related to the diencephalon, so those structures will be discussed here as well.

The **thalamus** serves as a relay station for all sensory information entering the brain from everywhere in the body, with the exception of the sense of smell. The thalamus sorts the information and relays it to the proper area of the cerebral cortex for interpretation and response.

The **hypothalamus** is located just inferior to the thalamus (hence its name) and is involved in maintaining homeostasis, hunger, and emotional responses. Because the hypothalamus regulates metabolism, body temperature, and water balance, it is the primary player in causing hunger, and it causes thirst through a process related to its release of antidiuretic hormone (ADH). ADH is released when receptors in the hypothalamus sense that the salt level in the blood is too concentrated, stimulating thirst and the kidneys to reabsorb more water. Finally, the hypothalamus plays a role in aggressive and sexual behaviors.

The posterior pituitary gland is the place where hypothalamic hormones enter the bloodstream, beginning the journey to their target organs. Oxytocin, also released by the hypothalamus, enters circulation via the posterior pituitary gland. The **pineal gland**, a small gland located posterior to the thalamus, is responsible for the body's circadian rhythms and releasing melatonin. Melatonin is produced in greater quantities in the dark and is believed to help us go to sleep.

Lateral to each lobe of the thalamus in each hemisphere of the brain are the **basal ganglia**. These structures are involved in coordinating movement so that posture is maintained and other coordinated movements are smooth and fluid. Damage or destruction to the basal ganglia results in Parkinson disease (PD).

Limbic System

The **limbic system** is a group of structures closely related to the diencephalon that are primarily associated with memory. The primary components include the septal nuclei, the amygdala, and the hippocampus.

The **septal nuclei** contain the pleasure centers of the brain. Stimulation of the septal nuclei is intensely pleasurable, and it is believed that these nuclei are responsible for addictive behaviors.

The **hippocampus** plays a vital role in memory formation and learning. It converts information into long-term memories and redistributes them to portions of the cerebral cortex associated with memory. The hippocampus is connected directly to the septal nuclei through a projection called the **fornix**. This connection between the memory formation processing center and the pleasure and emotional centers of the brain—the septal nuclei and anterior portion of the hypothalamus—explains why long-term memories of particularly emotional events, both positive and negative, are some of the most enduring of long-term memories. Damage to the hippocampus can cause the inability to form new long-term memories and is called **anterograde amnesia**. Previously formed memories usually remain intact. The opposite of anterograde amnesia is **retrograde amnesia**, in which memories prior to a brain injury are lost.

The **amygdala** is the fear and anger center of the brain, which is responsible for defensive and aggressive behaviors. Damage to or lesions within the amygdala result in a particularly docile and likely hypersexual person.

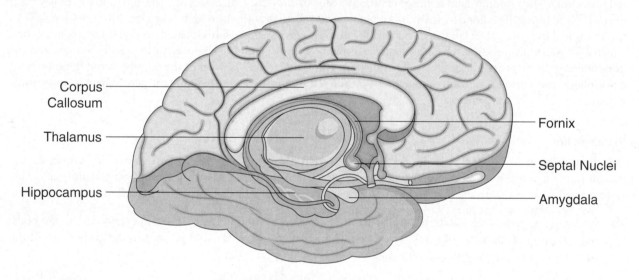

Figure 6-5. The Limbic System

Cerebellum

The **cerebellum** is the area of the brain found at the base of the posterior portion of the brain and appears different from any the other structure in the brain. The cerebellum is responsible for coordinated and smooth movements and for posture and balance. The cerebellum is closely related to the vestibulocochlear nerve, also known as cranial nerve VIII, which is responsible for hearing and balance. Damage to this area affects fine motor movements and causes slurred speech and overall poor balance. Alcohol impairs the cerebellum function.

Brainstem

The **brainstem** contains three distinct parts: the midbrain, the pons, and the medulla oblongata (referred to simply as the medulla). It is the most inferior part of the brain and is contiguous with the spinal column. Of the 12 cranial nerves, 10 arise directly from the brainstem. The brainstem then serves as a relay center to the appropriate areas of the cerebrum, or it handles autonomic functions directly. The **midbrain** is associated with involuntary reflexes and visual and auditory stimuli triggers. The **pons** lies between the midbrain and the medulla and contains nerve tracts that connect the midbrain to the medulla, the cerebellum, and the cerebrum. It contains centers that are associated with autonomic functions, including blinking, bladder control, changing from inhalation to exhalation, swallowing, and balance. The **medulla** regulates vital signs, including respiratory rate and depth, heart rate, and blood pressure. Damage to the medulla will eliminate these functions.

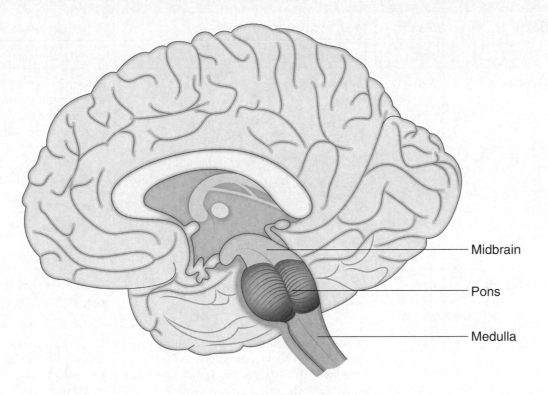

Figure 6-6. Brainstem Structures

Peripheral Nervous System

The PNS includes all the neurons outside the brain and spinal cord. These are further broken down into either the cranial nerves or spinal nerves, based on where they originate. Cranial nerves originate from the cerebrum, the diencephalon, the midbrain, the pons, or the medulla and reach their target organs without traveling down the spinal column. Spinal nerves, on the other hand, branch off the spinal cord and emerge from the space between the vertebrae.

Cranial Nerves

The 12 pairs of cranial nerves each have very specific functions. Some nerves have multiple functions, such as the vagus nerve that provides the parasympathetic innervation to all the visceral organs and motor control over most muscles in the pharynx; others have fewer functions, such as the trochlear nerve that controls exactly one muscle responsible for moving the eyeball toward the nose and down. Each of the 12 pairs of cranial nerves, an explanation of the functions, and methods to assess each are described in the table that follows.

Pro-Tip
Mnemonics exist to help you remember the cranial nerve names in order. For example: "Often Olga orders tasty treats and finally values growing voluptuous and happy." Other mnemonics can help you remember whether nerves are sensory, motor, or both. For example: "Some say money matters, but my brother says baking brownies matters more."

Table 6-1. Cranial Nerve Functions and Assessment

Nerve	Sensory or Motor	Function	Assessment
I. Olfactory	Sensory	Sense of smell	Not usually assessed.
II. Optic	Sensory	Sense of vision	Identify something.
III. Oculomotor	Motor	Levator palpebrae superioris—lifts upper eyelid Superior rectus—eyeball looks up Inferior rectus—eyeball looks down Medial rectus—eyeball looks toward the nose Inferior oblique—helps eye look up and laterally Sphincter pupillae—constricts the pupil Ciliary muscles—contracts, allowing for short-range vision	Have the patient follow your finger in the shape of a box with their eyes. Have the patient blink.
IV. Trochlear	Motor	Superior oblique—causes the eye to look down and in	Have the patient follow your finger in the shape of a box with their eyes.
V. Trigeminal	Both	Sensation to the face, forehead, eyelids, nose, nasal linings, cheeks, lips, gums, and teeth Movement of muscles of mastication (chewing) Spicy sensation in mouth	Touch the forehead, cheeks, and mandible gently with a sharp object to test all 3 branches of the nerve.
VI. Abducens	Motor	Lateral rectus of the eye—causes the eye to look laterally (away from the nose)	Have the patient follow your finger in the shape of a box with their eyes.
VII. Facial	Both	Controls facial expression Responsible for taste of the anterior 2/3 on the tongue Salivation from the submandibular salivary glands Lacrimation	Have the patient smile.
VIII. Vestibulocochlear (Auditory)	Sensory	Hearing from the cochlea and balance from the vestibular apparatus	Have the patient follow spoken word commands.
IX. Glossopharyngeal	Both	Sensation to the tongue, tonsils, pharynx, middle ear, and carotid body Taste from the posterior 1/3 of the tongue Salivation from the parotid gland Motor fibers to muscles of swallowing	Have the patient swallow.

(Continued)

Nerve	Sensory or Motor	Function	Assessment
X. Vagus	Both	Parasympathetic stimulation to all visceral organs, except the adrenal glands, and from the 3rd segment of the transverse colon through the rectum Muscles related to swallowing and the palatoglossus muscle of the tongue	Have the patient swallow.
XI. Accessory	Motor	Sternocleidomastoid muscle—rotates and tilts head Trapezius muscle—elevates the shoulders and abducts the arms.	Have the patient shrug their shoulders while pushing down on them to test symmetry.
XII. Hypoglossal	Motor	All muscles of the tongue except the palato-glossus (vagus).	Have the patient stick out their tongue.

Spinal Nerves

The 31 pairs of spinal nerves emerge from each side of the spinal column. The dorsal or posterior root is the afferent nerve bundle that carries sensory information from the body to the brain. Each set of afferent nerves services a specific area of the body, referred to as a dermatome. The ventral or anterior root carries the efferent or motor nerve fibers. Each set of efferent nerves supplies a specific set of muscles, known as the myotome.

Table 6-2. Myotomes

Level	Motor Function
C1–C6	Neck flexors
C1–T1	Neck extensors
C3, C4, C5	Supply diaphragm (mostly C4)
C5, C6	Move shoulder, raise arm (deltoid), and flex elbow (biceps)
C6	Externally rotate (supinate) the arm
C6, C7	Extend elbow and wrist (triceps and wrist extensors) and pronate wrist
C7, C8	Flex wrist and supply small muscles of the hand
T1–T6	Intercostals and trunk above the waist
T7–L1	Abdominal muscles
L1–L4	Flex thigh
L2, L3, L4	Extend leg at the knee and adduct thigh
L4, L5, S1	Abduct thigh, flex leg at the knee, dorsiflex foot (off gas pedal), and extend toes
L5, S1, S2	Extend leg at the hip, plantar flex foot (point foot), and flex toes

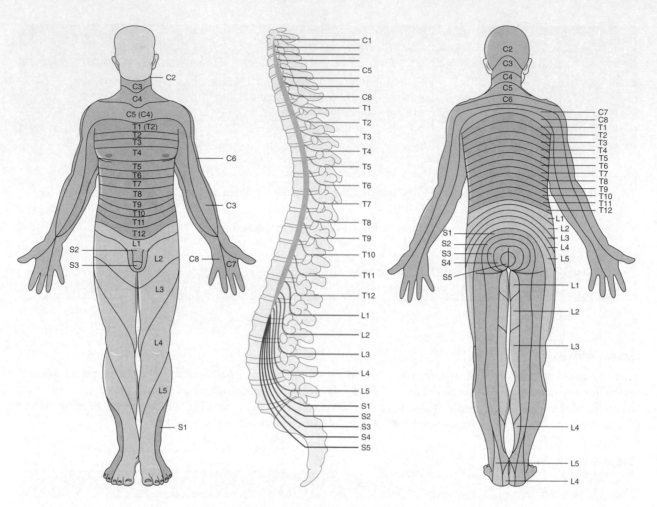

Figure 6-7. The Dermatomes

Cells of the Nervous System

Neurons are specialized cells capable of transmitting electrical impulses and then translating those electrical impulses to chemical signals. This section considers the structure of the neuron as well as how neurons communicate with other parts of the nervous system.

Neurons

Each neuron has a shape that matches its function, as dictated by the other cells with which that neuron interacts. A variety of different types of neurons are in the body, but they all share some specific features.

Like all other cells (besides mature red blood cells), neurons have nuclei. The nucleus is located in the **cell body**, also called the **soma**. The soma is also the location of the endoplasmic reticulum and ribosomes. The cell has many appendages emanating directly from the soma, called **dendrites**, that receive incoming messages from other cells. The information received from the dendrites is transmitted through the cell body before it reaches the **axon hillock**, which integrates the incoming signals. The axon hillock plays an important role in **action potentials**, or the transmission of electrical impulses down the axon. Signals arriving from the dendrites can be either excitatory or inhibitory; the axon hillock sums these signals; if the result is excitatory enough (reaching threshold, as discussed later in this chapter), it will initiate an action potential.

The **axon** is a long appendage that terminates in close proximity to a target structure (a muscle, a gland, or another neuron). Most mammalian nerve fibers are insulated by **myelin** to prevent signal loss or the crossing of signals. Just like insulation prevents wires next to each other from accidentally discharging each other, the **myelin sheath** maintains the electric signal within a single neuron. In addition, myelin increases the speed of conduction in the axon. Myelin is produced by **oligodendrocytes** in the CNS and **Schwann cells** in the PNS.

At certain intervals along the axon, small breaks in the myelin sheath with exposed areas of axon membrane are called the **nodes of Ranvier**. As will be explored in the discussion of action potentials to follow, the nodes of Ranvier are critical for rapid signal conduction. Finally, at the end of the axon is the **nerve terminal** or **synaptic bouton** (**knob**). This structure is enlarged and flattened to maximize neurotransmission to the next neuron and ensure the proper release of **neurotransmitters**, the chemicals that transmit information between neurons.

Neurons are not physically connected to each other. Between the neurons, there is a small space into which the terminal portion of the axon releases neurotransmitters, which bind to the dendrites of the postsynaptic neuron. This space is known as the **synaptic cleft**; together, the nerve terminal, the synaptic cleft, and the postsynaptic membrane are known as a **synapse**. Neurotransmitters released from the axon terminal traverse the synaptic cleft and bind to receptors on the postsynaptic neuron.

Multiple neurons may be bundled together to form a **nerve** in the PNS. These nerves may be **sensory**, **motor**, or **mixed**, which refers to the type(s) of information they carry; mixed nerves carry both sensory and motor information. The cell bodies of neurons of the same type are clustered together into ganglia.

In the CNS, axons may be bundled together to form **tracts**. Unlike nerves, tracts carry only one type of information. The cell bodies of neurons in the same tract are grouped into **nuclei**.

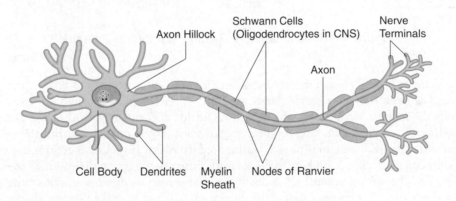

Figure 6-8. Structure of a Neuron

Transmission of Neural Impulses

Action Potential

After discussing the basic anatomy of the neuron, the focus turns to the physiology that underlies neuronal signaling. Neurons use all-or-nothing messages, called action potentials, to relay electrical impulses down the axon to the synaptic bouton. As will be explored in the following section, action potentials ultimately cause the release of neurotransmitters into the synaptic cleft.

Resting Potential

All neurons exhibit a resting membrane potential. This means that there is an electrical potential difference (voltage) between the inside of the neuron and the extracellular space. Usually, this is about −70 mV, with the inside of the neuron being negative relative to the outside. Neurons use selective permeability to ions and the **Na⁺/K⁺ ATPase** to maintain this negative internal environment.

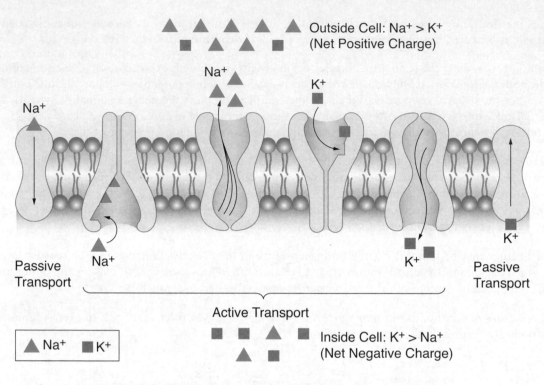

Figure 6-9. Maintenance of Resting Membrane Potential

Like any other cell, the neuronal plasma membrane is fairly impermeable to charged species. Because the plasma membrane contains a thick nonpolar barrier (fatty acid tails), it is not energetically favorable for ions to cross this barrier. Inside the neuron, K^+ is high and Na^+ is low. Outside of the neuron, Na^+ is high, whereas K^+ is low. The negative resting potential is generated by both negatively charged proteins within the cell and the relatively greater permeability of the membrane to K^+ compared with Na^+. If the cell membrane is more permeable to K^+ and the ion's concentration is higher inside, K^+ will diffuse down its gradient out of the cell. What does this mean in terms of charge movement? K^+ is positively charged, so its movement out of the cell results in a cell interior that is negative. Put another way, if the membrane starts at 0, and a positive charge is removed, the end result is a negative charge inside the cell: $0 - (+1) = -1$. Na^+ cannot readily enter at rest, so the negative potential is maintained.

The Na^+/K^+ ATPase is important for restoring this gradient after action potentials have been fired. It transports 3 Na^+ out of the cell for every 2 K^+ into the cell at the expense of 2 ATP (adenosine triphosphate). ATP is necessary because both Na^+ and K^+ are moved against their gradients by this process; thus, this qualifies as primary active transport. Each time the pump works, it results in the cell becoming relatively more negative: only two positive charges are moved in for every three that are moved out.

Axon Hillock

Neurons can receive both excitatory and inhibitory input. Excitatory input causes **depolarization** (raising the membrane potential, V_m, from its resting potential) and thus makes the neuron more likely to fire an action potential. Inhibitory input causes **hyperpolarization** (lowering the membrane potential from its resting potential) and thus makes the neuron less likely to fire an action potential. If the axon hillock receives enough excitatory input to be depolarized to the **threshold** value (usually in the range of −55 to −40 mV), an action potential will be triggered.

This implies that not every stimulus necessarily generates a response. A small excitatory signal may not be sufficient to bring the axon hillock to threshold. Further, a postsynaptic neuron may receive information from several different presynaptic neurons, some of which are excitatory and some of which are inhibitory. The additive effect of multiple signals is known as **summation**.

The two types of summation are temporal and spatial. In **temporal summation**, multiple signals are integrated during a relatively short period of time. A number of small excitatory signals firing at nearly the same moment could bring a postsynaptic cell to threshold, enabling an action potential. In **spatial summation**, the additive effects are based on the number and location of the incoming signals. A large number of inhibitory signals firing directly on the soma will cause more profound hyperpolarization of the axon hillock than the depolarization caused by a few excitatory signals firing on the dendrites of a neuron.

Ion Channels and Membrane Potential

A graph of membrane potential versus time during an action potential follows.

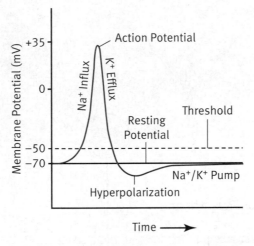

Figure 6-10. Action Potential Generation
Sufficient depolarization across the cell membrane to threshold leads to the generation of an action potential, followed by repolarization and hyperpolarization before returning to the resting membrane potential.

If the cell is brought to threshold, voltage-gated sodium channels open in the membrane. As the name implies, these ion channels open in response to the change in potential of the membrane (depolarization) and permit the passage of Na^+ ions. A strong **electrochemical gradient** promotes the migration of sodium into the cell. From an electric standpoint, the interior of the cell is more negative than the exterior of the cell, which favors the movement of positively charged Na^+ ions into the cell. From a chemical standpoint, the concentration of sodium outside the cell is higher than on the inside, which also favors the movement of sodium into the cell. As sodium passes through these ion channels, the membrane potential becomes more positive; that is, the cell rapidly depolarizes. Sodium channels not only open in response to changes in membrane potential but are also inactivated by them. When V_m approaches 35 mV, the sodium channels are **inactivated** and will have to be brought back near the resting potential to be **deinactivated**. Thus, these sodium channels can exist in three states: **closed** (before the cell reaches threshold and after inactivation has been reversed), **open** (from threshold to approximately 35 mV), and **inactive** (from approximately 35 mV to the resting potential).

The positive potential inside the cell triggers not only the voltage-gated sodium channels to inactivate but also the voltage-gated potassium channels to open. Once sodium has depolarized the cell, there is an electrochemical gradient favoring the efflux of potassium from the neuron. As positively charged potassium ions are driven out of the cell, there will be a restoration of the negative membrane potential called **repolarization**. The efflux of K^+ causes an overshoot of the resting membrane potential, hyperpolarizing the neuron. This hyperpolarization serves an important function: it makes the neuron refractory to further action potentials. There are two types of **refractory periods**. During the **absolute refractory period**, no amount of stimulation can cause another action potential to occur. During the **relative refractory period**, there must be greater than normal stimulation to cause an action potential because the membrane is starting from a potential that is more negative than its resting value.

The Na^+/K^+ ATPase acts to restore not only the resting potential but also the sodium and potassium gradients that have been partially dissipated by the action potential.

Impulse Propagation

So far, the movements of ions at one small segment of the axon have been discussed. For a signal to be conveyed to another neuron, the action potential must travel down the axon and initiate neurotransmitter release. This movement is called **impulse propagation**. As sodium rushes into one segment of the axon, it will cause depolarization in the surrounding regions of the axon. This depolarization will bring subsequent segments of the axon to threshold, opening the sodium channels in those segments. Each of these segments then continues through the rest of the action potential in a wavelike fashion until the action potential reaches the nerve terminal. After the action potential has fired in one segment of axon, that segment becomes momentarily refractory, as described previously. The functional consequence of this is that information can only flow in one direction.

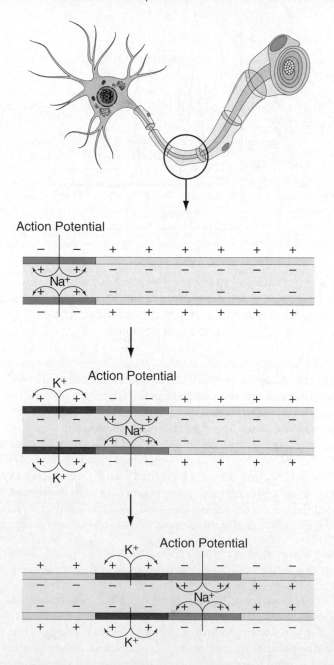

Figure 6-11. Action Potential Propagation

Action potentials are propagated down the axon when proximal sodium channels open and depolarize the membrane, inducing neighboring sodium channels to open as well; because of the refractory character of these channels, the action potential can move in only 1 direction.

The speed at which action potentials move depends on the length and cross-sectional area of the axon. Increased length of the axon results in higher resistance and slower conduction. Greater cross-sectional areas allow for faster propagation because of decreased resistance. The effect of cross-sectional area is more significant than the effect of length. To maximize the speed of transmission, mammals have myelin. Myelin is an extraordinarily good insulator that prevents the dissipation of the electric signal. The insulation is so effective that the membrane is permeable only to ion movement at the nodes of Ranvier. Thus, the signal "hops" from node to node—what is called **saltatory conduction**.

It is important to note that all action potentials within the same type of neuron have the same potential difference during depolarization. Increased intensity of a stimulus does not result in an increased potential difference of the action potential but rather an increased frequency of firing.

Synapse

As discussed previously, neurons are not actually in direct physical contact. There is a small space between neurons called the synaptic cleft into which neurotransmitters are secreted. To clarify the terminology, the neuron preceding the synaptic cleft is called the **presynaptic neuron**; the neuron after the synaptic cleft is called the **postsynaptic neuron**. If a neuron signals to a gland or muscle, rather than another neuron, the postsynaptic cell is termed an **effector**. Most synapses are **chemical** in nature; they use small molecules referred to as **neurotransmitters** to send messages from cell to cell.

Neurotransmitters

Prior to release, neurotransmitter molecules are stored in membrane-bound vesicles in the nerve terminal. When the action potential reaches the nerve terminal, voltage-gated calcium channels open, allowing calcium to flow into the cell. This sudden increase in intracellular calcium triggers fusion of the membrane-bound vesicles with the cell membrane at the synapse, causing exocytosis of the neurotransmitter.

Once released into the synapse, the neurotransmitter molecules diffuse across the cleft and bind to receptors on the postsynaptic membrane. This allows the message to be passed from one neuron to the next. As stated earlier, neurons may be either excitatory or inhibitory; this distinction truly comes at the level of the neurotransmitter receptors, which tend to be either ligand-gated ion channels or G protein-coupled receptors. If the receptor is a ligand-gated ion channel, the postsynaptic cell will either be depolarized or hyperpolarized. If it is a G protein-coupled receptor, it will cause either changes in the levels of cyclic AMP (cAMP; cyclic adenosine monophosphate) or an influx of calcium.

Neurotransmission must be regulated; there are almost no circumstances under which constant signaling to the postsynaptic cell would be desirable. Therefore, the neurotransmitter must be removed from the synaptic cleft. Three main mechanisms accomplish this goal. First, neurotransmitters can be broken down by enzymatic reactions. The breakdown of **acetylcholine (ACh)** by acetylcholinesterase (AChE) is a classic example.

Second, neurotransmitters can be brought back into the presynaptic neuron using **reuptake carriers**. The reuptake of **serotonin** is a classic example of this mechanism. **Dopamine** and **norepinephrine** also use reuptake carriers.

Third, neurotransmitters may simply diffuse out of the synaptic cleft. **Nitric oxide**, a gaseous signaling molecule, fits into this category.

General Assessment

As with any call, always begin by assuring that you arrive safely and have a safe scene for you and your partner to work. Once a secure scene has been reasonably established, form a general impression of the patient. This will help you determine early on the urgency of the situation: Is the patient seriously ill and requires rapid transportation or can some interventions be performed on scene before moving to the ambulance? Rapidly assess the ABCs and take appropriate steps to ensure a patent airway, adequate rate and depth of breathing, and adequate circulation.

When assessing the ABCs at this point, it is not essential to get numbers; merely ensuring that what they have will last to the ambulance, or until a time to fully evaluate respiratory and pulse rates, is sufficient.

Regardless of the chief complaint, every patient should be evaluated for their level of consciousness; however, this is especially true for neurological emergencies. Early and frequent assessment of the neurological status of any patient is essential to be able to track the progression of the issue. Several methods can be used to assess a patient's level of consciousness: AVPU, degree of orientation, and Glasgow Coma Scale (GCS).

AVPU

AVPU is a mnemonic that will help you remember the tenets of the most basic level of consciousness:

- **A = alert or awake** and indicates that the patient's eyes are open. It makes no assumptions about the patient's ability to converse, answer questions, or follow directions. The patient could be confused or even unable to communicate.

- **V = verbally responsive,** and the patient can respond in any fashion to such stimulus. If the patient's eyes cannot open or remain open throughout contact, the patient may be responsive only to verbal stimuli. Calling the patient's name may then cause them to open their eyes, perhaps look at you if only briefly, or possibly even have a conversation with you. This person is then said to be responsive to verbal stimuli only.

- **P = painfully responsive,** wherein the patient responds in any fashion to a painful or noxious stimulus. After calling the patient's name or speaking very loudly in their ear, attempt to elicit a response to pain. The key here is to cause the patient sufficient pain to respond but not enough to leave a mark or bruise. This can be successfully done in several ways. First, apply pressure to the finger nail bed with a pen pressing directly on the cuticle. (Keep in mind that this will not work for a person with a spinal lesion higher than T2 because the pain sensation will not reach the brain.) Next, pressure can be applied to the fleshy part of the hand between the thumb and the forefinger. Finally, another choice is to squeeze the trapezius muscle about 3 cm lateral to the neck. Although not painful, it evaluates the corneal reflex and provides insight into the patient's level of consciousness. This reflex protects the patient's eyes by tightly and quickly closing the eyelids. Even if the patient's eyes are already closed, the lids will twitch noticeably. When a patient's eyes are closed, lightly tapping the area of the forehead between the eyebrows or brushing a finger across the patient's eyelids will stimulate this reflex.

- **U = unresponsive**. Once the attempt to elicit a painful response has failed, the patient is not unresponsive to verbal and painful stimuli. It is important here to distinguish between unconscious and unresponsive. Unconscious is a diagnosis, whereas this patient is unresponsive to techniques used to this point.

Orientation

As already mentioned, the A in AVPU means only that a patient will perform spontaneous eye-opening. This should be coupled with the degree of orientation the patient can orally provide. Orientation is assessed by determining whether patients know who they are and where they are and can correctly describe a reference of time. Ask the patient the following 3 questions:

1. Person: "What is your name?"
2. Place: "Where are you currently?" Generic answers, such as "I am at a restaurant" or "at a park," can be correct because the person may not have known the specific name of the place.
3. Time: "What day/month/year is it?" Any one of these can be used, but an accurate response is important. A patient who answers incorrectly and fails to self-correct without being prompted is said to be disoriented to time.

Patients with neurological problems often lose orientation of time, place, and person—in that order. Orientation to time tends to be lost first. Time is the most transient of the three categories and thus the easiest to forget. (Even fully oriented people often need a calendar to remember whether today is Tuesday or Wednesday!) Place tends to "stick" longer unless the person is in an unfamiliar location. Someone who is at home, for example, is less likely to forget where they are. Person is generally the last degree of orientation to be lost; people tend to keep the same name (or at least the same first name) throughout their lives, making it the most consistent of the three categories.

Responding correctly on all 3 orientation questions means the patient is alert and oriented times 3 (A&O×3); if the patient misses a question, the patient is A&O×2, and so on. Some authorities recommend asking patients a fourth question to determine their orientation: What happened? A person who can successfully provide a detailed history of the present illness or complaint might then be described as A&O×4.

Glasgow Coma Scale

The **GCS** is a comprehensive tool that assigns a numeric value to a person's level of consciousness. During assessment of the patient, assign the patient a score in each of the categories and then add the numbers from each category. Generally, an adult with a total score <8 (<5 for children) is considered critical. The person is most likely unable to maintain a patent airway because the gag reflex is lost; the patient should be aggressively managed and frequently reassessed.

Table 6-3. Glasgow Coma Scale

Category	Score	Adult (≤7)	Pediatric (<5)
Eye opening	4	Spontaneous	Spontaneous
	3	Verbal stimulus	Verbal stimulus
	2	Painful stimulus	Painful stimulus
	1	Unresponsive	Unresponsive
Best verbal response	5	Oriented	Smiles/coos/babbles
	4	Confused	Consolable, inappropriate interactions
	3	Inappropriate words	Inconsolable, inappropriate cry
	2	Garbled	Grunting and ineffective whimpering
	1	None	None
Best motor response	6	Obeys commands	Obeys commands
	5	Localizes pain	Withdraws from touch
	4	Withdraws from pain	Withdraws from pain
	3	Decorticate posturing	Decorticate posturing
	2	Decerebrate posturing	Decerebrate posturing
	1	None	None

Neurological Assessment Points

Pupils

It has been said that the eyes are the windows to the soul. In more practical terms, the pupils are the window to the functional status of the brain. Examine the pupils for reactivity to light, size, and shape.

- **Shape.** The pupils should be round. Oval pupils could indicate glaucoma. Pupils in the shape of a keyhole are likely the result of cataract surgery. Other shapes are associated with birth malformations.

- **Size.** Estimating the size of the pupil can be helpful during reassessment to identify changes. Pupils should be roughly equal in size and should not be either extremely large (dilated) or pinpoint (constricted). Dilated pupils could indicate pressure on CN III, the oculomotor nerves, or stimulant overdose such as cocaine. Pinpoint pupils likely indicate opiate overdose or one of several signs and symptoms of organophosphate poisoning. Pupils should be equal in size. If pupils are unequal, it could be related to a head injury and pressure on one side of CN III. It also could be normal for the patient—called anisocoria—which occurs in about 10% of the population.

- **Reactivity.** Pupils should constrict to a light directed at them and dilate as the light is removed. This reaction should be brisk and happen in <1 second. Pupils that do not constrict at all (or dilate in the dark) could indicate a drug overdose or a head injury. Slowed constriction could indicate cerebral or medullary ischemia.

Speech

As noted in the GCS, verbal responses and the quality of them is an important assessment finding in the patient with neurological deficits. First evaluate the quality of the speech according to the GCS. Is it slurred or garbled? Are the words appropriate? There are several situations in which a person can have clear speech but incorrect word choice. Agnosia is when a patient is unable to tell you the correct name for a common object because of a breakdown in communication between the visual cortex in the occipital lobe of the brain and the temporal lobe where general knowledge is stored. Apraxia is a situation where the patient may be able to name the object in question (occipital to temporal lobe communication is intact); however, the patient is completely incapable of demonstrating how to use it. In this case, nerve tracts between knowledge in the temporal lobe and the motor cortex in the frontal lobe have been damaged.

A patient may have receptive aphasia, which is a condition where the patient is unable to understand what is communicated to them either written or verbally. Receptive aphasia results from damage to the Wernicke area located in the left hemisphere of the brain, whether from a medical event or a traumatic event. Patients with receptive aphasia are often able to speak clearly; however, the words they use are frequently nonsensical, made up words. Sentence structure appears intact, but the sentences are completely devoid of any meaning or ability to be interpreted. They also often talk continuously, though with seemingly appropriate intonation and inflection. Frequently, these patients also are completely unaware that the speech they are saying is nonsensical because they cannot understand their own words either.

The opposite of this is expressive aphasia, where the patient cannot form or select the words needed to complete a thought or a sentence. The patient understands completely what is happening around them and is able to understand spoken and written communication. The patient's speech is effortful but often visibly frustrating. The patient can follow commands because the speech interpretation area (Wernicke area) is intact; here, the Broca area is damaged or impaired, resulting in telegraphic speech—speech where only important words are spoken after some time of deliberate concentration on forming them. If the patient smiles when instructed to do so but cannot clearly state the action performed, the patient most likely has expressive aphasia.

Global aphasia is a complete disruption of verbal or written communication. The patient displays both expressive and receptive aphasia. The patient may blurt out incomprehensible words or syllables, but otherwise, any communication attempted cannot be interpreted. This patient is still able to think and interact with their environment through other senses; the patient just has no way of communicating this.

Pathophysiology, Assessment, and Treatment of Neurological Conditions

Stroke

Pathophysiology

Stroke is a condition where blood flow to an area of the brain is compromised. A stroke can be either ischemic or hemorrhagic in nature. **Ischemic strokes**, sometimes referred to as occlusive strokes, result from a blockage to an artery that services a part of the brain or possibly the entire hemisphere. Ischemic strokes can be further differentiated into thrombic or embolic. In a **thrombic stroke**, the clot formed right there in that artery. In an **embolic stroke**, the clot formed elsewhere in the body and traveled to its current location. The most common locations for clots to form that eventually release the embolus resulting in a stroke are the heart or carotid arteries. In cases of AF, clots can form as a result of blood stasis in the atria if the AF is not found early enough or if the patient is not properly anticoagulated. A piece of this clot or the entire thing may break loose and travel into the brain. If the leaflets to the aortic valve are damaged for any reason, clots will form on the leaflets, which can then embolize into the brain. The carotid arteries may become damaged after years of high blood pressure and arterial or atherosclerotic plaque can build up inside the artery. This, too, can break apart and embolize up to the brain.

In a **hemorrhagic stroke**, an artery in the brain has weakened and ruptured, compromising the blood-brain barrier. This bleeding will continue, leading to increasingly worsening symptoms over time and increased ICP; eventually, the brainstem will herniate out of the skull and compress the medulla. Once the medulla becomes compressed, vital sign regulation will become erratic and fail, resulting in certain death for the patient. The progressive worsening of symptoms seen in a hemorrhagic stroke is in stark contrast to an ischemic stroke, where symptoms typically come on suddenly and remain, rather than worsen. Between bleeding into the brain tissue and the increasing pressure inside the cranial vault, the damage resulting from a hemorrhagic stroke often is irreversible and pervasive.

Assessment of Stroke

Depending on the location of the lesion—the occlusion or hemorrhage—stroke symptoms are widely varied and affect multiple functions. Patients will often state that they are having the worst headache of their life, and, frequently, this headache is focused on one side of the head. The patient also may exhibit weakness, a loss of sensation, or paralysis to the side of the body opposite the side on which the headache is located. If the lesion includes the visual cortex or the auditory cortex, visual or hearing disturbances also may be noted.

To help prehospital providers determine the severity of the stroke, various scales can be used to guide assessment of a patient who has had a stroke. The Cincinnati Prehospital Stroke Scale and the Los Angeles Prehospital Stroke Screen are good examples of such scales. If a finding is abnormal in the Cincinnati Prehospital Stroke Scale, it predicts a stroke 72% of the time. If the criteria numbered 1–6 in the Los Angeles Prehospital Stroke Screen are all "yes," it predicts a stroke 97% of the time.

Table 6-4. Los Angeles Prehospital Stroke Screen

Criteria			
1. Age >45	Yes	No	Unknown
2. History of seizures or epilepsy absent	Yes	No	Unknown
3. Symptoms <24 hours	Yes	No	Unknown
4. Patient was not wheelchair or bed bound prior.	Yes	No	Unknown
5. Blood glucose level between 60 and 400 mg/dL	Yes	No	Unknown
6. Notable asymmetry in any 1 of the 3:	Yes	No	Unknown
Test	**Right**	**Left**	**Equal?**
Have patient smile	Moves less	Moves less	Equal
Have patient squeeze your fingers as tightly as possible	Weaker/None	Weaker/None	Equal
With palms up and eyes closed, hold patient's arms out in front of them. Ask the patient to hold up their arms	Drifts/Falls	Drifts/Falls	Both held up equally

Table 6-5. Cincinnati Prehospital Stroke Scale

Assessment Point	Clinical Test	Normal	Abnormal
Facial droop	Smile and show teeth.	Smile is symmetrical.	Smile is asymmetrical.
Arm drift	With palms up and eyes closed, hold the patient's arms out in front of the patient. Ask the patient to hold up their arms.	Arms remain in place.	One arm drifts down slowly or 1 arm falls down immediately.
Speech	Have the patient repeat any easy sentence.	Speech is clear and with correct words.	Speech is slurred, or the patient is completely unable to speak.

Minimizing the long-term effects of a stroke, or cerebrovascular accident (CVA), is time dependent. Similar to the saying "Time is muscle" in a heart attack, the saying "Time is brain" applies to a CVA. Rapid, thorough assessment, coupled with rapid transport to a facility capable of conducting a computerized tomography (CT) scan is critical. In the hospital, clots from an ischemic stroke can be physically removed in 1 of 2 ways: (1) using a surgical technique that goes into the vasculature, grabs the clot, and pulls it out of the body or (2) using "clot busting" medications called fibrinolytics. If time permits and the patient or their family is able to answer the necessary questions, assess the patient's ability to receive fibrinolytics at the hospital. Fibrinolytics need to be administered within 3 hours of the onset of symptoms, so if the paramedic can have this checklist filled out after arriving at the hospital, precious time can be saved. Assessment of a stroke should always include evaluation of a blood glucose level as well.

Table 6-6. Fibrinolytics Checklist

Fibrinolytics Checklist			
Patient 18 years or older?	Yes	No	Unknown
Facial droop?	Yes	No	Unknown
Slurred speech?	Yes	No	Unknown
Arm drift?	Yes	No	Unknown
Was there a seizure?	Yes	No	Unknown
Systolic blood pressure >185?	Yes	No	Unknown
History of structural nervous system disease? (stroke, arteriovenous malformation (AVM), aneurysm)	Yes	No	Unknown
Head or facial trauma within 6 weeks?	Yes	No	Unknown
MI within 6 weeks?	Yes	No	Unknown
Blood clotting disorder or on anticoagulants?	Yes	No	Unknown
Ulcers?	Yes	No	Unknown
Time signs and symptoms began or time last known to be well	Date/Time:		
Blood glucose reading	Value:		

Seizures

Pathophysiology

Seizures, regardless of type, are caused by an erratic misfiring of cerebral neurons. This excessive overstimulation of neurons can lead to several different presentations of seizures. The first and most common kind of seizure is the grand mal or tonic-clonic seizure. Next is the focal motor seizure, sometimes referred to as the partial seizure. Finally is the petit mal or absence seizure. A variety of reasons may lead a person to have a seizure, including the following:

- Brain abscess or infection
- Congenital cerebral malformation or organic brain syndrome
- Drug and/or alcohol use
- Brain injury, including stroke or brain tumor
- Electrolyte imbalance or kidney failure
- Fever—called a febrile seizure, which is particularly common in children
- Idiopathic—all of the preceding conditions have essentially been ruled out as causes

Generalized Seizures

The **generalized seizure** involves the entire brain and body and presents as forceful jerking movements of all the skeletal muscles. The seizure begins with the **tonic** phase, which is a brief tensing of all the muscles in the body. This precedes the **clonic** phase, which is the alternating forceful contraction of all the muscles with a relaxed phase of all the muscles. During this time, the patient is not breathing and is moving air in and out of the lungs only by virtue of the diaphragm and the intercostal muscles contracting along with the rest of the body. This is by no means effective. During the active part of the seizure, the patient also may be incontinent to both urine and feces. Many patients who have a history of seizures often are able to sense when they are about to have a seizure, called an aura, and prepare themselves by lying on the ground.

Following a seizure, patients enter a **postictal** state, which is essentially a recovery time for the brain to reset. A patient in the postictal state appears to be deeply asleep. After the postictal phase, frequently within about 10–15 minutes, a patient will slowly regain consciousness and become fully oriented after a period of confusion.

Status epilepticus is a genuinely life-threatening condition associated with generalized seizures that needs to be quickly recognized and aggressively managed. Either of two criteria in a patient constitutes status epilepticus:

- Tonic-clonic seizures lasting >5 consecutive minutes; or
- Failure to regain consciousness after a seizure.

Absence Seizures

Another form of generalized seizure that affects the entire brain is the **absence seizure.** This seizure does not involve tonic-clonic movements but rather a complete lack of movement. Patients afflicted with the absence seizure can stop all movement, including stopping mid-sentence, and pick up right where they left off without ever knowing anything happened. Often, these seizures last no more than a few seconds, and they are not regarded as life threatening unless they happen at a time when surrounding events can cause an injury, such as while the person is crossing a street.

Partial Seizures

Partial seizures differ from generalized seizures in that they involve only one part of the brain. A partial seizure may be classified as a simple partial seizure or a complex partial seizure. During a **simple partial seizure**, one area of the body will begin moving if the frontal lobe is involved, or 1 area will lose feeling if the parietal lobe is involved. This movement or loss of feeling will move in a wave-like fashion across and seemingly out of the body. For example, the patient's right hand may start shaking; the shaking will move to the arm, then shoulder and then the head before finally going down the left arm and hand and finally leaving the body. During a **complex partial seizure**, the effects of the simple partial seizure are seen; however, it is accompanied by hallucinations or changes in the patient's level of consciousness. The patient will not usually fully lose consciousness and may have a memory of the incident.

Assessment of Seizures

When called to assist a patient having a seizure, you may encounter a patient who is fully alert, postictal, or still seizing. The assessment of each type of individual, however, is largely similar. Witnesses may be the greatest source of valuable information because the patient may or may not be responsive. Even if alert when the paramedics arrive, the patient may have only a limited memory. It is important to try to first determine the type of seizure. Next, attempt to determine how long the patient was seizing and how long it has been since the patient's last seizure. Also, find out if the patient is compliant with their medication regimen or has had seizures in the past. With the above list as a reference, try to determine what caused the seizure by ruling out other causes, particularly if seizures have not previously occurred or if none of the bystanders are familiar with the patient's medical history.

Performing a thorough physical examination will help determine the cause in patients who are unable to talk or recall events leading up to the seizure. Although seizures may be preceded with an aura, injuries may have occurred if the patient was standing at the onset of the incident.

- **Head.** Assess for trauma to help rule out brain injury. Assess the pupils to see if they are equal and reactive; pinpoint pupils can indicate opiate overdose, dilated pupils can indicate amphetamine or cocaine overdose, and unequal pupils are a sign of head injury. Assess for facial droop and slurred speech as indicators of a stroke or a head injury. Patients also may bite their tongue during a tonic-clonic seizure.
- **Chest and Abdomen.** Assess for trauma. Assess lung sounds to ensure adequate ventilation.
- **Extremities.** Assess the arms and legs for equality in strength to look for a stroke.

Treatment of Seizures

Treatment is not usually necessary for either absence seizures or partial seizures, beyond ensuring the patient's safety during any seizure activity they may have in the presence of the paramedics. This discussion will therefore focus on the tonic-clonic seizure activity. If the patient is still seizing on arrival to the scene, do not restrain the patient. Allow the patient to continue the seizure without interference. Ensure that adequate space is around the patient to avoid injury during these convulsions. Do not make any attempts to force anything into the patient's mouth. Because the patient usually has their teeth clenched, this will do more harm than good. Because the patient is still seizing and attempting to start an intravenous could result in injury to the paramedic or the patient, consider administering intranasal midazolam, 0.2 mg/kg, up to 10 mg, to help the patient stop seizing. You also may consider giving 0.5 mg/kg diazepam rectally, up to 10 mg.

Once the seizure has stopped, work quickly to begin the necessary interventions in case this is merely an intermission of status epilepticus. Initiate cardiac monitoring and obtain a full set of vital signs. Remember that the patient was breathing ineffectively during the seizure, so initiate high-flow O_2 and consider providing BVM ventilation if necessary for long periods of apnea. Always check the blood sugar reading and administer 25 g D50 if it is <60 mg/dL. Initiate an intravenous line and provide a fluid bolus if the patient is hypotensive. If you suspect opiate drug overdose, administer 0.4–2 mg naloxone, titrated to adequate respirations. Arrange padding around the patient if possible in case the patient begins seizing again. If the patient does seize during transport, loosen the seat belts and protect them from hurting themselves as much as possible. Be prepared to administer benzodiazepine again if seizures begin again. The intravenous options are as follows:

- 5–10 mg diazepam
- 2–4 mg lorazepam
- 2–2.5 mg up to 0.1 mg/kg midazolam

Altered Mental Status

A common call the paramedic must be ready for is altered mental status. The mnemonic AEIOU-TIPS can help evaluate the possible reasons for a person to have an altered level of consciousness (LOC). Note that the reasons for altered mental status do not differ appreciably from those that cause seizures.

Table 6-7. Causes for Altered Mental Status: The AEIOU-TIPS Mnemonic

Letter	Cause	Onset	Additional Signs and Symptoms	Treatment Options
A	Alcohol, acute	Hours	Slurred speech, unsteady gait	Time, fluids
	Alcohol, chronic	Days	Slurred and garbled speech and abdominal pain	Fluids, thiamine, D50
	Acidosis, metabolic	Days	Eating without taking insulin, high blood sugar, and Kussmaul respirations	Fluids; bicarbonate in extreme circumstances
	Acidosis, respiratory	Minutes	Decreased respiratory effort and no breathing	Restoring adequate ventilation
E	Epilepsy	Seconds	Tonic-clonic activity	Diazepam or lorazepam
I	Insulin	Minutes	Unresponsiveness and low blood sugar	D50 or glucagon
O	Overdose	Minutes	Pupillary changes, needle track marks, and drug paraphernalia at scene	Naloxone for opiates; otherwise, drug dependent
U	Uremia (acute renal failure)	Days to weeks	Decreased urine output, failure to go to dialysis, and recent excessive exercise	Ensure adequate blood pressure, SpO$_2$, and blood glucose level
T	Trauma	Seconds	Multiple systems involvement	Varies with injury; treat for shock
I	Infection	Days	Hot, dry skin, foul smelling urine, and a productive cough	Maintain SBP >100; treat for shock
P	Psychosis	Seconds	Possible drug overdose, agitated or hypoactive, and delirium	Ensure adequate blood pressure, SpO$_2$, and blood glucose level
S	Stroke	Seconds	Unilateral weakness, facial droop, and slurred speech	Ensure adequate blood pressure, SpO$_2$, and blood glucose level

Assessment of Altered Mental Status

When evaluating the patient with altered mental status, focus on the time that the patient was last known to be at their baseline level of consciousness and how quickly the patient arrived at their current state. Assess the GCS level and document any changes to that level throughout transport; depending on the cause of the alteration, the patient may get better or worse as time goes on. The use of bystanders as part of the assessment technique here is essential because although the patient may be able to answer, there is no reliable way to know if what the patient is saying is accurate. Evaluate the patient for any trauma, especially of the head, but not necessarily only the head. Evaluate the patient on the basis of one of the previously mentioned stroke scales. Attempt to identify any overdose or poisoning agent.

Treatment of Altered Mental Status

There are some treatment options for each cause of an altered mental status; however, some global treatment options should be performed with any patient in this population. First, ensure adequate ABCs: secure the airway, ventilate with a BVM, and initiate CPR if needed above all else. If the ABCs are intact, consider O_2 to maintain an SpO_2 >94%. Check the blood sugar reading and administer 25 g D50 if it is <60 mg/dL. Initiate an intravenous line and provide a fluid bolus if the patient is hypotensive. If you suspect opiate drug overdose, administer 0.4–2 mg naloxone, titrated to adequate respirations.

Syncope

Pathophysiology

Also known as fainting, syncope or a syncopal episode results from a sudden temporary drop in blood flow to the brain, resulting in a brief period of unresponsiveness. The transient lack of O_2 and glucose causes the brain to shut down. Although this is the ultimate cause, the assessment goal will be to figure out why this happened in the first place. Standing up too fast from a seated or lying position, cardiac rhythm disturbance, a transient ischemic attack (TIA), a vasovagal response (i.e., straining too hard to have a bowel movement), and psychogenic shock are all possibilities that should be discussed with or evaluated on the patient.

Once blood returns to the brain in a sufficient quantity, the patient will regain consciousness, though frequently without recollection of the incident.

Assessment of Syncope

As with any patient, evaluate the ABCs and ensure that there is adequate ventilation, oxygenation, and circulation. Once this is assured, assess the patient for any trauma, particularly if there was a fall during the syncopal episode, paying close attention to the head. Finally ask the patient questions to attempt to isolate a cause from those listed above. It may not be obvious what caused the patient to pass out, and it may never be determined conclusively in the hospital.

Treatment of Syncope

Manage any derangement of the ABCs and any trauma the patient may have sustained. Evaluate the blood sugar level and treat with D50 as indicated for seizures and altered mental status. Continuously monitor the patient's cardiac rhythm and treat any disturbances that may have contributed to the syncope; these include excessive PVCs, couplets or runs of VT, bradydysrhythmias, and tachydysrhythmias, among others.

Headache

Pathophysiology and Assessment

The chief complaint of a headache is not one that usually strikes fear in the hearts of even the most novice paramedic. Fact is, most headache complaints are likely not life threatening or debilitating, with 2 glaring exceptions: meningitis and stroke. Strokes and the other symptoms were discussed earlier, which will help you differentiate a nominal headache from the life-altering headache of a CVA. Here, the discussion focuses on the other types of headaches, including the headache that is associated with meningitis.

- **Tension Headache.** This headache is the result of stress that manifests itself in continuous muscle contraction of the muscles of the face, neck, and temples. This is the most common kind of headache and generally not an emergency.
- **Cluster Headache.** An uncommon vascular headache that comes on suddenly and intensely around one eye or side of the face. The pain typically wanes in <60 minutes; however, when present, the pain can be so bad that the patient actually considers suicide to escape it.
- **Sinus Headache.** Another nonemergency version of a headache, this is caused by blockage and resulting inflammation of one or more of the sinus cavities in the face. Sinus headache pain often increases when the patient bends over.
- **Migraine.** Caused by spasming of the blood vessels at the base of the brain. In addition to the pain, patients also complain of photophobia (fear of light) or other visual disturbances. Patients also may have nausea, vomiting, or dizziness with the headache. This headache can last for days or weeks.

- **Meningitis.** Meningitis is an infection that can be caused by either a virus or bacteria. Fortunately, the viral form of meningitis typically comes and goes on its own. In fact, patients may have had viral meningitis and not even known it. Bacterial meningitis, on the other hand, is highly infectious and spreads relatively easily from one person to another, especially in tight living quarters such as dorms and prisons. This droplet-borne disease is most commonly caused by either *Neisseria meningitidis* or *Streptococcus pneumoniae*. It causes inflammation of the meninges surrounding the brain and can be deadly. Common signs and symptoms of meningitis include sudden onset fever and headache with a hallmark sign of a stiff neck that cannot be flexed to touch the chin to the chest. In addition, the patient may have a rash that starts pink and becomes purple. The patient also will almost certainly exhibit projectile vomiting and an altered mental status.

Treatment for Headaches

Typical headaches are rarely treated in the field. If the patient is in severe pain from a migraine or a cluster headache, consider giving 30 mg ketorolac intramuscularly, 2–4 mg morphine sulfate IV push, or 1 mcg/kg fentanyl (to a maximum of 100 mcg per dose) via slow IV push for analgesia. Headaches often are accompanied by nausea, so 4 mg ondansetron would be recommended. For a meningitis headache, analgesia can be considered, but medical control should be contacted first.

Initiating an intravenous line for fluid administration and being prepared in case of seizures or cardiac arrest is important in meningitis. That said, the most important treatment for a patient with meningitis may very well be to put a surgical mask on your own face if the patient does not wish to or for some reason cannot wear a mask. Although patient-to-provider transmission is rare, it is not a gamble worth taking. If the physician at the hospital believes that the provider was exposed, the physician will prescribe prophylactic antibiotics to the provider.

Dementia

Dementia refers to any number of disorders that result in chronic deterioration of the brain. These diseases can occur as quickly as weeks, such as in Wernicke encephalopathy, or over decades, such as Huntington disease. The degradation of the brain can affect memory, personality, and language skills. Patients can become aggressive when they were previously docile, or vice versa. Because none of these conditions are particularly acute, they do not usually represent a serious emergency. When presented with a patient that is afflicted with one of these diseases, it is important to ascertain the patient's baseline level of consciousness and degree of orientation. The patient may appear to have an altered mental status to the provider, even though this may simply be the new normal. If a caregiver or family member indicates to you that a person with dementia of any kind is not acting normally, then find out what the patient's baseline is. This change may represent a progression of the disease, or there may be another underlying reason for an altered mental status.

Other Nervous System Disorders

The paramedic should have a basic understanding of the following nervous system disorders; however, prehospital treatment of these disorders is limited in scope and primarily supportive (i.e., done to relieve symptoms). For example, if the patient is anxious, it may be worthwhile to give an anxiolytic, such as lorazepam; if the patient is in pain, consider ketorolac or fentanyl. The goal here is to ensure that the patient is comfortable because most of these disorders are chronic and require complex, continuous management beyond what a paramedic can accomplish.

Multiple sclerosis (MS) is an autoimmune disorder in which the body's immune system arbitrarily attacks the myelin sheath surrounding the axons of the neurons, particularly those within the CNS. This results in scarring and a decline in functioning of the body part those neurons innervated. Patients often complain of numbness in their extremities and visual disturbances as the initial presenting sign. Over time, an increasing number of neurons are compromised, leading to widespread functional declines across nearly all body systems: muscle weakness and paresthesias, perceiving light touch as painful, bowel and bladder dysfunction, cognitive changes including speech and comprehension changes, and depression, just to name a few.

Guillain-Barré syndrome is a demyelinating disease like MS, where the immune system attacks the myelin sheath; however, the progression of Guillain-Barré syndrome is much more rapid. Unlike MS, it is reversible, and a high percentage of patients make a full recovery. Although it is not fully understood, more than 60% of patients have experienced a recent respiratory illness, such as the flu, or a bout with diarrhea. Agents believed to cause Guillain-Barré syndrome include the bacteria *Campylobacter jejuni* and the influenza virus. The disease presents itself as weakness and tingling sensation in the legs that moves up the body, quickly moving to the abdomen, chest, and arms. The progression from normal to profound systemic weakness requiring a ventilator for breathing can take but a few hours. Treatment is largely supportive but be prepared to initiate aggressive interventions, including intubation, ventilation, and fluid infusions. Unlike complications arising in MS, where the patient is aware of the disease, patients with this condition are unaware because of the nature of its sudden onset.

Amyotrophic lateral sclerosis (ALS) (or Lou Gehrig's Disease) is a devastating and ultimately fatal disease. Little is understood even about what causes it in the first place, and there is no known cure. The best treatment is supportive, even after diagnosis. This disease attacks the voluntary motor nerves, causing them to die and the muscles they once innervated to atrophy. Disease progression will result in eventual failure of the muscles of speech and breathing. Patients will die within 3–5 years of the initial diagnosis.

Parkinson disease (PD) is associated with a decrease in the production of dopamine in the brain, often caused by damage to the area of the brain responsible for its production. The damage could be caused by a concussion or other injury or simply the result of overuse. Dopamine is a neurotransmitter that is necessary for muscles to contract in a smooth, coordinated fashion. The disease progresses over time, starting off with minor tremors that are often isolated to one side. Patients then start walking stooped over as their muscles of posture begin to be affected. Next, the patient starts to display highly uncoordinated exaggerated movements, where the muscles seem to go from fully relaxed to fully contracted with a loss of subtle fine motor control. In the later stages, patients are at risk for aspiration and pneumonia because of poor swallowing and gag reflexes. Patients also are at risk for injury from falls.

Peripheral neuropathy is a global term for a group of conditions that damage the peripheral, or spinal, nerves. Trauma, tumors, bacterial or environmental toxins, metabolic disorders such as diabetes, and autoimmune diseases are all possible causes for peripheral neuropathy. The most common form of peripheral neuropathy is diabetic neuropathy. Patients complain of a burning and tingling sensation; as the disease process continues, the patient may lose all feeling in the area. In the case of diabetic neuropathy, the feet and fingers are most generally affected.

REVIEW QUESTIONS

Select the ONE best answer.

1. A 28-year-old male patient presents with agitation and is physically combative after being struck in the head during a bar fight. He is particularly combative when he is unable to answer questions posed to him. His conversation consists of clear words but nonsensical sentences and phrases. Which of the following lobes of the brain has most likely been damaged?

    A. Frontal

    B. Occipital

    C. Parietal

    D. Temporal

2. Assessment of a 76-year-old male patient reveals that he is unable to move his right eye up, down, and medially. The pupil in his right eye also is dilated. Which cranial nerve is most likely affected?

    A. Oculomotor (CN III)

    B. Trochlear (CN IV)

    C. Trigeminal (CN V)

    D. Abducens (CN VI)

3. A 38-year-old female complains of dizziness and balance problems. Which of the following is the most likely explanation for the dizziness?

   A. Cerebellar infarct

   B. Inner ear infection

   C. Lesion of vestibulocochlear nerve (CN VIII)

   D. Any of these

4. To propagate a nerve impulse (action potential), _____ must enter the neuron at the nodes of Ranvier, starting at the cell body and continuing all the way along the _____ to the synaptic cleft.

   A. Potassium, axon

   B. Potassium, dendrite

   C. Sodium, axon

   D. Sodium, dendrite

5. An 88-year-old male patient deliberately overdosed on donepezil, an Alzheimer disease medication, about 45 minutes ago in an attempt to commit suicide. Donepezil is an inhibitor of AChE, the enzyme that breaks down ACh. Although currently symptom free, what medication do you prepare to give in anticipation of the drug's effects?

   A. Atropine

   B. Dextrose 50%

   C. Midazolam

   D. Naloxone

ANSWERS AND EXPLANATIONS

1. **The correct answer is (A).** The frontal lobe contains areas of impulse control. Damage to this area can lead to bizarre behavior, including combativeness and agitation or sedation and apathy. The frontal lobe also contains the Broca area, which is responsible for speech formation and control. Damage to this area can lead to an inability to put together words into sentences; however; clear words will still be spoken; slurring of speech comes from cerebellar damage. The occipital lobe (B) is responsible for vision interpretation. The parietal lobe (C) is responsible for peripheral sensation and motor impulses. The temporal lobe (D) is responsible for hearing interpretation.

2. **The correct answer is (A).** The oculomotor nerve is responsible for all of the listed actions and also responsible for movement of the upper eyelid and movement of the ciliary muscles, which change the shape of the lens to focus light on the retina. The trochlear nerve (B) is responsible for moving the eye down and medially only. The trigeminal nerve (C) is responsible for sensation of the mouth, eyelids, and cheeks and the movement of muscles of chewing. The abducens nerve (D) causes the eye to move laterally.

3. **The correct answer is (D).** Any of the listed areas of the neurological system could lead to a complaint of dizziness. The inner ear (B) senses a person's orientation in space; CN VIII (C) carries that information to the balance centers in the cerebellum; the cerebellum (A) interprets these data and controls fine muscle movements. All of these work together to help a person maintain balance. Lesions (cancer, infection, infarct, and/or bleeding) in any of these areas could have a similar impact.

4. **The correct answer is (C).** Sodium rushes into the neuron as potassium rushes out as the action potential moves along the axon. Axons are the only portions of the neuron that are covered with Schwann cells and myelin. Axons carry messages away from the cell body, whereas dendrites receive information from other neurons and bring it toward the cell body.

5. **The correct answer is (A).** Because donepezil is an AChE inhibitor, ACh will build up in the synapses of the parasympathetic nervous system. This amounts to a cholinergic overdose, which will eventually produce symptoms of SLUDGE: salivation, lacrimation, urination, diarrhea, GI upset (vomiting), and eyes (dilated pupils). The other medications listed would not likely benefit this patient.

ENDOCRINE EMERGENCIES

The **endocrine system** as a whole regulates the functions of the body and maintains homeostasis throughout the body. It consists of about half a dozen different glands scattered throughout the body. These endocrine glands manufacture and secrete hormones directly into the bloodstream, which carries the hormone to the cells of the target organ. Exocrine glands secrete hormones and other products through a duct directly to their site of action. Once the hormone arrives at the target organ, the hormone can exert its effects in one of two primary ways: (1) it can attach to a receptor on the cell membrane, and a secondary messenger inside the cell will carry the "message" of altering the cell's activity, or (2) it can pass through the cell membrane and directly exert its effects on the enzyme or protein in the cell.

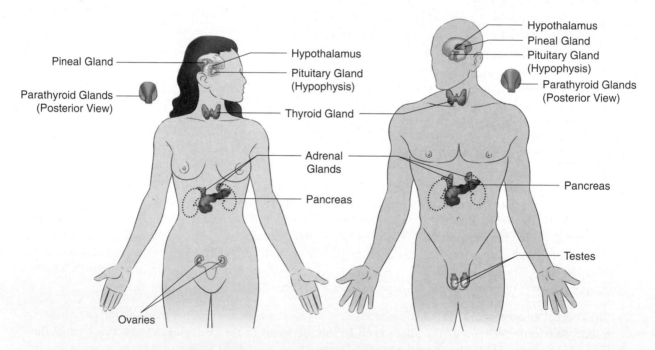

Figure 6-12. Organs of the Endocrine System
Endocrine organs produce hormones that are secreted into the bloodstream to act on distant target tissues.

This section of the chapter will discuss issues related to the glands of the endocrine system. Each gland will be presented in a similar manner. First, the anatomy and physiology of the gland, including the hormones that the gland primarily produces and their actions on the body, will be discussed. This is followed by syndromes resulting from dysfunction of that hormone or gland and the emergency treatment for that dysfunction as it relates to the paramedic. The most common endocrine emergency that paramedics must know how to treat is diabetes, particularly low blood sugar.

Endocrine Glands

Pituitary Gland

The **pituitary gland** hangs off the base of the brain and is attached directly to the hypothalamus. It is known as the master gland because the hormones it releases control the release of hormones from other endocrine glands. The two lobes of the pituitary gland are the posterior lobe and the anterior lobe.

The posterior lobe of the pituitary gland does not manufacture or secrete its own hormones; rather it stores and secretes oxytocin and antidiuretic hormone (ADH), both of which are made in the hypothalamus. Oxytocin is responsible for the initiation of contractions for and throughout childbirth, and it stimulates milk production in the breasts. ADH is released when the sodium concentration is too high and stimulates water reabsorption in the kidneys. It also stimulates thirst and increases blood pressure.

The anterior lobe of the pituitary gland manufactures and releases 6 hormones.

- **Growth Hormone (GH).** Responsible for the growth of muscle and bones and shunts glucose to those places.
- **Adrenocorticotropic Hormone (ACTH).** Directs the synthesis and release of glucocorticoids from the cortex of the adrenal gland.
- **Thyroid-Stimulating Hormone (TSH).** Directs the thyroid to manufacture and release two thyroid hormones, triiodothyronine and thyroxine.
- **Prolactin.** Stimulates milk production.
- **Follicle-Stimulating Hormone.** In females, it promotes the development of the ovarian follicle into an ovum; in males, it promotes the development of sperm.
- **Luteinizing Hormone.** In females, it causes ovulation; in males, it stimulates testosterone production.

Panhypopituitarism is the major syndrome associated with pituitary gland malfunction. Although often the result of an abnormal hypothalamus, this condition results in an inadequate or a complete lack of pituitary hormone production. This patient will be followed closely by a pediatric endocrinologist, and a paramedic will not likely see this patient for anything acute, and it will considerably alter the paramedic's course of treatment for other problems.

Pineal Gland

The **pineal gland** is located near the posterior portion of the thalamus in the brain. It is responsible for circadian rhythms. **Melatonin** is secreted from this gland when light entering the eye decreases, which helps us fall asleep. No significant medical conditions that the paramedic would encounter are associated with this gland.

Thyroid Gland

The **thyroid gland** is located in the neck, anterior to the trachea at the level of the thyroid cartilage. The thyroid produces **triiodothyronine** (T3) and **thyroxine** (T4), known collectively as **thyronines**, which are responsible for increasing metabolism. These hormones increase the basal metabolic rate at a cellular level and regulate fat, protein, and carbohydrate metabolism. An increase in these hormones increases body heat. These hormones are important in normal neurological and physical development in children.

The thyroid gland also produces **calcitonin**, which is responsible for decreasing the blood calcium level. Calcitonin decreases calcium levels in the following three ways: increases calcium excretion in the kidneys, increases calcium storage in the bones, and decreases the amount of dietary calcium that is absorbed in the intestines. Remember, calcitonin tones it down!

Medical conditions can result from too much or too little production of thyronines. Hyperthyroidism results from overproduction of thyroid hormones, and hypothyroidism comes from too little production.

Table 6-8. Comparison of Hypothyroidism and Hyperthyroidism

System	Hypothyroidism	Hyperthyroidism
Cardiovascular	Slow heart rate	Tachycardia and hypertension
Metabolic	Decreased metabolism and weight gain	Increased metabolism, hyperthermia, and weight loss
Muscular	Weakness	Tremor and hyperactive reflexes
Neurological	Decreased level of consciousness and sleepiness	Restlessness and irritability
Integumentary	Dry, cold skin	Hot, flushed skin and diaphoresis
Gastrointestinal	Constipated	Diarrhea

Graves disease or **hyperthyroidism** is the most common and most severe form of hyperthyroidism, which can be fatal if left untreated. In Graves disease, the thyroid increases in size as its activity increases. This enlarged thyroid is called a **goiter** and is visible on the anterior neck of the patient. Patients suffering from Graves disease have an increased appetite combined with weight loss, excessive thirst (polydipsia) from excessive sweating, and diarrhea. Another classic finding in Graves disease is **exophthalmos**, which is the protrusion of the eyeballs from their sockets, giving these patients a perpetual surprised look.

Graves disease is not usually treated by paramedics on its own because it tends to be a chronic condition. That said, Graves disease, among other causes including cancer and drug overdoses, can cause a condition known as **thyrotoxicosis** or **thyroid storm**. Excessive circulating thyroid hormones increase metabolism to unmaintainably high levels, resulting in a critically ill patient.

- Symptoms include extremely high fever, diaphoresis, tachycardia, and possible nausea/vomiting.
- Symptoms may also include irritability, agitated delirium, seizures, or unconsciousness.
- Hypoglycemia may be seen after initial treatments as a result of the hypermetabolic state.

Thyroid storm needs to be aggressively managed to avoid death. Monitoring and continuous treatment of low blood sugar should be a concern, especially during long transport times. Patients presenting with thyroid storm may require abnormally high doses of benzodiazepines to achieve sedation, sometimes in excess of 3 times the normal dose. Tachycardia could be a result of the agitation, excessive dehydration from the sweating and hyperpyrexia, or some combination of both. Therefore, fluid should be aggressively administered to these patients as long as they are normotensive or hypotensive. Initiating beta-blocker treatment is recommended where available. Atenolol or metoprolol may be used; however, 0.5–1 mg propranolol slow IVP over 10 minutes is the preferred choice. Finally, patients should be actively cooled using cold packs to the axillae and groin or intravenous cold saline to reduce their core temperature, especially if their temperature exceeds 103°F (39.4°C).

Hypothyroidism (sometimes called **myxedema coma**) is a slow-to-develop condition related to a decline in the production of thyroid hormones. Myxedema coma begins slowly and has subtle changes that may be mistaken for other problems or even just the general effects of aging.

- Early symptoms include fatigue, dry skin, weight gain, and feeling cold all the time.
- The continued decline in the thyroid hormone can lead to deterioration of the patient's mental status, at which point the family may call for an ambulance.
- If not treated, the patient can quickly decline further from altered mental status to unconsciousness and death.
- Once patients have reached the stage of myxedema coma heralded by an altered mental status, they are very likely to also be hypothermic, sometimes with core temperature <90°F (32.2°C).

Treatment for myxedema coma is largely supportive, with goals focused on maintaining oxygenation, cardiovascular function, and temperature. Patients should receive supplemental O_2 if the SpO_2 is <95%, and intubation and ventilation should be considered in those patients without a gag reflex who also are breathing inadequately. Monitor the ECG and blood glucose level and give D50 if <60 mg/dL. For patients who are hypothermic, begin passive rewarming methods, including blankets and hot packs to the groin, axillae, and neck. Patients who are severely hypothermic or are hemodynamically unstable and requiring aggressive cardiovascular management or CPR should receive warmed fluids as well.

Parathyroid Glands

Located on the posterior side of the thyroid gland are 4 small glands that make up the parathyroid gland. These glands produce a hormone aptly named the **parathyroid hormone** (**PTH**). PTH also is involved in regulation of the blood calcium level, but in opposition to calcitonin. Calcitonin tones calcium levels down, whereas PTH increases calcium levels. It accomplishes this by limiting the excretion of calcium in the kidneys and increasing reabsorption of bone (dissolving bone to its components of calcium and phosphate).

Hyperparathyroidism is a condition where the parathyroid glands secrete excess amounts of the hormone for long periods of time. Because of increased calcium levels, the patient can be prone to kidney stones resulting from the amount of calcium and phosphorus in the blood. Patients also can have pathologic fractures—fractures not caused by an obvious traumatic event such as standing up—caused by continuous bone reabsorption. Treatment for any of these conditions is largely supportive.

Thymus Gland

The thymus gland is located in the chest of children. During adolescence, the thymus atrophies and essentially disappears, so adults do not actually have a thymus. During childhood, this gland produces **thymosin**, which stimulates the development of T-lymphocytes, a family of white blood cells essential in cell-mediated immunity. Cytotoxic T-cells, or killer T-cells, attack the antigen—virus, fungus, parasite, tumor cell, or bacterium—directly by engulfing it through a process called phagocytosis and killing it. Helper T-cells secrete chemical mediators called **lymphokines** that alert other lymphocytes to the presence of an invader and signal the thalamus to raise the body temperature. After the invader is cleared from the body, suppressor T-cells contain the immune response. It is thought that the failure of suppressor T-cells is a factor in allergic reactions and autoimmune diseases. A paramedic will seldom encounter a thymus-related problem.

Adrenal Glands

The body has 2 adrenal glands, each perched atop a kidney. Each adrenal gland has 2 distinct regions: the outer part (adrenal cortex) and the central part (adrenal medulla).

The **adrenal cortex** produces hormones that have widely varied functions. The outermost layer of the adrenal cortex produces **mineral corticoids** that are responsible for maintaining the salt balance within the body. A decrease in salt concentration in the blood, a decrease in blood pressure, or an increase in potassium concentration stimulates the adrenal cortex to produce an important mineral corticoid called **aldosterone**. Aldosterone works on the kidneys to increase the reabsorption of sodium and instead increase the excretion of potassium. During times of stress, ACTH from the pituitary gland stimulates the middle layer of the adrenal cortex to produce the **glucocorticoids**. **Cortisol**, a prominent glucocorticoid, stimulates the body to increase its energy production and also increases the rate that fat is deposited in adipose tissue in the belly. Finally, the inner layer of the cortex is responsible for the production of the sex hormones estrogen and testosterone.

The adrenal medulla is the primary site of production in the body for epinephrine and norepinephrine, collectively known as catecholamines. These catecholamines aid in the fight-or-flight response to stress. The adrenal emergencies are adrenal insufficiency, Cushing syndrome, and congenital adrenal hyperplasia.

Adrenal insufficiency can be primary or secondary.

- In **primary** adrenal insufficiency (known as **Addison disease**), the patient's adrenal cortex is no longer functioning, resulting in a deficiency of all steroid hormones. The failure can be brought on by idiopathic atrophy, an infection such as tuberculosis, adrenal cancer, or an autoimmune disease where antibodies destroy the adrenal cortex.

- **Secondary** adrenal insufficiency is caused by a lack of production of ACTH, which results in a lack of production of all cortical steroids except aldosterone. Aldosterone is still produced because its secretion is not dependent on ACTH but rather potassium and sodium concentrations in the blood. Secondary adrenal insufficiency also may be seen in people who suddenly stop taking corticosteroid medications such as hydrocortisone or solumedrol. Because these medications suppress natural corticosteroid production by keeping blood concentrations high, the body does not catch up to the sudden drop quickly enough.

For the paramedic treating a patient in addisonian crisis, the goal is to support cardiovascular function and treat for the apparent shock with normal saline. Fluid volume expansion is usually the first line of treatment. This will help increase the sodium level in the blood and reduce the concentration of circulating potassium as well as address hypotension and dehydration. Administering several doses of 20 mL/kg NSS is not out of the question in this patient. Check the blood sugar level and administer D50 if <60 mg/dL. Consider administering 1 g calcium chloride or calcium gluconate if the cardiac rhythm reveals hyperkalemia; treat any other dysrhythmias encountered as if cardiac in nature.

Cushing syndrome is caused by an excess production of cortisol secondary to tumors of the pituitary or adrenal cortex. It is characterized by a rise in blood sugar. Protein synthesis is impaired, causing rhabdomyolysis (breakdown of skeletal muscle). Patients will complain of weakness, fatigue, depression, and mood swings. Patients also have a characteristic weight gain in Cushing syndrome. They gain weight in the belly but not the arms or legs. Fat deposits appear above the shoulders (supraclavicular), between the shoulder blades (buffalo hump), and in the face (moon face). Women will get notable facial hair in a pattern similar to that of men and will often start losing their scalp hair. Prehospital treatment involves symptomatic treatment and an evaluation of blood sugar levels.

Congenital adrenal hyperplasia (**CAH**) is the opposite of Cushing syndrome in that it is the inadequate production of cortisol as well as aldosterone. This is a lifelong problem and will require lifelong treatment with cortisol and/or aldosterone. Children with CAH appear masculine in nature, and female genitalia may resemble a penis. Male and female patients may exhibit signs of puberty as toddlers, including body hair and lowering of the voice.

Gonads

Testes

The **testes** are the main source of testosterone and other androgens in males. The androgens are responsible for the development of male secondary sex characteristics throughout life, especially during puberty.

Ovaries

The **ovaries** are located in the lower quadrants of the abdomen at the distal ends of the fallopian tubes. In females they are the primary source of estrogen, which is responsible for the development of female secondary sex characteristics.

Pancreas

The pancreas is centrally located in the abdomen, with part of it located in all 4 quadrants. It is both an exocrine and an endocrine gland because it delivers enzymes directly to the duodenum via the pancreatic duct and secretes hormones into the bloodstream. For our purposes here, only the endocrine properties will be addressed.

The endocrine component of the pancreas is in specific areas called the **islets of Langerhans**. These are groups of cells within the body of the pancreas whose sole purpose is to manufacture the hormones insulin, glucagon, and somatostatin.

Insulin is necessary for glucose in the bloodstream to be able to cross the cell membrane, where it can be properly used as cellular fuel. Insulin, which is secreted by the beta cells within the islets of Langerhans, also is required to move glucose from the blood into the liver, where it can be stored in long chains of molecules called glycogen. Once the blood glucose decreases to a normal level, the islets stop producing insulin. **Glucagon**, secreted by the alpha cells of the islets of Langerhans, on the other hand, stimulates the liver to convert the glycogen back to glucose during times of fasting or inadequate food consumption and release it back into circulation so it can be used by the other cells of the body. **Somatostatin** is released by the delta cells of the islets of Langerhans and is a potent inhibitor of both glucagon and insulin.

Diabetes Mellitus

Pathophysiology

Diabetes is the body's inability to metabolize glucose because it is not able to get into the cells. Insulin production in diabetes can either be nonexistent when no insulin is produced, inadequate when not enough insulin is produced to meet the needs of the body, or produced but unable to signal the cell properly to allow glucose to enter. Regardless of the reason, the glucose cannot enter the cell and cannot, therefore, be metabolized in the cells. As the glucose level continues to rise in the bloodstream, it will eventually reach a level where it spills into the urine so that it does not become a poison to the body. Diabetes is further classified into type 1 or type 2.

In type 1 diabetes, previously called juvenile diabetes because the initial onset is typically during childhood, the beta cells of the islets of Langerhans have been destroyed and no longer produce insulin. The cause still has not been conclusively determined; however, there may be a genetic cause or an autoimmune component. Because the patient no longer has functioning beta cells to produce insulin, these patients are dependent on daily insulin injections to regulate their blood sugar for the rest of their lives. The insulin prescribed to these patients is either fast acting or long acting. Fast-acting insulin is generally injected at about the time of the meal so that the increase in blood sugar is handled quickly, while the long-acting is taken once and exerts its effects equally throughout the day, resulting in fewer fluctuations of blood sugar level. For patients on long-acting insulin, they have to eat consistently throughout the day to maintain their blood sugar levels. Insulin also must be kept refrigerated when not in use to maintain its potency; if it is left out for more than approximately 28 of days, it will be as useful as injecting saline to control blood sugar.

Type 2 diabetes was once called adult onset diabetes because it begins in late adulthood. In most people with type 2 diabetes, the pancreas produces insulin; however, the insulin it produces is either not produced in high enough quantity to be able to effectively regulate blood sugar or is produced in sufficient quantity but unable to signal the cells to allow the glucose in. **Insulin resistance** occurs when insulin is produced but the body cannot effectively use it. These patients often are on medications called oral antihyperglycemics that help the body use the insulin it does produce more efficiently.

In both types of diabetes, the patient can have either critically high or critically low blood sugar levels, hyperglycemia or hypoglycemia, respectively. Most commonly, hypoglycemia results from too much insulin taken for the amount of food consumed, or not consuming food often enough or in great enough quantity to keep up with the type of insulin taken. Hypoglycemia generally comes on suddenly and without obvious warning signs; the patient is suddenly found unresponsive.

Normal blood sugar levels are generally accepted to be between 70 and 140 mg/dL; they will be higher if the blood sugar is taken within 2 hours of having eaten. Clinically significant hyperglycemia usually takes a few days to develop to the point where the patient shows signs and symptoms because blood sugar levels can easily swell to >200 mg/dL after a carbohydrate-heavy meal. Hyperglycemia is defined as sustained blood sugars despite fasting between 140 and 400 mg/dL; it is concerning when symptoms described in the next section are concurrently present. If blood sugar levels are not treated, the patient may progress to either **diabetic ketoacidosis (DKA)** in patients with Type I DM or a condition called **Hyperosmolar Hyperglycemic State (HHS)** in patients with Type II DM. Other terms for this state include **hyperosmolar hyperglycemic nonketotic coma (HHNC)**, also known as **hyperosmolar nonketotic coma (HONK)**.

DKA is typically associated with type 1 diabetes and can become a life-threatening condition as blood sugar levels rise and the acid levels in the blood exceed the body's capacity to neutralize the acid, lowering overall pH. As the patient's blood sugar continues to rise, the bloodstream will eventually become so concentrated that the kidneys will start to excrete the sugar in the urine, a condition known as **osmotic diuresis**. This requires large amounts of fluid to be able to safely excrete the glucose resulting in frequent, full bladder urination called **polyuria**. When a patient is in DKA, the patient's cells turn to fat for fuel instead of glucose. This emergent type of fat metabolism results in the production of ketones (a specific group of organic compounds) that can be eliminated in both the urine and during exhalation. These ketones have a sweet or fruit-like odor to them that can be smelled on the patient's breath.

HHS is most often found in patients with type 2 diabetes. These patients have the same metabolic situation of hyperosmolarity (spilling sugar into the urine) and hyperglycemia; however, they lack the ketone, fruity smell to their breath. Frequently, a concurrent illness, commonly pneumonia or a urinary tract infection, can precipitate HHS.

Assessment of Diabetic Emergencies

Patients with diabetes and either hypoglycemia or hyperglycemia present with an altered mental status, but that is about where the similarities end.

Table 6-9. Hyperglycemia versus Hypoglycemia

Assessment Point	Hyperglycemia	Hypoglycemia
Thirst	Excessive (polydipsia)	Normal
Hunger	Absent	Extreme
Vomiting	Frequently	Rarely
Urination frequency	Frequent (polyuria)	Normal
Insulin dose	Less than required	More than required
Onset timing	Slowly (over days)	Rapidly (minutes to hours)
Skin	Hot and very dry	Cool, pale, and diaphoretic
Respirations	Fast and deep (Kussmaul)	Normal
Blood pressure	Normal	Normal to low
Pulse	Full, bounding	Weak, thready
Blood sugar level	>140	<60

Treatment of Diabetic Emergencies

Hypoglycemia

Treatment for hypoglycemia focuses on restoring normal blood sugar levels. Depending on the patient's level of consciousness, this can be accomplished orally or parenterally. If the patient can protect the airway at a minimum, or better yet swallow, then provide medical oral glucose or drink orange juice or regular soda to raise the blood sugar level. Patients also should be encouraged to eat complex carbohydrates after the orange juice or soda so that their blood sugar levels are more likely to be maintained.

If the patient is unresponsive or unable to maintain an airway, the patient can be administered 1 mg glucagon intramuscularly if no intravenous access is readily available. If an intravenous line is available, give 25 g of D50 (1 amp) through a patent intravenous line and flush with saline. It is important to ensure that the intravenous line is not infiltrated into the soft tissue prior to administering the D50 because D50 is extremely hypertonic and could cause tissue necrosis if it extravasates.

Due to the hypertonicity of D50, an alternative treatment is now being recommended using D10. Administration of 250 mL of a D10 solution provides the same 25-gram dose of dextrose to the patient but does not increase the blood sugar as quickly, thus avoiding the need for the patient to take more insulin. Additionally, this administration can be stopped early if the patient regains consciousness, resulting in less rebound hyperglycemia.

Hyperglycemia

Although the in-hospital course of treatment for hyperglycemia focuses on lowering blood sugar levels, prehospital treatment focuses on fluid replacement and beginning to correct the prevalent metabolic acidosis. Begin by establishing at least 1 intravenous line of NSS and plan to deliver 1 L of fluid during the first half hour. As with any patient receiving a hefty fluid bolus, continually evaluate lung sounds and cardiac function throughout this infusion to ensure that the patient is not getting fluid overloaded, although this is extremely unlikely in the hyperglycemic patient. Monitor the ECG rhythm and note the presence of peaked T waves that could indicate hyperkalemia, a possible complication brought about by cellular death. If this is found, consider administering 1 g calcium chloride or calcium gluconate. Although it may seem like a good idea to administer bicarbonate for the acidosis, this decision should be left up to the physician because rapid reversal of this kind of acidosis with bicarbonate could have negative effects. If employed, it must be carefully controlled, which is beyond what is capable in the field.

REVIEW QUESTIONS

Select the ONE best answer.

1. A 44-year-old patient presents with restlessness and irritability that has been worsening during the past couple months. He has noted unintended weight loss over that period of time and states he is hungry all the time. His skin is flushed, and his eyes appear to be bulging. What endocrine problem do you suspect?

    A. Hyperpituitarism

    B. Hyperthyroidism

    C. Hypothyroidism

    D. Thyroid storm

2. A conscious 70-year-old male patient presents confused but alert. His spouse tells you that his blood sugar recently was 44 mg/dL and your glucometer confirms this. The next most appropriate treatment would be to administer:

    A. 25 g of D50.

    B. 4 LPM of O_2.

    C. 15 g of oral glucose.

    D. 20 mg/kg of crystalloid.

3. Which of the following is the paramedic's primary goal when treating a patient presenting with a blood glucose level >600 mg/dL, Kussmaul respirations, and excessive urination?

    A. Control the respiratory rate with overdrive BVM ventilations.

    B. Hydrate and dilute circulating glucose with 1 L NSS.

    C. Manage the hyperkalemia with 1 g calcium carbonate.

    D. Treat the metabolic acidosis with 1 mEq/kg sodium bicarbonate.

ANSWERS AND EXPLANATIONS

1. **The correct answer is (B).** The symptoms the patient is describing are consistent with hyperthyroidism. Thyroid storm (D) is an acute, sudden onset hyperthyroidism that can be fatal if not aggressively treated. Patients with thyroid storm may present with similar symptoms but also will be extremely hyperthermic, often in excess of 103°F (39.4°C), and hypertensive. Hypothyroidism (C) will present much the opposite and include decreased appetite, weight gain, and cold skin. Hyperpituitarism (A) is extremely rare and generally associated with excess production of growth hormone leading to gigantism.

2. **The correct answer is (C).** Because the patient is alert, oral replenishment of glucose is appropriate. The only option given here is oral glucose; however, a sandwich, pasta, or sugared orange juice are also appropriate options. D50 (A) would be necessary in a patient who is unresponsive or unable to protect the airway. There is no mention of hypotension or hypoxia, so (B) and (D) are not immediately appropriate.

3. **The correct answer is (B).** Replacing fluids lost during osmotic diuresis and coincidentally diluting the blood sugar levels are the paramedic's primary goals in treating hyperglycemic patients in DKA. Patients can lose liters of circulating volume through osmotic diuresis and the increased respiratory rate. The paramedic should never try to reduce the patient's respiratory rate (A) because this is the primary way the body has to increase pH. Managing hyperkalemia (C), if present, should be considered; however, it is not a primary goal. Treating the metabolic acidosis with bicarbonate (D) is seldom recommended because it could cause the patient to become alkalotic once the blood sugar level is reduced.

IMMUNOLOGIC EMERGENCIES

Each day, the human body is exposed to numerous bacteria, viruses, fungi, and even parasites. Yet our bodies are able to protect us from infection most of the time. Even when people do get sick, the immune system is usually able to contain and eliminate the infection.

To fight infection, the human body has two different divisions of the immune system: innate and adaptive immunity. **Innate immunity** is composed of defenses that are always active against infection, but they lack the ability to target specific invaders over others; for this reason, it is also called **nonspecific immunity**. **Adaptive** or **specific immunity** refers to the defenses that target a specific pathogen. This system is slower to act but can maintain immunological memory of an infection to be able to mount a faster attack in subsequent infections.

Anatomy

The immune system is not housed in a single organ. The structure and components that serve as nonspecific defenses often serve functions in other organ systems. The bone marrow produces all the leukocytes (white blood cells) that participate in the immune system through the process of **hematopoiesis**. The spleen functions as blood storage and activation of B-cells, which turn into plasma cells to produce antibodies as part of adaptive immunity. When B-cells leave the bone marrow, they are considered mature but naïve (because they have not yet been exposed to an antigen). Because these antibodies dissolve and act in the blood (rather than within cells), this division of adaptive immunity is called **humoral immunity**. T-cells, another class of adaptive immune cells, mature in the thymus, a small gland just in front of the pericardium, the sac that protects the heart. T-cells are the agents of cell-mediated immunity because they coordinate the immune system and directly kill virally infected cells. Finally, lymph nodes, a major component of the lymphatic system, provide a place for immune cells to communicate and mount an attack; B-cells can be activated here as well. Other immune tissue is found in close proximity to the digestive system, which is a site of potential invasion by pathogens. These tissues are commonly called **gut-associated lymphoid tissue** and include the tonsils and adenoids in the head, Peyer's patches in the small intestine, and lymphoid aggregates in the appendix.

Leukocytes are produced in the bone marrow through hematopoiesis. Leukocytes are divided into two groups of cells: granulocytes and agranulocytes. These names refer to the presence or absence of granules in the cytoplasm. These granules contain toxic enzymes and chemicals, which can be released by exocytosis, and are particularly effective against bacterial, fungal, and parasitic pathogens. Both granulocytes and agranulocytes come from a common precursor: hematopoietic stem cells. Hematopoietic stem cells also are the cell type that gives rise to red blood cells and platelets. Granulocytes include cells such as neutrophils, eosinophils, and basophils. The names of these cells actually refer to the way that the cells appear after staining with certain chemicals. Agranulocytes include the lymphocytes, which are responsible for antibody production, immune system modulation, and the targeted killing of infected cells. Monocytes, which are phagocytic cells in the bloodstream, are considered agranulocytes. They become macrophages in tissues; many tissues have resident populations of macrophages with specific names (such as microglia in the central nervous system, Langerhans cells in the skin, and osteoclasts in bone).

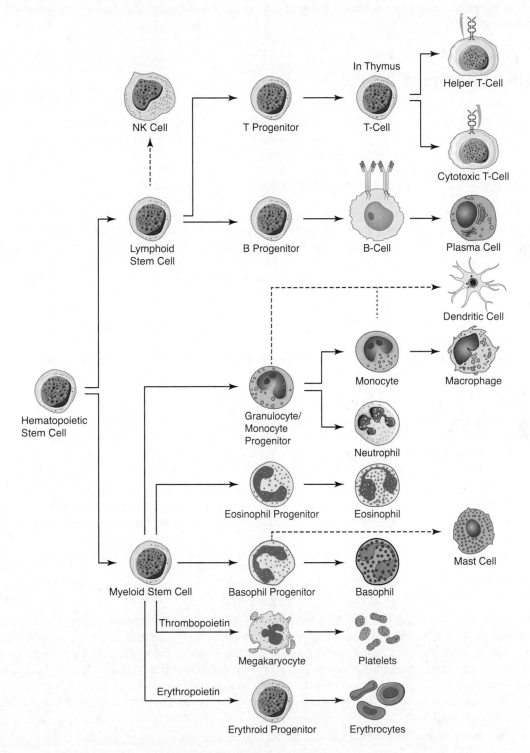

Figure 6-13. Hematopoiesis

Innate immunity refers to the responses that cells can carry out without learning; for this reason, it is also known as the nonspecific immune response. Conversely, adaptive immunity is developed as immune cells learn to recognize and respond to particular antigens and often is aptly referred to as the specific immune response. The specific immune system can be divided into humoral immunity (driven by B-cells and antibodies) and cell-mediated immunity (provided by T-cells).

Noncellular Nonspecific Defenses

The innate immune system consists of cells and structures that offer nonspecific protection. Our first line of defense is the skin (**integument**). The skin provides a physical barrier between the outside world and the body's internal organs, excluding most bacteria, viruses, fungi, and parasites from entering the body. In addition, antibacterial enzymes called **defensins** can be found on the skin. Sweat also has antimicrobial properties. The skin is an important first line of defense: a cut or an abrasion on the skin provides an entry point for pathogens into the body. Deeper wounds allow pathogens to penetrate deeper into the body.

The respiratory system also has mechanisms to prevent pathogens from entering the body. The respiratory passages are mucous membranes, lined with cilia to trap particulate matter and push it up toward the oropharynx, where it can be swallowed or expelled. Although mucus helps to trap particulates such as smoke and dirt, it also helps prevent bacteria and viruses from gaining access to the lung tissue below. Several other mucous membranes, including around the eye and in the oral cavity, produce a nonspecific bacterial enzyme called **lysozyme**, which is secreted in tears and saliva, respectively.

Gastrointestinal Tract

The **gastrointestinal (GI) tract** also plays a role in nonspecific immunity. First, the stomach secretes acid, resulting in the elimination of most pathogens. In addition, the gut also is colonized by bacteria. Most of these bacteria lack the necessary characteristics to cause infection. Because there is already such a large bacterial population in the gut, many potential invaders are not able to compete and are thus kept at bay. Many antibiotics reduce the population of gut flora, thus providing an opportunity for the growth of pathogens resistant to that antibiotic.

Complement

The **complement system** consists of a number of proteins in the blood that act as a nonspecific defense against bacteria. Complement can be activated through a classical pathway (which requires the binding of an antibody to a pathogen) or an alternative pathway (which does not require antibodies). The complement proteins punch holes in the cell walls of bacteria, making them osmotically unstable. Despite the association with antibodies, complement is considered a nonspecific defense because it cannot be modified to target a specific organism over others.

Interferons

To protect against viruses, cells that have been infected with viruses produce **interferons**, proteins that prevent viral replication and dispersion. Interferons cause nearby cells to decrease the production of both viral and cellular proteins. They also decrease the permeability of these cells, making it harder for a virus to infect them. In addition, interferons upregulate MHC (major histocompatibility complex) class I and class II molecules, resulting in increased antigen presentation and better detection of the infected cells by the immune system, as described in the next section. Interferons are responsible for many flu-like symptoms that occur during viral infection, including malaise, tiredness, muscle soreness, and fever.

Cells of the Innate Immune System

So, what happens when bacteria, viruses, fungi, or parasites breach these defenses? The cells of the innate immune system are always poised and ready to attack.

Macrophages

Macrophages, a type of agranulocyte, reside within the tissues. These cells derive from blood-borne monocytes and can become a resident population within a tissue (becoming a permanent, rather than transient, cell group in the tissue). When a bacterial invader enters a tissue, the macrophages become activated. The activated macrophage does 3 things. First, it phagocytizes the invader through endocytosis. Then, it digests the invader using enzymes. Finally, it presents little pieces of the invader (mostly peptides) to other cells using a protein called MHC. MHC binds to a pathogenic peptide (also called an antigen) and carries it to the cell surface, where it can be recognized by cells of the adaptive immune system. In addition, macrophages release cytokines—chemical substances that stimulate inflammation and recruit additional immune cells to the area.

MHC molecules come in 2 main classes: class I and class II. All nucleated cells in the body display MHC class I molecules. Any protein produced within a cell can be loaded onto MHC-I and presented on the surface of the cell. This allows the immune system to monitor the health of these cells and to detect if the cells have been infected with a virus or another intracellular pathogen; only those cells that are infected would be expected to present an unfamiliar (non-self) protein on their surface. Therefore, the MHC-I pathway often is called the endogenous pathway because it binds antigens from inside the cell. Cells that have been invaded by intracellular pathogens can then be killed by a certain group of T-cells (cytotoxic T-lymphocytes) to prevent infection of other cells.

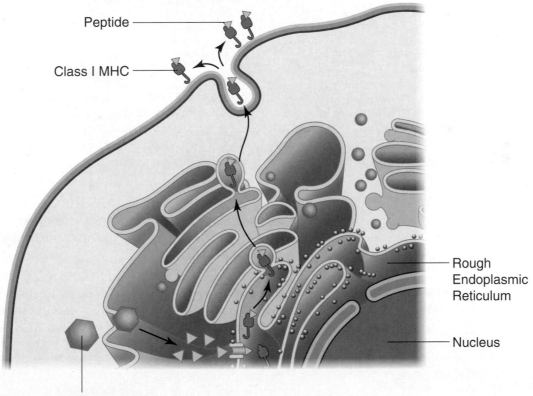

Figure 6-14. Endogenous Pathway for Antigen Presentation (MHC Class I)
MHC-I exists in all nucleated cells.

MHC class II molecules are mainly displayed by professional antigen-presenting cells such as macrophages. Remember that these phagocytic cells pick up pathogens from the environment, process them, and then present them on MHC-II. An **antigen** is a substance (usually a pathogenic protein) that can be targeted by an antibody. Although antibody production is the domain of the adaptive immune system, it is important to understand that cells of the innate immune system also present antigens. Because these antigens originate outside the cell, this pathway often is called the exogenous pathway. The presentation of an antigen by an immune cell may result in the activation of both the innate and adaptive immune systems. Professional antigen-presenting cells include macrophages, dendritic cells in the skin, some B-cells, and certain activated epithelial cells.

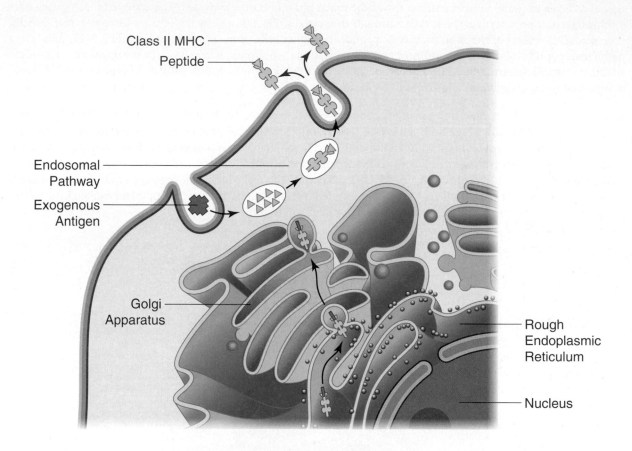

Figure 6-15. Exogenous Pathway for Antigen Presentation (MHC Class II)
MHC-II exists only in professional antigen-presenting cells, such as macrophages, dendritic cells, some B-cells, and some activated epithelial cells.

Macrophages and dendritic cells also have special receptors known as **pattern recognition receptors** (**PRRs**), the best described of which are **toll-like receptors** (**TLRs**). PRRs are able to recognize the category of the invader (bacterium, virus, fungus, or parasite). This allows for the production of appropriate cytokines to recruit the right type of immune cells; each immune cell has different weapons that can target particular groups of pathogens.

Natural Killer Cells

In the arms race between the human immune system and pathogens, some pathogens have found ways to avoid certain defenses. For example, some viruses cause downregulation of MHC molecules, making it harder for T-cells to recognize the presence of an infection. **Natural killer** (**NK**) cells, a type of nonspecific lymphocyte, are able to detect the downregulation of MHC and induce apoptosis in these virally infected cells. Cancer cells also may downregulate MHC production, so NK cells offer protection from the growth of cancer as well.

Granulocytes

In addition to macrophages, the granulocytes, which include neutrophils, eosinophils, and basophils (and closely related mast cells) also are involved in nonspecific defense. **Neutrophils** are the most populous leukocyte in blood and are very short lived (a bit more than 5 days). These cells are phagocytic, like macrophages, and target bacteria.

Neutrophils can literally follow bacteria using **chemotaxis**—the sensing of certain products given off by bacteria and the migration of neutrophils to follow these products back to the source (the bacterium itself). Neutrophils also can detect bacteria once they have been opsonized (marked with an antibody from a B-cell). Other cells, such as NK cells, macrophages, monocytes, and eosinophils, also contain receptors for antibodies and can attack opsonized bacteria. Dead neutrophil collections are responsible for the formation of pus during an infection.

Eosinophils contain bright red-orange granules and are primarily involved in allergic reactions and invasive parasitic infections. Upon activation, eosinophils release large amounts of histamine, an inflammatory mediator. This results in vasodilation and increased leakiness of the blood vessels, allowing additional immune cells (especially macrophages and neutrophils) to move out of the bloodstream and into the tissue. Inflammation is particularly useful against extracellular pathogens, including bacteria, fungi, and parasites.

Finally, **basophils** contain large purple granules and are involved in allergic responses. Under normal conditions, they are the least populous leukocyte in the bloodstream. **Mast cells** are closely related to basophils but have smaller granules and exist in the tissues, mucosa, and epithelium. Both basophils and mast cells release large amounts of histamine in response to allergens, leading to inflammatory responses.

Cells of the Adaptive Immune System

The adaptive immune system can identify specific invaders and mount an attack against that pathogen. The response is variable and depends on the identity of the pathogen. The adaptive immune system can be divided into two divisions: humoral immunity and cell-mediated (cytotoxic) immunity. Each involves the identification of the specific pathogen and organization of an appropriate immune response.

The adaptive immune system consists mainly of two types of lymphocytes: B-cells and T-cells. B-cells govern the humoral response, whereas T-cells mount the cell-mediated response. All cells of the immune system are created in the bone marrow, but B- and T-cells mature in different locations. B-cells mature in the bone marrow (although the B in their name originally stood for the bursa of Fabricius, an organ found in birds), and T-cells mature in the thymus. When exposed to a pathogen, it may take a few days for the physical symptoms to be relieved. This occurs because the adaptive immune response takes time to form specific defenses against the pathogen.

Humoral Immunity

Humoral immunity, which involves the production of antibodies, may take as long as a week to become fully effective after the initial infection. These antibodies are specific to the antigens of the invading microbe. Antibodies are produced by B-cells, which are lymphocytes that originate and mature in the bone marrow and are activated in the spleen and lymph nodes.

Antibodies (also called **immunoglobulins [Igs]**) can carry out many different jobs in the body. Just as antigens can be displayed on the surface of cells or float freely in blood, chyle (lymphatic fluid), or air, so too can antibodies be present on the surface of a cell or secreted into body fluids. When an antibody binds to an antigen, the response will depend on the location. For antibodies secreted into body fluids, there are three main possibilities. First, once bound to a specific antigen, antibodies may attract other leukocytes to phagocytize those antigens immediately. This is called opsonization, as described earlier. Second, antibodies may cause pathogens to clump together or agglutinate, forming large insoluble complexes that can be phagocytized. Third, antibodies can block the ability of a pathogen to invade tissues, essentially neutralizing it. For cell-surface antibodies, the binding of antigen to a B-cell causes activation of that cell, resulting in its proliferation and the formation of plasma and memory cells, as described later in this chapter. In contrast, when antigen binds to antibodies on the surface of a mast cell, it causes degranulation (exocytosis of the granule contents), allowing the release of histamine and causing an inflammatory allergic reaction.

Antibodies are Y-shaped molecules that are composed of two identical heavy chains and two identical light chains. Each antibody has an antigen-binding region at the end of what is called the **variable region** (domain), at the tips of the Y. Within this region, specific polypeptide sequences will bind one, and only one, specific antigenic sequence. Part of the reason it takes so long to initiate the antibody response is that each B-cell undergoes hypermutation of its antigen-binding region, trying to find the best match for the antigen. Only those B-cells that can bind the antigen effectively survive. The remaining part of the antibody molecule is known as the **constant region** (domain). It is this region that cells such as NK cells, macrophages, monocytes, and eosinophils have receptors for and that can initiate the complement cascade.

Each B-cell makes only one type of antibody; because the human body has many B-cells, the body's immune system can recognize many antigens. Further, antibodies come in five different isotypes (IgM, IgD, IgG, IgE, and IgA). Although knowing the specific purposes of each antibody is not necessary for the paramedic, you should know that the different types can be used at different times during the adaptive immune response, for different types of pathogens, or in different locations in the body. The antibody IgE is the antibody involved in allergic reactions. Cells can change which isotype of antibody they produce when stimulated by specific cytokines in a process called **isotype switching**.

Not all B-cells that are generated actively or constantly produce antibodies. Antibody production is an energetically expensive process, and there is no reason to expend energy producing antibodies that are not needed. Instead, naïve B-cells (those that have not yet been exposed to an antigen) wait in the lymph nodes for their particular antigen to come along. After exposure to the correct antigen, a B-cell will proliferate and produce two types of daughter cells. Plasma cells produce large amounts of antibodies, whereas memory B-cells stay in the lymph node, awaiting reexposure to the same antigen. This initial activation takes approximately 7–10 days and is known as the **primary response**. The plasma cells will eventually die, but the memory cells may last the lifetime of the organism. If the same microbe is ever encountered again, the memory cells jump into action and produce the antibodies specific to that pathogen. This immune response, called the **secondary response**, will be more rapid and robust. The development of these lasting memory cells is the basis of the efficacy of vaccinations.

Cytotoxic Immunity

Whereas humoral immunity is based on the activity of B-cells, cell-mediated immunity involves the T-cells. T-cells mature in the thymus, where they undergo both positive and negative selection. Positive selection refers to maturing only those cells that can respond to the presentation of antigen on MHC (cells that cannot respond to MHC undergo apoptosis because they will not be able to respond in the periphery). **Negative selection** refers to causing apoptosis in cells that are self-reactive (activated by proteins produced by the organism itself). The maturation of T-cells is facilitated by thymosin, a peptide hormone secreted by thymic cells. Once the T-cell has left the thymus, it is mature but naïve. After exposure to an antigen, T-cells also will undergo clonal selection so that only those with the highest affinity for a given antigen proliferate.

The 3 major types of T-cells are helper T-cells, killer (cytotoxic) T-cells, and suppressor T-cells.

- **Helper T-cells** (Th), also called CD4+ T-cells, coordinate the immune response by secreting chemicals known as lymphokines. These molecules are capable of recruiting other immune cells (such as plasma cells, cytotoxic T-cells, and macrophages) and increasing their activity. The loss of these cells, which occurs in a human immunodeficiency virus (HIV) infection, prevents the immune system from mounting an adequate response to infection; in advanced HIV infections, also called acquired immunodeficiency syndrome (AIDS), even weak pathogens can cause devastating consequences as opportunistic infections. CD4+ T-cells respond to antigens presented on MHC-II molecules. Because MHC-II presents exogenous antigens, CD4+ T-cells are most effective against bacterial, fungal, and parasitic infections.

- **Cytotoxic T-cells** (Tc or CTL, for cytotoxic T-lymphocytes), also called CD8+ T-cells, are capable of directly killing virally infected cells by injecting toxic chemicals that promote apoptosis into the infected cell. CD8+ T-cells respond to antigens presented on MHC-I molecules. Because MHC-I presents endogenous antigens, CD8+ T-cells are most effective against viral (and intracellular bacterial or fungal) infections.

- **Suppressor or regulatory T-cells** (Treg) also express CD4 but can be differentiated from helper T-cells because they also express a protein called Foxp3. These cells help to tone down the immune response once an infection has been adequately contained. These cells also turn off self-reactive lymphocytes to prevent autoimmune diseases; this is termed **self-tolerance**.

Finally, memory T-cells can be generated. Similar to memory B-cells, these cells lie in wait until the next exposure to the same antigen. When activated, they result in a more robust and rapid response.

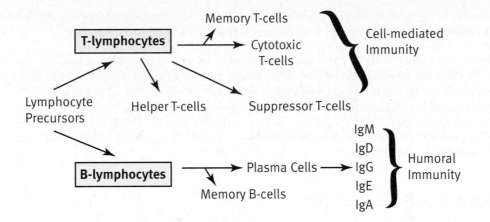

Figure 6-16. Lymphocytes of Specific Immunity
This diagram shows the differentiation of lymphocyte precursors and the cell types involved in specific immunity.

Activation of Adaptive Immune System

When the human body encounters an antigen, the immune system must be able to respond. It is important to note that the innate and adaptive immune systems are not really disparate entities that function separately. The proper functioning of the entire immune system depends on the interactions between these two systems. There are five types of infectious pathogens: bacteria, viruses, fungi, parasites (including protozoa, worms, and insects), and prions (for which there are no immune defenses). Although the immune system's response depends on the specific identity of the pathogen, two classic examples are presented: a bacterial (extracellular pathogen) infection and a viral (intracellular pathogen) infection. Keep in mind that this categorization is imperfect; for example, some bacteria, such as *Mycobacterium tuberculosis* and *Listeria monocytogenes*, actually live intracellularly.

Bacterial (Extracellular Pathogen) Infections

Macrophages are like the sentinels of the human body, always on the lookout for potential invaders. Let's say a person suffers a laceration, and bacteria are introduced into the body via this laceration. First, macrophages (and other antigen-presenting cells) engulf the bacteria and subsequently release inflammatory mediators. These cells also digest the bacteria and present antigens from the pathogen on their surfaces in conjunction with MHC-II. The cytokines attract inflammatory cells, including neutrophils and additional macrophages. Mast cells are activated by the inflammation and degranulate, resulting in histamine release and increased leakiness of the capillaries. This augments the ability of the immune cells to leave the bloodstream to travel to the affected tissue. The dendritic cell then leaves the affected tissue and travels to the nearest lymph node, where it presents the antigen to B-cells. B-cells that produce the correct antibody proliferate through clonal selection to create plasma cells and memory cells. Antibodies then travel through the bloodstream to the affected tissue, where they tag the bacteria for destruction.

At the same time, dendritic cells also are presenting the antigen to T-cells, activating a T-cell response. In particular, CD4+ T-cells are activated. These cells come in two types: Th1 and Th2. Th1 cells release interferon gamma (IFN-γ), which activates macrophages and increases their ability to kill bacteria. Th2 cells help activate B-cells and are more common in parasitic infections.

After the pathogen has been eliminated, the plasma cells die, but the memory B- and T-cells remain. These memory cells allow for a much faster secondary response during reexposure to the pathogen at a later time.

Viral (Intracellular Pathogen) Infections

In a viral infection, the virally infected cell will begin to produce interferons, which reduce the permeability of nearby cells (decreasing the ability of the virus to infect these cells), reduce the rate of transcription and translation in these cells (decreasing the ability of the virus to multiply), and cause systemic symptoms (malaise, muscle aching, fever, and so on). These infected cells also present intracellular proteins on their surface in conjunction with MHC-I; in a virally infected cell, at least some of these intracellular proteins will be viral proteins.

CD8+ T-cells will recognize the MHC-I and antigen complex as foreign and will inject toxins into the cell to promote apoptosis. In this way, the infection can be shut down before it is able to spread to nearby cells. In the event that the virus downregulates the production and presentation of MHC-I molecules, NK cells will recognize the absence of MHC-I and will accordingly cause apoptosis of this cell.

Again, once the pathogen has been cleared, the memory T-cells will be retained to allow a much faster response to be mounted during a second exposure.

Recognition of Self and Nonself

Self-antigens are the proteins and carbohydrates present on the surface of every cell of the body. Under normal circumstances, these self-antigens signal to immune cells that the cell is not threatening and should not be attacked. However, when the immune system fails to make the distinction between self and foreign, it may attack cells expressing particular self-antigens, a condition known as **autoimmunity**. Note that autoimmunity is only one potential problem with immune functioning: another problem arises when the immune system misidentifies a foreign antigen as dangerous when, in fact, it is not. Pet dander, pollen, and peanuts are not inherently threatening to human life, yet some people's immune systems are hypersensitive to these antigens and become overactivated when these antigens are encountered, in what is called an allergic reaction. Allergies and autoimmunity are part of a family of immune reactions classified as **hypersensitivity reactions**.

The human body strives to prevent autoimmune reactions very early in T-cell and B-cell maturation processes. T-cells are educated in the thymus. Part of this education involves the elimination of T-cells that respond to self-antigens, called negative selection. Immature B-cells that respond to self-antigens are eliminated before they leave the bone marrow. However, this process is not perfect, and occasionally a cell that responds to self-antigens is allowed to survive. Most autoimmune diseases can be treated with a number of therapies; a common example is the administration of glucocorticoids (modified versions of cortisol), which have potent immunosuppressive qualities.

Immunization

Often, diseases can have significant, long-term consequences. Infection with the poliovirus, for example, can leave a person disabled for the remainder of their life. Polio used to be a widespread illness; however, today, polio is rarely heard about beyond the Indian subcontinent because of a highly effective vaccination program, which led to the elimination of polio from the Western hemisphere.

Immunization can be achieved in an active or a passive fashion. In **active immunity**, the immune system is stimulated to produce antibodies against a specific pathogen. The means by which people are exposed to this pathogen may either be natural or artificial. Through natural exposure, antibodies are generated by B-cells once an individual becomes infected. Artificial exposure (through vaccines) also results in the production of antibodies; however, the individual never experiences a true infection. Instead, the patient receives an injection or intranasal spray containing an antigen that will activate B-cells to produce antibodies to fight the specific infection. The antigen may be a weakened or killed form of the microbe, or it may be a part of the microbe's protein structure.

Immunization also may be achieved passively. **Passive immunity** results from the transfer of antibodies to an individual. The immunity is transient because only the antibodies, not the plasma cells that produce them, are given to the individual. Natural examples are the transfer of antibodies across the placenta during pregnancy to protect the fetus and the transfer of antibodies from a mother to her nursing infant through breast milk. In some cases of exposure, such as the rabies virus or tetanus, intravenous immunoglobulin may be given to prevent the pathogen from spreading.

Lymphatic System

The immune system and the lymphatic system are intimately related. B-cells proliferate and develop within the lymphatic system, especially the lymph nodes. This system also serves other necessary functions for the body.

The **lymphatic system**, along with the cardiovascular system, is a type of circulatory system. It is made up of one-way vessels that become larger as they move toward the center of the body. These vessels carry lymphatic fluid (**lymph**), and most join to comprise a large **thoracic duct** in the posterior chest, which then delivers the fluid into the left subclavian vein (near the heart).

Lymph nodes are small, bean-shaped structures along the lymphatic vessels. Lymph nodes contain a lymphatic channel, as well as an artery and a vein. The lymph nodes provide a space for the cells of the immune system to be exposed to possible pathogens.

The lymphatic system serves many different purposes in the body by providing a secondary system for circulation.

Equalization of Fluid Distribution

At the capillaries, fluid leaves the bloodstream and goes into the tissues. The quantity of fluid that leaves the tissues at the arterial end of the capillary bed depends on both hydrostatic and oncotic pressures (**Starling forces**). Hydrostatic pressure exists at the arteriole end of the capillary bed and is caused entirely by the pressure of the blood on the arterial walls, essentially the blood pressure. The oncotic pressure is pressure that is caused primarily by the presence of proteins (instead of ions or sugars) and exists at the venule end of the capillary bed. Remember that the oncotic pressure of the blood draws water back into the vessel at the venule end, once hydrostatic pressure has decreased. Because the net pressure drawing fluid in at the venule end is slightly less than the net pressure pushing fluid out at the arterial end, a small amount of fluid remains in the tissues. Lymphatic vessels drain these tissues and subsequently return the fluid to the bloodstream.

The lymphatics offer some protection against pathology. For example, if the blood has a low concentration of albumin (a key plasma protein), the oncotic pressure of the blood is decreased, and less water is driven back into the bloodstream at the venule end. Thus, this fluid will collect in the tissues. Provided that the lymphatic channels are not blocked, much of this fluid may eventually return to the bloodstream via the lymphatics. Only when the lymphatics are overwhelmed does **edema** occur—swelling caused by fluid collecting in tissue.

Transportation of Biomolecules

The lymphatic system also transports fats from the digestive system into the bloodstream. **Lacteals**, small lymphatic vessels, are located at the center of each villus in the small intestine. Fats, packaged into chylomicrons by intestinal mucosal cells, enter the lacteal for transport. Lymphatic fluid carrying many chylomicrons takes on a milky white appearance and is called **chyle**.

Immunity

As stated previously in this chapter, lymph nodes are a place for antigen-presenting cells and lymphocytes to interact. B-cells proliferate and mature in the lymph nodes in collections called **germinal centers**.

Anaphylactic Reactions

Pathophysiology

Anaphylaxis is a result of the body's overreaction to an otherwise harmless invader. At some time prior, the patient was exposed to the allergen, which, for the duration of this section, will be a peanut. So, the patient ate a few peanuts a while back and had no problem with them, but inside, the body was sensitized to this allergen so that the next time the body had this allergen introduced into it, it was prepared. Now, the patient has a peanut again and the body's defense system—the immune system—short circuits.

First, the mast cells remember this invader from before and begin to release large quantities of **histamine**, which is a chemical mediator the body uses to signal a problem and begin the inflammatory response. The histamine release causes immediate swelling in the area of the security breach, which, in times of bacteria introduced through the skin in a laceration, is a very good thing; in the case of a peanut, however, it is now a system-wide problem. With systemic histamine overproduction in anaphylaxis, the capillaries dilate and become leaky, leading to edema. This swelling is seen as urticaria (hives) on the skin and swelling of the tongue, lips, and eyelids on the face. Histamine also causes constriction of smooth muscles, which is seen as laryngospasm, bronchospasm, and abdominal cramping, in addition to the edema of the upper and lower airways. Histamine also has a negative inotropic effect on the heart, which in the presence of dilated, leaky capillaries will lead to potentially profound hypotension.

The presence of histamine causes white blood cells to produce **leukotrienes**, which compound the effects of the histamine, worsening edema and capillary leakiness, bronchoconstriction, vasodilation, and smooth muscle contraction. Leukotrienes also can cause coronary vasoconstriction, possibly leading to myocardial ischemia or MI. This entire process can happen in minutes to hours depending on the body's sensitivity to the allergen.

Assessment

Anaphylaxis leaves no body system completely unaffected; in some way, every body system bears the effects of the histamine flood in anaphylaxis. The following represents the signs and symptoms of anaphylaxis, and the physiological reason for it is in parentheses:

- **Skin.** Warm and flushed (vasodilation); swelling of the face, tongue, lips (histamine); itching and hives (histamine)
- **Respiratory.** Shortness of breath secondary to bronchoconstriction and increased secretions in the bronchial tree (histamine and leukotrienes); hoarseness and stridor (upper airway swelling and laryngospasm)
- **Cardiovascular.** Hypotension and tachycardia (peripheral vasodilation, negative inotropy from leukotrienes); cardiac dysrhythmias (coronary artery vasoconstriction from leukotrienes)
- **GI.** Abdominal cramping, nausea, vomiting, diarrhea (histamine smooth muscle contraction)
- **Nervous System.** Dizziness, altered mental status, anxiety, and restlessness (secondary to hypotension from histamine and leukotrienes)

Treatment of Anaphylaxis

Anaphylaxis can be lethal very shortly after symptoms start to appear, sometimes resulting in full airway closure in >30 minutes. To be considered in anaphylaxis, a patient should have signs of airway compromise or swelling, such as stridor or wheezing and hypotension. Many things need to be accomplished in a fairly short amount of time for the patient to achieve an optimal outcome. What follows is a list of treatments in the order in which they should be completed.

1. Remove the offending agent from the patient. If there is still a stinger embedded in the patient, remove it by scraping a credit card or something similar across it. Trying to tweeze it out may inadvertently inject more venom. If the agent is something injected or inhaled, remove the patient from the area to fresh air. Some patients may be so sensitive to an allergen that just being in the vicinity of the allergen is enough to start a reaction.

2. Initiate cardiac monitoring. Whenever possible, this should be done before epinephrine is administered; however, this step should not delay the administration of epinephrine. Epinephrine can be hard on the heart, so early cardiac monitoring will allow you to catch cardiac dysrhythmias should they occur, whether from the epinephrine or hypoxemia.

3. The primary goal in anaphylaxis is the administration of 0.3 mg epinephrine 1:1,000 subcutaneously or intramuscularly. This can be accomplished by drawing up 0.3 mg epinephrine from an ampule and injecting it or using an Epi-Pen. Epinephrine will reverse the effects of the histamine and leukotrienes, including increasing cardiac output by reversing the histamine's negative inotropic effects, increasing peripheral vascular resistance, accelerating the heart rate, and reversing the bronchoconstriction. Note: For patients under the age of 8, reduce the epinephrine dose to 0.15 mg or use the Epi-Pen Jr.

4. Initiate at least 1 intravenous line with the largest bore (smallest gauge number) possible. The patient will have moved a substantial amount of fluid into the interstitial space that will not return to the vasculature as quickly as it left. This will potentially leave the patient hypovolemic if the fluid is not replaced. The intravenous line should be run wide and up to 1 L can be delivered easily; many times up to 2 L are needed to normalize blood pressure and heart rate after an anaphylactic event.

5. Only after epinephrine has been administered and the intravenous line has been initiated should antihistamines be considered. Antihistamines, such as diphenhydramine, block histamine receptors, blunting the effects of the histamine that is present and still being released. The recommended dose is 25–50 mg diphenhydramine IVP.

6. Corticosteroids can be administered at this time. Although they do not have an immediate effect on the patient's current condition, they can prevent late-phase reactions.

In addition to the above, some treatments to consider include aggressive airway management, inhaled beta-agonists, beta-blockade reversal agents, and blood pressure support. Patients may go into anaphylaxis quickly, so be prepared to manage an airway that is closing, either with early intubation or later with a cricothyrotomy. For patients who are on beta-blockers, consider administering 1–2 mg glucagon IV push every 5 minutes. This can help minimize beta receptor antagonism, resulting in increased cardiac contractility and heart rate. Treat refractory bronchoconstriction with inhaled beta-agonists such as albuterol. Albuterol can be essentially continuous. Intramuscular or subcutaneous epinephrine can be repeated if necessary. In the event that the transport time is extended, and the patient is not improving after at least 2 L of NSS or lactated Ringer solution has been administered (some case studies indicate fluid resuscitation exceeding 4 L), the paramedic should consider administering a pressor. Mix 1 mg of 1:1,000 epinephrine in a 1,000 mL bag of NSS and run this mix at 0.1 mcg/kg/min. Most likely, pharmacologic pressure support will be used only during interfacility transports because it should take a couple of hours to get 4 L of fluid into the patient.

Systemic Lupus Erythematosus

Systemic lupus erythematosus (lupus or SLE) is a multisystem autoimmune disease that affects the entire body. It should be suspected in women of child-bearing age who complain of joint pain, rash, and a fever. The assessment and treatment of these patients focuses on addressing life threats and other acute problems.

Organ Transplant Disorders

Paramedics will, at some point in time, likely encounter a patient who has had an organ transplanted. The most common organs to be transplanted are the heart, liver, kidney, lung, and pancreas. Treatment for any problem with an organ transplant patient should be completed as per normal. The only major difference in treatment for the paramedic would be in a heart transplant patient. Because the new heart is not connected to the vagus nerve, atropine will not work to increase the heart rate. In the case of a bradycardic heart transplant patient, consult medical control.

If the patient's body begins to reject these organs, the initial signs are subtle and can be confused for the flu—general malaise, weakness, and fever. Treatment for patients suspected of organ transplant rejection should be transported to the nearest facility. Consider contacting their organ transplant facility for guidance.

Leukemia

Leukemia literally means "white blood" and is a form of cancer that causes white blood cells to develop abnormally and excessively. Leukemia can cause anemia and thrombocytopenia (low platelet count), and the chemotherapy used to cure it often will often cause leukocytopenia (low white blood cell count). If caught early, leukemia is one of the more curable cancers.

Assessment of the patient with leukemia often is related to a problem other than the leukemia itself. For example, paramedics may be called to treat a patient with leukemia who has had excessive vomiting after chemotherapy; or perhaps the patient is short of breath owing to the anemia. How the patient presents will be wholly the result of the complaint and the overall state of the cancer. Therefore, management of this patient will generally be based on the presenting symptoms. Some overarching guidelines would be to provide supplemental O_2 in the event the patient is having a bout with anemia and to treat the patient as positively as possible. The patient may not have the most positive outlook on life at the moment the paramedic arrives, so even a smile can go a long way to brighten the patient's day. If it is possible to know, try to find out if the patient is leukocytopenic at the time. If so, consider putting a surgical mask on the patient to minimize the chances of another infection on top of everything else.

Lymphomas

Lymphoma is any of a group of cancers that involves the lymphatic cells. The most common lymphoma is called **non-Hodgkin's lymphoma**. Other common types of lymphomas include **Hodgkin's lymphoma** and **multiple myeloma**. These cancers are treatable depending on how early they are found and based on how aggressive they are. More aggressive cancers are generally found later, have already moved to other organs or body systems, and require a more complicated course of cytotoxic chemotherapy to treat. This makes successfully battling the cancer highly difficult. With any of these cancers, the initial signs are insidious, including vague complaints such as night sweats, chills, and a persistent cough. Some patients may note swelling of the neck lymph nodes, loss of appetite, and weight loss. Any treatment a paramedic will render for these patients is largely supportive and aimed at relieving symptoms.

REVIEW QUESTIONS

Select the ONE best answer.

1. The primary role of mast cells in anaphylactic reactions is to:

   A. Release IgE.

   B. Release histamine.

   C. Produce antibodies.

   D. Proliferate and attack foreign substances.

2. The term for the immunity a person would possess as a result of receiving a vaccination is:

   A. Active immunity.

   B. Acquired immunity.

   C. Herd immunity.

   D. Passive immunity.

3. The most appropriate first treatment for a 45-year-old male presenting with only urticaria and tingling of the lips after being stung by a bee is:

   A. Albuterol, 2.5 mg in 3 mL, inhaled.

   B. Diphenhydramine, 50 mg intravenously.

   C. Epinephrine, 1:1,000, 0.3 mg intramuscularly.

   D. Remove the stinger.

ANSWERS AND EXPLANATIONS

1. **The correct answer is (B).** Mast cells initially and primarily produce histamine, which is largely responsible for airway swelling, bronchoconstriction, urticaria, and facial swelling common in anaphylaxis. Plasma cells release antibodies (C) including IgE (A), which is an antibody specific to allergic reactions. Mast cells are part of the immune system but are not circulating white blood cells; therefore, they do not proliferate (D) in times of anaphylaxis or infection.

2. **The correct answer is (B).** This is the definition of acquired immunity. Active immunity (A) also is known as natural immunity, and it is the immunity conferred by actually getting the illness and fighting it off. Herd immunity (C) is the immunity a person has as a benefit of being surrounded by people who are immune to a disease. Although the person is not immune individually, the likelihood of them catching a particular disease is reduced to zero because no one around the person can get it. This type of immunity can be weakened in areas with low pediatric vaccination rates. Passive immunity (D) is the immunity passed from the mother to child while in utero or breastfeeding. After birth and when no longer breastfeeding, the child is typically no longer immune to those diseases.

3. **The correct answer is (D).** In this case, the stinger could be continuing and prolonging the reaction. Scrape it out with a credit card before considering the other treatment options listed. Because the patient is not in severe distress and is not displaying any airway compromise, epinephrine (C) can be held off until the stinger is removed.

INFECTIOUS DISEASES

This section talks about a variety of infectious diseases that the paramedic should be concerned about when encountering patients. It also will discuss ways to prevent the transmission of these diseases from patient to provider and from patient to patient.

Protections for Providers and the Public

Agencies at all levels of government—federal, state, and local—exist for the protection of the public. The **Occupational Safety and Health Administration (OSHA)** is a national agency responsible for establishing rules to ensure the safety of employees. One of the more important rules for EMS agencies is the Blood Borne Pathogen Standard, which establishes an exposure control plan and preexposure education requirements for all healthcare facilities and agencies. The Ryan White Act, among other things, requires that hospitals notify emergency response personnel whenever they have been exposed to any of a wide array of diseases, particularly those that are airborne or droplet borne. The **Centers for Disease Control and Prevention (CDC)** keeps tabs on disease statistics and works with state and local health departments to ensure that prevention and follow-up activities are implemented and working. They often will intervene if there is an increase beyond the endemic number of cases in an area. A rise in the number of cases above the endemic, or expected, number of cases may signal an epidemic. If the disease spreads worldwide with a great number of new cases all over, it is called a pandemic.

Paramedics need to be a part of the protection of their patients, through community education whenever possible; they also have an obligation to prevent or minimize the chances of **nosocomial** infections—infections spread in the healthcare environment. To achieve this, after every call ensure that the ambulance is cleaned to OSHA standards, which includes sterilizing any reusable equipment that comes in contact with patient fluids, such as laryngoscope blades with chemical sterilants. Clean other equipment that comes in contact with skin, such as stethoscopes, the stretcher, and blood pressure cuffs, with a bleach and water mixture whenever the equipment is used.

Modes of Transmission

Patient-to-provider transmission is rare, but understanding modes of disease transmission and taking steps for protection against those modes of transmission is crucial to being able to protect yourself from getting sick. Pathogens are spread from person to person in any of 4 ways:

- **Airborne Transmission.** Pathogens are capable of surviving in air for an extended period of time without being supported in a medium such as a droplet. They have the ability to go long distances on air currents.

- **Direct Contact.** This is where transmission of the disease comes from intimate contact with the individual who carries it. Direct contact includes casual contact with the person, accidental needle stick transmission, or transfusion of contaminated blood.

- **Droplet Transmission.** Infection occurs when a person inhales droplets contaminated with the pathogen. These microscopic droplets are released when a person coughs or sneezes. They tend to fall after 3–6 feet.

- **Indirect Contact.** Touching something that the infected person also handled is called indirect contact. The objects that are contaminated with pathogens that are still capable of causing disease are called **fomites**. The fact that some microorganisms can survive for long periods on fomites is a good reason to conduct thorough cleanings after every patient.

Paramedics need to protect themselves from potential transmission of diseases from the patient. The agency for which the paramedic works is responsible for providing personal protective equipment (PPE), based on OSHA and CDC recommendations. PPE protects providers from getting any potentially contaminated material on their hands.

Gloves should be the bare minimum of PPE worn for every patient contact. Gloves are the first-line defense against blood-borne pathogens of the patient and surfaces. Other PPE that the provider will need to use on a much less frequent basis includes gowns, face and eye shields, and surgical masks or respirators. These PPE should be employed anytime there is risk of splashing or squirting bodily fluids, including blood, amniotic fluid, or vomit.

After the call and throughout the day, providers should ensure proper handwashing with soap and water. The CDC identifies handwashing as the ideal way to clean hands when they are visibly soiled. When hands are not visibly soiled or if soap and water are not immediately available, the CDC recommends using a waterless alcohol cleaner rubbed over all areas of the hands until dry. One of these 2 methods should be employed after every patient contact. Handwashing with regular soap and water or the regular use of a waterless alcohol based cleaner can break the infection cycle immediately.

Exposures

Not every patient you encounter with an infectious disease constitutes an exposure; simply being on scene with a patient or having a patient in the ambulance who has pneumonia does not necessarily mean an exposure has occurred. An exposure to a blood-borne pathogen has occurred when a potentially infectious material—such as blood, vomit, saliva, semen, vaginal fluids, amniotic fluid, feces, or urine from a person who is known to have or has later been proven to have a communicable disease—comes in contact with a mucous membrane; splashes into the eyes, nose, or mouth; or comes in contact with an open wound on the provider. Under this set of circumstances, the employer is responsible for having the potential source of the transmission tested. Under the **Ryan White Comprehensive AIDS Resources Emergency Act**, the medical facility must release these test results back to the infection control officer for the requesting agency, who will then share the information with the employee. At this point, the affected provider can receive proper care and counseling as needed.

For airborne or droplet borne diseases, the agency's designated infection control officer will consider the circumstances surrounding the possible exposure. The circumstances include the amount of time with the patient and the proximity of the provider to the patient. The infection control officer also will consider the possible organism involved and the task(s) the provider performed on the patient. For example, if the provider needed to intubate the patient and the patient with bacterial pneumonia coughed, this may constitute an exposure. Alternatively, if a patient with TB was wearing a mask during a routine transport and never took off the mask, and the provider was never in close contact with the patient, an exposure likely did not happen.

Whether a person becomes infected depends on a lot of factors. Exposure to a pathogen must meet or exceed the following requirements for an infection to be possible:

- The organism needs to be present.
- The organism needs to be capable of causing an infection in humans. There are literally hundreds of thousands of different strains of bacteria, viruses, and fungi that do not in any way affect humans.
- The person needs to be exposed to a quantity of pathogen that will exceed the body's ability to eliminate it before fully exerting its effects. For example, for *Vibrio cholera* to cause the syndrome of symptoms associated with the disease it causes (cholera), a person would need to receive a dose in excess of 10,000 organisms. Whereas for *Shigella* to cause disease, a person needs to come in contact with fewer than 50 live bacteria.
- The **virulence** of the organism is a relative term for the ability of an organism to cause disease in a host, as measured by the degree of disease it causes.
- For the disease to occur, the pathogen must enter the host through the correct route. The pathogen must successfully navigate the environment and the body's defenses to arrive at the spot where it can reproduce. For example, swallowing bacteria that would cause pneumonia if it got into the lungs will not result in pneumonia.
- The host's defenses must not be so strong that they fight off the pathogen invasion before the pathogen can cause the infection.

Specific Infectious Diseases

This section will discuss a variety of diseases with which the paramedic could come in contact. Rather than focusing on treatment as in previous sections, the pathophysiology and symptoms associated with the infection will be presented.

Unless otherwise noted, prehospital treatment and management of these infections are supportive and focused on relieving the associated symptoms.

Tuberculosis

Tuberculosis (TB) is a droplet-borne disease and comes in 3 forms. Only one form is communicable—typical TB—so that will be discussed here. (The other 2 types are atypical TB and nonpulmonary TB, which infects kidney, bone, etc.)

TB can be active or latent. For TB to be transmitted, the disease must be active.

- In the **latent form**, the bacterium that causes TB lives in the patient's lungs, yet there are no symptoms. The patient cannot spread the disease, and oftentimes active disease never develops even though the test is positive.
- In the **active form**, the patient has active, live bacteria in the sputum, and the chest x-ray shows consolidations consistent with TB.

Because TB is a droplet-borne disease, a paramedic should use the following guidelines:

- Adequate protection is provided by placing a surgical mask on the patient and opening the windows of the ambulance.
- Only paramedics who are in extremely close contact to the patient for an extended period of time or who perform mouth-to-mouth on TB patients are at increased risk of transmission.
- TB is spread more readily in school dormitories, prisons, and nursing homes, where people remain in close contact for extended periods of time.

Whether active or latent, TB is detected with a skin test and confirmed to be "active" with a chest x-ray.

Symptoms of active TB typically include persistent cough >3 weeks, night sweats, fever, unexplained weight loss, and bloody sputum (hemoptysis). Respiratory distress and nonreproducible localized chest pain are also common.

Tuberculosis: Droplet Borne or Airborne?

TB prevention methodologies vary from one reliable medical text to another:

- Paramedic texts and National Registry materials for the paramedic exam describe TB as a droplet-borne bacillus. According to these sources, a mask on the patient and open windows are all that is needed to adequately prevent disease transmission to a paramedic who is not otherwise in close contact with a person infected with pulmonary TB.
- Other reliable sources describe TB as an airborne disease requiring the paramedic to wear a mask with high particulate filtration (HEPA or N95) to prevent transmission.

It is recommended that you follow EMS-specific texts for the paramedic exam and use your best judgment and local protocols in the field.

Pneumonia

Pneumonia is an all-encompassing term for any infection that causes inflammation of the lungs. Pneumonia caused by the bacteria *Staphylococcus* or *Streptococcus* is communicable, whereas pneumonia caused by viruses or fungi is not. Communicable pneumonia is transmitted via droplets sneezed or coughed out. Patients will complain of respiratory distress and have a productive cough of a colored sputum, fever, chills, and possible chest pain. The paramedics should wear a mask or place the patient on a high-flow O_2 via a mask to protect themselves from transmission.

Influenza

Annually, millions are infected with **influenza** (the flu), and >36,000 die each year. The flu is a droplet-borne virus that is primarily transmitted by indirect contact, such as getting it on the hand and then touching one's mouth, nose, or eyes. Patients often complain of a runny nose, muscle pain, fever, chills, and loss of appetite. The course of the infection tends to be about 3–4 days, but the patient is infectious one day before and one day after the symptoms present. For these patients, supporting the blood pressure and pulse oximetry are the goals of prehospital treatment.

Sexually Transmitted Diseases

For our purposes here, **sexually transmitted diseases** are primarily diseases that are not only transmitted sexually but also directly affect the genitals. This includes genital herpes, chlamydia, syphilis, gonorrhea, and the human papillomavirus. Paramedics will rarely need to assess the genitals of any patient, including the patient who complains of genital sores. This type of infection generally poses little threat of transmission to a paramedic.

Scabies

Scabies is a parasite that is transmitted through direct or indirect skin-to-skin contact, including during sexual contact or sharing towels or clothing. Scabies causes a body-wide or localized rash of small red bumps on the skin, where the parasite has burrowed into the skin. Patients often complain of intense itching, especially at night, and can scratch so feverishly that they lacerate the skin or develop larger sores. To prevent transmission, only routine cleaning of the ambulance and changing of bed linens is necessary.

Lice

Lice are parasites that are spread only by being in close physical contact with or through sharing hats or clothing of an infected person. Lice cannot live for >24 hours off a person and can be located anywhere on the body. Common symptoms include intense itching because lice bite the skin in the infested area. Eggs, called nits, and the lice can be seen clinging to hair follicles. Prevention requires usual cleaning and changing bed linens.

Lyme Disease

Lyme disease, a tick-borne disease, is contracted when a tick infected with *Borrelia burgdorferi* bites a person, injecting this bacterium into the new host. Lyme disease causes widely varied symptoms that come in phases. Common symptoms include any or all of the following: fever, chills, muscle pain, and joint pain (especially in the knees). Headache is another common symptom of Lyme disease; it results from meningoencephalitis (swelling of the brain and meninges) and can often be mistaken for a migraine.

Patients also have a characteristic bull's eye rash somewhere on the body, not necessarily related to where the bite is; it appears as a red central area surrounded by a white ring and outer red ring. It is possible to have more than one of these rashes called **erythema migrans**. After the initial diagnosis, patients may also experience relapses with similar symptoms, though a new bite is not necessary. This disease is not transmitted from person to person.

Prehospital treatment is supportive while an in hospital course may be extensive based on associated neurological findings. Paramedics should support blood pressure and manage pain as needed.

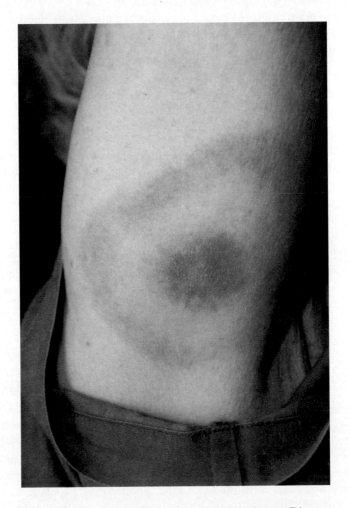

Figure 6-17. Classic Bull's Eye Rash in Lyme Disease

Rabies

Rabies is transmitted through the bite of an infected animal, most commonly raccoons, skunks, and foxes. The virus that causes it is shed in the saliva of the animal and essentially injected into the bloodstream.

- Symptoms are usually nonspecific and flu-like, but numbness in the area of the bite is a common complaint.
- As the disease progresses into the neurologic phase, patients can display hyperactive delirium, seizures, and bizarre behavior. Patients may experience hydrophobia (fear of water) because water causes severe spasms of the throat muscles and the muscles of mastication.
- If left untreated, symptoms can worsen; coma and death are possible.

Treatment is driven by the presenting symptoms and includes management of the ABCs and sedation for seizures or delirium.

Hepatitis

All forms of **hepatitis** caused by a viral infection result in inflammation and failure of the liver. Hepatitis types B, C, and D are all blood borne and are transmitted by coming in direct contact with blood and fluids containing blood. They also can be transmitted via needlestick injuries and transfusions. Hepatitis B and C are primary infections. Hepatitis D only occurs if the patient is already infected with hepatitis B.

Hepatitis A and E are not blood borne but rather are transmitted via the fecal-oral route. At some point, the infected person ate something contaminated with feces from an infected person or animal or consumed contaminated water.

The signs and symptoms for hepatitis, regardless of type, are basically the same. They include loss of appetite, jaundiced or yellow skin color, a low grade fever, general malaise, and gray feces. There may even be a yellowing of the whites of the eyes, called icterus. Patients who previously smoked often have a sudden distaste for cigarettes. The use of gloves during routine patient contact and routine cleaning of all patient contact areas is all that is needed to prevent transmission.

Human Immunodeficiency Virus

The pathophysiology of **HIV** at the cellular level is highly complicated, involving changes in cellular markers. A deeper discussion here is not included; however, HIV invades and kills helper T-cells required for both cellular and humoral immunity. Patients with HIV often are asymptomatic for a long period of time when HIV is in a latent period. Patients will then **seroconvert**, which means that they have detectable levels of antibodies to HIV in the blood.

- Transmission of blood-borne HIV primarily occurs from needlestick injuries and contact with blood on an open wound or through transfusion.
- HIV is not transmitted through casual contact or saliva.
- The virus also can be found in vaginal and seminal fluids, so sexual transmission is likely as well.

AIDS (**acquired immunodeficiency syndrome**) is the end-stage of HIV infection and is characterized by an overall failure of the immune system to fight off any infections. Patients become susceptible to opportunistic infections rarely seen in the patient with a normal immune system, including pneumocystis pneumonia, atypical TB, and Kaposi sarcoma (a purplish skin cancer). Care for the patient infected with HIV is supportive and related to other diseases the patient may have. HIV does not survive for long on hard surfaces once the fluid it was in has dried. Regular cleaning procedures are all that is required to rid the ambulance of the virus.

Medication-Resistant Pathogens

The overuse and misuse of antibiotic medications for decades have resulted in the creation of bacterial infections that are resistant to currently available antibiotics on the market. These so-called superbugs are very difficult to manage and generally require hospitalization for aggressive intravenous antibiotic therapy. The following list is not exhaustive but includes the most common bacteria that paramedics may encounter. Fortunately for the provider, these infections are relatively difficult to transmit from person to person, especially in people with normal immune systems; typically, gloves and handwashing are all that is required for protection because none of these are air or droplet borne.

- **Methicillin-Resistant *Staphylococcus aureus* (MRSA).** Commonly found on the skin, once these organisms enter the skin through an abrasion or laceration, they can cause skin infections and cellulitis.

- **Vancomycin-Resistant *Enterococcus* (VRE).** Commonly found in the intestinal tract, these organisms become a problem when the other natural and more numerous species of bacteria also naturally found in the intestines are killed off during long courses of antibiotic treatment. As these other species are killed off, VRE can take over, leading to diarrhea.

- *Clostridioides difficile* (*C. diff*). Similar to VRE, it causes diarrhea and is allowed to develop when other bacteria in the gut are killed off from excessive courses of antibiotic usage. It presents with copious amounts of watery green, foul-smelling diarrhea. Gloves and good handwashing after contact are generally enough to prevent spreading of the infection.

Practical Point

Pandemics are not specifically tested on the National Registry Paramedic exam, so the following discussion is for informational purposes only.

Pandemics

In 2020, the world experienced the infectious disease pandemic known as **SARS-CoV-2 or Covid-19**. In recent decades, several notable infectious diseases have arisen quickly and left variable paths of morbidity and mortality in their wakes.

It is worth noting here the difference between pathogenicity and virulence. **Pathogenicity** is the ability of a pathogen (bacteria, virus, or fungus) to infect a host and cause disease. It can be thought of as the infectiousness, or the dose of pathogen needed to cause disease. **Virulence** is the severity of disease that the pathogen causes, once it has established an infection.

There is no correlation between pathogenicity and virulence. Some diseases may have a low pathogenicity requiring very few bacteria, viruses, or spores to cause a disease, and those may cause only relatively minor symptoms. In addition, virulence may depend on the host rather than the pathogen, i.e., the same pathogen may cause severe symptoms and even death in one person while barely affect another person.

Coronaviruses are a family of viruses that, when viewed under a microscope, appear to have a solid core surrounded by a "crown" (or corona) similar to that surrounding the sun during a total solar eclipse. Members of the coronavirus family typically cause upper respiratory infections including runny nose, cough, sore throat, and sometimes fever and shortness of breath.

Since the early 2000s, new coronaviruses have been liberated from animal reservoirs (specifically bats) and have successfully infected humans. These include the following viruses and diseases.

- SARS-CoV, which causes severe acute respiratory syndrome (SARS)
- MERS-CoV, which causes Middle East respiratory syndrome (MERS)
- SARS-CoV-2, which causes coronavirus disease 2019 (Covid-19)

SARS-CoV

Originally discovered in 2002, SARS-CoV infected more than 8,000 people in 26 countries and resulted in 774 deaths attributed to the virus, or nearly 10% of infections. No new infections have been reported since 2004.

MERS-CoV

First reported in late 2012 in Saudi Arabia, this virus is thought to have moved from bats to camels to humans. It infected over 2,500 people and resulted in over 850 deaths, or about 33% of those infected.

SARS-CoV-2

First identified in China in December 2019, SARS-CoV-2 has spread worldwide. As of the time of writing, it had infected more than 35 million people and caused more than 1.1 million fatalities worldwide. Unique to this virus compared to its predecessors is its variability of presentation: SARS-CoV-2 can cause severe illness and death in some, yet others who are infected can remain completely asymptomatic. There also seems to be an extended **incubation period** (the time it takes for an infection to reach a concentration within the host high enough to show symptoms and become infectious), resulting virus shedding and infection spread through individuals who are unaware that they are disease hosts.

Stopping the spread of the previous coronaviruses was comparatively easy because those infected showed symptoms in about 2 days after exposure. Quick isolation and quarantine were effective in controlling spread of those pathogens. Achieving the same with SARS-CoV-2 has proven much more difficult, requiring much more routine testing in order to identify the asymptomatic among the infected.

SIRS and Sepsis

Systemic Inflammatory Response Syndrome (SIRS)

SIRS is the body's system-wide response to insult or infection. A person experiencing SIRS needs specific care, so the SIRS criteria were developed to identify these patients.

It is important to note that SIRS can arise from noninfectious conditions; these include pancreatitis, burns, and trauma. In practice, however, when SIRS criteria are present in a patient, you should suspect an infection until this possibility has been ruled out. For the paramedic who first encounters a sick patient, SIRS = sepsis. A patient presenting with 2 or more of the clinical findings listed in the SIRS criteria is considered positive for SIRS.

SIRS criteria:

- Temperature: <96.8°F (36°C) *or* >100.4°F (38°C)
- Respiratory rate >20
- Heart rate >90
- pCO_2: <32 mmHg
- White blood cell count: <4,000 *or* >12,000 *or* >10% bands

Paramedics are generally without the benefit of a complete blood count, so presentation of any 2 (or more) of the first 4 bullets constitutes SIRS in the prehospital setting. This highlights the need for continuous waveform capnometry in the prehospital setting; it should be included in any patient presenting with a fever, lethargy, or suspected infection.

Sepsis

When 2 or more of the SIRS criteria and a suspected or confirmed infection are present, the patient is now said to have **sepsis**. Sepsis, at least initially, is not a life-threatening event. If allowed to progress beyond the body's ability to compensate, however, it can develop into **severe sepsis** and, eventually, **septic shock**.

Sepsis has progressed to the severe sepsis stage if the patient has signs of end-organ damage, systolic BP below 90 mmHg, and serum lactate >4 mmol. The lactate level is a marker for organ dysfunction relating to hypoperfusion in severe sepsis. While point-of-care lactate machines do exist, they are often costly, and lactate is not typically checked in the field at this time. For prehospital providers, a useful stand-in measurement is end-tidal CO_2 ($EtCO_2$): There is a strong inverse correlation between rising lactate levels and falling levels of $EtCO_2$. Therefore, paramedics should regard an $EtCO_2$ level below 26 mmHg as an indication of severe sepsis or septic shock.

Pro-Tip

Lactate is also known as lactic acid. A buildup of lactic acid leads to acidosis. The body's primary mechanism to correct acidosis is increased respiration rate: Increasing respirations result in decreasing end-tidal CO_2. Therefore, an increase in lactate directly leads to 2 observable SIRS criteria: increased respiratory rate and low $EtCO_2$.

If the blood pressure remains low despite fluid resuscitation efforts, it is an indication that the patient has progressed to the stage of septic shock. Altered mental status is another indication: Mild or severe altered mental status, or even unresponsiveness, is likely as the patient progresses through the stages of sepsis. In later stages, the body may no longer be able to maintain an elevated temperature. Be on the alert for the patient presenting with signs of sepsis and end-organ failure combined with body temperature that is normal or low.

Early recognition, early intervention, and early notification to the hospital are crucial steps in prehospital treatment of the septic patient. The paramedic should identify the presence of any of the SIRS criteria in a patient and record a Glasgow Coma Score (GCS). If any of the criteria are present, give the patient normal saline in 500 mL doses until the criteria have resolved, the max infusion of 2 liters has been reached, or arrival has been made at the hospital. If systolic BP remains less than 90 mmHg after 2 liters of fluids have been infused, vasopressors should be initiated, if available (dopamine, epinephrine, or norepinephrine). Definitive treatment includes antibiotics (outside the current scope of practice for paramedics in most systems).

The table records clinical findings for SIRS versus sepsis. Note that only the metrics that can be obtained in the prehospital assessment are considered in the table.

Table 6-10. SIRS and Sepsis Classifications

Criteria	SIRS	Sepsis	Severe Sepsis	Septic Shock
Temperature <96.8°F (36°C) *or* >100.4°F (38°C)	X	X	X	X
Respiratory rate >20	X	X	X	X
Heart rate >90	X	X	X	X
pCO_2: <32 mmHg	X	X	X	X
Known or suspected infection		X	X	X
$EtCO_2$: <26 mmHg			X	X
Altered mental status (GCS <15)			X	X
SBP <90			X	X
SBP improves with fluid			X	

REVIEW QUESTIONS

Select the ONE best answer.

1. Rabies is transmitted when an infected animal bites a person and saliva gets in the broken skin. This is an example of which of the following forms of communicable disease transmission?

    A. Direct contact

    B. Indirect contact

    C. Airborne transmission

    D. Droplet transmission

2. Transmission from patient to paramedic of which of the following diseases can be reasonably prevented if the paramedic wears a surgical mask?

    A. Hepatitis B

    B. Fungal pneumonia

    C. Scabies

    D. Tuberculosis

3. A 58-year-old female patient is complaining of a recent history of frequent episodes of watery, green diarrhea. She has been on levofloxacin for several weeks for a recurrent upper respiratory infection and denies being out of the country in the past year. She further denies any significant past medical history or other medications. Which of the following is most likely the cause of her diarrhea?

    A. Amoebic dysentery

    B. *C. diff*

    C. VRE

    D. MRSA

4. The patient from the previous question has the following vital signs: HR: 124; BP: 88/60; RR: 26; EtCO$_2$: 28; Temp: 102.8°F (39.3°C). Which of the following is the most appropriate treatment?

    A. 1 L normal saline solution

    B. 1 L Ringer lactate

    C. 5 mcg/kg/min dopamine

    D. 2 mcg/kg/min epinephrine

5. Which of the following SIRS criteria is most closely associated with an elevated lactate?

    A. Altered mentation

    B. Decreased end tidal CO$_2$

    C. Elevated heart rate

    D. Elevated temperature

ANSWERS AND EXPLANATIONS

1. **The correct answer is (A).** The transmission of rabies occurs from direct contact with a pathogen-containing substance, often blood. Indirect contact (B) would be when you touch a contaminated surface and then your own mucous membranes. Airborne transmission (C) is when the pathogen is transmitted directly on the air. Droplet transmission (D) is when the pathogen is contained within a droplet of mucus or saliva. This is different than airborne transmission.

2. **The correct answer is (D).** TB is a droplet-borne infection caused by a bacterium that can be transmitted from one person to the next when a person with the disease coughs or sneezes. Hepatitis B (A) is transmitted only through direct contact. Fungal pneumonia (B) is not communicable (spread from one person to the next). Scabies (C) is a parasite and can be transmitted only through direct or indirect contact with the patient. A surgical mask will not prevent transmission.

3. **The correct answer is (B).** *C. diff* is the most common and severe form of antibiotic-related diarrhea. It is known for its particularly watery consistency. Although VRE (C) can be caused by the overuse of antibiotics, fluoroquinolone use, such as levofloxacin, is more closely correlated with a *C. diff* infection than VRE. Because the patient did not travel out of the country, amoebic dysentery (A) is highly unlikely. MRSA (D) is not typically associated with infections leading to diarrhea and is more common as a skin infection.

4. **The correct answer is (A).** NSS of up to 1 L in a patient without signs of CHF is the initial treatment because the patient is showing signs of dehydration. Lactated Ringer solution (B) is not preferred because it may raise already elevated potassium levels. Pressors (C) and (D) are not appropriate until after at least 2 L of NSS has failed to raise the blood pressure, or the patient begins showing signs of fluid overload.

5. **The correct answer is (B).** Lactate, or lactic acid, production leads to acidosis. The first way the body works to fix acidosis is to breathe faster in order to lower carbon dioxide levels. This in turn will lead to a reduced ETCO$_2$. Refer to Chapter 1 for a full review on the bicarbonate/CO$_2$ buffer system. The remaining answers are not closely tied to elevated lactate.

TOXICOLOGICAL EMERGENCIES

The paramedic will need to, at some point, treat a patient who has overdosed on some form of drug. The drug could be alcohol, prescription/over-the-counter medication, illicit street drugs such as heroin, or any other substance that alters the mind, produces euphoria, or could result in death as the desired outcome.

Practical Point

A **drug** is any substance that, in appropriate quantities, can bring about a therapeutic effect. A **poison** is a substance that is toxic in some capacity, regardless of dose and route of entry.

Toxicologic emergencies can be intentional or unintentional.

- Examples of **intentional intake** include attempted suicide and deliberate overuse based on flawed logic ("if some is good, more must be better").
- Examples of **unintentional intake** include unawareness of accumulated intake (e.g., taking acetaminophen tablets plus a cold remedy containing acetaminophen); forgetfulness (e.g., an older person with poor memory takes the same medication multiple times); environmental exposure (e.g., working in proximity to poisonous chemicals); and mistaking drugs for harmless materials (e.g., candy).

Practical Point

Young children are particularly susceptible to accidental poisoning because they explore the world with their mouths.

As a provider, it is nearly impossible to keep up with the amount of poisons and drugs available to the public, their **toxidromes**—the signs and symptoms associated with a particular drug or poison or class of drugs or poisons—and steps to take when a patient has taken them. Some bottles will say drink water, some drink milk; still others advise to induce vomiting, whereas others advise against it. Even in this book, only some of the more common drugs and poisons a paramedic may encounter will be highlighted. Some major toxidromes and classes of drugs and poisons will be referred to during the discussion of specific poisons later. Don't worry, however. The **Poison Control Centers** are available to help with the paramedics' diagnosis of what poison was taken or to what the patient was exposed. Always call the Poison Control Center, 1-800-222-1222, and solicit their help. Identify who you are and provide all the information possible to the toxicologist on the other end of the line.

Table 6-11. Toxidromes

Drug Class	Examples	Signs and Symptoms
Anticholinergic	Atropine, antihistamines, and antipsychotics	Dry flushed skin, hyperthermia, tachycardia, hallucinations, and dilated pupils
Cholinergics	Fertilizers, sarin gas, VX gas, and insecticides	Salivation, lacrimation, urination, diarrhea, vomiting, and pinpoint pupils
Narcotics (opiates)	Heroin, morphine, oxycodone, fentanyl, and hydromorphone	Pinpoint pupils, respiratory depression or coma, and bradycardias
Sedatives/hypnotics	Zolpidem, phenobarbital, and benzodiazepines	Drowsiness, slurred speech, confusion, and CNS depression
Stimulants and sympathomimetics	Amphetamine, methamphetamines, pseudoephedrine, cocaine, diet pills, and nasal decongestants	Agitated delirium, insomnia, anorexia, tachypnea, dilated pupils, seizures, tachydysrhythmias, hypertension, and paranoia

Routes of Absorption

When a poison is **ingested**, it is consumed in the same way as food. Depending on the poison, the damage to the body can begin immediately, such as in the consumption of strong acids or bases or petroleum products. Conversely, the effects of the poison can be delayed if the toxin must first be digested and absorbed into the bloodstream. In this case, the medical team may have a bit more time to prevent a negative outcome for the patient. The paramedic may be able to prevent it from being digested and absorbed by inducing vomiting or administering activated charcoal. Because the effects will come on slowly, paramedics and physicians may be able to administer an antagonist (antidote) for what was ingested until it can be safely eliminated from the body.

When a poison is **inhaled**, poisoning occurs in one of 2 ways.

- The toxin can cross the alveolar wall and get into the bloodstream, where it can be carried to the brain, heart, or other organs to exert its effects (e.g., carbon monoxide poisoning).
- The toxin can simply take the place of O_2 in the atmosphere, effectively suffocating the patient in air (e.g., closed environments where other gases are present, as in a farm silo, a walk-in refrigerator with a refrigerant leak, a room where bottled gases are stored).

When a poison is **injected**, the toxin is placed directly into the body where absorption and time to onset of the effects are the fastest. This involves the injection of street drugs, such as cocaine or heroin, but it also includes snake, spider, scorpion, and jellyfish bites and stings. The effects of injection are directly related to what was injected. Street drugs cause wide-ranging systemic effects, including death. Insect and animal bites cause localized effects initially, at the area of the bite, and then over several hours cause systemic problems.

Toxins that can cross the skin can be absorbed. **Absorption** often is the slowest of all routes. Pesticides, petroleum products, and some prescription medications can be absorbed through the skin.

Terms Related to Toxicology

The following terms are related to toxicology:

- **Antagonist.** One medication acts in opposition to another drug or system.
- **Drug Abuse.** The recurrent use of illegal street drugs or the intentional misuse of prescription or over-the-counter medications for purposes other than what is described on the label.
- **Drug Addiction.** The compulsive use of a medication or street drug despite the harm that may happen (or is happening) to the user, the user's family, job status, or social status.
- **Habituation.** A conditioned decrease in response to a stimulus resulting from repeated exposures. Also the act of becoming part of the routine.
- **Physical Dependence.** A physiological addiction to a drug such that suddenly stopping the medication or drug will cause physical signs and symptoms.
- **Potentiation.** One drug or medication increases the effect of another drug.
- **Psychological Dependence.** The emotional attachment to the way a drug makes the user feel. Alternatively, thinking that the drug is what is responsible for the feelings experienced.
- **Synergism.** Two drugs when taken together have a greater effect than the sum of each individual drug. In other words, the two drugs work together to create a greater effect.
- **Tolerance.** Needing an ever-increasing quantity or dose of a drug to achieve the same effect.
- **Withdrawal Syndrome.** Predictable signs and symptoms that occur when a drug is suddenly stopped.

Assessment of Toxicological Emergencies

In addition to typical assessment points, including OPPQRST, SAMPLE, and vital signs, the paramedic needs to assess specific factors related to drug overdose and poisonings. The questions below can help determine the severity of the overdose and the treatment to prepare for the patient.

- **What was the agent?** This may not always be obviously known and may require sleuthing. Recently filled but empty prescription bottles could provide a clue if it was a prescription overdose. A spoon and a lighter nearby could indicate heroin or some other cooked drug, including methamphetamines; crack cocaine can be inhaled when heated. The police are great resources for this because they can look around while the paramedic begins treatment.
- **How was it taken?** Refer to the routes of absorption earlier in this section. Some routes are faster to circulation than others, and, therefore have a faster onset of effects.
- **How long ago was it taken?** Here again is a question that may not have a definitive answer, especially if the patient was alone at the time. If it was taken orally and it is within an hour, the Poison Control Center may advise you to induce vomiting or have the patient drink an activated charcoal slurry if the person is capable of maintaining their own airway. In some cases, the paramedic may be able to insert a nasogastric tube to provide a route of administration for the activated charcoal if the patient is obtunded.
- **How much was taken?** This may be an estimate only if it was a prescription medication or if the patient is unable to relate this information. Street drugs may be even more difficult to quantify.

- **Were any other drugs taken?** This can include washing down the poison or the medication with lethal amounts of alcohol, but it also can be an overdose where multiple medications are taken in a desperate attempt to either get high or die trying.
- **Has the patient vomited?** If the agent was ingested, vomiting may limit the effects.
- **Why did the patient take the medication?** This is another question that may garner an unreliable answer. Whatever the answer, simply document what was said.

Toxicological Emergencies

Alcohol (Ethanol)

Pathophysiology

Three pathophysiologies are to be considered when talking about alcohol, the most abused drug in the United States. The first is acute intoxication, the second is the chronic effects on the body as a result of alcoholism, and the last is withdrawal and delirium tremens (DTs) associated with a sudden stop of alcohol consumption in a long-term alcoholic.

Acute alcohol intoxication can be just as lethal as an overdose of just about any other drug. Alcohol has the effect of being a CNS depressant, which can cause slowed breathing and heart rate. The patient also may become unconscious as a result of the intoxication and is no longer able to protect their airway. Vomiting is common as the body reflexively tries to get rid of the poison in the stomach. If the patient vomits while unconscious, there is a high likelihood of aspirating the vomit. Death is a very real possibility when the blood alcohol content exceeds 400 mg/dL.

For patients believed to have acute alcohol intoxication, it is best to treat them as patients with an altered mental status. Evaluate their vital signs and perform a thorough physical assessment. Although it is easy to chalk a patient's behavior up to alcohol, it may not be the only issue at hand. Furthermore, it may not be the most life-threatening issue. With this in mind, take steps to rule out other causes of altered mental status, particularly hyperglycemia or hypoglycemia, head injury, hypoxia, or other drug use. Establish an intravenous line and run it by keeping the vein open (KVO). Check the blood sugar level and treat the value appropriately. Be prepared to manage the airway if the patient vomits, passes out, or does both. If available, administer 100 mg thiamine intravenously to help the body process the alcohol.

Chronic Alcohol Use (Alcoholism)

Alcohol dependence is still one of the top five causes of death in the United States. Typically, dependence begins as a psychological dependence, where the consumer enjoys the feeling drinking provides. The person feels the need to have alcohol to function properly, particularly in social situations. Eventually, needing alcohol this frequently evolves into a physical dependence heralded by the fact that when the person stops consuming alcohol, withdrawal symptoms begin, including restlessness, anxiety, agitation, and muscle tremors. To relieve these symptoms, the person returns to alcohol, further deepening the dependence and volume of consumption. Chronic abuse leads to damage to multiple different organs of the body, including the liver, the esophagus, the stomach, the pancreas, and the brain.

Alcohol has a direct effect on the entire digestive system, particularly the stomach. Alcohol causes **alcoholic gastritis**, which is an irritation and inflammation of the lining of the stomach and sometimes the small intestine. This leads to pain; reflux; and, in more extreme cases, hematemesis, or bloody vomit. The accessory organs to the digestive system also are taxed in heavy drinkers. The pancreas is prone to inflammation called **pancreatitis**, which can be either acute, lasting a few days, or chronic, repeating over and over again with no extended wellness period between episodes. Chronic pancreatitis can lead to diabetes or the highly lethal pancreatic cancer.

The liver is the site of detoxification in the body, so it is where alcohol will go to be metabolized and removed from the body, eventually through the kidneys. The chronic abuse of alcohol will lead to inflammation of the liver followed by fatty deposits throughout the liver cells. Eventually, this will lead to **hepatitis**, **cirrhosis**, and liver failure. Cirrhosis causes venous vascular pressures to build up within the liver, and in the veins leading to it, causing them to distend and possibly turn into varicose veins. These varicose veins are most concerning when they occur in the lining of the esophagus. Here, **esophageal varices** are subject to the abrasion of food passing by, increasing their likelihood of rupturing. The rupture of esophageal varices can be lethal because of the amount of blood stored in those veins and the pressure to which they are subjected.

The brain and the peripheral nerves are not immune from the destructive effects of chronic alcohol consumption. The brain will sustain damage to the cerebrum and the cerebellum. Damage to the cerebrum will lead to problems with the memory, motor coordination, and speech areas of the brain. This combination of ataxia, memory, and speech problems is called **Wernicke encephalopathy** and is a result of chronic thiamine deficiency. In addition, the brain may actually shrink in size from neuronal destruction. This shrinking from alcoholism combined with the natural shrinking caused by aging predisposes a patient to serious head injuries and intracranial bleeding from falls. In this situation, the brain has more room to shake around the cranial vault, allowing for the increased possibility that blood vessels will tear as the brain sloshes back and forth. As if the motor coordination problem from cerebral damage was not enough, cerebellum damage diminishes the patient's ability to balance, resulting in more falls.

Delirium Tremens and Alcohol Withdrawal

Suddenly stopping alcohol consumption in the long-term alcoholic can be fatal. Over time, however damaging, the body essentially comes to need the alcohol to function; stopping it suddenly can be similar to eliminating a nutrient from the diet. Initial alcohol withdrawal symptoms begin within 6–12 hours of the last drink and can include sweating, nausea and vomiting, and headache. Heavier drinkers who stop drinking may experience visual, auditory, or tactile hallucinations beginning within 24 hours after the last drink. Unlike the hallucinations associated with DTs discussed later, the patient is usually aware that the sensations felt are not real. Throughout the first two days after the last drink, the patient is at risk of having withdrawal seizures. Symptoms of DTs peak within five days and can be characterized with any of the following: profuse sweating, seizures, intense visual hallucinations that the patient cannot distinguish from reality, continuous full body tremors, high blood pressure, and a low-grade fever. In DTs, the hallucinations and disorientation can become so intense and disturbing that the patient may opt for suicide to escape the situation.

Treatment for alcohol withdrawal and seizures can be difficult because of the realism of the hallucinations possibly increasing the patient's agitation. Make every attempt to reassure the patient that you are there to help them feel better and work to keep the patient calm. Although restraints may be necessary, they should be a last resort because this can be more agitating to the patient who is hallucinating. Once it is safe, initiate cardiac monitoring, establish vascular access, and consider volume replacement with normal saline. If available, administer 100 mg thiamine via a slow IV push or infusion. Be prepared to administer benzodiazepines for seizures as they occur.

Stimulants

Stimulants have the highest potential for abuse and the lowest chances for recovery because of the feelings of excitement they tend to cause. Stimulants can be smoked, snorted, injected, or taken orally. Patients who have taken any stimulant are excited or hyper, often with tachycardia, hypertension, and dilated pupils. Patients also may be in a state of agitated delirium. As the dose increases, patients can have seizures, high fevers, or suddenly collapse in cardiac arrest from either the increased workload on the heart or the coronary artery spasms these drugs often cause. The stimulant abuser also can appear jittery or on edge and hypersensitive to touch. In this state, the patient could easily be set off and become combative or even violent.

Common drugs in this class include cocaine and amphetamines. Cocaine can be taken in any of the ways previously mentioned, but it is most often snorted or smoked. If the patient snorted the cocaine, the effects are felt within 2 minutes, and the peak high will last for about 20–30 minutes, at which point the high begins to fade. When smoked, the effects are felt within seconds, and the high is much more intense but shorter lasting. This results in a person wanting to redose much more quickly. As the high fades and the effects of cocaine are no longer felt, the patient "crashes," which is characterized by depression with sleeplessness, irritability, and exhaustion.

Amphetamines, methamphetamines, and amphetamine-like drugs have legitimate clinical applications as nasal decongestants and in medications for attention deficit disorder (ADD) and attention deficit with hyperactivity disorder (ADHD). Methamphetamines can be made relatively easily in the home from the nasal decongestant pseudoephedrine and other household chemicals, making it easier and cheaper to use than cocaine but with the added benefit that the high from methamphetamine can last up to 12 hours, compared with 30 minutes for cocaine. Although treatment for the amphetamine abuser is largely supportive, patients can become violent with little notice.

Treatment for Stimulants

EMS systems do not typically carry an antidote to any of the stimulant classes of drugs, so treatment is limited to symptoms. As with any patient, ensure an adequate airway and oxygenation; these patients may be necessarily tachypneic to keep up with myocardial and skeletal O_2 demands. Titrate supplemental O_2 to a pulse oximetry of 95% or higher and initiate cardiac monitoring. Appropriately treat any dysrhythmias found. For seizures, violent behavior, combativity, or anxiety, administer a benzodiazepine and be prepared to manage the airway. The patient may have a very high fever, sometimes in excess of 106°F (41.1°C), which will require aggressive cooling measures, including ice packs to the groin, axillae, and neck.

Opiates

Opiates are drugs derived directly from the poppy seed, whereas opioids are typically synthetic medications. The term *opiate* will be used to refer to any narcotic drug. Opiates act on opiate receptors found primarily in the brain to produce euphoria and analgesia. They can be absorbed through the nasal mucosa (snorted); smoked, entering the bloodstream through the alveoli; taken orally; or injected. Oral opiates are subjected to first-pass metabolism and, therefore, have their effects lessened compared with absorption via other routes. Heroin, for example, when injected, does not appreciably change when first metabolized in the liver. This means that heroin can outlast the antidote naloxone.

Patients who have taken opiate derivatives present as being sedated, sometimes with respiratory depression, hypotension, and pinpoint pupils. Sometimes, the patient's respiratory status can be depressed to the point of bradycardia. Narcotics also are well known for affecting the GI tract by slowing overall transit. This can present as nausea, vomiting, and constipation.

Treatment for opiates is primarily the administration of the reversal agent, naloxone. Naloxone can be given intravenously, intraosseously, intranasally, or endotracheally, but the onset of reversal is fastest via the intravenous or intraosseous route. Naloxone should be given slowly and titrated to the improvement of the respirations rather than waking the patient all the way up. It is recommended to draw up 2 mg in a 10 mL syringe, creating a 0.2 mg/mL concentration and giving 2 mL at a time until the respiratory rate improves. If the patient is given all of it at once, vomiting will likely occur, possibly creating an airway problem, but, at the very least, a dirty ambulance problem. The patient also may get very agitated that their expensive high is now gone, creating a safety issue for the paramedics and the hospital staff.

Sedatives and Hypnotics: Barbiturates and Benzodiazepines

Barbiturates were once commonly prescribed as antiseizure medications; however, they were frequently combined with alcohol in successful suicides because of the combined CNS depressant effects of both drugs. There are long- and short-acting versions of barbiturates. Benzodiazepines have largely replaced barbiturates for seizure control and other medical applications for a variety of reasons. Benzodiazepines have a lower possibility for abuse and a significantly lower chance for toxicity. They also have a wider range of uses, including general sedation and anxiolysis, none of which are possible with barbiturates.

Both barbiturates and benzodiazepines have a similar mechanism of action in the CNS. Both bind to the gamma-aminobutyric acid (GABA) receptor and exert their effects by hyperpolarizing the postsynaptic cell. Because the cell is now hyperpolarized, it takes a larger stimulus for it to depolarize, resulting in sedation and the cessation of seizure activity.

Patients who overdose on benzodiazepines, or low doses of barbiturates, will appear intoxicated with alcohol: slurred speech, drowsy, ataxic gait, and decreased mentation. Even in high doses of benzodiazepines, the assessment will be similar. However, in high doses of barbiturates, increasing lethargy followed by unconsciousness and possible apnea may occur in the patient. If a patient who is suspected of a benzodiazepine overdose is suffering from severe respiratory depression or is unresponsive, it is very likely that the patient took other depressants, alcohol, or opiates with the benzodiazepine.

Overdoses of either benzodiazepines or barbiturates are symptom-based for the most part. Manage the airway as for any other unresponsive or minimally responsive patient and consider intubation and ventilation. Respiratory depression is far more likely in barbiturate overdoses but could be significant with barbiturates when other drugs are involved. Establish vascular access and administer a fluid bolus if hypotension is present. Fluid resuscitation is the first-line treatment for hypotension; only after about 1–2 L have been administered should dopamine be considered for continued hypotension.

Marijuana

Classified as a hallucinogen despite not actually producing true hallucinations, marijuana does sometimes cause the user to have a distorted sense of time, space, and reality. Its principal psychoactive compound is tetrahydrocannabinol (THC). Marijuana is most commonly smoked; however, it can be eaten as well. If ingested, the onset of effects can take several hours, whereas the onset of the relaxing effects starts within a few minutes if smoked. Either way, the effects tend to last about 2–4 hours before waning.

Rarely will smoking marijuana result in an emergency visit to the hospital, unless it is laced with some other drug. Patients who have smoked marijuana will have bloodshot eyes, drowsiness, and euphoria. Patients will occasionally have a bad reaction and feel paranoid or anxious. Low-dose benzodiazepines are recommended here; alternatively, simply talk to the patient to calm the person.

Hallucinogens

Any substance that causes changes in senses of perception, including vision, hearing, and touch, is called a **hallucinogen**. Hallucinations of taste and smell are extraordinarily uncommon. Effects and sensations can be impacted by the user's social setting, history of drug use, and mere expectations of what the drug will do. For this section, the effects of each will be discussed, which will be followed by general treatment guidelines for patients who have taken hallucinogens.

Ketamine

Until recently, **ketamine** was not commonly used in human medicine; it was primarily used in veterinary medicine as a tranquilizer or anesthetic. However, now it is being used in pediatrics and adults to control seizures. Street ketamine often is snorted or taken orally and is physically and psychologically addicting. Low doses result in patients who seem intoxicated but have a reduction of inhibitions and slurred, dreamy speech. At higher doses, patients may appear anesthetized and have difficulty moving.

LSD

LSD saw its use peak in the 1960s, with a brief resurgence in the 1990s. It is a highly potent hallucinogen, with users achieving the desired effects with <100 mcg. It often is taken orally or sublingually, and the effect typically lasts between 3 and 4 hours, with effects occasionally lasting in excess of 12 hours with larger doses. Patients often report synesthesias with LSD, which are total changes in perception, such as hearing colors or touching sounds. The hallucinations are very real and can cause anxiety for the patients during so called "bad trips."

Peyote and Mescaline

Found in the dried flower "buttons" of the peyote cactus in the American Southwest, native tribes have used **peyote** and **mescaline** for religious purposes for centuries. People typically ingest the "buttons" and vomit them back up after a short while (because it is a powerful gastric irritant) to begin the hallucination. Hallucinations have been described as a psychedelic experience complete with bright flashes of color often in geometric shapes being reported, thus people also experience out-of-body sensations and floating feelings.

Phencyclidine

Phencyclidine (**PCP**) often is referred to as angel dust on the streets and is occasionally used to lace other drugs, such as marijuana. In smaller doses, it can cause symptoms similar to alcohol intoxication: slurred speech, a staggering gait, and horizontal gaze nystagmus (bouncing of the eyes when the person looks as far right or left as possible). With larger doses, patients can experience what is known as mind-body separation or violent outbreaks that PCP is reputed to cause. Patients at this level of overdose are extremely combative and violent. They often have no response to attempts at physical containment, including being hit with tasers. These patients combine an almost complete lack of sensation of pain with superhuman strength and now pose a significant threat to law enforcement and EMS on scene until they can be subdued.

Psilocybin Mushrooms

Certain species of "shrooms" contain a psychoactive drug called **psilocybin**. The patient eats these mushrooms and after about 30 minutes to an hour, begins to have hallucinations similar to those experienced with LSD. Though less intense, the hallucinations last slightly longer, up to 6 hours. It is rare to need emergent medical care directly related to a shroom overdose.

Treatment for Hallucinogens

Most hallucinogens rarely cause life-threatening problems, so treatment is symptom related. Providing a calm environment for the patient is important. If there is extensive anxiety from the hallucinations, anxiolysis with benzodiazepines is recommended in low doses sufficient to bring about a state of relaxation. Do not play into the patient's hallucinations because that confirms the experience and increases anxiety or agitation. If the patient is or becomes combative, higher doses of benzodiazepines may be required, likely via the intramuscular route first until an intravenous line can be safely established.

Organophosphate and Cholinergic Poisoning

Insecticides, pesticides, and fertilizers fall into a chemical category called organophosphates. The most common causes for overdose of these materials are intentional for purposes of suicide or accidentally during regular agricultural use and pesticide applications. ACh is the neurotransmitter of the PNS. Organophosphates inhibit AChE, an enzyme responsible for the breakdown of ACh in the synapse. With AChE no longer able to break down and remove the ACh from the synapse, the parasympathetic nerve will continuously produce its parasympathetic response. This is systemic. Consequently, in organophosphate poisoning, the patient will show symptoms consistent with parasympathetic stimulation, including marked bradycardia and bradypnea and other symptoms contained in the mnemonic SLUDGE:

- Salivation: continuous drooling
- Lacrimation: excessive tear production
- Urination: urine incontinence
- Defecation/diarrhea: continuously moving the bowels
- GI upset: excessive continuous vomiting and GI cramping if conscious
- Eyes: pinpoint pupils (Some have emesis for the "E.")

To treat the patient poisoned by organophosphates, first ensure that the patient has been completely decontaminated and is not going to share the organophosphate with the ambulance crew and the entire emergency department. Once the patient is no longer a direct threat to the paramedics, assess and treat the ABCs as appropriate, including endotracheal intubation. Monitor the ECG, SpO_2, and capnography. Administer 2 mg atropine as soon as an intravenous line is available and flush the line. Repeat this every 3–5 minutes until the secretions dry up. In the case of poisoning, the 0.3 mg/kg limit that is imposed during cardiac arrest or other bradycardic situations is not in play because atropine is the primary antidote for organophosphate poisoning. Fluid resuscitation sometimes in excess of 1 L is recommended for hypotension. If available, administer 2 mg pralidoxime chloride over 5 minutes.

Anticholinergic Overdose

Overdoses of drugs that inhibit the parasympathetic side of the CNS also are possible. Anticholinergic medications are available both over the counter and by prescription. Examples of anticholinergics include diphenhydramine and other antihistamines, certain cough suppressants, medications for overactive bladder such as oxybutynin, among others. Anticholinergic drugs competitively inhibit the ACh receptors in the synapse and prevent ACh from stimulating the postsynaptic nerve, essentially allowing the sympathetic side of the CNS to run amok. The symptoms of anticholinergic overdose are listed, along with a common memory aid for such overdoses.

- Blind as a bat (dilated pupils)
- Red as a beet (vasodilation/flushing)
- Hot as a hare (hyperthermia)
- Dry as a bone (dry skin and mucous membranes/no secretions)
- Mad as a hatter (hallucinations/agitation)

Management of this overdose is rooted in relieving and treating symptoms. Give benzodiazepines for any seizures that may happen. Be prepared to manage the patient's airway. Because of decreased systemic secretions, it is recommended to judiciously lubricate the ETT before insertion. Monitor the ECG, establish an intravenous line, and observe the patient for changes during rapid transport to the nearest appropriate facility.

Carbon Monoxide

Carbon monoxide (**CO**) is a colorless, odorless, and tasteless gas that is produced during the incomplete combustion of hydrocarbon fuels, including oil, natural gas, and wood. CO can be found in gases from a malfunctioning furnace, a blocked chimney, or car exhaust. CO is a poison because it attaches to red blood cells at the same spot of attachment as O_2; however, the CO attaches 200 times more strongly than O_2. This means two things: (1) Once attached, it takes a long time for it to detach and make space for the O_2 again; and (2) in the presence of both O_2 and CO, the red blood cell will attach to the CO.

Patients with CO poisoning may be difficult to identify if it is early in the poisoning process. Early on a patient's complaints are general and flu-like: nausea, vomiting, headache, confusion, and weakness. Having multiple people in the same location with similar complaints is characteristic of CO poisoning. Late in CO poisoning, usually near death, the patient will have a cherry red appearance to their face, though at that point the poisoning is seldom survivable. The patient who has CO poisoning will have an SpO_2 of 100% because it will read that the hemoglobin is saturated, but the sensor cannot tell if it is CO or O_2.

Treatment of CO poisoning is primarily high-flow O_2, regardless of the SpO_2 reading. Evaluate the ECG and consider intubation if the patient is unresponsive or has severe altered mental status. Check the blood sugar level to rule out hypoglycemia. Transport the patient to a hospital where the patient can receive emergent hyperbaric O_2 therapy.

Cyanide

Cyanide is used in chemical and industrial processes and also is produced when certain plastics burn, which can happen in house fires. It is found in the pits and seeds of certain fruits, though not in any quantity that could inflict harm on a person. It is an extremely fast-acting poison that works by shutting down cytochrome oxidase, a cellular enzyme responsible for more than 80% of cellular energy production, and blocks the use of O_2 at the cellular level.

The patient will present as being weak and lethargic. Breathing will initially be rapid but will slow and eventually stop as the muscles are no longer able to function. As lactic acid builds up in the cell's last ditch effort to make energy, the patient becomes increasingly acidotic and will have a decreasing level of consciousness. Eventually, the patient will become unresponsive. It has been reported that patients have a smell of bitter almonds; however, nearly 60% of the population cannot smell that.

Treatment for known or suspected cyanide poisoning includes the following:

1. Establish an airway and provide 100% supplemental O_2. Intubate and ventilate if necessary.
2. If available, begin the administration of the antidote.
   - Hydroxocobalamin: 5 g infusion over 15 minutes
   - Amyl nitrite: inhaled for 20 seconds out of every minute for 5 minutes, alternating with 40 seconds of high-flow O_2
   - Sodium nitrite: 10 mL of a 3% solution infused over 5 minutes. This is the second medication to be given after hydroxocobalamin
   - Sodium thiosulfate: 12.5 g over 5 minutes
3. Treat seizures with benzodiazepines.
4. Rapidly transport to the nearest medical facility, especially if EMS does not have access to the above antidotes.

Hydrogen Sulfide

Hydrogen sulfide has a distinctive rotten egg smell. It is a highly toxic, colorless gas. It can be created by reacting household chemicals, and its use in suicide attempts is on the rise. People are locking themselves in cars, mixing the chemicals that react to form the lethal hydrogen sulfide, and dying there. EMS should not open the car door, and the people have been known to put up signs in the car's window that will say something like, "Chemical suicide in progress. Do not open the door." Obey the sign, unless a full hazardous material suit is available. Even ventilating a patient with hydrogen sulfide poisoning may cause exposure to the toxic gas (by inhaling the patient's exhalation) sufficient to sicken or kill the paramedic. There is no proven antidote for hydrogen sulfide poisoning.

Synthetic Cannabinoids

Synthetic cannabinoids are a group of chemicals that, once in the body, act on the same receptors in the brain as THC, the active compound in marijuana. These are variously called **K2, spice**, or **"synthetic marijuana"** and are generally available as liquids that can be sprayed on dried plant material (such as regular marijuana or tobacco) and smoked or inhaled directly through vape pens and e-cigarettes. Some people will even brew it as tea.

Synthetic cannabinoids are psychoactive, mind-altering chemicals that produce wildly different effects in different people. These differences can be attributed to the variable chemical composition of the liquid from one brand to another, and even batch to batch of the same brand or type. The effects can mimic those of regular marijuana or produce paranoia, hallucinations, or extreme anxiety, any of which can lead to violent behavior.

Treatment for the patient who has used K2/spice/synthetic marijuana varies according to the presenting syndrome and symptoms. For the relaxed patient, no treatment may be needed beyond observation for worsening sedation. However, for those exhibiting severe psychosis and violent behaviors, sometimes referred to as excited delirium, more aggressive management may be required.

Excited (or agitated) delirium is a combination of symptoms most commonly including psychomotor agitation, hallucinations or generalized confusion, diaphoresis, violent and erratic behavior, unexpected strength, and occasionally hyperthermia. Whether induced by K2 or a serotonin reuptake inhibitor (overdose of which can lead to serotonin storm), this syndrome can make the patient especially hard to control and dangerous to be around. Aggressive physical restraint may be required to maintain the physical safety of the responders as well as the patient. Untreated, excited delirium can lead to death of the patient.

First and foremost, maintain scene safety and security as well as situational awareness; a person who has used synthetic marijuana may be calm one moment and become aggressively agitated the next. Physical restraints of the wrists and ankles, using proper techniques, should be employed in the physically aggressive patient. Chemical restraint may also be considered in the patient exhibiting agitated delirium, ideally ketamine. The advantages of ketamine over other options are its much faster onset of action and the fact that it seldom requires maintaining an airway (unlike benzodiazepines). Often ketamine is the only necessary therapy. Although it can be combined with other sedatives, that is usually not required. Ketamine can be administered either intravenously or intramuscularly.

- IV route: dosage 1–2 mg/kg of patient's body mass, given rapidly; onset <1 minute
- IM route: dosage 4–5 mg/kg of patient's body mass; onset 3–4 minutes

Treatment considerations in the patient with excited delirium include acidosis and rhabdomyolysis. Acidosis—and the extracellularized potassium resulting from the rhabdomyolysis—could lead to cardiac dysrhythmias. Consider infusing a bolus of 500–1,000 mL NSS. If hyperkalemia is suspected, calcium chloride or calcium gluconate would also be appropriate. Also consider bicarbonate for acidosis as needed.

REVIEW QUESTIONS

Select the ONE best answer.

1. The ambulance has been called to the scene of an agitated person. The police have restrained the 32-year-old male so you can assess vital signs: HR: 140; RR: 28; BP: 190/110; SpO$_2$: 100%. The patient only indicates that he took a full 20 pills of some medication that came in a box. To which of the following classes of drugs could this patient have overdosed?

    A. Stimulant or cholinergic
    B. Anticholinergic or sympathomimetic
    C. Anticholinergic or benzodiazepine
    D. Cholinergic or hypnotic

2. You are called to an unconscious patient who presents with bradypnea (RR: 8, HR: 68) and pinpoint pupils. The patient has track marks on the right arm. The optimal treatment for this patient is:

    A. Insertion of Combitube and positive pressure ventilation.
    B. Positive pressure ventilation with BVM.
    C. Naloxone intravenously in 0.4 mg increments until breathing improves.
    D. Naloxone 2 mg followed with 4 mg ondansetron for nausea.

3. All of the following are signs and symptoms of an anticholinergic overdose EXCEPT:

    A. Hypertension.
    B. Hyperthermia.
    C. Pinpoint pupils.
    D. Tachycardia.

4. You have 15 LPM oxygen flowing on a 52-year-old male patient suspected of having cyanide poisoning. Assuming you have all of these options available to you, which is the first-line medication for this patient?

    A. Amyl nitrite
    B. Sodium nitrite
    C. Hydroxocobalamin
    D. Sodium thiosulfate

ANSWERS AND EXPLANATIONS

1. **The correct answer is (B).** Anticholinergics and stimulants and sympathomimetics produce similar symptoms. Stimulants and sympathomimetics work primarily by accelerating the sympathetic side of the nervous system. Anticholinergics work by eliminating the parasympathetic tone, resulting in unopposed sympathetic stimulation. Treatment for overdose of either class of drugs is basically the same: increase the sympathetic tone.

2. **The correct answer is (C).** Intravenous naloxone titrated to the effect of improving the patient's respiratory rate is the preferred treatment for what should be presumed as an opiate overdose. Option (D) is not ideal because it is likely to suddenly and violently remove the opiate effects, leading to nausea, vomiting, and possible airway compromise. Management of the airway, as suggested in (A) and (B), would be appropriate in situations where naloxone is not readily available or if naloxone did not work.

3. **The correct answer is (C).** Patients on stimulants often have dilated pupils. The other symptoms listed are common with stimulant use.

4. **The correct answer is (C).** Hydroxocobalamin is the 1st-line medication in known or suspected cyanide poisoning. Amyl nitrite (A) is used as a temporizing agent until hydroxocobalamin can be administered. Sodium nitrite (B) and sodium thiosulfate (D) are used in combination as a 2nd-line medication. In cyanide poisonings, oxygen also should be liberally administered regardless of pulse oximetry.

GASTROINTESTINAL EMERGENCIES

The acute abdomen is a common complaint that patients offer to paramedics. This can involve everything in the abdomen, including abdominal aortic aneurysms or ovarian cysts, but for our purposes here, the focus will be on GI emergencies.

Anatomy and Physiology

Two types of digestion can occur. **Intracellular digestion**, as a part of metabolism, involves the oxidation of glucose and fatty acids for energy. However, our diets do not consist of pure glucose and fatty acids; rather, these substances must be extracted from our food. **Extracellular digestion** is the process by which these nutrients are obtained from food occurs within the lumen of the alimentary canal. This is technically "outside" the body, as it occurs outside cell borders.

The human digestive tract has specialized sections with different roles. The most basic functional distinction is between digestion and absorption.

- **Digestion** involves the breakdown of food into its constituent organic molecules: starches and other carbohydrates into monosaccharides, lipids (fats) into free fatty acids and glycerol, and proteins into amino acids.
  - **Mechanical** digestion is the physical breakdown of large food particles into smaller food particles, but it does not involve breaking chemical bonds.
  - **Chemical** digestion is the enzymatic cleavage of chemical bonds, such as the peptide bonds of proteins or the glycosidic bonds of starches.
- **Absorption** involves the transport of the products of digestion from the digestive tract into the circulatory system for distribution to the body's tissues and cells.

Practical Point

The **alimentary canal** runs from the mouth to the anus and is sectioned off by sphincters, or circular smooth muscles around the canal that can contract to allow compartmentalization of function.

The digestive tract begins with the **oral cavity** (mouth) and is followed by the **pharynx**, a shared pathway for both food entering the digestive system and air entering the respiratory system. From the pharynx, food enters the **esophagus**, which transports food to the **stomach**. From the stomach, food travels to the **small intestine** and then the **large intestine**. Finally, waste products of digestion enter the **rectum**, where feces are stored until the appropriate time of release. In addition to the actual organs of the digestive tract, the **salivary glands**, **pancreas**, **liver**, and **gallbladder** help provide the enzymes and lubrication necessary to aid the digestion of food.

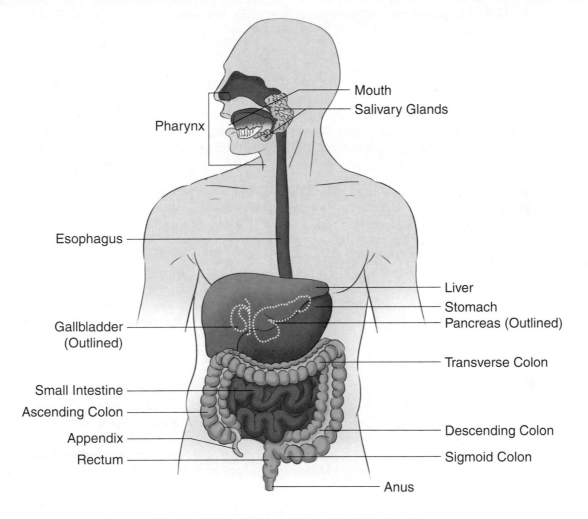

Figure 6-18. Anatomy of the Digestive System

The **enteric nervous system** is a collection of 100 million neurons that govern the function of the GI system. These neurons are present in the walls of the digestive tract and trigger **peristalsis**, or rhythmic contractions of the gut tube, to move materials through the system. This system can function independently of the brain and spinal cord, although it is heavily regulated by the autonomic nervous system. The parasympathetic division is involved in the stimulation of digestive activities, increasing secretions from exocrine glands and promoting peristalsis. The sympathetic division is involved in the inhibition of these activities. The fact that so often people feel sleepy and lethargic after eating a big meal (often called a *food coma* colloquially) is caused, in part, by parasympathetic activity. On the other hand, during periods of high sympathetic activity, blood flow is decreased to the digestive tract, and gut motility slows significantly.

Ingestion and Digestion

To supply the body with nutrients, people must **ingest** (eat) food. Several hormones are involved with feeding behavior, including antidiuretic hormone (ADH or vasopressin), aldosterone, glucagon, ghrelin, leptin, and cholecystokinin. ADH and aldosterone trigger the sensation of thirst, encouraging the behavior of fluid consumption. Glucagon, secreted by the pancreas, and ghrelin, secreted by the stomach and the pancreas, stimulate feelings of hunger. Leptin and cholecystokinin do the opposite, stimulating feelings of satiety. Digestion begins in the oral cavity and continues in the stomach and the first part of the small intestine, known as the duodenum.

Oral Cavity

The oral cavity plays a role in both the mechanical and chemical digestion of food. Mechanical digestion in the mouth involves the breaking up of large food particles into smaller particles by using the teeth, tongue, and lips. This process is called **mastication** (chewing). Chewing helps to increase the surface-area-to-volume ratio of the food, allowing for more surface area for enzymatic digestion as it passes through the gut tube. It also moderates the size of food particles entering the lumen of the alimentary canal; food particles that are too large create an obstructive risk in the tract.

Chemical digestion begins the breakdown of chemical bonds in the macromolecules that make up food. This relies on enzymes from **saliva** produced by the 3 pairs of **salivary glands**. Saliva also aids mechanical digestion by moistening and lubricating food. The salivary glands, like all glands of the digestive tract, are innervated by the PNS. The presence of food in the oral cavity triggers a neural circuit that ultimately leads to increased parasympathetic stimulation of these glands. Salivation also can be triggered by signals that food is near, such as smell or sight. Saliva contains salivary amylase, also known as ptyalin, and lipase. **Salivary amylase** is capable of hydrolyzing starch into smaller sugars (maltose and dextrins), and **lipase** catalyzes the hydrolysis of lipids. The amount of chemical digestion that occurs in the mouth is minimal, though, because the food does not stay in the mouth for long. Our muscular tongue forms the food into a **bolus**, which is forced back to the pharynx and swallowed.

Pharynx

The pharynx is the cavity that leads from the mouth and posterior nasal cavity to the esophagus. The pharynx connects to not only the esophagus but also the larynx, which is a part of the respiratory tract. The pharynx can be divided into 3 parts: the nasopharynx (behind the nasal cavity), the oropharynx (at the back of the mouth), and the laryngopharynx (above the vocal cords). Food is prevented from entering the larynx during swallowing by the epiglottis, a cartilaginous structure that folds down to cover the laryngeal inlet. Failure of this mechanism can lead to the aspiration of food and choking.

Esophagus

The esophagus is a muscular tube that connects the pharynx to the stomach. The top third of the esophagus is composed of skeletal muscle, the bottom third is composed of smooth muscle, and the middle third is a mixture of both. What does this mean in terms of nervous control? Although the top of the esophagus is under somatic (voluntary) motor control, the bottom—and most of the rest of the GI tract, for that matter—is under autonomic (involuntary) nervous control. The rhythmic contraction of smooth muscle that propels food toward the stomach is called peristalsis. Under normal circumstances, peristalsis proceeds down the digestive tract. However, certain conditions, such as exposure to chemicals, infectious agents, physical stimulation in the posterior pharynx, and even cognitive stimulation, can lead to a reversal of peristalsis in the process of emesis (vomiting).

Swallowing is initiated in the muscles of the oropharynx, which constitute the upper esophageal sphincter. Peristalsis squeezes, pushes, and propels the bolus toward the stomach. As the bolus approaches the stomach, a muscular ring known as the lower esophageal sphincter (cardiac sphincter) relaxes and opens to allow the passage of food.

Stomach

The 3 main energy sources are carbohydrates, fats, and proteins. As mentioned earlier, the chemical digestion of carbohydrates and fats is initiated in the mouth. No mechanical or chemical digestion takes place in the esophagus, except for the continued enzymatic activity initiated in the mouth by salivary enzymes. Thus, digestion that occurs prior to the entrance of the bolus into the stomach is minimal compared with digestion that occurs in the stomach and small intestine.

The stomach is a highly muscular organ with a capacity of approximately 2 L. In humans, the stomach is located in the upper left quadrant of the abdominal cavity, under the diaphragm. This organ uses hydrochloric acid and enzymes to digest food, creating a fairly harsh environment, and its mucosa is quite thick to prevent autodigestion. The stomach can be divided into four main anatomical divisions: the fundus and body, which contain mostly gastric glands, and the antrum and pylorus, which contain mostly pyloric glands. The internal curvature of the stomach is called the lesser curvature; the external curvature is called the greater curvature. The lining of the stomach is thrown into folds called rugae.

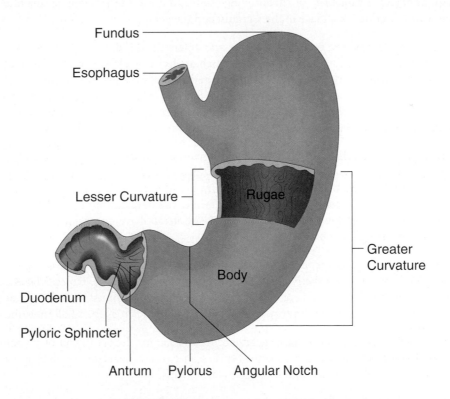

Figure 6-19. Anatomy of the Stomach

The mucosa of the stomach contains gastric glands and pyloric glands. The **gastric glands** respond to signals from the **vagus nerve** of the PNS, which is activated by the brain in response to the sight, taste, and smell of food. Gastric glands have 3 different cell types: mucous cells, chief cells, and parietal cells. **Mucous cells** produce the bicarbonate-rich mucus that protects the muscular wall from the harshly acidic (pH = 2) and proteolytic environment of the stomach.

Gastric juice is a combination of secretions from the other two cell types in the gastric glands. The **chief cells** secrete **pepsinogen**, which is the inactive, **zymogen** form of pepsin, a proteolytic enzyme. Hydrogen ions in the stomach, secreted by **parietal cells** as hydrochloric acid, cleave pepsinogen to pepsin. **Pepsin** digests proteins by cleaving peptide bonds near aromatic amino acids, resulting in short peptide fragments. Because pepsin is activated by the acidic environment, it follows that pepsin is most active at a low pH. This is a unique characteristic among human enzymes because most human enzymes are most active at physiological pH. Stomach acid also kills most harmful bacteria (with the exception of *Helicobacter pylori*, infection with which is usually asymptomatic but can cause inflammation, ulcers, and even certain gastric cancers). The acidic environment also helps denature proteins and can break down some intramolecular bonds that hold food together. In addition to HCl, parietal cells secrete **intrinsic factor**, a glycoprotein involved in the proper absorption of vitamin B_{12}.

The **pyloric glands** contain **G-cells** that secrete gastrin, a peptide hormone. **Gastrin** induces the parietal cells in the stomach to secrete more HCl and signals the stomach to contract, mixing its contents. The digestion of solid food in the stomach results in an acidic, semifluid mixture known as **chyme**. The combined mechanical and chemical digestive activities of the stomach result in a significant increase in the surface area of the now unrecognizable food particles, so when the chyme reaches the small intestine, the absorption of nutrients from it can be maximized. A few substances can be absorbed directly from the stomach (such as alcohol and aspirin), but the stomach is mainly an organ of digestion.

Duodenum

The **small intestine** (quite long, up to 7 m) consists of 3 segments: the duodenum, the jejunum, and the ileum. The duodenum is responsible for the majority of chemical digestion and has a minor role in absorption, but most of the absorption in the small intestine takes place in the jejunum and the ileum.

Food leaves the stomach through the **pyloric sphincter** and enters the duodenum. The presence of chyme in the duodenum causes the release of brush-border enzymes such as disaccharidases (maltase, isomaltase, lactase, and sucrase) and peptidases (including dipeptidase). **Brush-border enzymes** are present on the luminal surface of cells lining the duodenum and break down dimers and trimers of biomolecules into absorbable monomers. The duodenum also secretes enteropeptidase, which is involved in the activation of other digestive enzymes from the accessory organs of digestion. Finally, it secretes hormones such as secretin and cholecystokinin (CCK) into the bloodstream.

The **disaccharidases** digest disaccharides. **Maltase** digests maltose, **isomaltase** digests isomaltose, **lactase** digests lactose, and **sucrase** digests sucrose. The lack of a particular disaccharidase causes an inability to break down the corresponding disaccharide. Then bacteria in the intestines are able to hydrolyze that disaccharide, producing methane gas as a byproduct. In addition, undigested disaccharides can have an osmotic effect, pulling water into the stool and causing diarrhea. This is why people who are lactose intolerant have symptoms of bloating, flatulence, and possibly diarrhea after ingesting dairy products.

Peptidases break down proteins (or peptides, as the name implies). **Aminopeptidase** is a peptidase secreted by glands in the duodenum that removes the N-terminal amino acid from a peptide. **Dipeptidases** cleave the peptide bonds of dipeptides to release free amino acids. Unlike carbohydrates, which must be broken down into monosaccharides for absorption, dipeptides and even tripeptides can be absorbed across the small intestine wall.

Enteropeptidase (formerly called **enterokinase**) is an enzyme critical for the activation of **trypsinogen**, a pancreatic protease, to **trypsin**. Trypsin then initiates an activation cascade, as described later in this chapter. Enteropeptidase also can activate **procarboxypeptidases A** and **B** to their active forms.

Secretin is a peptide hormone that causes pancreatic enzymes to be released into the duodenum. It also regulates the pH of the digestive tract by reducing HCl secretion from parietal cells and increasing bicarbonate secretion from the pancreas. Secretin also is an **enterogastrone**, a hormone that slows motility through the digestive tract. Slowing of motility allows increased time for digestive enzymes to act on chyme—especially fats.

Finally, **CCK** is secreted in response to the entry of chyme (specifically, amino acids and fat in the chyme) into the duodenum. This peptide hormone stimulates the release of both bile and pancreatic juices and also acts in the brain, where it promotes satiety. **Bile** is a complex fluid composed of bile salts, pigments, and cholesterol. **Bile salts** are derived from cholesterol. They are not enzymes and therefore do not directly perform chemical digestion. However, bile salts serve an important role in the mechanical digestion of fats and ultimately facilitate the chemical digestion of lipids. Bile salts have hydrophobic and hydrophilic regions, allowing them to serve as a bridge between aqueous and lipid environments. In fact, bile salts are much like the common soaps and detergents used to wash our hands, clothes, and dishes. In the small intestine, bile salts **emulsify** fats and cholesterol into **micelles**. Without bile, fats would spontaneously separate out of the aqueous mixture in the duodenum and would not be accessible to pancreatic lipase, which is water soluble. In addition, these micelles increase the surface area of the fats, increasing the rate at which lipase can act. Ultimately, proper fat digestion depends on both bile and lipase. Bile gets the fats into the solution and increases their surface area by placing them in micelles (mechanical digestion). Then, lipase can come in to hydrolyze the ester bonds holding the lipids together (chemical digestion).

CCK also promotes the secretion of pancreatic juices into the duodenum. **Pancreatic juices** are a complex mixture of several enzymes in a bicarbonate-rich alkaline solution. This bicarbonate helps neutralize acidic chyme, as well as provides an ideal working environment for each of the digestive enzymes, which are most active around pH 8.5. Pancreatic juices contain enzymes that can digest all 3 types of nutrients: carbohydrates, fats, and proteins. The identities and functions of these enzymes will be discussed in the next section of this chapter.

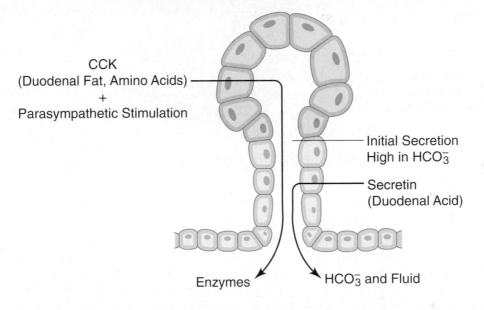

Figure 6-20. Hormonal Control of the Exocrine Pancreas

Accessory Organs of Digestion

Digestion is a complex process that requires the release of enzymes from not only the cells directly lining the alimentary canal but also the pancreas, liver, and gallbladder. Collectively, these organs—which all originate as outgrowths of endoderm from the gut tube during development—are called accessory organs of digestion.

Pancreas

The **pancreas** serves 2 quite different roles in the body, reflecting its exocrine and endocrine functions. The endocrine functions of the pancreas include the release of insulin, glucagon, and somatostatin—peptide hormones necessary for the maintenance of proper blood sugar levels. The hormonal function of the pancreas is limited to cells residing in the islets of Langerhans scattered throughout the organ. The bulk of the pancreas, however, is made of exocrine cells called **acinar cells** that produce pancreatic juices. As mentioned earlier, pancreatic juices are bicarbonate-rich alkaline secretions containing many digestive enzymes that work on all 3 classes of biomolecules. **Pancreatic amylase** breaks down large polysaccharides into small disaccharides and is therefore responsible for carbohydrate digestion. The pancreatic peptidases (**trypsinogen**, **chymotrypsinogen**, and **carboxypeptidases A** and **B**) are released in their zymogen form, but once activated are responsible for protein digestion. Enteropeptidase, produced by the duodenum, is the master switch. It activates trypsinogen to trypsin, which can then activate the other zymogens, and also activates procarboxypeptidases A and B to their active forms. Finally, the pancreas secretes **pancreatic lipase**, which is capable of breaking down fats into free fatty acids and glycerol.

Pancreatic juices are transferred to the duodenum via a duct system that runs along the middle of the pancreas. Like all exocrine cells, acinar cells secrete their products into ducts. These ducts then empty into the duodenum through the **major** and **minor duodenal papillae**.

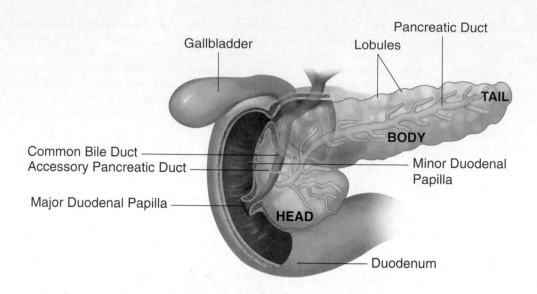

Figure 6-21. Anatomy of the Pancreas

Liver

The **liver** is located in the upper right quadrant of the abdomen and contains two unique structures for communicating with the digestive system. First, **bile ducts** connect the liver with both the gallbladder and small intestine. Bile is produced in the liver and travels down these ducts, where it may be stored in the gallbladder or secreted into the duodenum. The liver also receives all blood draining from the abdominal portion of the digestive tract through the **hepatic portal vein**. This nutrient-rich blood can be processed by the liver before draining into the inferior vena cava on its way to the right side of the heart. For example, the liver takes up excess sugar to create **glycogen**, the storage form of glucose, and stores fats as **triacylglycerols**. The liver also can reverse these processes, producing glucose for the rest of the body through **glycogenolysis** and **gluconeogenesis** and mobilizing fats in **lipoproteins**. The liver detoxifies both endogenous compounds (those made in the body) and exogenous compounds (those brought in from the environment). For example, the liver modifies ammonia, a toxic waste product of amino acid metabolism, to urea, which can be excreted by the kidneys. The liver also detoxifies and metabolizes alcohol and medications. Some drugs actually require activation by the enzymes of the liver. In addition, some drugs cannot be taken orally because modification of these drugs by the liver renders the drugs inactive.

Bile production is one of the most significant jobs of the liver vis-à-vis the digestive system. As mentioned earlier, bile is composed of bile salts, pigments, and cholesterol. Bile salts are amphipathic molecules that can emulsify fat in the digestive system. The major pigment in bile is **bilirubin**, which is a byproduct of the breakdown of hemoglobin. Bilirubin travels to the liver, where it is **conjugated** (attached to a protein) and secreted into the bile for excretion. If the liver is unable to process or excrete bilirubin (from liver damage, excessive red blood cell destruction, or blockage of the bile ducts), **jaundice** or yellowing of the skin may occur.

In addition to bile production, processing of nutrients, detoxification, and drug metabolism, the liver also synthesizes certain proteins necessary for proper body function. These proteins include albumin, a protein that maintains plasma oncotic pressure and also serves as a carrier for many drugs and hormones as well as clotting factors used during blood coagulation.

Gallbladder

The **gallbladder** is located just beneath the liver and both stores and concentrates bile. After the release of CCK, the gallbladder contracts and pushes bile out into the **biliary tree**. The bile duct system merges with the pancreatic duct before emptying into the duodenum.

The gallbladder is a common site of cholesterol or bilirubin stone formation. This painful condition causes inflammation of the gallbladder. The stones also may travel into the bile ducts and may get stuck in the biliary tree. In some cases, stones can get caught just before entering the duodenum, resulting in blockage of not only the biliary tree, but the pancreatic duct as well, causing pancreatitis.

Absorption and Defecation

The absorption of nutrients primarily occurs in the small intestine, especially in the jejunum and the ileum. The large intestine largely absorbs water.

Jejunum and Ileum

The small intestine consists of 3 segments: the duodenum, the jejunum, and the ileum. As discussed previously, the **duodenum** is primarily involved in digestion. The **jejunum** and **ileum** are involved in the absorption of nutrients. The small intestine is lined with **villi**, which are small, fingerlike projections from the epithelial lining. Each villus has many **microvilli**, drastically increasing the surface area available for absorption. In addition, at the middle of each villus is a capillary bed for the absorption of water-soluble nutrients and a **lacteal**, a lymphatic channel that takes up fats for transport into the lymphatic system.

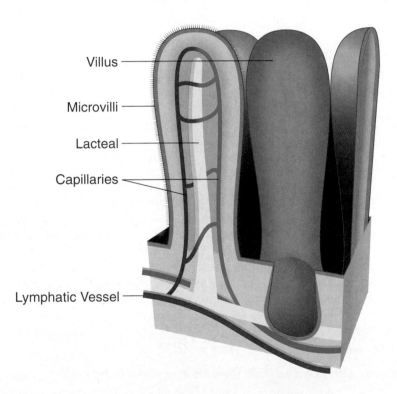

Figure 6-22. Structure of a Villus

Simple sugars, such as glucose, fructose, and galactose, and amino acids are absorbed by secondary active transport and facilitated diffusion into the epithelial cells lining the small intestine. Then, these substances move across the epithelial cells into the intestinal capillaries. Blood is constantly passing by the epithelial cells in the capillaries, carrying the carbohydrate and amino acid molecules away from the epithelial cells. This creates a concentration gradient, such that the blood always has a lower concentration of monosaccharides and amino acids than inside the epithelial cells. Thus, simple carbohydrates and amino acids diffuse from the epithelial cells into the capillaries. The absorbed molecules then go to the liver via the hepatic portal circulation.

What about fats? Small fatty acids will follow the same process as carbohydrates and amino acids by diffusing directly into the intestinal capillaries. These fatty acids do not require transporters because they are nonpolar, so they can easily traverse the cellular membrane. Larger fats, glycerol, and cholesterol move separately into the intestinal cells but then reform into triglycerides. The triglycerides and esterified cholesterol molecules are packaged into **chylomicrons**. Rather than entering the bloodstream, chylomicrons enter the lymphatic circulation through **lacteals**, small vessels that form the beginning of the lymphatic system. These lacteals converge and enter the venous circulation through the **thoracic duct** in the base of the neck, which empties into the left subclavian vein.

Vitamins also are absorbed in the small intestine. Vitamins can be categorized as fat-soluble or water-soluble.

- **Fat-soluble:** there are only 4 fat-soluble vitamins (A, D, E, and K), so these can be easily memorized; dissolve directly into chylomicrons to enter the body
- **Water-soluble:** all other vitamins (B complex and C); absorbed (along with water, amino acids, and carbohydrates) across the endothelial cells of the small intestine, passing directly into the plasma

Practical Point

A failure to digest and absorb fat properly, which can be caused by pathologies in the liver, gallbladder, pancreas, or small intestine, may lead to deficiencies of fat-soluble vitamins.

In addition to fats, carbohydrates, amino acids, and vitamins, the small intestine also absorbs water. Much of the water in chyme is actually the result of secretions. The average person may consume up to 2 L of fluid per day, but secretions into the upper GI tract may total up to 7 L of fluid per day. To maintain proper fluid levels within the body, much of this fluid must be reabsorbed by osmosis. As solutes are absorbed into the bloodstream, water is drawn with it, eventually reaching the capillaries. Water passes not only **transcellularly** (across the cell membrane) but also **paracellularly** (squeezing between cells) to reach the blood.

Large Intestine

The final part of the GI tract is the large intestine. It is primarily involved in water absorption. The large intestine has a larger diameter but shorter length than the small intestine. It is divided into 3 major sections: the cecum, the colon, and the rectum. The **cecum** is simply an outpocketing that accepts fluid exiting the small intestine through the **ileocecal valve** and is the site of attachment of the **appendix**. The appendix is a small, fingerlike projection that was once thought to be **vestigial**, although recent evidence suggests that it may have a role in warding off certain bacterial infections and repopulating the large intestine with normal flora after episodes of diarrhea. Inflammation of the appendix (**appendicitis**) is a surgical emergency.

Practical Point

Appendicitis is the most common reason for unscheduled surgery in the United States.

The **colon** itself is divided into the ascending, transverse, descending, and sigmoid colons. Its main function is to absorb water and salts (such as sodium chloride) from the undigested material left over from the small intestine. While the small intestine actually absorbs much more water overall than the colon, the colon primarily concentrates the remaining material to form feces with just the right amount of residual water. Too much water absorbed from the feces and constipation will result; too little water absorbed and it's off to the races with diarrhea.

Finally, the rectum serves as a storage site for feces, which consists of indigestible material, water, bacteria (*Escherichia coli* and others), and certain digestive secretions that are not reabsorbed (enzymes and some bile). The **anus** is the opening through which wastes are eliminated and consists of two sphincters: the internal and external anal sphincters. The **external anal sphincter** is under voluntary control (somatic), but the **internal anal sphincter** is under involuntary control (autonomic).

The large intestine—and even the small intestine—is home to many different species of bacteria. In fact, 30% of the dry matter in stool consists of bacteria. Most of these bacteria are anaerobes, but the cecum also is home to many aerobic bacteria. This relationship is symbiotic: the bacteria are provided with a steady source of food, and the byproducts produced by the bacteria are beneficial to humans. For example, bacteria in the gut produce vitamin K, which is essential for the production of clotting factors, and biotin (vitamin B_7), which is a coenzyme for many metabolic enzymes.

Assessment of Acute Abdomen

As with any patient, the assessment begins with evaluating the patient for conditions that are more serious and more likely to be associated with death. Evaluating a patient's ABCs and treating any problems with that should be of the highest priority. For example, acute coronary syndromes could present as pain in the upper abdomen, yet the patient may never complain of any chest-related problems. Nervous, respiratory, and cardiovascular problems are rarely directly related to an abdominal problem. Findings related to these systems may not leave time for a thorough evaluation of the abdomen, even if that is the patient's chief complaint. If there are no discernible derangements of the heart, breathing, blood pressure, level of consciousness, or CNS functions (such as CVA or syncope), completing a secondary survey related to the abdominal complaint is now appropriate.

The history of the present illness is a very valuable aspect to the acute abdomen assessment. OPPQRST and SAMPLE can provide some of the most important information to your assessment. Last oral intake can be important in assessing new or unusual foods the person may have eaten, and the patient's list of medications can provide information about preexisting GI problems. Asking some other questions, including evaluating any changes in bowel or bladder habits, any blood in the stool or vomit, and the overall color of recent bowel movements, can help clarify the possible problems the patient is experiencing.

Auscultation, observation, palpation, and percussion are the primary tools that will be used to assess the acute abdomen, in addition to a thorough verbal history of the present illness. By discussing the components of a thorough physical examination of the abdomen, these components can then be applied to any of the conditions described later. During the discussion on the specific pathologies that the paramedic may encounter, the assessment section of each will contain only abnormal findings associated with that pathology. It is understood and expected that the patient will receive a full assessment to rule out other possible conditions.

Auscultation

Although not often performed in the prehospital world, **auscultating** the abdomen should be performed, especially if the patient complains of diarrhea or not having had a bowel movement in several days. This should be done before palpating the abdomen because palpation may artificially increase the bowel sounds. Auscultation is done by placing the bell of the stethoscope anywhere on the abdomen, preferably over the lower quadrants, and listening for the presence or absence of bowel sounds. The absence of bowel sounds is most concerning because it may indicate paralysis of the bowel and severe constipation and obstruction.

Observation

Observe the surface of the abdomen and evaluate the skin and the shape of the abdomen while also being alert for bruising. The skin may have striae, which are stretch marks that can indicate a relatively rapid change in weight in a short period of time. This can be from fat, fluid, or pregnancy. The abdomen can be extremely large, called protuberant, most commonly from fluid buildup. Fluid in the abdomen is called ascites and happens most commonly from hepatic hypertension and results in an abdomen that is hard to the touch. Bruising may be found over the abdomen as well. The Cullen sign is bruising around the umbilicus and indicates intraperitoneal bleeding. This is a late sign of bleeding in the area. Bruising on 1 or both flanks indicates retroperitoneal bleeding and is called Grey Turner sign.

> **Pro-Tip**
>
> Remember the Cullen and Grey Turner signs with this play on words.:
>
> - **Cullen sign:** think of the made-up word *umbili-cullen*
> - **Grey Turner sign:** remember to "turner" the patient over to evaluate the flank

Palpation

The abdomen is divided into 4 quadrants.

- **Left Upper Quadrant (LUQ).** Stomach, spleen, a portion of the transverse colon and the descending colon, and the tail of the pancreas
- **Right Upper Quadrant (RUQ).** Liver, gall bladder, head of the pancreas, and a portion of the transverse colon and the ascending colon
- **Left Lower Quadrant (LLQ).** Descending and sigmoid colon, small intestine, and left ovary (females)
- **Right Lower Quadrant (RLQ).** Appendix, ascending colon, small intestine, and right ovary (females)

The upper half of the abdomen lies superior to a horizontal line drawn at the level of the umbilicus, and the lower half is below that line. The abdomen is divided into right and left halves at the midline. When performing palpation, be sure to assess all 4 quadrants. It is not uncommon to miss the lower quadrants because the provider is uneasy with getting too close to the genitalia. Missing the lower quadrants could mean missing issues such as an appendicitis or a large bowel obstruction.

To palpate the abdomen, place the fingers of one hand over the flat fingers of the other and firmly depress about 2–4 inches posteriorly. This should not be painful to the patient with a normal abdomen. Note any rigidity, discomfort, or masses in the area depressed. Also note any muscular or physical guarding in the area. Muscular guarding occurs when the patient tenses the abdominal muscles over an area of the abdomen to prevent pain already in that area from being made worse; physical guarding is when the patient actually holds their hands or arms over the location for the same reason.

Palpate this way over all 4 quadrants, noting differences as they are found. In addition, if the patient has complained about abdominal pain in one or more quadrants, assess the most painful area last. Palpating the most painful area last will minimize the chance of the patient feeling pain in a larger area, which might happen if the painful quadrant is palpated first. Pain can be a sign of infection, bleeding, trauma, or obstruction.

Some special assessment points are to be evaluated during palpation. When palpating over the liver (RUQ) in the supine patient, observe the jugular veins as pressure is applied. If they engorge or become visible, it is possible the patient is fluid overloaded and narrowly avoiding going into pulmonary edema. This is a particularly important assessment point when providing any patient aggressive fluid resuscitation, especially those with a history of CHF. Also when palpating this area, the patient may complain of an increase in pain in their right shoulder. This could be referred pain often found with gall bladder problems.

As the abdomen is assessed, be alert for signs of rebound tenderness. When the hands are quickly pulled off the abdomen after applying light pressure, the abdominal wall briefly bounces. This bouncing of the abdominal wall is the rebound. If this causes the patient pain, the peritoneum, the membrane lining the cavity of the abdomen and covering the abdominal organs, is irritated either from blood or infection. Rebound tenderness, once discovered, should not be checked for again because it is extremely uncomfortable for the patient.

Percussion

Percussion is the least used assessment tool the paramedic can employ because it requires the greatest amount of practice and experience with normal to master. To percuss an area of the patient, in this case the abdomen, lay one hand over the area to be percussed. With the dominant hand, firmly tap the middle finger of the hand on the abdomen. Note the sound produced. A solid sound could indicate fluid or blood buildup in that area or it could be a normal finding if over one of the solid organs of the abdomen—the liver, spleen or pancreas. A hollow sound could indicate air, though it is a usual sound to hear during percussion of the abdomen. Percussion is also discussed in the Patient Assessment chapter.

Physiology, Assessment, and Treatment of Abdominal Problems

Gastrointestinal Bleeding

GI bleeding can be classified as upper GI or lower GI, depending on the location of the bleed. Generally speaking, **upper GI** is considered everything through the small intestine. **Lower GI** is the large intestine, rectum and anus. The appearance of blood from a GI bleed can present in any of 4 forms.

- The patient vomiting may vomit frank red blood, where the blood is vomited back up before it can be digested. This is called **hematemesis**.
- If the blood has a chance to be digested before it irritates the stomach lining, the vomit will resemble coffee grounds, often with some undigested red blood still visible.
- Fully digested blood that is not removed via emesis will be excreted from the body in the stool. Stools containing fully digested blood are called **melena** and are sticky and very dark, almost black.
- Lower GI bleeds will cause bloody diarrhea with red blood present and a smell unlike any other.

Upper GI Bleeds

Esophageal varices are veins found in the inferior portion of the esophagus that are larger than normal. This occurs as a result of an increase in pressure in those veins, often the result of hepatic portal hypertension caused primarily by alcohol abuse or hepatitis C. Very often, the patient is unaware of the esophageal varices until one of them ruptures. Rapid bleeding from one of the veins usually results in hematemesis, frequently in copious amounts. Slower bleeds may result in coffee-ground vomit, and even slower bleeds may present with melena.

Prehospital treatment for esophageal varices is aimed at maintaining the person's blood pressure and rapid transport. The patient may lose or have lost a large percentage of the circulating volume, resulting in hypotension and hypovolemia. Decreased hematocrit and hemoglobin also can result in reduced O_2-carrying capacity plus signs and symptoms of shortness of breath or hypoxia. Patients should receive supplemental O_2, even with saturations in the high 90s. Patients should at least have a saline lock started if they are normotensive and fluid run if there is even borderline hypotension. Because the vomiting is caused by stomach lining irritation secondary to the bleeding, antiemetic medications will not usually work and are generally not recommended in the case of bleeding.

Mallory-Weiss syndrome is a tear in the junction between the esophagus and the stomach, often as a result of forceful, protracted vomiting. This tends to occur more in older adults but has been seen in pregnant women with severe **hyperemesis gravidarum**, commonly known as morning sickness. The condition can be life threatening. Bleeding with this condition is significantly less than with varices. Prehospital treatment includes treatment for hypotension because of dehydration from the protracted vomiting. Ondansetron may be given to attempt to minimize the vomiting and retching. Treatment for this condition involves rapid transport for surgical intervention at the hospital.

In **gastroesophageal reflux disease** (**GERD**), the cardiac sphincter, the circular muscle that separates the esophagus from the stomach, is not strong enough to prevent the flow of gastric contents superiorly. The patient will have a chronic complaint of heartburn, especially after lying down. The continued effect results in distal esophageal bleeding because acid from the stomach erodes the esophagus. Bleeding can occur from the damaged, weaker areas of the esophagus. As with previous conditions, prehospital treatment is largely related to preservation of the blood pressure. GERD may be difficult to distinguish from ACS; when in doubt, obtain a 12-lead ECG and treat as if it is a heart problem.

Peptic ulcer disease (**PUD**) is caused primarily by the bacteria *Helicobacter pylori*, which has the ability to survive the extremely acidic conditions in the stomach and overcome the lining of mucus that protects the stomach from digesting itself. Once the mucus layer is gone, the acid can now erode the stomach lining itself, causing bleeding and LUQ pain. This also can be caused by erosive gastritis, most commonly by excessive use of nonsteroidal anti-inflammatory drugs (NSAIDs), such as acetaminophen, naproxen, and ibuprofen. Here again, erosion of the stomach lining causes pain and bleeding. Smoking and alcohol use can increase gastric acidity, worsening already existing ulcers.

Eating often mitigates the pain somewhat, only to return later after the food leaves the stomach, so asking about how the pain is before and after eating can help lead to a working diagnosis of PUD. If left untreated, the ulcer can bleed heavily, leading to hematemesis, coffee-ground vomit, and/or melena. Treatment for the paramedic is again focused on maintaining blood pressure if the patient is hypotensive or tachycardic.

Lower GI Bleeds

Hemorrhoids are swelling and inflammation of the blood vessels surrounding the rectum. They can develop over time as a result of straining at stool, chronic constipation, or pregnancy. Irritation can cause them to rupture, and the bleeding can be quite profuse. Anal fissures are an actual tearing of the tissue in and around the anus. The causes for this are unknown, but anal intercourse or trying to pass large hard stools are believed to be the most common reasons. Patients seldom bleed heavily with either of these conditions, and treatment is therefore symptomatic. Only in rare cases will the bleeding be sufficient enough to cause a drop in blood pressure.

Inflammatory Conditions

Appendicitis is inflammation of the appendix, a small, tube-like structure at the proximal end of the cecum of the large intestine. It can occur at any age and most often is the result of fecal matter blocking the lumen of the appendix. Once in there, the appendix is unable to flush out the fecal matter, and an infection begins. The bacteria and toxins irritate the lining of the appendix, and it begins to get inflamed. If left untreated, the appendix can burst, allowing bacteria and toxins to permeate the abdominal cavity. This will, in turn, irritate the peritoneum, leading to peritonitis. At this point, the profound infection can lead to sepsis and death.

Early on in appendicitis, the patient will present with periumbilical pain (pain in the area of the umbilicus), accompanied by a low-grade fever, nausea, and vomiting. As the infection and inflammation worsen, the periumbilical pain moves and centers over the LRQ and intensifies. If the appendix is not removed before this, rupture is likely. If the appendix has ruptured, the patient will actually report a transient decrease in pain; however, the pain the patient does have will be diffuse throughout the abdomen and be accompanied by rebound tenderness. When assessing these patients, repeated palpation over the area of the appendix could accelerate rupture, so care should be taken not to do this more than is needed to adequately assess the area.

Treatment for appendicitis involves treatment for shock if it is present. Establish an intravenous line and give fluid. Transport the patient in the position of maximal comfort, which may be on their left side with the knees drawn up. Drawing up the knees relieves tension in the abdominal wall and can substantially lessen any discomfort the patient would feel in other positions. If the patient is nauseous or vomiting, administer 4 mg ondansetron and consider analgesia.

Cholecystitis is the inflammation of the gall bladder. It may occur for a variety of reasons; however, little is known about why it occurs. Frequently, calcifications, called gall stones, occur within the gall bladder and block the outflow of the bile when it is needed. Bile is needed when fatty foods enter the duodenum to aid in the digestion of these fatty foods. If the gall stones block the duct leading to the small intestine, the patient will feel extreme pain when the gall bladder contracts to try and inject the bile into the small intestine.

The patient will complain of pain in the RUQ, often about 2–3 hours after a meal, especially if it is high in fat. The patient also may complain of nausea, vomiting, and fever and appear jaundiced. Treatment for this patient will center on getting the patient to the hospital; the patient will likely need gall bladder surgery. Analgesia seems like the humane thing to do during transport; however, morphine is believed to cause the sphincter of Oddi to contract, actually worsening pain. Meperidine is recommended in the case of cholecystitis, if it is available pre-hospital.

Diverticulitis is an inflammation of the diverticula. A **diverticulum** is an outward bulge, or pouch, in the digestive tract, usually of the large intestine. It is believed that these pouches form as a result of stools becoming harder. As they become harder, it becomes more difficult for the peristaltic movements of the colon wall to push the feces out. Consequently, pressure on the wall builds up with each contraction, and, eventually, a weak area gives way. In diverticulitis, this pouch (diverticulum) becomes inflamed, typically as a result of an infection caused by trapped fecal matter.

Patients will complain of pain, often in the LLQ, along with fever, malaise, and possibly vomiting. Patients can become septic very easily with diverticulitis. The patient who is septic needs large amounts of fluid to maintain blood pressure and may even require pressors such as dopamine. Patients will likely require surgery for the diverticulum and any adhesions that may have developed.

Pancreatitis is inflammation of the pancreas, and can be chronic or acute. Acute pancreatitis is most commonly caused by gall stones and cholecystitis. The most common cause of chronic pancreatitis is heavy alcohol use. It causes intense, diffuse pain throughout the upper abdominal quadrants that is sometimes described as a burning pain that radiates to the back. Treatment for pancreatitis is largely symptomatic. Avoid morphine for the same reason as in cholecystitis.

Chronic Inflammatory Conditions

For chronic inflammatory conditions, prehospital treatment is the same: treat symptomatically and provide fluid if hypotensive. If the hypotension is refractory to fluid administration, consider pressors. Pain management should be nonnarcotic only to prevent opioid-induced constipation and an inadvertent worsening of the patient's symptoms.

In **Crohn disease,** it is believed that the immune system attacks the GI tract, most commonly the area of the small intestine called the ileum (the last 11 feet of the small intestine). Genetics and heredity are also suspected of playing a role. The disease may be present in the colon but only in certain areas in addition to or instead of the ileum. Symptoms include:

- Skin rashes and other extraintestinal symptoms (not always)
- LRQ abdominal pain with diarrhea that may be bloody if the disease is extensive and the ulcerations are actively bleeding

Irritable bowel syndrome (IBS) is a chronic condition characterized by a hypersensitivity of colonic pain receptors. Normal degrees of stretch in these receptors, which people without this condition would not otherwise notice, is responded to with spasms in the colon of the patient with IBS. These spasms can be isolated, leading to bloating and constipation, or they may be wave-like and resemble peristalsis, leading to diarrhea and faster transit of stool through the colon. Patients will present with lower quadrant abdominal pain and either have not had a bowel movement recently or have had intractable diarrhea.

Ulcerative colitis (UC) is similar to Crohn disease in that it is an inflammatory bowel syndrome, but it is seen exclusively in the colon and has no systemic symptoms. In addition, Crohn disease affects the entire wall (transmural) of the colon and small intestine, whereas UC involves only the inner lining of the colon. As the lining gets ulcerated, the ulcers may start to bleed, leading to bloody stools and diarrhea. Infection also can be an issue in the ulcers, so the patient may have a fever, general malaise, and weakness. This is seldom a true emergency, and little can be done in the field to treat UC.

Obstructive Conditions

Small bowel obstruction (SBO) is any of a family of conditions that either narrow the diameter of the small intestine or prevent it from dilating when a larger amount of food moves through it. Postoperative adhesions, Crohn disease, cancer, and foreign bodies are the most common reasons for SBO. Patients will present with diffuse abdominal pain and often will be vomiting. The vomit or the patient's breath may smell like feces caused by the backup of food at the point of the obstruction. Patients also may present with weakness, lethargy, and fever. Treatment is supportive until surgery at the hospital. Vomiting in this patient is therapeutic, so it should be allowed to happen; therefore, antiemetics are not recommended.

Large bowel obstructions can be caused by a mechanical obstruction or a constriction of the colon. Adults age 65 and older are more susceptible to a mechanical obstruction because of an increased prevalence of cancer and diverticulitis in this age group. Meanwhile, the pediatric population can have a large bowel obstruction caused by intussusception or volvulus, both of which narrow the diameter of the large bowel. **Intussusception** is a condition where the bowel telescopes over itself, and **volvulus** is a twisting of the colon that causes a kink where fecal matter cannot pass. Presentation and treatment are similar to that of SBO.

A **hernia** is when an organ pushes through a potential opening or ligament into a different body cavity. The 3 common types of hernias are hiatal, inguinal, and umbilical hernias.

- In a **hiatal hernia,** the stomach pushes superiorly through the diaphragm alongside the esophagus.
- In an **inguinal hernia** (more common in men), the small intestine pushes through the inguinal ligament and often can be felt inside the scrotum.
- In an **umbilical hernia** (common among older adults and those who have had abdominal surgery), part of the small intestine pushes through the abdominal wall and into the retroperitoneal space.
- In an **incisional hernia** (uncommon), abdominal contents push through the abdominal wall and either out of the body in extreme cases or into the retroperitoneal space (similar to a traumatic evisceration).

Hernias can be described as reducible, incarcerated, or strangulated. A **reducible hernia** is able to freely move back into its original anatomic position on its own or with manipulation. An **incarcerated hernia,** conversely, is trapped in its herniated position usually because the amount of intestine that has pushed through the opening is now larger than the opening, or the intra-abdominal pressure is high enough to keep it there. In a **strangulated hernia** (true surgical emergency), the blood supply to the portion of the organ that has herniated is diminished or occluded. This can lead to necrosis of that area of tissue in relatively short order if not relieved quickly.

Symptoms include pain (varying amounts, from an unusual feeling to extreme debilitating pain) and small bowel obstruction if the hernia appreciably decreases the lumen of the small intestine. Pain management and rapid transport in the position of comfort are the prehospital care goals.

Practical Point

In a hernia, the amount of pain, the location of the pain, and the radiation/referral of the pain is almost entirely caused by the size of the hernia and degree of strangulation.

REVIEW QUESTIONS

Select the ONE best answer.

1. Initial digestion of proteins begins in which structure?

    A. Mouth

    B. Stomach

    C. Small intestine

    D. Large intestine

2. A patient is experiencing steatorrhea, which is diarrhea with a high fat content typically caused by poor fat digestion and decreased absorption. Which other nutrient may the patient be having difficulty absorbing?

    A. Glucose

    B. Amino acids

    C. Vitamin A

    D. Vitamin B

3. RUQ pain could be a complaint in patients with which one of the following problems?

    A. Appendicitis

    B. Gastric ulcer

    C. Hepatitis

    D. Ovarian cyst

4. You are on scene with a 67-year-old male patient who is complaining of a single episode of vomiting blood accompanied by RUQ pain. He has a history of alcoholism. He has jaundiced skin and sclera and also has noted black and tarry stools over the past several days. Which of the following is most likely causing this patient's bleeding problem?

    A. GERD

    B. Peptic ulcers

    C. Mallory-Weiss tears

    D. Esophageal varices

ANSWERS AND EXPLANATIONS

1. **The correct answer is (B).** Protein digestion begins in the stomach, where the food mixes with HCl and pepsin. The pepsin is the first of many enzymes involved in protein breakdown. Carbohydrate digestion begins in the mouth (A) and continues in the small intestine (C), with the enzyme amylase in both locations. The small intestine is the primary location for the digestion of fats and a secondary location for protein digestion. The large intestine (D) is the primary site of water absorption.

2. **The correct answer is (C).** Vitamins A, D, E, and K are fat-soluble vitamins. If the patient is having difficulty absorbing fats, then there may be trouble absorbing fat-soluble vitamins. Vitamin C and all the vitamins of the B complex (D) are water soluble and easily absorbed. Glucose (A) and amino acid (B) absorption is not often affected in patients with steatorrhea.

3. **The correct answer is (C).** The liver lies almost entirely within the RUQ, so this should be a consideration for a patient presenting with pain in this quadrant. A patient with an appendicitis (A) would present with periumbilical pain in the early stages or RLQ pain as it progresses. Gastric ulcers (B) would present with LUQ pain. Ovarian cysts (D) could present with pain in either lower quadrant, depending on which ovary is affected.

4. **The correct answer is (D).** This patient's history is consistent with liver disease, which is the primary cause of esophageal varices. GERD (A) can cause esophageal bleeding in extreme conditions, so it would not be at the top of the differential list. Peptic ulcers (B) are most likely going to present with LUQ pain, so this is not the most likely option. Mallory-Weiss tears (C) are common in adults age 65 and older and pregnant women who experience intractable vomiting. A single episode of vomiting, as in this case, is not the most likely option.

GENITOURINARY EMERGENCIES

Much of this section will center on the kidneys and problems associated with their failure. It has been said that if the kidneys die or fail, so does the organism. With dialysis, the rate of kidney failure has been slowed; however, without dialysis, a patient in kidney failure would not be able to survive more than a week or so because of the buildup of toxins in the bloodstream.

Anatomy and Physiology

The **excretory system** serves many functions, including the regulation of blood pressure, blood osmolarity, acid–base balance, and the removal of nitrogenous wastes. The kidneys play an essential role in these functions.

The excretory system consists of the kidneys, ureters, bladder, and urethra. The kidneys are two bean-shaped structures located behind the digestive organs at the level of the bottom rib. The functional unit of the kidney is the nephron; each kidney has approximately 1 million nephrons. All the nephrons eventually empty into the renal pelvis, which narrows to form the ureter. Urine travels through the ureter to the bladder. From the bladder, urine is transported through the urethra to exit the body.

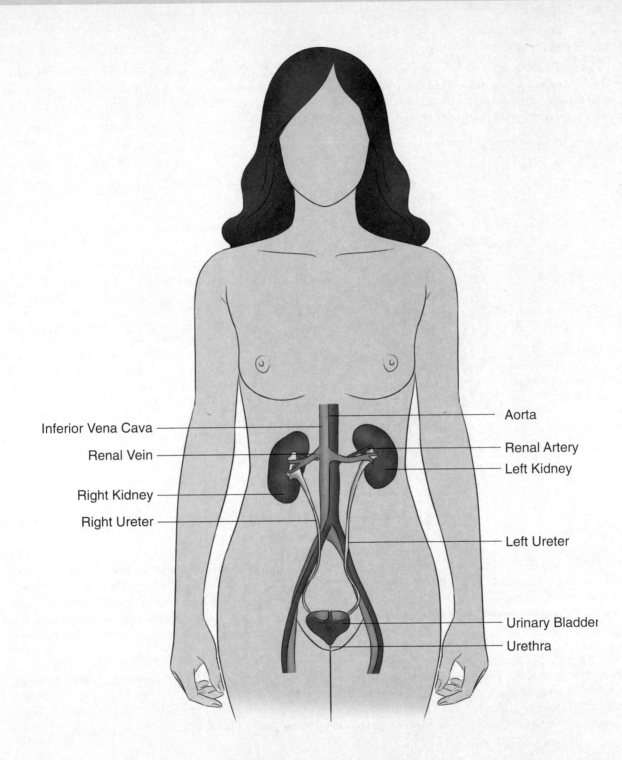

Figure 6-23. The Excretory System
Once it leaves the kidneys, urine moves through the ureters to be stored in the urinary bladder until it is excreted through the urethra.

Kidney Structure

Each **kidney** is subdivided into a cortex and a medulla. The **cortex** is the kidney's outermost layer, and the **medulla** of the kidney sits within the cortex. Each kidney also has a renal **hilum**, which is a deep slit in the center of its medial surface. The widest part of the ureter, the **renal pelvis**, spans almost the entire width of the renal hilum. The **renal artery**, **renal vein**, and **ureter** enter and exit through the renal hilum.

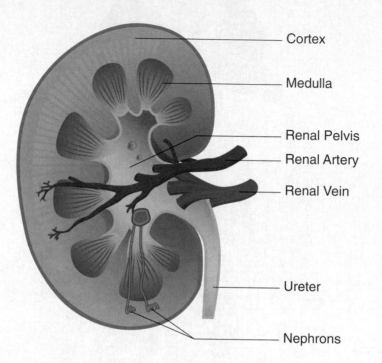

- Cortex
- Medulla
- Renal Pelvis
- Renal Artery
- Renal Vein
- Ureter
- Nephrons

Figure 6-24. Gross Anatomy of the Kidney

The kidney has one of the few portal systems in the body. A **portal system** consists of two capillary beds in series through which blood must travel before returning to the heart. The renal artery branches out, passes through the medulla, and enters the cortex as **afferent arterioles**. The highly convoluted capillary tufts derived from these afferent arterioles are known as **glomeruli**. After blood passes through a glomerulus, the **efferent arterioles** then form a 2nd capillary bed. These capillaries surround the loop of Henle and are known as **vasa recta**.

Around the glomerulus is a cup-like structure known as the **Bowman capsule**. The Bowman capsule leads to a long tubule with many distinct areas; in order, these are the proximal convoluted tubule, the descending and ascending limbs of the Loop of Henle, the distal convoluted tubule, and the collecting duct. The kidney's ability to excrete waste is intricately tied to the specific placement of these structures and their physiology.

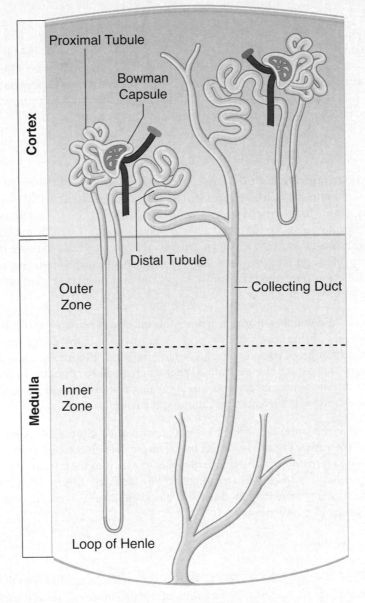

Figure 6-25. Nephron

Bladder Structure

The bladder has a muscular lining known as the **detrusor muscle**. Parasympathetic activity causes the detrusor muscle to contract. However, to leave the body, urine must pass through two sphincters: the internal and external urethral sphincters. The **internal urethral sphincter**, consisting of smooth muscle, is contracted in its normal state. Because the internal sphincter is made of smooth muscle, it is under involuntary control. The **external urethral sphincter** consists of skeletal muscle and is under voluntary control. When the bladder is full, stretch receptors convey to the nervous system that the bladder requires emptying. This causes parasympathetic neurons to fire, and the detrusor muscle contracts. This contraction also causes the internal sphincter to relax. This reflex is known as the **micturition reflex**. The next step is up to the individual. The person can choose to relax the external sphincter to urinate or can maintain the tone of the external sphincter to prevent urination. This can cause a few moments of discomfort, but the reflex usually dissipates in a few minutes. However, if the bladder is not emptied, then the process will begin anew shortly thereafter. Urination itself is facilitated by contraction of the abdominal musculature, which increases pressure within the abdominal cavity, resulting in compression of the bladder and an increased urine flow rate.

Osmoregulation

The kidney filters the blood to form urine. The composition and quantity of urine are determined by the present state of the body. For example, if blood volume is low and blood osmolarity is high, then it is most beneficial to the body to maximally retain water. This results in low-volume, highly concentrated urine. Likewise, a patient receiving large amounts of intravenous fluids is likely to produce a larger volume of less concentrated urine. Thus, the primary job of the kidneys is to regulate blood volume and osmolarity. To do this, kidney function may be divided into three different processes: filtration, secretion, and reabsorption.

Filtration

The nephron's first function is **filtration**. In the kidneys, approximately 20% of the blood that passes through the glomerulus is filtered as fluid into the Bowman capsule. The collected fluid is known as the **filtrate**. The movement of fluid into the Bowman capsule is governed by **Starling forces**, which account for the pressure differentials in both hydrostatic and oncotic pressures between the blood and the Bowman capsule. The hydrostatic pressure in the glomerulus is significantly higher than that in the Bowman capsule, which causes fluid to move into the nephron. On the other hand, the osmolarity of blood is higher than that of the Bowman capsule, resulting in pressure opposing the movement of fluid into the nephron. However, hydrostatic pressure is much larger than oncotic pressure, so the net flow is still from blood into the nephron.

Under most circumstances, fluid will flow from the glomerulus into the Bowman capsule. However, various pathologies can cause derangements of this flow. Consider what might happen if the ureter was obstructed by a kidney stone. An obstruction would result in a buildup of urine behind the stone. Eventually, enough fluid will build up and cause distention of the renal pelvis and the nephrons. What will happen to filtration in this case? The hydrostatic pressure in the Bowman capsule would increase to the point that filtration could no longer occur because there would be excessive pressure opposing movement of fluid into the nephron.

The filtrate is similar in composition to blood but does not contain cells or proteins because of the filter's ability to select based on size. In other words, molecules or cells that are larger than glomerular pores will remain in the blood. As described earlier, the blood remaining in the glomerulus then travels into the efferent arterioles, which empty into the vasa recta. The filtrate is isotonic to blood so that neither the capsule nor the capillaries swell. Our kidneys filter about 180 L per day, which is approximately 36 times our blood volume. This means that the entire volume of a person's blood is filtered about every 40 minutes.

Secretion

In addition to filtering blood, the nephrons are able to **secrete** salts, acids, bases, and urea directly into the tubule by either active or passive transport. The quantity and identity of the substances secreted into the nephron are directly related to the needs of the body at that time. For example, a diet heavy in meat results in the intake of large amounts of protein, which contains a significant amount of nitrogen. Ammonia is a byproduct of the metabolism of nitrogen-containing compounds and, as a base, can disturb the pH of blood and cells. The liver converts the ammonia to **urea**, a neutral compound, which travels to the kidney and is secreted into the nephron for excretion with the urine. The kidneys are capable of eliminating ions or other substances when present in relative excess in the blood, such as potassium cations, hydrogen ions, or metabolites of medications. Secretion also is a mechanism for excreting wastes that are simply too large to pass through glomerular pores.

Reabsorption

Some compounds that are filtered or secreted may be taken back up for use via **reabsorption**. Certain substances are almost always reabsorbed, such as glucose, amino acids, and vitamins. In addition, hormones such as ADH (vasopressin) and aldosterone can alter the quantity of water reabsorbed within the kidney to maintain blood pressure.

Nephron Function

The kidney uses mechanisms such as filtration, secretion, and reabsorption to produce urine and regulate the blood volume and osmolarity. However, the function of the nephron isn't quite that simple. In fact, renal physiology often is considered one of the most difficult topics covered in medical school.

To simplify this topic, it is important to understand that the kidney has two main goals: (1) keep what the body needs and lose what it doesn't and (2) concentrate the urine to conserve water. The kidney allows the human body to reabsorb certain materials for reuse while also selectively eliminating waste. For example, glucose and amino acids are not usually present in the urine because the kidney is able to reabsorb these substances for later use. By contrast, waste products such as hydrogen and potassium ions, ammonia, and urea remain in the filtrate and are excreted. Finally, water is reabsorbed in large quantities to maintain blood pressure and adequate hydration.

To understand this complex organ, the nephron will be studied piece by piece, which will include a discussion of exactly what is occurring in each segment. Follow along with the nephron diagram. As a theme, note that segments that are horizontal in the diagram (the Bowman capsule, the proximal convoluted tubule, and the distal convoluted tubule) are primarily focused on the identity of the particles in the urine (keep what the body needs and lose what it doesn't). In contrast, the segments that are vertical in the diagram (the loop of Henle and collecting duct) are primarily focused on the volume and concentration of the urine (concentrate the urine to conserve water).

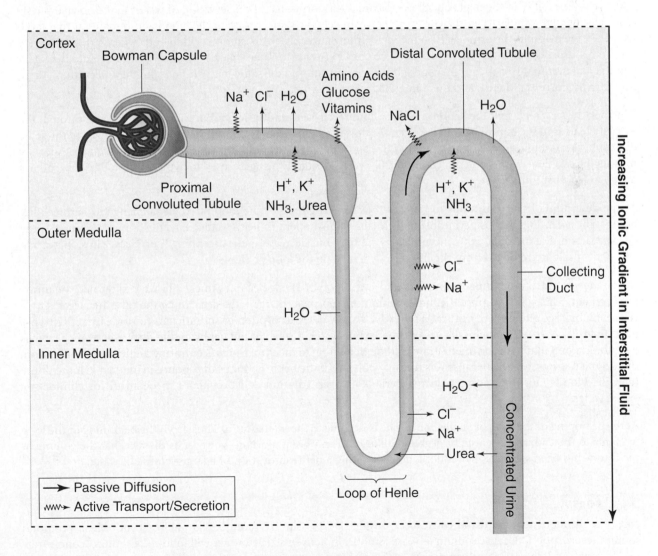

Figure 6-26. Reabsorption and Secretion in the Nephron

Proximal Convoluted Tubule

The filtrate first enters the **proximal convoluted tubule** (PCT). In this region, amino acids, glucose, water-soluble vitamins, and the majority of salts are reabsorbed along with water. Almost 70% of filtered sodium will be reabsorbed here, but the filtrate remains isotonic to the **interstitium** (connective tissue surrounding the nephron), as other solutes and a large volume of water also are reabsorbed. Solutes that enter the interstitium are picked up by the vasa recta to be returned to the bloodstream for reuse within the body. The PCT also is the site of secretion for a number of waste products, including hydrogen ions, potassium ions, ammonia, and urea.

Loop of Henle

Filtrate from the proximal convoluted tubule then enters the **descending limb of the loop of Henle**, which dives deep into the medulla before turning around to become the **ascending limb of the loop of Henle**. The descending limb is permeable only to water, and the medulla has an ever-increasing osmolarity as the descending limb travels deeper into it. Think for a moment how this would affect the flow of water. As the descending limb traverses deeper into the medulla, the increasing interstitial concentration favors the outflow of water from the descending limb, which is reabsorbed into the vasa recta.

The kidney is capable of altering the osmolarity of the interstitium. This creates a gradient that, coupled with the selective permeability of the nephron, allows maximal reabsorption and conservation of water. In the normal physiological state, the osmolarity in the cortex is approximately the same as that of the blood and remains at that level. Deeper in the medulla, the osmolarity in the interstitium can range from isotonic with blood (when trying to excrete water) to 4 times as concentrated (when trying to conserve water). Water will move out of the tubule, into the interstitium, and eventually back into the blood. If the concentration is the same in the tubule and the interstitium, there is no driving force (gradient), and the water will be lost in urine.

Together, the vasa recta and the nephron create a **countercurrent multiplier system**: The flow of filtrate through the loop of Henle is in the opposite direction from the flow of blood through the vasa recta. If the two flowed in the same direction, they would quickly reach equilibrium, and the kidney would be unable to reabsorb as much water. By making the two flow in opposite directions, the filtrate is constantly being exposed to hypertonic blood, which allows maximal reabsorption of water.

As the descending limb transitions to become the ascending limb of the loop of Henle, a change in permeability occurs. The ascending limb is permeable only to salts and is impermeable to water. Here, the opposite occurs: At the deeper parts of the medulla, salt concentrations are high but decrease as the ascending limb rises. Thus, increasing amounts of salt are removed from the filtrate as it travels up the loop of Henle.

At the transition from the inner to outer medulla, the loop of Henle becomes thicker, in what is termed the **diluting segment**. This is not because the lumen within the tube has enlarged; the cells lining the tube are larger. These cells contain large amounts of mitochondria, which allow the reabsorption of sodium and chloride by active transport. Indeed, because so much salt is reabsorbed while water is stuck in the nephron, the filtrate actually becomes hypotonic compared with the interstitium. Although tending to focus on the concentrating abilities of the nephron, this segment is noteworthy because it is the only portion of the nephron that can produce urine that is more dilute than the blood. This is important during periods of overhydration and provides a mechanism for eliminating excess water.

At the beginning of the loop of Henle, the filtrate is isotonic to the interstitium. Thus, from the beginning of the loop of Henle to the end, there is a slight degree of dilution. Far more important, however, is the fact that the volume of the filtrate has been significantly reduced, demonstrating a net reabsorption of a large volume of water.

Distal Convoluted Tubule

Next, the filtrate enters the **distal convoluted tubule** (DCT). The DCT responds to aldosterone, which promotes sodium reabsorption. Because sodium ions are osmotically active particles, water will follow the sodium, concentrating the urine and decreasing its volume. The DCT also is the site of waste product secretion, like the PCT.

Collecting Duct

The final concentration of the urine will depend largely on the permeability of the collecting duct, which is responsive to both aldosterone and ADH (vasopressin). As the permeability of the collecting duct increases, so too does water reabsorption, resulting in further concentration of the urine. The reabsorbed water enters the interstitium and makes its way to the vasa recta, where it reenters the bloodstream to once again become part of the plasma. The collecting duct almost always reabsorbs water, but the amount is variable. When the body is very well hydrated, the collecting duct will be fairly impermeable to salt and water. When in conservation mode, ADH and aldosterone will each act to increase reabsorption of water in the collecting duct, allowing for greater water retention and more concentrated urine output.

Ultimately, anything that does not leave the tubule by the end of the collecting duct will be excreted; the collecting duct is the point of no return. After that, there are no further opportunities for reabsorption. As the filtrate leaves the tubule, it collects in the renal pelvis. The fluid, which carries mostly urea, uric acid, and excess ions (sodium, potassium, magnesium, and calcium), flows through the ureter to the bladder, where it is stored until voiding.

Functions of Excretory System

The kidneys use osmolarity gradients and selective permeability to filter, secrete, and reabsorb materials in the process of making urine. However, these processes have larger implications for the human body as a whole. The selective elimination of water and solutes allows the kidneys, in conjunction with the endocrine, cardiovascular, and respiratory systems, to control blood pressure, blood osmolarity, and the acid–base balance.

Blood Pressure

The hormones aldosterone and ADH (vasopressin) are very important for maintaining proper blood pressure.

Aldosterone is a steroid hormone that is secreted by the adrenal cortex in response to decreased blood pressure. Decreased blood pressure stimulates the release of **renin** from **juxtaglomerular cells** in the kidney. Renin then cleaves **angiotensinogen**, a liver protein, to form **angiotensin I**. This peptide is then metabolized by **angiotensin-converting enzyme** in the lungs to form **angiotensin II**, which promotes the release of aldosterone from the adrenal cortex.

Aldosterone works by altering the ability of the DCT and collecting duct to reabsorb sodium. Remember that water does not move on its own but rather travels down an osmolarity gradient. Thus, if more sodium is reabsorbed, water will flow with it. This reabsorption of isotonic fluid has the net effect of increasing blood volume and therefore blood pressure. Aldosterone also will increase potassium and hydrogen ion excretion.

ADH (also known as **vasopressin**) is a peptide hormone synthesized by the hypothalamus and released by the posterior pituitary gland in response to high blood osmolarity. It directly alters the permeability of the collecting duct, allowing more water to be reabsorbed by making the cell junctions of the duct leaky. Increased concentration in the interstitium (hypertonic to the filtrate) will then cause reabsorption of water from the tubule. Alcohol and caffeine both inhibit ADH release and lead to the frequent excretion of dilute urine.

In addition to the kidneys, the cardiovascular system also can vasoconstrict or vasodilate to maintain blood pressure. Constriction of the afferent arteriole will lead to a lower pressure of blood reaching the glomeruli, which are adjacent to the juxtaglomerular cells. Therefore, this vasoconstriction will secondarily lead to renin release, which also will help raise blood pressure.

Osmoregulation

The osmolarity of the blood must be tightly controlled to ensure correct oncotic pressures within the vasculature. A note on terminology: **osmotic pressure** is the "sucking" pressure that draws water into the vasculature caused by all dissolved particles. **Oncotic pressure**, on the other hand, is the osmotic pressure that is attributable to dissolved proteins specifically. Blood osmolarity is usually maintained at approximately 290 milliosmoles (mOsm) per liter. As described earlier, the kidneys control osmolarity by modulating the reabsorption of water and filtering and secreting dissolved particles. When blood osmolarity is low, excess water will be excreted, whereas solutes will be reabsorbed in higher concentrations. In contrast, when blood osmolarity is high, water reabsorption increases and solute excretion increases.

Acid–Base Balance

The **bicarbonate buffer system** is the major regulator of blood pH. Remind yourself of the buffer equation:

$$CO_2 \ (g) + H_2O \ (l) \rightleftharpoons H_2CO_3 \ (aq) \rightleftharpoons H^+ \ (aq) + HCO_3^- \ (aq)$$

The respiratory system can contribute to acid–base balance by increasing or decreasing the respiratory rate. If the blood pH is too low, then increasing the respiratory rate blows off more CO_2 and favors the conversion of H^+ and HCO_3^- to water and CO_2, increasing the pH. If the blood pH is too high, then decreasing the respiratory rate causes the opposite effects. The respiratory system can react to derangements of pH quickly. What can the excretory system do to contribute? The kidneys are able to selectively increase or decrease the secretion of both hydrogen ions and bicarbonate. When blood pH is too low, the kidneys excrete more hydrogen ions and increase reabsorption of bicarbonate, resulting in a higher pH. Likewise, when blood pH is too high, the kidneys can excrete more bicarbonate and increase reabsorption of hydrogen ions. This is slower than the respiratory response, but it is a highly effective way for the body to maintain its acid–base balance.

Pro-Tip

The order the bicarbonate buffer system equation is written in does not matter. It can be written with the CO_2 and H_2O on the left or the H^+ and HCO_3^- on the left. When evaluating the equation, such as in an examination question, observe how it is written and answer the question accordingly. Do not memorize it, or the rules presented here, regarding the equation as it has been written. It may not be written the same way on an examination. Rather, understand what is meant when it is said that the equation proceeds to the left or right.

Renal Emergencies

Acute and Chronic Renal Failure

Acute renal failure (**ARF**) is a sudden decrease of filtration of blood entering the kidneys and can be fatal in up to about 80% of cases. ARF could present as **oliguria**, which is a reduction in urine output to <500 mL per day, or anuria, which literally means without urine and is a complete lack of urine production. ARF can be further characterized into prerenal, intrarenal or postrenal causes.

Prerenal causes are those that prevent blood from entering the glomeruli within the kidneys or significantly reduce the pressure in the glomeruli to the point where filtrate cannot be collected in the capsule. Such causes include profound hypotension from hemorrhage, dehydration, trauma, shock of any kind, or sepsis. This is typically the easiest ARF cause to treat because it should resolve itself once kidney perfusion is restored.

Intrarenal ARF is far more complicated and is ultimately caused by damage to any of the glomerular capillaries and arterioles, the renal tissue itself or the cells of the nephron. These issues can be brought on by such widely varying conditions as diabetes mellitus (blood vessel damage), heavy metals (nephron damage), or certain medications or street drugs (renal cells surrounding nephrons and vasculature).

Postrenal ARF is caused by inhibition of urinary outflow from the renal pelvis. If urinary outflow fails, urine will back up through the collecting ducts and eventually all the way back to the capsule, thus preventing filtrate from entering the capsule from the glomerulus. Failure of the kidneys in this case to filter the blood will quickly lead to the retention of toxins, potassium ions, and hydrogen ions, any of which can alter the blood chemistry and lead to altered mental status and death relatively quickly.

Although all the ARF causes can be reversed with time and appropriate treatments, **chronic renal failure** (**CRF**) is a progressive and irreversible failure of the kidneys caused by destruction of the nephrons. This situation usually takes years to develop and often is found in late stages of uncontrolled or poorly controlled hypertension and diabetes. Nephron destruction has something of a domino effect on the kidney as a whole. First, one or several nephrons are damaged and cease to function and are replaced by scar tissue. This scarring then causes surrounding tissue to waste away and shrink, damaging other neighboring nephrons. This leads to renal mass loss and eventually irreversible kidney failure.

ARF and CRF can present with similar findings, including fatigue, weight loss, and sleep disturbances. ARF just occurs over a shorter time frame and will likely also be a result of a bigger problem, such as hemorrhage, sepsis, and trauma to the mid-back or flanks (such as what might result from a football player being tackled from behind). Evaluation of the patient's recent urinary output will be helpful information. Sudden oliguria or anuria likely indicates ARF. Patients in both cases may present with altered mental status caused by toxin buildup in the blood. Patients also frequently have cardiac dysrhythmias, including tachycardias, ectopic beats, VT, and indications of hyperkalemia (peaked T waves and absent P waves).

Treatment for ARF is primarily related to restoring kidney perfusion and removing anything that may be causing the kidney failure. For example, if the patient is hypotensive, restoring renal blood flow can be accomplished with aggressive fluid resuscitation or pressor administration. If a pressor is needed, dopamine is preferred to epinephrine. The removal of offending agents could mean stopping certain antibiotics or clearing the body of street drugs. Patients may need dialysis to accomplish this; however, for ARF, many patients will not need that aggressive of a treatment. For CRF, on the other hand, dialysis is almost always needed. Once patients start on dialysis for CRF or end stage renal disease, they will remain on that for life, unless a kidney becomes available and they receive a transplant. For patients in any of these conditions, it is recommended to not give any medications based solely on protocol. Seek advice from medical control before administering any medications to a patient on dialysis; with the kidneys unable to remove the medication, it may build up to overdose or even toxic levels.

Dialysis

Two types of dialysis are performed on a routine basis in an outpatient setting: peritoneal dialysis and hemodialysis. **Peritoneal dialysis** involves bathing the entire abdominal cavity with special dialysis fluid by injecting it through the abdominal wall, usually near the umbilicus. The fluid is allowed to remain in the abdominal cavity for about 2 hours, and then it is allowed to drain back out of the body. During the time it spent in the body, waste products diffuse into the fluid as they would in the kidneys. This is as effective as hemodialysis.

Hemodialysis is what is commonly thought of when thinking of dialysis. It involves the patient being connected to a machine that draws blood out of the body and functions much the same way as the kidneys. The patient is connected to the machine 3 days a week for about 4 hours per session. To be on dialysis, the patient has a shunt somewhere in the body that connects an artery and a vein that not only allows for repeated needle punctures but also can handle the pressures of the machine removing and returning the blood. Commonly, the shunt is placed near the anterior surface of the elbow and can be seen under the skin as a bump that looks like a large vessel. If there is a shunt in the arm, blood pressure cannot be measured in that arm. Alternatively, the shunt may be located in the anterior thigh or in the lateral anterior chest.

Patients undergoing dialysis are more vulnerable to conditions the general population also experience. They are more likely to experience hypertension and CHF as a result of the hypertension. Patients undergoing dialysis also are more likely to have an MI and life-threatening dysrhythmias caused in large part by potassium not being removed from the body consistently. They also may get a condition known as **uremic pericarditis**, which is caused by high levels of blood urea nitrogen (BUN) in the blood, although exactly how it causes pericarditis is not well understood. Patients on dialysis also experience several issues directly related to the act of receiving dialysis to which paramedics are frequently called.

- **Air Embolism.** This can happen if the machine the patient is connected to has loose tubes that allow air to enter the system. This air can then be pumped back into the patient. If this is suspected, transport immediately, supine or with the legs slightly elevated if the patient can tolerate the position and rapidly transport to the nearest medical facility.

- **Disequilibrium Syndrome.** During dialysis, fluid, electrolytes, and BUN are removed from the blood; however, the same concentration remains in the CSF. Briefly, these two fluids have unequal concentrations of salts in them, resulting in a fluid shift of water by osmosis from blood into the CSF. If this shift of water into the CSF is significant enough (electrolytes dialyzed off the patient too quickly), the ICP can increase. The patient will complain of nausea and vomiting or have an altered mental status and in extreme cases possibly pass out or seize. After a couple of hours, the fluids equilibrate, and the symptoms resolve themselves.

- **Hypokalemia or Hyperkalemia.** Patients on dialysis are given a list of foods that they should not eat because of their high potassium content. In between dialysis sessions, potassium will build up in the blood, possibly leading to hyperkalemia, which can be worsened by eating foods such as bananas and spinach. This can then be seen as peaked T waves on the ECG, and the patient may complain of chest pain, dizziness, or weakness. Hypokalemia can occur as a result of removing too much from the patient as indicated above.

- **Hypotension and Shock.** During or shortly after hemodialysis, the patient may suddenly become hypotensive, likely as a result of either drawing off too much fluid or the sudden alteration of blood electrolyte chemistry. Initiate cardiac monitoring and continue for the duration of contact, treating any dysrhythmias as it presents. Initiating a peripheral intravenous line in the patient often is difficult, so it should be attempted only if it is essential to give the patient fluids or medications and the shunt is not available for some reason. Paramedics can access the shunt if needed, but medical control should be contacted first for any reason other than cardiac arrest. Although electrolyte imbalances are the most likely reason for a sudden drop in blood pressure, rule out bleeding from the GI tract or the shunt as well.

Other Urinary Conditions

Kidney Stones

Kidney stones form when insoluble salts or uric acid precipitate out of solution in the renal pelvis and form large stones, sometimes filling the entire renal pelvis. These stones can be composed of various chemicals and most often are attributable to an insufficient intake of water. As long as the stone stays in the renal pelvis and does not move around, it generally is not a problem, unless it blocks urinary outflow, leading to ARF. Once the stone begins to move, it will quickly enter the ureter. Here, the diameter narrows considerably and the stone gets stuck. Urine then backs up behind it, forcing it further and further down the ureter, sometimes lacerating the ureter as it travels. This is where the excruciating pain originates. This pain will continue until the kidney stone is "passed" or removed from the body through the urethra.

Patients will complain of extreme pain on one flank. Tapping the back lightly in the area of the costovertebral angle with a closed fist will elicit a spike in pain as the kidney is briefly squeezed like a sponge, sending a surge of urine down the ureter, jarring the lodged stone. The patient will not be able to find a comfortable position and may vomit from the sheer amount of pain. Treatment with 0.1 mcg/kg fentanyl IV push would bring welcome relief to the patient with a kidney stone.

Urinary Tract Infections

Urinary tract infections (UTIs) are common infections throughout the life span. UTIs can be classified as either an upper UTI or a lower UTI. Upper UTIs can become a much more serious infection called **pyelonephritis**, which can lead to kidney failure and sepsis. Lower UTIs are typically isolated to the urethra and bladder. If left untreated, the infection can move up the one or both ureters and become an upper UTI.

A patient will be at heightened risk of UTI if there is an indwelling urinary catheter in place for the treatment of chronic urinary retention, incontinence, or being in a bed-ridden state. An indwelling catheter can harbor bacteria that can be delivered directly to the bladder if urine is permitted to backflow from the Foley bag or tubing and into the body. To prevent this, it is essential to keep the bag, and as much of the tubing as possible, at a height lower than the patient's pelvis.

Patients will complain of pain on urination and possibly an increase in frequency and urgency of urination. There also could be lower midline pelvic pain or discomfort in both men and women. Patients may note that the urine has a strong, foul odor. Depending on the degree to which the infection has progressed, the patient may not display any other physical symptoms. On the other hand, the patient may be in septic shock, where the skin will be either warm or cool to the touch, have dry skin, and have an altered mental status. Patients should be treated based on their level of consciousness. If the patient has altered mental status, check blood sugar level and treat if hypoglycemic, initiate an intravenous line and cardiac monitoring, give fluids at least at a KVO rate and consider a 200 mL fluid bolus.

Urinary Incontinence

Loss of voluntary control over urination is known as **incontinence**. There are three types of incontinence, the first two of which are clinically significant: urge incontinence, overflow incontinence, and stress incontinence. **Urge incontinence** is when the patient gets the urge to urinate, as all people do, but the patient is unable to hold it beyond a few seconds, resulting in involuntary urine loss. Urge incontinence can be a sign of UTI, Parkinson disease, Alzheimer disease, stroke, or neuropathies. **Overflow incontinence** is a continuous trickle of urine out the urethra. It is associated with diabetic neuropathy and prostate problems. **Stress incontinence** is a common condition where a person involuntarily allows some urine to dribble out when there is an increase in intra-abdominal pressure, such as during a cough, a sneeze, or hearty laughing.

Male Genitalia Conditions

The three conditions listed here are for your information and will seldom require anything more for the patient beyond courteous transport to the hospital. On certain occasions, analgesia would make you that man's favorite person on Earth.

- **Epididymitis and Orchitis.** Inflammation and swelling of the epididymis and testes, respectively. The patient will complain of pain in the groin that may worsen with bowel movements, and urine may have a foul odor. Transport respectfully and provide analgesia if necessary.
- **Testicular Torsion.** A testicle spontaneously spins on the spermatic cord, which effectively diminishes or cuts off its own blood supply. This is a genuine emergency because the testicle could be lost. Provide analgesia.

REVIEW QUESTIONS

Select the ONE best answer.

1. Which of the following is true of the kidney's role in blood pressure?

    A. Produces renin.

    B. Releases aldosterone.

    C. Controls acid–base levels.

    D. Converts angiotensin I to angiotensin II.

2. All of the following are prerenal causes of ARF EXCEPT:

    A. Sepsis.

    B. Dehydration.

    C. Heavy metal toxicity.

    D. Hemorrhage/trauma.

3. About an hour into her dialysis, a 79-year-old female becomes confused and has a brief seizure. The dialysis technician reports normal blood pressure and heart rate readings throughout treatment. The most likely cause for this seizure is:

   A. An air embolism.

   B. Disequilibrium syndrome.

   C. Hypokalemia.

   D. Hyponatremia.

ANSWERS AND EXPLANATIONS

1. **The correct answer is (A).** When the blood pressure in the glomerulus drops, the juxtaglomerular cells in the capsule release renin. Renin causes angiotensinogen to be cleaved into angiotensin I. Angiotensin converting enzyme I converts angiotensin I into angiotensin II (D) in the lungs. Angiotensin II then stimulates the adrenal gland to release aldosterone (B). Although the kidney does play a role in maintaining acid–base levels (C), this does not play a particular role in controlling blood pressure.

2. **The correct answer is (C).** Heavy metal toxicity is considered an intrarenal cause of acute renal failure. Anything that can prevent blood from flowing into the glomerulus would be a prerenal cause of ARF. All other answers are prerenal causes of ARF.

3. **The correct answer is (B).** This is the most likely reason for a change in mental status during or shortly after dialysis. If salts are taken off suddenly, this can result in an internal fluid shift into the CSF via osmosis, which could potentially lead to all the same symptoms seen with increases in ICP. Hyponatremia (D) is not likely to be significant enough at any time to cause seizures. Hypokalemia (C) does not usually lead to seizures. An air embolism (A) may cause the patient to have chest pain or difficulty breathing but is not likely to cause a neurological problems.

HEMATOLOGICAL EMERGENCIES

Hematological emergencies fall into 2 categories: hemolytic disorders and hemostatic disorders.

- In **hemolytic disorders**, blood cells break down or fail to function properly, and transport of O_2 is impaired.

- **Hemostatic disorders** refer to any problem related to abnormal clotting, which could mean both prolonged bleeding and clots forming in places they are not needed.

This section discusses the physiology of the blood and the clotting cascade. It will focus on problems related to the red blood cells and clotting; issues of the white blood cells and the immune system were covered in the section on immunological emergencies. Continuous movement of blood throughout the body is essential to the health of the body.

What does blood do?

- Transports O_2 from the lungs to all tissues.
- Carries nutrients dissolved in the plasma for use in cells.
- Carries wastes such as CO_2 and urea away from cells to the lungs and kidneys, respectively, for excretion.
- Contains defense mechanisms including antibodies and white blood cells.
- Carries hormones from the endocrine gland in which they are produced to their target organs.

Anatomy and Physiology

Blood is composed of primarily two components: the plasma and the formed elements. The plasma is the watery fluid in which the formed elements are carried and makes up about 55% of the circulating volume. The plasma contains dissolved O_2, CO_2, proteins, hormones, glucose, and electrolytes. The formed elements and information about each follows.

- **Red Blood Cells.** These cells make up about 44% of the circulating volume. They do not contain a nucleus (except in mononucleosis), so they have as much room as possible inside to carry as much hemoglobin as possible. Hemoglobin is the O_2-carrying molecule, all of which is found within red blood cells. The **hematocrit** is the term given to the proportion of the circulating red blood cells in the blood. Hematocrit should be roughly 3 times the value of the hemoglobin number.
  - Normal Hemoglobin: Women: 12–16; Men: 14–18
  - Normal Hematocrit: Women: 35–45; Men: 40–50
- **White Blood Cells.** Larger than red blood cells, white blood cells make up approximately 1% of the circulating volume overall. They are responsible for the immunity of the body to foreign invaders of all kinds. See the immunological emergencies section earlier in this chapter for more information.
- **Platelets.** Also called **thrombocytes**, they are integral in clot formation.

ABO Classification System and Rh factor

The red blood cells have on the exterior surface of the plasma membrane markers called **antigens**. Antigens cause antibodies to be formed. Here is a way to remember that: ANTIGENS are ANTIbody GENerating. These antigens can have the designation A or B. The cells can have any combination of antigen on their surface. People who have only A antigens are said to have the A blood type; people who have only B antigens have the B blood type; people who have both A and B antigens have the AB blood type; and, finally, people who have neither A nor B antigens on their blood cells have the O blood type.

For those with type A blood, the antibodies are anti-B, which means that if the patient's blood comes in contact with type B blood, antibodies will attack it like a foreign invader. People with type AB blood do not have antibodies to either anti-A or anti-B blood, so they can receive any blood type from a donor. People with type O blood can donate to any other blood type because there are no antigens on the surfaces of their red blood cells for the antibodies of the recipients to attack.

Table 6-12. Blood Types and Donors

Blood Type	Surface Antigen	ABO Antibody	Donor Blood Type Accepted
A	A	Anti-B	A and O
B	B	Anti-A	B and O
AB	A and B	None	A, B, AB, and O
O	None	Anti-A and Anti-B	O

Blood also may contain a second antigen called the **Rh factor**. This antigen is located on the surface of the red blood cells. People either have the antigen Rh positive (Rh+) or Rh negative (Rh−). The Rh designation is needed as well to ensure full compatibility of the blood donor with the recipient. Here, the Rh− person can donate to either Rh+ or Rh−; however, an Rh+ person can donate only to other Rh+ people.

Determining the Rh factor is of particular importance in pregnant women and the unborn fetus to prevent hemolytic disease of the newborn. If an RH− mother has an Rh+ fetus, the mother's body may develop antibodies to the Rh+ blood. If at any time the baby's blood comes in contact with the mother's blood during gestation, the mother will get sensitized to the Rh+ blood and produce antibodies against it. Those antibodies can cross the placental barrier and attack the baby's red blood cells as a foreign invader. The baby's red blood cells would be lysed or broken down, resulting in hemolytic disease, also called **hemolytic anemia**. This results in an inability to transport O_2 in the infant, leading to illness, brain damage, or death of the fetus.

Hemostasis

Hemostasis is a highly complex process of stopping bleeding anywhere in the body. The first step in this process is localized **vasoconstriction**, which clamps off a large amount of the blood flow heading to that area. The 2nd step is the action of platelets plugging the hole. The blood is exposed to collagen fibers surrounding the vessel. When platelets come in contact with the collagen, they become activated. Activated platelets become sticky and release other chemicals that begin aggregation of more platelets at the site of the injury. Finally, about a dozen different clotting factors arrive at the area of injury to further seal off the wound. There are two pathways: the intrinsic pathway initiated by damage to the vessel itself, and the extrinsic pathway activated when blood comes in contact with tissues outside the lumen of the vessel.

Coagulopathies are any of a variety of problems that interfere with the body's ability to form a clot. They can lead to heavy or prolonged bleeding, even from a wound that should not otherwise be life threatening.

Hemolytic Emergencies

Sickle Cell Crisis

Sickle cell disease is an inherited disorder that affects the shape of red blood cells. The mutation is on the gene that codes for adult-type hemoglobin, designated HbA. The disease has to be inherited from both parents to exhibit symptoms of the disease; therefore, both parents must have at least one copy of the gene (be a carrier but not express symptoms of the disease) to pass it on. In this disease, the malformed hemoglobin causes the cells to change shape from a smooth biconcave disk to a curved shape resembling a gardener's sickle. These cells are no longer capable of transporting O_2, and their shape now causes them to get stuck trying to transit the smallest capillaries, leading to a clot in the area. If enough capillaries in that area get clogged with sickled cells and clots form, necrosis and tissue death could begin in that area.

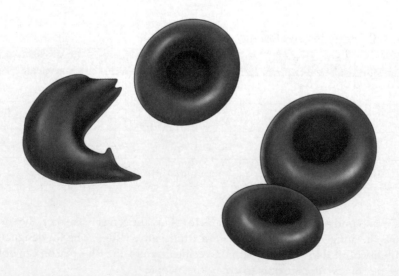

Figure 6-27. Sickle-Shaped and Normal Red Blood Cells

Sickle cell crisis can occur in any of a variety of ways:

- **Aplastic Crisis.** Suspension of the production of red blood cells leads to the patient becoming weak, pale, and short of breath.
- **Hemolytic Crisis.** Excessive red blood cell destruction in the liver leads to an overproduction of bilirubin, which is characterized by a jaundice in a patient.
- **Vaso-occlusive Crisis.** This most common complication of sickle cell disease, it occurs when capillaries clot off and tissue starts to become ischemic. This presents as often intractable pain in the area of the clotted capillaries, which typically lasts about a week.
- **Splenic Sequestration Crisis.** Red blood cells get trapped in the spleen, which results in painful enlargement of the spleen. The organ can swell to the point it ruptures. Patients present with a sudden onset of LUQ pain, weakness, pallor, tachycardia, and shortness of breath with tachypnea.
- **Acute Chest Syndrome.** This is a specific type of vaso-occlusive crisis associated with pneumonia. In addition to shortness of breath and a productive cough from pneumonia, the patient also may have severe chest pain.

Patients in sickle cell crisis often are in serious condition. The patient may be in severe systemic pain from areas being clotted off now getting hypoxic. The patient may be short of breath from pneumonia, systemic hypoxia, or clots forming in the lungs or any combination of all 3. Patients also will complain of pain in the joints.

It is important for these patients to administer high-flow O_2 to help prevent further destruction of red blood cells. In this case, the SpO_2 reading is not helpful because it is impossible to know how many normal-shaped red blood cells the patient has. Have the patient remain as comfortable as possible while initiating an intravenous line and running fluids to help flush out the sickled cells and prevent further dehydration. Keep the patient warm because that may help prevent further sickling of the cells, whereas cold can accelerate it. Provide analgesia as needed, beginning with 0.1 mcg/kg fentanyl. Patients may have built-in tolerance to pain medications, so doses may need to be repeated.

Anemia

Anemia is a deficiency in red blood cells or hemoglobin. **Iron deficiency anemia** is the most common and is most frequently associated with some other disease process. It can be from slow, long-term blood loss, a decrease in overall production of cells, or an increase in red blood cell recycling in the liver or spleen. Red blood cells also can be destroyed in an autoimmune disorder.

Patients with anemia will complain of feeling weak, tired, and possibly short of breath, especially with even minimal exertion. They may appear pale in color. Patients also may have chest pain, depending on the few red blood cells they have and the ongoing myocardial O_2 demand. Treat these patients with high-flow O_2, and if it is not possible to completely rule out ACS concurrently with the anemia, treat the patient as you would for an ischemic cardiac event. Closely monitor the vital signs and ECG throughout transport and treat other symptoms as they arise.

Polycythemia

Polycythemia is a condition where the patient has an excess of red blood cells. The overproduction could be caused by external conditions of hypoxia, such as what might happen at high altitudes. Internal conditions of hypoxia, such as in COPD, also could lead to an increased production of red blood cells. Another possible reason is that the patient is overproducing or is "doping" with erythropoietin (EPO)—the hormone produced in the kidneys that tells the bone marrow to make more red blood cells—to gain a competitive advantage, particularly in endurance sports. The overall result is a thickening of the blood. Because of the thicker blood, several problems can develop. The patient becomes more prone to abnormal clotting, which puts them at risk for strokes, MI, and DVT, and PE.

Essentially, the patient the paramedic will treat is not the one who complains of polycythemia, but rather the CVA or MI. There is no prehospital treatment directly targeting the condition, so proper treatment of the patient's other symptoms, such as chest pain and headache, would be most appropriate for the patient. Short of having red blood cell count paperwork along with the patient, which may be available at a skilled nursing facility, no particular symptom would indicate that a patient has this condition.

Disseminated Intravascular Coagulopathy

Disseminated intravascular coagulopathy (DIC) is a life-threatening event that involves systemic activation of the clotting cascade in all areas of the body, not just those with blood vessel damage. It does not typically occur as its own distinct condition but rather is a complicating factor of other disease processes. DIC may occur as a result of massive trauma accompanied by massive blood loss, severe late stage sepsis, and obstetrical hemorrhage. In the first stage of the condition, fibrin and thrombin in the blood cause platelets to begin to get sticky and form clots throughout the body. Now that some, if not all, of the body's thrombin and fibrin have been used up in what amounts to pointless clots, severe, uncontrollable hemorrhage worsens because of the lack of clotting factors.

Treatment for these patients begins with aggressive fluid therapy and rapid transport to the most appropriate medical facility, in many cases, a trauma center. Early administration of O_2 and treatment for shock is essential in these patients. Monitor the ECG and treat any dysrhythmias.

Bleeding in Hemophilia

Hemophilia is a genetic disorder that results in poor or no clotting. It is far more common in men than in women because it is X-linked. Any bleeding in a hemophiliac should be treated as severe until proven otherwise because even small lacerations or abrasions can bleed them into a life-threatening situation. Falls and other accidents can be catastrophic for a person with hemophilia. Spontaneous intracranial hemorrhage is a relatively common problem and often leads to death.

Assessment of the hemophiliac is related to the symptoms found and centers on working to control bleeding. Bleeding will not likely stop until a hemostatic agent is introduced or the patient receives clotting factors at the hospital, so the paramedic should be dedicated to the manual control of external hemorrhage. Missing an intravenous line on these patients could mean that a crew member is dedicated to holding pressure on the failed intravenous site, so use every precaution before attempting a line. Even an intramuscular or subcutaneous injection can have unintended consequences of bleeding. Treatment is otherwise symptomatic.

REVIEW QUESTIONS

Select the ONE best answer.

1. A blood test reveals that a patient has anti-A antibodies. Which type(s) of blood can the patient receive when a transfusion is needed?

    A. A only

    B. B only

    C. A and O

    D. B and O

2. You are at the home of a 9-year-old male patient who has a known history of sickle cell disease. The patient is complaining of a several day history of increasing pain in the LUQ and diffuse rebound tenderness. The patient is weak and pale. The parents had been trying to control the pain with tramadol at home, but it is not working. What is the most likely cause of this patient's pain?

    A. Aplastic crisis

    B. Hemolytic crisis

    C. Splenic sequestration crisis

    D. Vaso-occlusive crisis

3. The patient in the previous question has the following vital signs: HR: 128, BP: 108/60; RR: 28; SpO_2: 99%; $EtCO_2$: 32 mmHg. What is the most appropriate treatment for the patient?

    A. 1 mcg/kg fentanyl

    B. 500 mL crystalloid

    C. 2–4 mg morphine

    D. 325 mg chewable baby aspirin

ANSWERS AND EXPLANATIONS

1. **The correct answer is (D).** If this patient has anti-A antibodies, it means that this person has type B blood. Persons with type B blood can receive their own type—in this case B—and type O blood. If this patient received type A blood, the patient's anti-A antibodies would attack those cells as foreign and cause widespread hemolysis.

2. **The correct answer is (C).** The LUQ pain suggests that the spleen is the site of the coagulation, which could lead to swelling of the spleen and increasing pain. Splenic rupture is possible and is suggested by the rebound tenderness resulting from irritation of the peritoneum from internal hemorrhage. Aplastic crisis (A) occurs when the body is no longer manufacturing red blood cells, resulting in anemia. Hemolytic crisis (B) is more likely to present with symptoms of liver failure, particularly jaundice, because of the overdestruction of red blood cells in the liver. Vaso-occlusive crisis (D) is a term for any vessel occlusion anywhere in the body; however, this generally refers to any capillary in the body.

3. **The correct answer is (A).** Management of the pain in a person with sickle cell crisis should be the first priority for the paramedic. Online medical direction also is recommended for pain control in these patients because they may require much higher amounts than anticipated. Fluid (B) should be considered but not as a primary treatment. Fentanyl is preferred to morphine (C). Aspirin (D) is never recommended in any patient under the age of 20 because of the risk of Reye syndrome, despite this being a coagulopathy problem.

PSYCHIATRIC EMERGENCIES

Behavioral and psychiatric emergencies can be some of the most difficult calls a paramedic will need to handle. These are emergencies where the behavior of the patient interferes with activities of daily living (ADLs) primarily caused by depression or anxieties. Psychiatric emergencies exist when the abnormal behavior threatens a person's safety, whether that person is the patient or someone else. Ultimately, however, the person calling for the ambulance has determined that this situation is beyond their ability to handle and has become an emergency. Now the paramedic will enter an already escalated situation that must be sorted out and handled safely for everyone on the scene. Skills with psychiatric emergencies are arguably more important than any of the other skills discussed thus far in the paramedic training because they can be the difference between calming the patient down and maintaining a safe, secure scene and having the scene escalate out of control and becoming increasingly dangerous and possibly putting the crew, patient, and bystanders at unnecessary risk.

This section first discusses the pathophysiologies and presentations of abnormal behavior and specific behavioral emergencies. Toward the end of the section, global assessment guidelines will be discussed for psychiatric patients, including communication techniques and crisis intervention skills. Medicolegal considerations for the psychiatric patient also will be discussed here. Finally, the section rounds out with a discussion on chemical and physical restraints for patients.

Pathophysiology and Presentations of Abnormal Behavior and Psychiatric Illnesses

Most of the psychiatric illnesses or diagnoses that follow have their causes rooted in one of the following four broad categories.

- **Neurologic Disease.** This category involves destruction or alteration of the brain tissue itself. This can include atrophy, chronic hypoxia, dementias, seizures, and tumors. These conditions cause a derangement of normal functioning of the brain and cause the patient to display abnormal behaviors. These conditions can lead to suicide, agitation, anger and rage issues, or alterations in perception, depending on the area of the brain affected.

- **Personal Experiences.** The life the person has led can directly influence their behavior. For a child growing up in a home where verbal or physical abuse was accepted or tolerated, for example, it can lead that child to display the same kind of behavior in adulthood; it was normal for them. Experiencing extensive bullying throughout childhood can lead a person to be withdrawn or take inappropriate action in other nonthreatening social situations. This can then lead to depression because the feeling of not being accepted becomes overwhelming. Posttraumatic stress disorder can fall into this category; generally, no physical brain injury occurs to lead to this diagnosis, but repeated emotional experiences typically do.

- **Injuries and Illnesses.** Minor repeated head injuries over time, or a single large traumatic brain injury, can permanently alter the brain's ability to carry out everyday functions. This can lead to inappropriate behaviors, violent outbursts, and even suicidal ideations. Illnesses and infections also can change the brain's functioning. Syphilis, Creutzfeldt-Jakob disease, bovine spongiform encephalopathy, and multiple sclerosis are examples of diseases that alter brain function over time, resulting in abnormal behavior.

- **Toxicities.** Patients can display psychoses when they are under the influence of street drugs, alcohol, or medications. As seen in the toxicology section, the long-term effects of alcoholism can resemble psychiatric problems because destruction of brain tissue.

Acute Psychosis

Acute psychosis is characterized by a person being out of touch with reality in such a way that the person has their own internal, personal reality. The interaction of the common reality and the personal reality of a psychotic episode can either make the patient act out toward others in a violent or combative way or act withdrawn and possibly mute. Any of the reasons listed above can contribute to the onset of a psychotic episode. Patients present with disorganized thought and disorientation to any person, place, or time; however, these can be symptoms of any of a variety of ailments, not just the patient with psychosis.

A thorough assessment, particularly the part of the assessment that involves evaluation of the history of present illness and interrogation, is usually very difficult to obtain because of the disorganized thought patterns in a patient experiencing psychosis. The COASTMAP mnemonic is helpful to assess patients with any level of mental disorder, particularly psychosis.

- **Consciousness.** The patient is usually awake and alert but easily distracted. The patient may be struggling to focus on the paramedic (reality) and concurrent hallucinations (personal reality).

- **Orientation.** Severely psychotic patients often are only oriented to person and often will lose place and time into their own personal reality.

- **Activity.** Activity can be accelerated, haphazard, bizarre, or violent as in agitated delirium, or slowed to nonexistent as in hypoactive delirium.

- **Speech.** Speech can be slurred, garbled, or completely unintelligible. The patient also may use words, speech, or sounds they invented.

- **Thoughts.** Disturbed in progression and concentration. The person may have rapid bouncing from one thought to another. For the person with the psychosis, the connection between one thought and another is completely logical, but for the listener, there may not be any obvious connection. The person could show thought broadcasting, thought insertion, or thought withdrawal. **Thought broadcasting** is where the person thinks that their thoughts can be heard by others, **thought insertion** is the belief that the person is being programmed by another person or another's thoughts, and **thought withdrawal** is that the person's thoughts are being actively taken away.

- **Memory.** May be completely or partially intact.
- **Affect.** Patients can be euphoric, flat, or sad or have swings in between any of these presentations.
- **Perception.** Patients hear voices most often commenting on their behavior or directing them to do something. Sidebar conversation is a common observation with psychotic patients.

Delirium

Delirium differs from dementia in that dementia is a chronic, often irreversible problem. Delirium, on the other hand, tends to be acute; reversible; and tied to substance abuse, infection, or nutrient or electrolyte imbalance. Delirium can be agitated (sometimes referred to as hyperactive) or hypoactive in nature. The delirium is said to be agitated whenever the patient is active; this can be violent or combative actions, seizures, or simply walking around but unaware of surroundings. Some causes for this type of delirium include hypoxia, hypoglycemia, hallucinations, brain injuries, and often stimulant drug overdoses. Hypoactive delirium is generally an acute onset of altered mental status accompanied by a decrease in activity. Some conditions where hypoactive delirium may be seen include hyperglycemia, fever or hyperthermia, sedative or opiate overdoses, and hypothermia.

Suicidal Ideation

Suicide is the taking of one's own life. Below is a list of factors that, if present, particularly if more than one is present, increases a person's risk for attempting suicide. Patients contemplating suicide will develop a plan; if a patient ever communicates a clear plan, an attempt is nearly certain to happen. Evaluate every patient who complains of depression for suicidal ideation. Although it may seem like a bad idea to bring up suicide to the patient who is depressed, rest assured that the person most likely has already contemplated it, if not actually made an attempt at it; asking the person about it will give the person an opportunity to open up and possibly face the problems that are leading them down this pathway in the first place. When in the presence of these patients, remember to carefully evaluate the scene and continually be aware of the surroundings; if the person is willing to take their own life, there is often little hesitation in taking someone else along with them.

The risk factors for suicide are as follows:

- Depression
- Males >45 years old
- White
- Single, divorced, or widowed
- Recent significant loss—loved one, job, ending of marriage
- Chronic illness
- Alcohol or drug abuse
- Achievable plan
- Family history
- Previous unsuccessful attempts

Specific Psychiatric Diagnoses

This section will discuss the diagnoses a patient may have in their medical history that may impact the paramedic's patient assessment.

Mood Disorders

Everyone has had their moments of extreme elation and joy accompanied by long bouts of sadness. But the person is not said to be manic or depressed, respectively, during these times. When it comes to mood disorders, people experience sadness with depression, for example, but they also have other symptoms accompanying the sadness or the elation, which together impact the person's ability to function in society. Mood disorders can be unipolar, such as major depression or mania, or bipolar, where patients bounce back and forth between clinically significant mania and depression.

Manic Behaviors

Mania is characterized by extreme joy or exaggerated happiness, which sounds like a great way to be except that it often is accompanied with hyperactivity and insomnia. These patients often are hyperactive to the point of not being able to concentrate, so they become easily distracted. They display nonlinear or tangential thinking, where thoughts and speech jump wildly from one topic to another, likely without a discernible connection.

For these patients, it is not always wonderful. They can get into trouble by becoming promiscuous, spending wildly, and often picking fights with people who question them or try to pull them down. This behavior is typically so boisterous and over the top that an ambulance is called at that time. The patient likely will not think anything is wrong, so you will need to talk to the person removed from any other distractions while avoiding a power struggle or being confrontational. If the patient will not agree to go, medical control can be contacted to see if the patient can be taken against their will because the patient is still usually well oriented to person, place, and time. No major treatment needs to be considered at this time.

Major Depression

Depression is far more common than mania and is a cause of disability in a broad swath of the population. Depression can sometimes be linked to one adverse event, or a couple of negative events in the patient's life that happened in close succession; however, most clinically diagnosed depression is without identifiable cause. Symptoms of depression can be summarized with the mnemonic DEPRESSED:

- **Disinterest.** The patient loses interest in things that once were important to them. This can include favorite sports teams or sex.
- **Energy.** The patient is listless and tired. This is closely related to disinterest.
- **Psychomotor Abnormalities.** The person who is depressed will often move slowly overall but also may at the same time engage in compulsive behaviors such as hand wringing or pacing.
- **Regret.** This can often manifest as guilt, feelings of worthlessness, or as a failure in some aspect of their life.
- **Eating.** The depressed person can go either way on this one. Some will eat all the time, almost as a compulsion, whereas others completely lose their appetite.
- **Sleep.** Another symptom that can go either way. Most often, the person who is depressed will report insomnia, but a minority may report sleeping far more than usual. In some cases, sleeping excessively contributes to the development of depression and vice versa.
- **Suicidal Thoughts.** Depressed patients often will report some degree of suicidal ideation of varying degree. Some will say that it only crossed their mind, whereas others have developed and begun to execute a plan.
- **Escapes Reality.** People who are depressed often go to great lengths to be alone, which only further contributes to their depression by reinforcing the idea that they are isolated.
- **Distracted.** Patients with depression often are not able to concentrate for extended periods on any topic or activity.

Bipolar Disorder

Patients diagnosed with **bipolar disorder** often swing from one extreme to the other: manic for a period of time then back to normal for a period of time, then either back to manic or over to depression. Although there are some medications for this, triggers for each are not well understood. As a paramedic, understanding what this may mean for the overall treatment of the patient can help. Patients will not typically swing from one extreme to the other in the short period of time they are with the paramedics.

Neuroses

Neurotic disorders are a group of disorders characterized by excessive reactions to fear and apprehension. Anxiety or stress can help the average person through difficult situations or issues with unknown outcomes. Writing this book gave the author anxiety about finishing on time, but it did not prevent the author from working or living.

People with neurotic disorders are completely unable to face fears and panic easily. Neurotic disorders include generalized anxiety disorder, panic disorder, and phobias.

In **generalized anxiety disorder**, the patient has anxiety or intense worry that is difficult to control and impacts day-to-day life. The patient finds it difficult to turn off the level of worry, resulting in an inability to make a decision because each possible result brings with it separate anxieties. For these patients, the best thing the paramedic can do for them is to approach them in a calm, reassuring, and confident manner. Seeing another person in control of the situation and receiving constant assurance that the outcome will be favorable will help temper the patient's fears.

Phobias are fears that prevent people from behaving in a predictable fashion when encountered with the source of their phobia. Typically, the patient has a phobia of a particular object or situation, and the phobia tends to be isolated and not transmitted to other situations. As long as the patient does not encounter the phobia during interaction with the paramedics, the duration of contact should be appropriate. The ambulance, however, can be enough of an enclosed space for claustrophobics (those with a fear of enclosed spaces) to have an exacerbation of fear and anxiety. They may be able to be coached into accepting the space they are in by being told to look out the windows or to close their eyes and imagine an open field. They also may need a small dose of an anxiolytic, such as lorazepam, to make it through the trip.

Panic disorders are the ultimate form of anxiety-related issue. Panic attacks can come on out of the blue and prevent a person from performing ADLs; in extreme cases, it can prevent the patient from even leaving their home or another place of security because of an intense fear of the unknown. The signs and symptoms of a panic attack are rooted in sympathetic nervous system effects, which makes sense because the patient is preparing themselves for flight, though usually in a situation that would not be threatening to a person who does not suffer from panic attacks. The signs and symptoms include sweating, nausea (sometimes with vomiting, though less common), palpitations, chest pain, dizziness, weakness, shortness of breath and/or tachypnea, shakiness, and tension. When treating a patient having a panic attack, provide them with a quiet, stress-free environment where the patient and paramedic can talk quietly and calmly. Use the word *safe* often; frequently this is the most important thing a person with a panic attack needs to know. The patient may need to hear it over and over again during the transport, but this will help the patient gain control without needing pharmacologic intervention.

Eating Disorders

The two major types of eating disorders are bulimia nervosa and anorexia nervosa. Both disorders are largely seen in women, particularly of affluent communities where stereotypes of perfection are rewarded and need to be maintained. The woman does everything she can to achieve the thin appearance that is perceived and often competed for in such places.

Bulimia nervosa is a condition where the person eats as much as possible, often in a short amount of time. The consumption is seldom of a particularly nutritive variety—usually junk food. The patient will then purge their system, most often intentionally vomiting the entire contents back up within a relatively short period of time after eating. Some bulimics will use excessive amounts of laxatives or diuretics to help the purge.

Anorexia nervosa is characterized by a patient who eats extremely low quantities of food because of an intense fear of becoming overweight or an intense belief of already being overweight. Career anorexics appear emaciated and have a body weight well below average for their age. They consume so few calories and often do not take vitamin supplements, so their health is compromised. They often can have weaker, thinner bones than others because of the lack of calcium in their diets. Women also experience amenorrhea (no menstrual periods).

Other Disorders

Somatoform and Factitious Disorders

In **somatoform disorders**, the patient is so convinced of being sick that even a physician cannot convince the person otherwise after running every test possible. Hypochondriacs fall into this category because they have an intense anxiety that they have a serious disease. Here, anxiety is the root of the problem, even though the person is concerned with the symptoms. In **somatization disorder**, another variety of somatoform disorders, the patient will offer multiple complaints but is concerned with meaning to their health. Finally, in patients with **conversion disorder**, the patient actually manifests a physical problem that has no other identifiable cause beyond the patient extensively believing it is happening.

Factitious disorder, also called **Munchausen syndrome**, is a condition where a person fakes actual symptoms, including physical signs of a problem. Although there is no physiologic reason for the symptoms, the patient is actually in control over the symptoms being displayed. The patient does this typically to try to get out of trouble with the law or get attention from people around them. There also is Munchausen syndrome by proxy, where a parent intentionally makes a child sick to gain attention. After a child is born, the attention bestowed on the mother subsides, and the child now garners the attention directly. The mother, essentially jealous, makes the child sick so that people can pity her and her situation.

Impulse control disorders are a family of disorders where the patient compulsively behaves in a generally unacceptable way where the patient cannot keep themselves from acting on an impulse. These include intermittent explosive disorder, kleptomania, pyromania, and pathologic gambling.

Assessment of the Psychiatric Patient

Assessment of the psychiatric patient during a behavioral emergency can test even the most skillful of paramedics because the assessment of this type of patient involves strong communication skills and getting the patient to open up to what is bothering them. It also can be a challenge to gain permission to treat the patient or take the patient to the hospital. Throughout the assessment, do not forget to be alert to clues of other problems that may be present that could be of serious consequence to your patient, such as shortness of breath, chest pain, or altered mentation beyond what caregivers identify as baseline for the patient based on their psychiatric history. This section will focus on communication techniques to use to not only assess the patient but also deescalate potentially explosive scenes or combative patients.

Psychiatric patients can present in a wide variety of ways. With that in mind, there can be a higher degree of unpredictability in their behavior, so it is worth taking some time to set ground rules for the patient's behavior. This will help everyone be on the same page about what is and is not acceptable; it also helps the paramedic assert who is in charge in a friendlier manner. Once ground rules have been established, begin the assessment as for any other patient with open-ended, free response questions. The questions should be geared to allow the patient to tell the story in their own way and at their own pace. The patient then can begin to gain control over the situation while still providing valuable information. Open-ended questions also do not hint at possible answers that the patient can then select from.

Communication

Make the patient and their story the overall priority by demonstrating active listening skills. This can be accomplished by summarizing what the patient has already relayed while avoiding injecting personal feelings, biases, or judgment. The paramedic should be positioned to be able to look at the patient and so that the patient can see the paramedic; this can help decrease the patient's anxiety and discomfort. Acknowledge the patient's feelings displayed and help the patient express their feelings in a controlled and appropriate manner. Facilitation of further communication can be accomplished with simple phrases such as "I see," or "go on," and asking more nonleading questions such as "How did that make you feel?" or "What did you do then?"

The patient may stop and start the conversation, and silence on the part of the patient is not necessarily something that needs to be avoided or broken. Sometimes, the paramedic may be able to restart the conversation by commenting on something that was said earlier of particular concern or interest. If the conversation needs to be continued, try to accomplish that without sounding intrusive, nagging, or judgmental. The patient may say some things with which the paramedic does not agree or are simply untrue. These may be the result of the altered reality the patient is facing and should not be contradicted or argued; that said, the patient should not necessarily be substantiated or played into either. For example, perhaps there is an intravenous bag hanging from the ceiling of the ambulance, and the patient remarks about the bag, "It looks like that big condor is going to swoop down and kill us!" It may be tempting, in an effort not to play into the patient's delusions, to simply say, "That's just an intravenous bag. It's not a condor!" This can spark an argument and escalate the situation. Perhaps it would be better to say, "I can see how that might look like a large bird, but it is an intravenous bag. Let me take it down and put it away so it cannot hurt us." This legitimizes what the patient may, in fact, be seeing, provides them with real context to help establish common reality, and minimizes the patient's fear overall.

Restraints

Many patients will go to the hospital willingly, cooperating the whole time whether they request to be carried on the stretcher or walk to the ambulance themselves. A small number of patients present a problem for the responders. Patients who need to go to the hospital for a psychiatric evaluation and become combative with the paramedics may need to be restrained for transport. Restraint should be performed only if the patient poses an immediate risk of harm to himself, herself, or others, not simply as a matter of course for the routine treatment of psychiatric patients. The minimum amount of force should be employed to restrain the patient.

Ensure that you have enough staff to accomplish the task at hand. There should be one person for each limb at a minimum. The mere presence of that many people may be enough to have the patient acquiesce; other times it just hypes the person up even more. Law enforcement personnel should be involved in restraining a patient because they have had special training in this that EMS does not typically receive. Ensure that the patient cannot get a hold of any weapons, either on your person or in the area where the restraint application will take place. This includes the police officer's sidearm; whenever possible, ensure that it is not accessible by the patient. When the team is ready to approach the patient, there should be at least one restraint for each extremity ready to be applied within reach of the patient.

Secure the patient in the supine position *only*. Patients have died in the hands of EMS when they have been secured to the stretcher in the prone position, hog-tied, or hobble tied (ankles tied together). Tie each leg and each wrist independently to the stretcher. Always use 4-point restraints in the prehospital environment. Once the restraints are secure, leave them tied until it comes time to move the patient at the hospital. During the act of restraining the patient, be aware of the behavior of the patient to prevent any attempt to bite you or a team member. If the patient is spitting, place a surgical mask over their mouth or sometimes, more appropriately, an O_2 mask with O_2 flowing.

Once the patient is restrained, continually monitor the patient's status, especially the ABCs. The patient will not be able to move well if vomiting occurs, so always be prepared to suction the airway if needed. Recheck the restraints to make sure that they are tight enough to maintain restraint but not so tight that they are serving as a venous or, worse, an arterial tourniquet. Generally, the dorsalis pedis pulse and the radial pulse will be accessible to check.

Patients also may be restrained chemically in lieu of or in addition to the physical restraint method above. Employing a chemical restraint should be used only on the order of the medical control physician. Haloperidol is frequently used in patients older than 14 years old who are not known or suspected to be pregnant, but it comes with an increased possibility of side effects compared with benzodiazepines. The most common drugs used for chemical restraint include short-acting benzodiazepines, preferably lorazepam or midazolam, although diazepam is used whenever a patient may need to be sedated for a longer period of time.

Lorazepam can be administered 1–2 mg intramuscularly or intravenously, but in a patient who is combative, the intramuscular route is preferred for the initial route of administration. Midazolam also can be administered intramuscularly or intranasally at 0.2 mg/kg up to 10 mg total. Once adequately sedated, the patient can have an intravenous line established, and sedatives can be administered via the intravenous line. After a benzodiazepine is given to a patient, continuously monitor the patient for respiratory depression or compromise and be prepared to assist with ventilations.

Some patients having a psychiatric or medical emergency may need exceedingly high doses of a benzodiazepine to achieve sedation. **Serotonin syndrome** and **neuroleptic malignant syndrome** can each present as extremely violent patients requiring doses of benzodiazepines in excess of 5 times the normal dose to even begin to sedate the patient.

REVIEW QUESTIONS

Select the ONE best answer.

1. A 58-year-old female with a history of substance abuse has threatened to kill herself and actively attempted to do so. Police have restrained her in handcuffs, and she is refusing care. She is conscious, alert, and oriented, and there is no evidence of intoxication or recent substance abuse. Her husband on scene has agreed to sign involuntary commitment papers. Can she be allowed to refuse?

    A. No, because she needed to be placed in handcuffs to be controlled.

    B. No, because a witness to the behavior offered to sign an involuntary psychiatric commitment.

    C. Yes, because she is alert and oriented and therefore capable of making her own decisions.

    D. Yes, because she has not admitted to, nor is there evidence of, recent substance abuse or intoxication.

2. A person who swings from mania to depression most likely suffers from which of the following disorders?

    A. Bipolar disorder

    B. Generalized anxiety disorder

    C. Panic disorder

    D. Schizophrenia

3. Which of the following is NOT required before deciding to restrain someone against their will?

    A. Perception that the patient poses a threat to themselves

    B. Perception that the patient poses a threat to crew or others

    C. Recent substance abuse or intoxication

    D. Sufficient resources to control patient

ANSWERS AND EXPLANATIONS

1. **The correct answer is (B).** As long as a person has a reason to involuntarily commit a person for psychiatric treatment, in this case suicidal ideation, the patient may be restrained. The patient must then actually be committed to the psychiatric facility. Ideally, police witness the behavior. In this case, because the threat was made, sobriety (D) and degree of orientation (C) are not sufficient to allow a person to refuse care.

2. **The correct answer is (A).** Bipolar disorder is characterized by a person who can display unpredictable manic behavior at one time and at other times symptoms consistent with severe depression. Generalized anxiety disorder (B) and panic disorder (C) are both neuroses. Neither cause a person to swing between depression and mania; however, both can prevent a person from participating in ADLs. Schizophrenia (D) is a condition where a patient is unable to differentiate between what is real and what is not.

3. **The correct answer is (C).** Recent substance abuse or intoxication is not, by itself, a reason to restrain a patient. The patient needs to pose a threat to themselves (A) or others (B) to be restrained against the person's will for their own protection and that of the crew and bystanders. To do this successfully, sufficient resources should be present to adequately and safely control the patient's extremities and torso (D).

ENVIRONMENTAL EMERGENCIES

Environmental emergencies encompass all issues that people can encounter as a result of the environment they are in. This includes heat- and cold-related emergencies, such as heat exhaustion and frostbite. It also includes animal bites and stings, such as spiders, snakes, and scorpions. The bee sting is covered in the immunologic section about allergic reactions. Injuries related to height or depth also will be addressed in this section, such as diving injuries, near drowning, and altitude sicknesses.

Anatomy and Physiology

The body always works to maintain an internal environment within a narrow range for all electrolytes, pH, and glucose, and it also regulates internal temperature to stay within a narrow band of 98.6°F (37°C). The hypothalamus in the brain is central to thermoregulation. When the **core body temperature** (**CBT**) declines, the hypothalamus will send signals to initiate **thermogenesis**, the process by which the body generates its own heat internally. Similarly, if the CBT increases too much, the hypothalamus initiates **thermolysis**, or the intentional liberation of excess body heat. The hypothalamus receives input from the body from warm and cold receptors located peripherally and centrally. Peripheral heat sensors are located in the skin and in muscles located near the surface of the skin and respond to environmental changes in temperature, whereas central heat sensors constantly measure the temperature of the circulating blood and are believed to be located within the hypothalamus itself. Central temperature receptor mechanisms are not yet well understood.

Thermogenesis is the production of heat and energy for the body. Increasing thermogenesis is the primary way the body will attempt to maintain CBT. The hypothalamus will signal for an overall increase in the systemic **basal metabolic rate**, which will generate heat through chemical bond breaking. This body also will increase the basal metabolic rate by stimulating increased muscle activity, which is experienced as shivering. Increasing the metabolism also is combined with shunting blood away from the cold periphery and toward the core. Starting with the most distal areas first, the body will shunt away from feet and hands, then as heat loss continues, it will shunt away from the lower legs and forcarms, and so on, until there is no way to shunt away from the cold areas of the body. Once the ability of the body to prevent heat loss and internally generate heat is exceeded, the CBT begins to fall and hypothermia sets in.

Thermolysis is the body's ability to dissipate excess heat. This is an ongoing process as the body tends to, under normal circumstances, generate more heat than is necessary to maintain CBT and ongoing body functions. Heat will always move from the area where heat is concentrated to the area where it is less concentrated. Put another way, heat will always move from the hotter object or area to the cooler object or area. When you grab a metal object in the winter, it is common to say it feels cold. But a shift in thinking about this process leads to a realization of how this happens: It obeys the rule that heat moved from the hotter area to the colder area. The reason the object feels cold is because the cold object is stripping heat from your body! Thinking about this further, what happens if the hand is kept there longer? Eventually, assuming the body's thermogenic mechanisms are not overwhelmed, both the metal object and your hand will be the same temperature.

There are 4 ways the body, or any object for that matter, can dissipate heat.

- **Conduction.** The direct removal of heat from one object to another because of direct contact. The transfer of heat to the metal object in the above example is an illustration of conduction.
- **Convection.** Heat carried away because of surrounding wind or water currents. Blowing on food helps cool it down because it continually introduces cooler air around the food. Like a conveyor belt of heat transfer, the air over top of the food gets a little warmer, cooler air replaces that air and gets warmed, and the process repeats. The same happens when a person is in water: not only is heat conducted from the body to the water, but the motion of the water removes heat through convection.
- **Evaporation.** The primary purpose of sweating is for the body to transfer heat energy to the water and cause it to evaporate. It takes a tremendous amount of energy to cause water to evaporate, so this should be a highly effective way to remove heat from the body. It is most effective when the atmospheric humidity is low; as humidity increases, evaporation becomes less effective.

- **Radiation.** This is the conversion of heat to infrared light. It is a constant, uncontrollable method of heat dissipation. This concept is what allows night vision goggles or thermal imaging cameras to work. They take the ordinarily invisible light things—and people—emit by virtue of their relative temperature and make it visible as an array of colors.

Thermolysis is always happening and always dependent on the ambient (surrounding) temperature gradient. Remember the main concept here: Heat will always move from the hotter area to the colder area. This means that even if a person is in a pool in the summer, and the temperature of that pool is, say, 88°F, the person will lose heat by all four mechanisms listed above to the pool water. Therefore, the person's CBT could drop, and thermogeneration mechanisms within the body—shivering, keeping arms close to the core, etc.—will begin. The temperature of the pool is by no means cold, but relative to the CBT, it is.

A similar process takes place in a sauna or a hot tub. Here the ambient temperature generally exceeds the CBT by a few degrees or more, causing the body to be the cooler area into which heat will move. After an extended period in such heat, thermolysis of the internal body heat will be initiated. Sweating begins, and peripheral vasodilation happens (seen as flushing of the body, particularly in the face) to enhance conductive cooling and radiation. In this situation of a warmer ambient temperature, vasodilation will actually enhance the absorption of heat from the environment, further increasing the CBT. In addition, the basal metabolic rate decreases to slow internal generation of heat. These factors can combine to cause the patient to pass out as peripheral vasodilation becomes so profound that the patient becomes hypotensive, and the basal metabolic rate drops to the point that the brain shuts down. This is why it is recommended to stay in these places for <15 minutes at a time.

Heat Emergencies

Heat emergencies occur whenever a patient is not able to regulate their internal body temperature by getting rid of excess heat. There are many situations where a person cannot decrease body temperature, resulting in any of three heat illnesses. The temperature of the patient's surroundings is perhaps the most obvious risk factor for heat-related illnesses; however, it is by no means the only thing that will affect a person's likelihood of getting sick from heat. The following is a list of factors to consider in a patient who presents with any of the heat-related illnesses.

- Cardiovascular disease
- Confined space
- Dehydration for any reason (illness, alcoholism, vomiting, hemorrhage)
- Fever
- Firefighter as job/career
- Heavy or constricting clothing
- High ambient temperature
- High humidity
- Hyperthyroidism
- Medications, particularly beta-blockers, diuretics, antidepressants, and antihistamines
- Obesity
- Physical activity of any kind
- Poor ventilation
- Stimulant use (caffeine, nicotine, cocaine, or methamphetamines)

In addition to these, the very old and the very young are at increased risk from heat-related problems. Adults age 65 and older often are on medications that interfere with the body's ability to regulate heat dissipation. The chronic disease processes themselves also may impact their ability to feel temperature changes, initiating peripheral vasodilation or sweat to begin with. Also, in some cases, impaired mobility may reduce how often a patient rehydrates. Limited resources may prevent the patient from having access to air conditioning and fans to keep them cool.

Children have primitive thermoregulatory centers that prevent them from responding as older children do. Ever seen a sweaty infant? Probably not. An infant's primary thermoregulatory mechanism is radiation of heat so you may see a flushed infant. Otherwise, infants rely on external factors to assist in thermoregulation, especially convection. Under most circumstances, an infant's high surface-area-to-volume ratio is usually enough to keep them cool in warmer areas and present a heat maintenance issue in colder environments.

Heat Cramps

Heat cramps are involuntary, painful muscle contractions, most commonly in the muscles of support and posture in the legs, abdomen, and back. The following factors contribute to a person getting heat cramps:

- **Salt Depletion.** Heat cramps are primarily dependent on the sodium balance in the body. An active person who consumes nothing but plain water during exercise can possibly make the sodium imbalance worse because the water is being replaced but not the sodium. Lightly salted water or commercial sports drinks with sodium and potassium are recommended over plain water on hot days during and after physical activity. When a person sweats, salt as well as water is lost, altering this balance.

- **Dehydration.** A person who is actively working or doing an activity in the heat can lose up to a liter of fluid an hour through sweating.

- **Muscle Fatigue.** This alone can contribute to cramping.

Heat cramps usually begin during exercise, and the pain can be so bad as to be incapacitating. Patients may be nauseous but usually will not vomit. Hypotension is rare because the patient is still able to accelerate the heart rate to compensate for the fluid loss.

Treatment for heat cramps involves getting the patient out of the hot environment and into a cooler one, preferably one where there are air currents. Encourage the patient to drink a commercial sports drink or add a half teaspoon of salt to at least 8 ounces of juice or water, as long as the patient is not nauseous. If the patient is nauseous, avoid a salt solution or ice cold drinks because this can worsen nausea and possibly cause the patient to vomit. Consider intravenous normal saline solution (NSS) run wide and expect to deliver about a liter of fluid. This will help correct the fluid and the salt issue at one time.

Heat Exhaustion

Heat exhaustion is more severe in the progression of heat-related illnesses. It may stem from sodium depletion, fluid depletion, or both. Sodium-depleted heat exhaustion can be caused by the loss of sodium through sweat and urine or by replacing water and not sodium, as seen with heat cramps. In heat exhaustion, the patient is not hypovolemic to the point where tachycardia is not enough to fully maintain blood pressure. Patients with heat exhaustion usually exhibit **orthostatic hypotension**, which is characterized by a change in systolic blood pressure (SBP) of 20 mmHg even with a compensatory increase in heart rate as the patient goes from lying down to standing up. Initial symptoms are similar to heat cramps: nausea, occasionally with vomiting and headache. As the exhaustion worsens, neurological changes are noted, including dizziness, confusion, mental status changes, and possibly seizures and syncope.

The patient is usually still capable of sweating, although it is diminished in volume. If available, measure the person's temperature and correlate it to CBT. It will likely be elevated though not higher than 106°F (41.1°C). The heart rate will be elevated, blood pressure may be normal or low, and the patient may have positive orthostatic changes in blood pressure.

To treat the patient with heat exhaustion, remove from heat and take precautions not to cool the patient so quickly to cause shivering. Initiate cardiac monitoring, and have the patient consume sports drinks or lightly salted water or juice as long as it is tolerable and doesn't worsen nausea or inducing vomiting. Initiate an intravenous line and administer at least 1 L of fluid over the first half-hour. Administering 4 mg ondansetron can help with nausea and prevent further fluid loss through vomiting.

Heat Stroke

Heat stroke is the ultimate form of heat illness. It is fortunately the least common because it is the most deadly. Heat stroke's hallmark signs are a CBT >106°F (41.1°C) and neurological dysfunction, most notably, altered mental status. There are two forms of heat stroke: exertional and nonexertional. **Exertional heat stroke** is generally associated with younger people who are active in a hot environment for a prolonged period, and **nonexertional heat stroke** more often affects older adults and people who are more sedentary and have a greater amount of comorbidities, such as obesity, a cardiovascular history, a psychiatric history (because of their medications), and peripheral neurovascular changes such as that seen in diabetes.

Excessive heat for prolonged periods can be devastating to the body. Temperatures in excess of 106°F (41.1°C) can begin to denature proteins, change the cellular membrane structure, cause breakdown of skeletal muscle, and prevent normal enzyme functioning at a cellular level, leading to altered cellular metabolism.

Patients with heat stroke will present with altered mental status and will be very hot to the touch. Patients with non-exertional heat stroke are likely to be red, hot, and dry, whereas patients with exertional heat stroke will be pale and diaphoretic. If this has set in over time, the urine may be very concentrated, foul smelling, and possibly even tea colored, indicating skeletal muscle breakdown (rhabdomyolysis).

Treatment for heat stroke should include aggressive fluid resuscitation with NSS after getting the patient to a cool environment. Infuse cold saline if available but stop if the patient begins to shiver. In heat stroke, cool the patient actively with cold packs to the groin, axillae, and neck. Monitor the ECG and treat any cardiac dysrhythmia as usual.

Cold Injuries

Frostnip and Frostbite

Local cold injuries, such as frostbite, often affect the extremities or exposed areas, including the fingers and toes, ears, cheeks, and the tip of the nose. **Frostnip** is a mild or early warning sign of possible frostbite if warmer areas are not sought out soon. In frostnip, the aforementioned areas begin to dull sensation and are sometimes described as numb and may appear red. Body parts with frostnip can be warmed by placing fingers or hands in warmer areas of the body such as the armpits or groin; other areas, such as the nose or ears, can be warmed by covering them with a warm hand.

Frostbite generally involves actual freezing of a body part. As part of the body's routine process of conserving heat, blood flow to the distal extremities is minimized and even completely shut down to shunt it back to the core. This allows the extremity to cool even faster. Ice crystals can form in the tissues, and eventually the entire area will be completely frozen. Frostbite can be accelerated if the area is wet because that accelerates cooling.

Assessment

Superficial frostbite involves only the outermost layers of the skin. The superficial layers are frozen, but the deeper tissues are not frozen. Symptoms usually include numbness and tingling or a burning sensation to the affected areas. Deep frostbite can be thought of as full thickness frostbite and includes the muscles, nerves, vessels, and possibly even the bone. On light-skinned people, the frozen areas will be darker or even black, whereas in dark-skinned people, the same areas will have a more waxy, gray-white appearance.

Treatment

Move the patient indoors or to a warmer area and remove any wet or constricting clothing. Avoid the temptation to rub or massage the affected area. Rubbing the area will cause the ice crystals in the tissue to move around, essentially becoming like little knives that lacerate the tissue and possibly cause extensive cellular level damage. If the transport time will be extensive, wrap the area with warm, dry sterile dressing, placing gauze between the fingers and toes to help prevent rubbing of the areas together. Consider rewarming on the way to the hospital if there is no danger of refreezing by using water that is about body temperature to a few degrees warmer and is easily tolerable to a person with normal sensation in their fingers. Remember, the patient will not be able to feel heat or pain, so it is possible, if the water is too hot, to actually cause burns to the affected, numb area. As the area defrosts, it will become extremely painful, so intravenous analgesics can be given as needed for pain.

Trench Foot and Chilblains

Trench foot was first systematically documented in soldiers who served in trenches during World War I. The cold water at the bottom of the trenches would cause essentially localized hypothermia of the feet. This can occur in temperatures as warm at 65°F (18°C). The affected area will lose circulation because of the local vasoconstriction, and the affected foot would be painful and appear blotchy. If allowed to be in the cold water for a long enough period of time, some areas of the foot can die and possibly require amputation. Treatment involves removal of the wet and constricting clothing and active rewarming of the area; once again, avoid rubbing it or walking on it.

Chilblains are similar to trench foot and usually occur after exposure to nonfreezing temperatures and are not associated with that area being wet. They can occur anywhere on the body, usually the fingers, toes, face, and ears. Chilblains appear as reddish-purple spots after the patient has come in out of the cold and rewarmed. The spots can become blisters or open sores, putting the patient at risk for infection. They will generally heal and disappear within about a week or so, although the area may remain sensitive to cold for life.

Hypothermia

Hypothermia is defined as a drop in CBT to <95°F (35°C) resulting from exposure to cold environments. In hypothermia, the body's ability to prevent heat loss and generate internal heat is ultimately overwhelmed, and body temperature begins to drop and will continue to drop until the patient can get to warmer environments.

The risk factors for hypothermia are as follows:

- Bleeding or trauma
- Cold water
- Dehydration
- Hypoglycemia and general malnutrition
- Metabolic disorders such as anorexia nervosa, diabetes, or hypothyroidism
- Paralysis
- Peripheral neuropathies like that seen in diabetes
- Sepsis
- Vasodilation from alcohol or drugs
- Wet or sweaty clothing
- Windy environment

Hypothermia can be classified as mild, moderate, or severe. Many outlets warn to be aware of the "umbles." This should remind us that as cognition declines, the patient will start to *fumble*, *tumble*, and *stumble* as coordination declines. Cognitive decline also includes mumbling and grumbling because the patient becomes confused and develops an altered mental status. This can begin after the CBT drops just a few degrees below physiologic normal.

- **Mild Hypothermia.** CBT between 95°F (35°C) and 90°F (32°C). The patient is still conscious, though usually lethargic and "umbling." If the patient has any degree of an altered mental status, assess the patient thoroughly to rule out causes other than the currently obvious hypothermia. Assessment for altered mental status should include evaluating for trauma, drug and alcohol use, and especially hypoglycemia. Even if the patient does not have diabetes, thermogenesis and shivering can possibly deplete the glucose stores in the body. Treatment includes the removal of wet clothing and active external rewarming—when there is no risk of cooling again—with blankets and hot packs. Initiate cardiac monitoring and warmed intravenous NSS. Also, treat hypoglycemia if present and be prepared to manage seizures should they develop. (Seizures are not common in this temperature range but become more common the more hypothermic a person becomes.)

- **Moderate Hypothermia.** CBT between 90°F (32°C) and 82.4°F (28°C). Here, the CNS depression worsens, and the patient may be comatose. Patients lose their ability to shiver around 87.8°F (31°C), allowing heat loss to accelerate. As the CBT continues to drop, arrhythmias can develop, including both atrial and ventricular dysrhythmias. Osborne waves or J waves can be seen on the ECG in coordinated rhythms. As the body's overall metabolism slows, so does the cardiac rhythm; bradycardias are the most common rhythm type seen in hypothermia. Active rewarming is essential in these patients. Use hot packs to the axillae, the groin, the nape of the neck, and the lower back. Use space blankets, if possible, directly against the patient's skin after first removing clothing. Then wrap the patient in blankets and make the ambulance as hot as possible. Initiate at least one intravenous infusion of warmed saline and administer a fluid bolus in 500 mL increments, checking vital signs between each bolus, especially breath sounds.

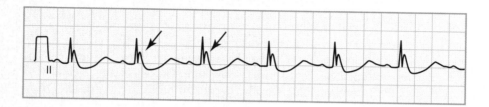

Figure 6-28. Sinus Bradycardic Rhythm with a First-Degree Atrioventricular Block with Osborne Waves (arrows).

- **Severe Hypothermia.** The CBT is <82.4°F (28°C). Patients rarely have a pulse at these temperatures, and VT is a common presenting rhythm. All the body's processes are slowed or nonexistent if the patient does, in fact, still have a perfusing rhythm. Treatment for this patient involves active rewarming and rapid transport to the nearest hospital. The patient will require active external rewarming where blood is rewarmed outside the body and then returned to the body. CPR and other resuscitative efforts should be initiated, with the understanding that the patient's response to medications will be much slower than usual and that the resuscitation will continue until the patient's CBT reaches physiologic temperatures >95°F (35°C). It is always recommended to attempt resuscitation because the effects of hypothermia are to protect the brain and other essential organs.

Water-Related Emergencies

Drowning

Drowning is a process resulting in respiratory impairment from submersion in a liquid medium, which ultimately prevents the patient from taking in O_2. Other terms related to drowning (near, wet, dry, active, and passive drowning, among others) should not be used because it can create confusion. Drowning can, however, be classified based on the temperature of the water the person was in. Temperatures higher than 68°F (20°C) are considered warm water drowning, and temperatures less than that are considered cold water drowning. It is believed that cold water drowning can have a protective effect on the body similar to hypothermia, although hypoxic time can eliminate the effect of the temperature.

Drowning can be further classified by the type of water in which the patient was submerged. A person can drown in fresh water, such as ponds and lakes; saltwater in oceans; or artificial bodies of water such as pools or bathtubs. The type of water has no impact on initial treatments and resuscitative efforts; however, once the patient is resuscitated, the type of water can have widely varying effects on the electrolyte balance in the body, particularly if a lot of water was inhaled or swallowed.

The drowning sequence usually begins with a person becoming tired in a body of water. The thrashing and splashing of a person trying to remain above water does not happen as often as Hollywood would have us believe. The patient starts with breath-holding as the body becomes submerged. When water enters the mouth and nose, the patient initially chokes on the water, invariably swallowing a considerable amount. Water hitting the larynx triggers

laryngospasm. Known as the diver's reflex, this is an attempt by the body to keep water out of the lungs and is the reason why bodies will float initially after a drowning. As part of the standard progression of death, the muscles of the body relax, including those responsible for laryngospasm. Water then is allowed to rush into the lungs, resulting in the body sinking. Resuscitation of the patient after the laryngospasm has released often is difficult because the water has washed away surfactant produced by the lungs. This will make them exceedingly difficult to inflate, resulting in an even worsened outcome.

Assessment and treatment of the drowning patient is really no different from assessing any other patient in cardiac or respiratory arrest. As in any "dry" cardiac arrest, administer antidysrhythmic and pressor medications, defibrillate, and do CPR. If the patient is hypothermic as a result of the drowning, continue resuscitation efforts until the patient has reached a physiologic temperature.

In the patient who regains consciousness and spontaneous breathing, aggressive treatment must be continued. The patient is at risk for severe lung complications, including **adult respiratory distress syndrome** (**ARDS**) and pulmonary edema. The patient may have prolonged difficulty breathing because of a lack of surfactant in addition to the ARDS and pulmonary edema, which could cause the patient to stop breathing again. Monitor the ECG, EtCO$_2$, and pulse oximetry throughout treatment. Administer albuterol for wheezing. Even if the patient is breathing, be prepared to intubate.

Diving Injuries

General Background and Pathology

At sea level, a person—every person—is subjected to 1 atmosphere (atm) of pressure, which also can be denoted as 14.7 pounds per square inch (psi) or 760 mmHg. One atmosphere is the pressure exerted by the weight of the gaseous atmosphere above. This does not change appreciably at most inhabitable altitudes. Divers experience an increase of pressure on their bodies equal to 1 atm for every 33 feet of seawater (fsw) above them. Gases, unlike liquids, are compressible and therefore behave according to the following laws:

- **Boyle's Law.** This law relates pressure and volume. It says that when the temperature of a gas is held constant, as the pressure on a gas increases, the volume decreases, and vice versa. If you take an empty, sealed soda bottle and squeeze it, its volume will be decreased. As the volume is decreased, the pressure the gas exerts back against the walls of the container increases. This concept helps explain barotrauma that can occur in a diver who came up from depth too quickly. Suppose this diver takes a breath at 33 fsw and then ascends holding their breath until reaching the top, never exhaling. The pressure decreased during the ascent by 1 atm of pressure in that distance. The volume of that breath has more than doubled in size as a result of the change in pressure!

- **Charles's Law.** When the pressure of a gas is held constant, the volume of the gas is directly proportional to the temperature of the gas. That is, as the temperature of the gas increases, the volume will increase if the pressure remains constant.

- **Dalton's Law.** The law of partial pressures of gases. This law states that the total pressure of a gas mixture is proportionally dependent on the proportion of each gas in the mixture.

- **Henry's Law.** This law states that the concentration of gas dissolved in a liquid is proportional to the partial pressure of the gas in the atmosphere above the liquid. This law helps us understand the idea of nitrogen narcosis and decompression sickness, also known as "the bends." Because the compressed air that divers breathe is generally atmospheric air under pressure, which contains about 78% nitrogen, nitrogen can then be predicted to be dissolved in blood according to Henry's Law. Some proportion of the nitrogen will make it into the bloodstream; if not given sufficient time for the nitrogen to escape as the partial pressure drops during ascent, the nitrogen will form bubbles in the bloodstream, much like a newly opened bottle of soda has bubbles of CO$_2$ form on the inner walls of the container. These bubbles can then form air emboli and get trapped in the capillaries.

General Assessment for Divers

Paramedics will need to get information regarding the dive from the patient or those who accompanied the patient on the dive. These questions can be made into a questionnaire for services that are near common diving locations, such as shore points and lakes or quarries.

- When did the symptoms start? During ascent, descent, or at depth?
- What type of diving was done? Not all diving requires a tank. In breath-hold diving, people will take a deep breath at the surface and then submerge for as long as they can hold their breath. Helmet divers are connected via a tube to an O_2 source located on the surface. In saturation diving, highly trained and exceptionally fit individuals hyperventilate at the surface and then stay underwater for an extended period.
- What type of equipment was used?
- What type of tank/gas was used during the dive? Divers who plan to go to depths in excess of 100 fsw will use a tank that contains nitrox, which is a special gas mixture that reduces the amount of nitrogen and increases the amount O_2. Nitrox also allows for longer dive times compared with standard compressed air.
- What was the water temperature?
- Were there any complications during the dive?
- What were the patient's pre- and postdive activities?
- Collect information about the amount of total dives within the prior 72 hours, including length of dive, depth of dive, surface interval, and gas used.

Specific Diving Emergencies

Nitrogen narcosis is a problem with dives of depths >100 ft, particularly those that used regular compressed air, not nitrogen. Excessive nitrogen in the bloodstream can cause a person to pass out while underwater, and it can be worsened if the patient is brought up to the surface too quickly. Divers afflicted with nitrogen narcosis at depth often engage in risky behavior and may even spit out the regulator and surface too quickly. Patients will present confused and also may complain of pain in their joints. Patients will likely need to be transported to a facility that has a hyperbaric chamber. They will need to be artificially taken back down to the approximate depth they were at when the problem started and then brought back up to the "surface" in a more controlled manner.

Barotrauma occurs when there is a pressure difference between the air-filled areas in the body and the external atmosphere. These spaces include the middle ear, the lungs, the joints, and the sinuses. During descent, the pressure outside increases, causing the gas-filled areas to be compressed. As long as these areas are given time to equilibrate with the surroundings during both descent and ascent, there should not be any issue. Problems arise when there are blockages, such as a sinus or middle ear infection that prevents or hinders equilibration. Rupture of the membranes or structures in the ear can lead to dizziness or disorientation in the water. This can further progress to panic and rapid ascent, leading to other injuries. In addition, nausea and vomiting can ensue after the onset of dizziness and further add to complications and panic underwater.

Perhaps the most aptly named of barotrauma syndromes because that is exactly what happens to the lung: it POPS! In **pulmonary overpressurization syndrome** (**POPS**), a person holds their breath during ascent as described in the Boyle's Law example above. This causes one or multiple ruptures in the lung from the decrease in pressure and a commensurate increase in volume that happens to gas held within the lungs. This can lead to a pneumothorax, pneumomediastinum, and profound **subcutaneous emphysema**—a feeling of bubbles popping under the skin.

Patients present with signs of a pneumothorax, including dyspnea, tracheal deviation, absent or diminished breath sounds on 1 side, and JVD. If air escaped the lungs and entered the mediastinum, the patient may complain of difficulty swallowing, fullness in the throat, and chest pain. Occasionally, the patient will have a crunching sound with each heartbeat, indicating air surrounding the heart. The physical examination findings, in addition to those above, may include muffled heart sounds, an increasing heart rate and respiratory rate, and a decreasing pulse oximetry reading.

Treatment should include high-flow O_2. Perform a needle decompression of the affected side. If sounds from both sides of the lung are diminished or the pulse oximetry does not improve significantly after the first needle decompression, decompress the other side of the chest as well. Pneumomediastinum cannot be treated in the prehospital environment and warrants immediate and rapid transport to the hospital. Initiate an intravenous line and continuous cardiac monitoring.

An **arterial gas embolism** is one of the most lethal complications of POPS. When the alveoli rupture in POPS, bubbles can enter the bloodstream and lodge anywhere in the circulatory system. If they find their way into the coronary arteries, they will cause the patient to suffer all the same symptoms as an MI. The more likely place for them to travel is the brain and head because this is generally the highest place in the body. Here, the bubbles can cause cerebral ischemia and symptoms similar to a head injury or stroke.

In either case, be prepared to treat cardiac arrest or any dysrhythmias if there are cardiac complications. Also be prepared to treat altered mental status, combativity, and seizures should the bubbles travel to the brain. Treatment for this patient will ultimately be to undergo hyperbaric pressure treatment, which will cause the bubbles to go back into solution. The patient will then be brought back to sea level in a controlled fashion. If the patient needs to be intubated, fill the cuff with saline rather than air so that when the patient is receiving hyperbaric therapy, the cuff does not deflate.

Decompression sickness is any of a range of conditions that the patient may experience as a result of nitrogen bubbles in the bloodstream caused by ascending too rapidly. Decompression sickness often mimics arterial gas embolism in symptoms but not in pathology. Treatment is the same and will involve recompression in a hyperbaric chamber.

Shallow water blackout is a condition often seen in boys who compete to see who can hold their breath the longest underwater. Holding their breath for a long period could lead to cerebral hypoxia toward the end of the period of time underwater, leading to syncope. This is generally a diagnosis of exclusion; in other words, after all other possibilities for the loss of consciousness have been ruled out, this is the only plausible explanation left.

High-Altitude Illnesses

A paramedic should be familiar with the common altitude sicknesses: **acute mountain sickness (AMS)**, **high-altitude cerebral edema (HACE)**, and **high-altitude pulmonary edema (HAPE)**. People are at risk for these illnesses based not only on how high they go but how quickly they got there. High-altitude illnesses can be seen at altitudes as low as 6,500 feet above sea level but become much more common at altitudes >8,000 feet. The primary issue in any high altitude illness is the decline in O_2 concentration. The body is capable of acclimatizing to the drop in O_2; however, it will take a day or so of rest for this to happen. Patients will often take acetazolamide to counteract the effects of high altitude sickness and help the body acclimatize faster. Acetazolamide forces the kidneys to excrete bicarbonate, establishing metabolic acidosis in the body. This allows the climber to hyperventilate to bring in more O_2 without causing respiratory alkalosis.

In **AMS**, patients will present with a headache and at least one of the following: fatigue or weakness, nausea, vomiting or loss of appetite, dizziness, or insomnia. This often can be completely cured by descending until the symptoms resolve and allowing time for the body to acclimatize to that altitude before continuing.

In **HAPE**, the symptoms include shortness of breath at rest and with exertion, a cough, a frothy sputum, chest tightness, and at least two of the following: tachycardia, tachypnea, rales/crackles, and/or central cyanosis. Descent and high-flow O_2 are the most important treatments for HAPE. Most patients will improve with rest and O_2; nifedipine and acetazolamide are recommended as first-line medications. Dexamethasone prophylaxis and administration upon descent also can help the patient improve from HAPE.

HACE is characterized by any of the symptoms listed with AMS, in addition to the presence of altered mental status and ataxia or clumsiness, which indicate that AMS has worsened to HACE. HACE can appear in a person who continues to ascend despite symptoms of AMS or in people who ascend so rapidly that symptoms of AMS do not actually have time to appear. HAPE also occurs concurrently with HACE.

Other Environmental Emergencies

Snake Bites

Pit Vipers

As members of the family Viperidae, pit vipers include the rattlesnake, cottonmouths, diamondbacks, and copperhead snakes. They have distinctive pits located between the eye and the nostril on each side and vertical pupils. This group is responsible for the greatest number of snake bites in the United States, primarily in the southeastern portion of the country. Pit viper venom is a toxic mixture of hemolytic and proteolytic enzymes. Hemolytic enzymes break down red blood cells and stimulate clot formation, and proteolytic enzymes break down proteins of all kinds. These work together to cause local tissue damage, swelling, necrosis, systemic bleeding, and clotting.

Pit viper bite symptoms are largely localized to the bite site and include swelling and bleeding from the fang marks. No bleeding from the bite site may indicate that a "dry," or venomless, bite has occurred. In mild envenomations, swelling will start at the site of the bite and slowly progress up the extremity, but the patient will lack systemic symptoms. In severe envenomations, extensive soft-tissue damage occurs locally, and extensive systemic effects develop, including spontaneous bleeding and coagulopathies, usually followed by shock, cardiovascular collapse, and death. Moderate envenomations fall somewhere in between with little systemic bleeding noted.

Treatment for a pit viper bite involves immobilization of the extremity and rapid transport for antivenin. Remove any constricting clothing and jewelry because swelling can be dramatic. Constricting bands and tourniquets are not recommended in pit viper bites, as they are in elapid bites.

Coral Snakes

As members of the Elapidae family, the coral snake is primarily found across the southern United States from southern California to Florida. The venom of coral snakes contains a neurotoxin that will lead to respiratory failure and death. Fortunately, coral snakes have comparatively small fangs, making it difficult for them to inject their venom. For an elapid bite to be of serious threat to the patient, the snake would have to remain attached for a reasonable amount of time to inject enough venom to be deadly.

Treatment for the elapid bite begins by applying a constriction dressing to slow the spread of the neurotoxin. The constriction dressing should be applied just proximal to the bite over the next major joint and back down to where it was started. Immobilize the extremity. All patients who have been bitten by a coral snake should be taken to the hospital, even if there is no evidence that the snake was able to inject the toxin. During transport, be prepared to aggressively manage the airway and provide ventilatory support.

Spider Bites

In the United States, three spiders pose a threat to humans when they bite: the black widow (female), the brown recluse, and the hobo spider.

The black widow lives primarily in the southeastern United States but can be found throughout the country. It prefers damp and dark areas, such as sheds, woodpiles, and outhouses. It is one of the most venomous spiders. Its venom is a neurotoxin that triggers the release of neurotransmitters. In less than an hour after the bite, it causes local pain and swelling, followed by muscle spasms and paralysis, both locally to the bite and systemically. Nausea and vomiting can occur. As the diaphragm becomes paralyzed from the venom, respiratory arrest can develop.

Treatment for a black widow spider bite is aimed at preventing paralysis and pain relief. Benzodiazepines can be used to calm the patient as well as relieve any spasms and paralysis from the venom. Narcotic pain medications should be used for pain. An antivenin is available but is generally reserved for the extremes in age. Most symptoms can be managed symptomatically until the venom wears off.

The brown recluse spider is known as the fiddleback spider, owing to the dark pattern on its thorax that resembles a violin. It makes its home primarily in the southeastern United States, extending into the Midwest and Texas. Brown recluse spider bites are typically painless and rarely cause any major problems of any kind for the patient. In a rare subset of patients, however, the patient will develop what is known as loxoscelism. This begins within hours of the bite and starts off as a fluid-filled vesicle at the location of the bite. This progresses to gangrene and a larger necrotic area after about a week or so that often will require skin grafting. The area will then take months to heal fully. Any systemic symptoms are far rarer. When a systemic reaction does occur, it is generally caused by coagulopathies and hemolysis that often lead to death.

The hobo spider is very similar in all aspects to the brown recluse except that it calls the Pacific Northwest home. The bite and sequelae of the hobo spider resemble that of the brown recluse.

There is no known treatment for bites from the brown recluse spider or the hobo spider.

Scorpion Stings

Scorpions of the genus *Centruroides* are the only ones whose sting poses a genuine threat to humans. Fortunately, it is the least common scorpion sting in the United States. Other scorpion stings cause only a local painful reaction. Scorpions of this species, called the bark scorpion, live primarily in the southwestern United States and northern Mexico. It is not aggressive and is active only at night.

A vast majority of scorpions produce only localized reactions similar to that of bee stings. The area around the scorpion sting will be red and itchy, and a burning pain similar to a strong electrical shock has been described. Local effects tend to subside within a few hours of the bite, and local tissue necrosis has not been reported.

Bark scorpion sting symptoms, on the other hand, rarely include local symptoms. The toxin in this scorpion's sting causes sodium channels in the nerves of both the parasympathetic and sympathetic autonomic nervous system to remain open. This leads to continued stimulation of these nerves. The symptoms depend entirely on which side of the autonomic nervous system is dominating—sympathetic or parasympathetic. If the sympathetic nervous system dominates, then the patient will have tachycardia, hypertension, dry mouth, and elevated temperature. Conversely, if the parasympathetic nervous system is running the show, symptoms are similar to that of organophosphate poisoning and include everything in the SLUDGE mnemonic.

Treatment for the bark scorpion sting involves maintaining the ABCs and is otherwise supportive. Intubate if necessary and treat any cardiac dysrhythmias. Applying a constricting band to slow lymph return to the heart is recommended. Rapid transport to the hospital is essential for careful management of the autonomic symptoms. There is an antivenin available in the Southwest, but it is rather hard to come by outside that region.

REVIEW QUESTIONS

Select the ONE best answer.

1. All of the following are internal methods of thermogenesis EXCEPT:

    A. Shivering.
    B. Shunting blood to the core.
    C. Increasing the basal metabolic rate.
    D. Dilation of the peripheral blood vessels.

2. You have a patient who fell while ice skating and is still lying on the ice when you arrive. During your assessment, she begins to shiver and complains that it is making the pain worse. You and your partner decide to move her off the ice before continuing the assessment and starting treatment because you know that she is most likely losing heat primarily by:

    A. Conduction.
    B. Convection.
    C. Evaporation.
    D. Radiation.

3. The following warning often can be found on the doors to saunas, steam rooms, and hot tubs. Use this for questions 3 and 4.

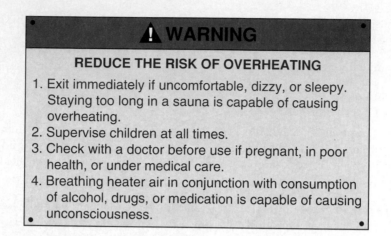

⚠ WARNING

REDUCE THE RISK OF OVERHEATING

1. Exit immediately if uncomfortable, dizzy, or sleepy. Staying too long in a sauna is capable of causing overheating.
2. Supervise children at all times.
3. Check with a doctor before use if pregnant, in poor health, or under medical care.
4. Breathing heater air in conjunction with consumption of alcohol, drugs, or medication is capable of causing unconsciousness.

Overheating in a steam room is most likely caused by overwhelming which of the body's methods of expelling heat?

A. Conduction

B. Convection

C. Evaporation

D. Radiation

4. Patients taking which of the following medications should pay particular attention to warning number 4 in the above sign?

A. Lisinopril, an ACE inhibitor

B. Loratadine, an antihistamine

C. Metoprolol, a beta-blocker

D. Omeprazole, a proton pump inhibitor.

5. Use this scenario to answer questions 5–7.

A 27-year-old female patient who was found by police stuck on the side of the road in a snowstorm for approximately 24 hours presents to you unresponsive with a weak central pulse, HR: 39, BP: 62/18, RR: 7. Her fingers, toes, nose, and ears are white and waxy. Her ECG is as follows:

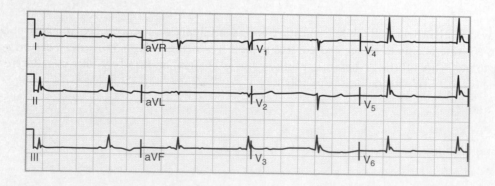

Based on the description, this patient is suffering from what degree of hypothermia?

A. Mild hypothermia

B. Moderate hypothermia

C. Severe hypothermia

D. Irreversible hypothermia

6. You have removed the patient's clothes once in the ambulance and covered her with warm blankets. What is the most appropriate next treatment?

A. Initiate an intravenous line with warmed saline.

B. Wrap the patient in a space blanket.

C. Place hot packs at the groin, axilla, back, and neck.

D. Vigorously rub the patient's arms and legs to generate heat through friction.

7. The white and waxy areas of skin found when examining this patient most likely indicate which of the following?

A. Chilblains

B. Cold necrosis

C. Frostbite

D. Frostnip

8. What is the best explanation for why the body of an ocean drowning victim tends to float at first?

A. Air gets trapped in the lungs because of diver's reflex.

B. Body fat causes the body to float like oil on water.

C. The human body overall is less dense than seawater.

D. Drowning tends to occur near the surface when the body is not waterlogged yet.

9. A person ascends from a 100-foot dive while holding their breath. Which answer correctly pairs the gas law with what will happen to the gas in the person's lungs as the pressure decreases?

A. Boyle's Law: Volume will increase.

B. Charles' Law: Volume will increase.

C. Dalton's Law: The partial pressure of nitrogen will increase.

D. Henry's Law: Volume will decrease as air enters the bloodstream.

10. A bite from which of the following can cause loxoscelism, a fluid-filled vesicle that forms within a couple of hours of the bite and can lead to gangrene in the area?

A. Bark scorpion

B. Black widow spider

C. Brown recluse spider

D. Coral snake

ANSWERS AND EXPLANATIONS

1. **The correct answer is (D).** Dilation of the peripheral blood vessels is a method of thermolysis or decreasing internal body temperature. All the other items in the list are ways the body works to increase the CBT in hypothermic conditions.

2. **The correct answer is (A).** Because the patient is lying in direct contact with the ice, she is most likely losing heat through conduction. By this method, heat moves directly from a warmer body to a colder body by virtue of direct contact. See question 3 for the other definitions of the remaining options.

3. **The correct answer is (C).** The extremely high heat in a steam room will prevent the evaporation of sweat from the body, and therefore the cooling effect that goes along with it. The body then would have to rely on other, less efficient methods to expel the excess heat. Conduction (A) is the removal of heat from the body through direct contact with another surface. Convection (B) is the removal of heat from a body by moving air or water currents. Radiation (D) is the conversion of heat energy to light energy and is a constant process—the reason thermal imaging cameras work.

4. **The correct answer is (B).** Antihistamines belong to the broader class of medications called anticholinergics. Anticholinergics can cause the internal body temperature to be set higher to begin with and also inhibit other thermoregulatory mechanisms, including sweating. This combined with the heat of the sauna can be a lethal prescription. Other medication classes with anticholinergic effects include antipsychotics, antidepressants (tricyclics are of particular concern), antiemetics, antidiarrheals, anti-Parkinsonians, diuretics, and muscle relaxants. The remaining medications listed do not have an appreciable effect on a person's thermoregulation.

5. **The correct answer is (B).** This patient is most likely in moderate hypothermia with a CBT between 90°F (32°C) and 82.4°F (28°C). This is known primarily by the presence of Osborne waves or J waves in the ECG. Osborne waves begin to be present once the CBT is <90°F (32°C). Below this range, severe hypothermia (C), VF or asystole are the most common presenting ECGs. Above this range, mild hypothermia (A), the patient often is still responsive and shivering. Irreversible hypothermia (D) is not a description of hypothermia.

6. **The correct answer is (C).** Hot packs are the first step in the initiation of active rewarming and should be placed in the areas indicated. A space blanket (B) if available, should be placed under the blankets directly against the patient's skin. An intravenous line of warmed saline (A) should be initiated, however, not before the hot packs are placed. Vigorously rubbing a patient (D) with possible areas of frostbite is never a recommended therapy.

7. **The correct answer is (C).** White and waxy most likely indicates frostbite, where the soft tissues have completely frozen. Frostnip (D) is when the area in question has altered sensation, often as a burning sensation despite being in the cold. Chilblains (A) are reddish-purple splotches in areas that were previously frostnipped or nearly frostbitten and have since been rewarmed. This patient may experience them but not so soon after being removed from the cold. Although the areas in question may become necrotic (B), there is no diagnosis of cold necrosis.

8. **The correct answer is (A).** Diver's reflex causes sudden and severe laryngospasm. This serves the purpose of keeping water out of the lungs; however, it also traps existing air in the lungs for a time. The body is typically denser than seawater (C) and regardless of body fat content (B), the body will eventually sink. Ordinary clothing (D) is not buoyant enough to prevent a drowning victim from sinking.

9. **The correct answer is (A).** Boyle's Law states that volume and pressure are inversely proportional when temperature is held constant. This means that as the pressure on a diver decreases during ascent, the volume in the lungs will increase. Charles' Law (B) states that temperature and volume are directly proportional when pressure is held constant. Dalton's Law (C) is concerned with partial pressures of a gas and does not apply here. Henry's Law (D) states that the volume of a gas dissolved in a liquid increases as pressure increases. This causes gases dissolved in blood to bubble out of solution—but not necessarily—and, in fact, rarely into the lungs. Therefore, it has a negligible impact on the volume within the lungs.

10. **The correct answer is (C).** This condition is unique to the brown recluse spider and often requires skin grafts and months to heal.

Gynecology, Obstetrics, and Newborn Resuscitation

7

Learning Objectives

❏ Describe the anatomy and physiology of the female reproductive system and the changes a pregnant woman's body undergoes during pregnancy.

❏ Identify and describe the cardinal movements of labor, the events associated with the three stages of labor, and complications associated with abnormal deliveries.

❏ Differentiate, assess, and treat various gynecological emergencies.

❏ Identify the steps for newborn resuscitation in any newborn and components of the APGAR score.

❏ Differentiate, assess, and treat emergencies related to the newborn.

This chapter addresses female reproductive anatomy and physiology, including gynecological conditions that the paramedic should be familiar with, then discusses conception, fetal development, and birth. Problems that may be encountered during gestation, birth, and the postnatal period are then presented. Finally, the chapter discusses the newborn child and resuscitation of the child under normal circumstances as well as during an emergency.

GYNECOLOGY

Female Reproductive Anatomy

Female reproductive anatomy is both external and internal. The **external anatomy** is collectively known as the **vulva**. Working posteriorly from the **mons pubis**, which overlies the symphysis pubis of the pelvis, the first specific structure of the vulva is the **clitoris**, which is a mass of erectile tissue and nerve fibers that is covered with the **prepuce** and becomes engorged with blood during sexual arousal. Dividing laterally and posteriorly from the prepuce are the labia. The **labia majora** are the most lateral and are immediately visible. The **labia minora** are thinner and lie medial to the labia majora.

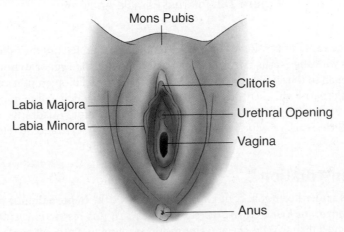

Figure 7-1. External Female Anatomy

The area between the 2 labia minora is known as the **vestibule**. At the anterior fold of the labia minora and within the vestibule is where the urethral opening, which drains urine from the bladder, is found. At the posterior end of the vestibule is the vaginal opening. The vagina serves 3 purposes:

- Receive the penis during intercourse
- Provide a conduit for menstrual flow
- Allow passage for an infant leaving the uterus

Within the vagina are 2 openings for the Bartholin glands. These glands secrete lubricant into the vagina during intercourse. Finally, posterior to the vaginal opening and anterior to the anus is the perineum. The perineum can tear during normal vaginal deliveries. A thin membrane called a hymen may cover or partially cover the vaginal opening.

The **internal anatomy** includes the vagina, the uterus, the fallopian tubes, and the ovaries. The vagina extends from the vestibule outside the body superiorly and ends at the inferior opening of the uterus called the **cervix**. The opening of the cervix is called the **os**. The **uterus** is a very muscular organ in which the fetus develops from conception to birth. The walls are almost entirely muscle, sometimes called the **myometrium**, and are internally lined with highly vascular tissue called **endometrium**, which sloughs off during menstruation. The uterus is responsible for contractions during birth.

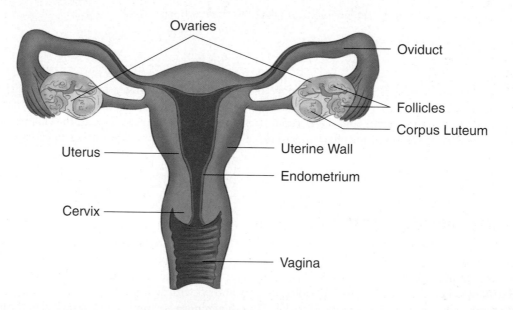

Figure 7-2. Internal Female Anatomy

Extending laterally from the superior portion of the uterus on the right and left are the **fallopian tubes**. The fallopian tubes connect the **ovaries** with the uterus and serve as a passageway for the egg, or **ovum**. The end of the fallopian tube nearest the ovary is open to the abdominal cavity; the ovaries and the fallopian tubes are not directly connected. Fertilization of the egg with sperm will likely occur in the fallopian tubes, which will then travel to and implant in the endometrium within the uterus. The ovaries lie within the lower abdominal quadrants, one on each side. In each ovary are thousands of follicles, each of which can mature to become an oocyte and be released as an ovum.

Ovulation and Menstruation

The ability to reproduce is under hormonal control. Prior to puberty, the **hypothalamus** restricts the production of **gonadotropin-releasing hormone (GnRH)**. At the start of puberty, this restriction is lifted as the hypothalamus releases pulses of GnRH, which then triggers the **anterior pituitary gland** to synthesize and release **follicle-stimulating hormone (FSH)** and **luteinizing hormone (LH)**. These hormones trigger the production of other sex hormones that develop and maintain the reproductive system.

Female Sexual Development

The ovaries, which are derived from the same embryonic structures as the testes, also are under the control of FSH and LH secreted by the anterior pituitary gland. The ovaries produce estrogens and progesterone.

Estrogens are secreted in response to FSH, and they result in the development and maintenance of the female reproductive system and female secondary sexual characteristics (breast growth, widening of the hips, and changes in fat distribution). In the embryo, estrogens stimulate development of the reproductive tract. In adults, estrogens lead to the thickening of the lining of the uterus (endometrium) each month in preparation for implantation of a zygote.

Progesterone is secreted by the **corpus luteum**—the remnant follicle that remains after ovulation—in response to LH. Interestingly, progesterone is involved in the development and maintenance of the endometrium but not in the initial thickening of the endometrium, which is the role of estrogen. This means that both estrogen and progesterone are required for the generation, development, and maintenance of an endometrium capable of supporting a zygote. By the end of the first trimester of a pregnancy, progesterone is supplied by the placenta, and the corpus luteum atrophies and ceases to function.

Menstrual Cycle

During the reproductive years (from menarche to menopause), estrogen and progesterone levels rise and fall in a cyclic pattern. In response, the endometrial lining will grow and be shed. This is known as the **menstrual cycle** and can be divided into 4 events: the follicular phase, ovulation, the luteal phase, and menstruation.

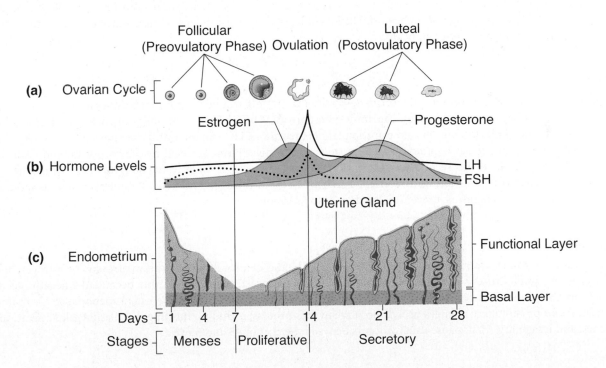

Figure 7-3. Menstrual Cycle
(a) FSH facilitates the maturation of a single ovum. (b) The peak of LH around day 14 marks ovulation, the release of the oocyte from the follicle. (c) The endometrial lining of the uterus reaches its peak in the luteal phase and is shed at the beginning of the next cycle.

Follicular Phase

The **follicular phase** begins when the **menstrual flow**, which sheds the uterine lining of the previous cycle, begins. GnRH secretion from the hypothalamus increases in response to the decreased concentrations of estrogen and progesterone, which fall off toward the end of each cycle. The higher concentrations of GnRH cause increased secretions of both FSH and LH. These hormones work in concert to develop several ovarian follicles. The follicles begin to produce estrogen, which has negative feedback effects and causes the GnRH, LH, and FSH concentrations to level off. Estrogen works to regrow the endometrial lining, stimulating vascularization and glandularization of the **decidua**.

Ovulation

Estrogen is interesting in that it can have both negative and positive feedback effects. Late in the follicular phase, the developing follicles secrete higher and higher concentrations of estrogen. Eventually, estrogen concentrations reach a threshold that paradoxically results in positive feedback, and GnRH, LH, and FSH levels spike. The surge in LH is important; it induces **ovulation**, the release of the ovum from the ovary into the abdominal (peritoneal) cavity.

Luteal Phase

After ovulation, LH causes the ruptured follicle to form the corpus luteum, which secretes progesterone. Remember that estrogen helps regenerate the uterine lining, but progesterone maintains it for implantation. Progesterone levels begin to rise, but estrogen levels remain high. The high levels of progesterone again cause negative feedback on GnRH, FSH, and LH, preventing the ovulation of multiple eggs.

Menstruation

Assuming that implantation does not occur, the corpus luteum loses its stimulation from LH, progesterone levels decline, and the uterine lining is sloughed off. The loss of high levels of estrogen and progesterone removes the block on GnRH so that the next cycle can begin.

Pregnancy

On the other hand, if fertilization has occurred, the resulting zygote will develop into a blastocyst that will implant in the uterine lining and secrete **human chorionic gonadotropin** (**hCG**). This hormone is an analog of LH, meaning that it looks very similar chemically and can stimulate LH receptors. HCG maintains the corpus luteum and is critical during first trimester development because estrogen and progesterone secreted by the corpus luteum keep the uterine lining in place. By the second trimester, hCG levels decline because the placenta has grown to a sufficient size to secrete progesterone and estrogen by itself. The high levels of estrogen and progesterone continue to serve as negative feedback mechanisms, preventing further GnRH secretion.

Menopause

As a woman ages, her ovaries become less sensitive to FSH and LH, resulting in ovarian atrophy. As estrogen and progesterone levels drop, the endometrium also atrophies, and menstruation stops. Also, because the negative feedback on FSH and LH is removed, the blood levels of these hormones rise. This is called **menopause**. Profound physical and physiological changes usually accompany this process, including flushing, hot flashes, bloating, headaches, and irritability. Menopause usually occurs between the ages of 45 and 55 years.

General Gynecological Assessment

Assessment of the patient with a gynecological problem can be a sensitive issue. On the part of the paramedic, it requires asking some personal questions that may result in emotional answers. Remember, you are a stranger asking about the patient's sexual history. Explain why the information is needed.

- Maintain the most professional and sensitive manner possible, as this is essential to being able to complete a thorough and appropriate assessment. The answers to the questions you pose can help you to rule out problems that could impact immediate treatment (e.g., administration of certain medications) or to ensure that the patient is taken to an appropriate facility. It also could simply be medically necessary. Whatever the reason, good communication about it can make for a better experience for the paramedic and the patient.

- Any patient deserves dignity and respect, especially the gynecological patient. The teenage patient likely will not want to answer such sensitive questions in the presence of her parents, for fear of getting into trouble, for example. Questions such as those that follow should be asked in privacy after ensuring the patient understands why they are being asked. Rarely are such patients such a dire emergency that the sensitive history and physical cannot wait until the patient is in the relative privacy of the ambulance.

- If the patient is a minor, you may ask the questions away from a parent, but you must share the information with the parent as part of informed consent for any treatment that you determine is needed unless the patient is pregnant and this has been confirmed.

- Once the patient is pregnant, or has been pregnant, the patient is considered legally emancipated and is capable of making her own decisions regarding healthcare without the usually requisite approval from a parent or guardian. In addition, the parent or guardian may not be informed about the treatment or condition without written consent from the emancipated minor; the patient is permitted all the same privacy concerns as any other competent adult.

- As with any patient, a thorough SAMPLE and OPPQRST as appropriate should be completed. However, this may leave some important questions unanswered, particularly for the gynecological and potentially pregnant patient. Following that, as part of the history of present illness interrogation, more direct questions need to be asked and answered.

What follows are some question types that should be asked of any known or suspected gynecological patient.

Menstruation Questions

- **When was your last menstrual period? Are your periods regular?** Together, these questions can help guide the paramedic whether the patient is or could be pregnant. A menstrual period that was previously occurring at regular, predictable intervals that is now >2 weeks late could mean that the patient is pregnant.

- **Was your last period's flow typical of your regular periods?** A patient who notes that her most recent period was considerably lighter than usual—either producing less blood or bleeding for fewer days—could have had what is known as breakthrough bleeding. Breakthrough bleeding occurs when the fertilized ovum, now called a zygote, implants in the endometrium. This generates some bleeding usually at about the time the patient would be expecting her period. In each case, if the periods were regular and are now late or the most recent period had lighter than usual flow, more investigation is needed into possible pregnancy.

- **Have you had any pain with menstruation?** This could indicate a host of issues (discussed later in the chapter).

Sexual History Questions

- **Could you be pregnant?** Many patients will answer *no* to this question, appropriately. However, many people do not realize the most probable time for a woman to become pregnant is to have unprotected intercourse approximately 14 days after the start of the previous menses, with most literature indicating the highest time being 12–17 days after the start of menses. Many will also answer no because they are on birth control and believe that such products or devices eliminate all possibility of pregnancy. If the woman is of childbearing age, the next question should be an automatic follow-up.

- **When was the last time you had unprotected intercourse?** This question should be asked when pregnancy is suspected, even if the patient answers "No" to the above question. After doing some math, if the last time she had unprotected intercourse falls within the 12–17 day window, pregnancy is highly likely, though still not certain. Notice also the use of the term *unprotected intercourse*. It is important here to not use slang or euphemisms. Professionalism is paramount here.

- **What forms of birth control were used?** A remarkable number of people believe that taking birth control eliminates the possibility of becoming pregnant. It is worth suggesting some forms in a nonjudgmental way. If the patient has not used any forms of birth control and still insists she is not pregnant, it is worth taking a few moments to ask about other symptoms, including tender or swollen breasts.

- **Have you had unprotected intercourse with multiple partners?** This could indicate the possibility of the patient having a sexually transmitted disease (STD), especially if the patient has an associated complaint of vaginal discharge.

Vaginal Discharge

- **What is the texture?** Is there an odor associated with it? Women are much more susceptible to getting a sexually transmitted infection than are men, and because of the dark, wet internal environment, the female is more likely to have a significant infection that can have a symptom that includes a vaginal discharge.
- **Was it bloody?** This could indicate problems other than infection, including cancer and trauma.

During the physical examination, direct observation or evaluation of the vulva is rarely necessary for a paramedic's assessment to be considered thorough. In most cases palpation of the lower quadrants of the abdomen can provide enough information about the internal anatomy of the gynecological patient, especially when combined with a good history of the present illness. In addition, do not omit the rest of a physical examination just because the complaint is gynecologic in nature; there could still be systemic effects, as will soon be seen.

Gynecological Conditions and Emergencies

There are various gynecological conditions that can be seen by the paramedic. For gynecological emergencies and transports to the hospital, the basic treatment includes the following:

- Maintain the patient's dignity and provide emotional support if needed.
- Transport the patient in the position of comfort, which can include transporting the patient in the captain's chair or on the bench seat if she is stable. Never transport a patient in the cab of the ambulance.
- If the patient is unstable or may be unstable, provide low-flow oxygen via a nasal cannula to maintain a pulse oximetry rating >95%.
- The patient should be able to be transported to the hospital of choice in most circumstances.

Vaginal Bleeding

Vaginal bleeding can occur for a variety of reasons, many of which the paramedic will not be able to thoroughly evaluate or assess. In patients of childbearing age, vaginal bleeding could be related to their menses. Alterations of menstruation include the following:

- **Hypermenorrhea** (or **menorrhagia**) is abnormally heavy bleeding during a period that lasts longer than usual or contains a larger amount of blood than usual.
- **Polymenorrhea** is a condition where a woman has a period more frequently than once every 24 days and is usually brought on by physical or mental stress.
- **Dysmenorrhea** is painful menses that can be so bad as to interfere with daily life. The patient experiences lower abdominal pain and cramping similar to that of childbirth.
  - Primary dysmenorrhea occurs early in life shortly after menarche, which is a girl's first menses.
  - Secondary dysmenorrhea occurs later in life after previously normal relatively painless menses. It often indicates a genuine gynecological problem.
- **Metrorrhagia** is spotting that occurs in between periods and often is related to hormonal problems or can be a harmless part of ovulation.

Vaginal bleeding that is spontaneous, unrelated to the menstrual cycle, or does not stop is always an abnormal finding. It could indicate cervical or uterine cancer, a new pregnancy, or a serious infection. Vaginal bleeding that presents during a known pregnancy is very ominous and likely indicates a spontaneous abortion if the gestational age is <20 weeks. After 20 weeks, it could still indicate spontaneous abortion, but it also may indicate **placenta previa**, or **abruptio placenta**, which is discussed at length later in this chapter.

Assessment of the patient who complains of vaginal bleeding is highly dependent on history taking.

- Evaluate if there has been any internal or external trauma.
- With empathy, determine whether the patient knows if she is pregnant. Reassure her that just because there is vaginal bleeding does not mean that the pregnancy is terminating, though it could negatively impact it.
- If the patient is not pregnant but of childbearing age, determine if this is in relation to her menses.

Blood loss can be evaluated without requiring the patient to undress: ask how many pads she has used in the past hour or past 24 hours.

The basic treatment discussed earlier applies here. If the patient is not currently wearing a pad, offer her a 5 × 9 dressing or allow her to place a pad before transporting the patient. Encourage the patient not to place a tampon or anything else into the vagina. Evaluate the vital signs as for any patient, and treat hypotension with volume expansion of 500–1,000 mL.

Endometritis

Endometritis is an inflammation of the inner uterine lining, the endometrium. It is most commonly caused by an STD, specifically chlamydia and gonorrhea. Symptoms include lower abdominal pain and pelvic pain. Pain can increase on palpation of the lower abdomen. If the swelling is bad enough, it can lead to constipation and abdominal distension. The patient also will have malaise, fever, and lethargy. Basic gynecological care applies.

Endometriosis

Endometriosis is a condition where the endometrial lining, normally confined to the uterus, grows outside the uterus on the ovaries and abdominal organs. In rare cases, it can even be found in the lungs and other parts of the body as well. It responds to hormones in much the same way that regular endometrium does, so during menstruation, it sloughs off and bleeds in much the same way. Without a clear path out of the body, it causes pain because of the irritation it causes to the peritoneum, called **peritonitis**.

Although it is painless in some women, it can be excruciatingly painful in others. In patients who complain of symptoms, the most common complaint is generalized lower abdominal pain that sometimes spreads around to the back and into the pelvis. Other patients may complain of painful intercourse and bowel movements. Some patients may have increased pain on palpation of the lower quadrants and also have rebound tenderness. Treatment includes basic gynecological care. Pain can be so intense that it may need to be managed with intravenous analgesics if medical control approves.

Ectopic Pregnancy

A pregnancy that occurs anywhere other than within the uterus is called an **ectopic pregnancy**. The most common location for an ectopic pregnancy is within one of the fallopian tubes, with >95% of them occurring within the tube. The other locations include the abdominal cavity and sometimes even on the surface of the ovary. Patients who have had pelvic inflammatory disease (PID), tubal ligation reversal, or previous ectopic pregnancies are at greatest risk. This population of patients is at risk because of scar tissue that may be present in the tubes, blocking the passage of the fertilized oocyte to the normal implantation location in the uterus. The patient may know she is pregnant because all of the usual changes associated with pregnancy occur, including increased progesterone, a positive pregnancy test, and sore and swollen breasts.

Patients will complain of unilateral lower abdominal pain that gradually worsens over a couple of days. The pain may come from the stretching and eventual rupture of the fallopian tube or the spontaneous abortion of the fetus. The patient also may have vaginal bleeding. Blood may accumulate in the abdominal cavity, causing rebound tenderness and diffuse abdominal pain. If the bleeding is excessive in the abdomen, the patient also may have the Cullen sign or the Grey Turner sign.

Patients will very likely need emotional support as well as medical treatment. After performing a complete assessment and ensuring the ABCs are secure, initiate cardiac monitoring and an intravenous line. Administer fluid as needed if hypotension is present. Consult medical control for pain management. Keep the patient warm and treat for shock.

Pelvic Inflammatory Disease

Pelvic inflammatory disease (PID) is an infection of the internal reproductive organs, specifically the uterus, fallopian tubes, and ovaries that occurs almost exclusively as a result of a sexually transmitted infection (STI) in women who are sexually active. The most common organisms causing PID are chlamydia, gonorrhea, candidiasis, and bacterial vaginitis; they infect the lining of the organs and can cause long-lasting reproductive problems such as infertility or scarring in the fallopian tubes, thus increasing the likelihood of an ectopic pregnancy. PID itself is rarely life threatening unless sepsis occurs and the patient goes into shock. Risk factors include frequent sexual activity with multiple sexual partners.

Patients most often will complain of diffuse bilateral lower quadrant achy pain. The patient often will note that the pain gets worse with walking and possibly with intercourse. Patients may state that they have vaginal discharge, fever, chills, and pain or burning on urination. An infection that has spread outside the reproductive tract and into the abdominal cavity may be characterized by rebound tenderness. Treatment includes the basic gynecological care mentioned earlier and symptomatic treatment for pain and hypotension. Septic shock is possible, so be prepared to treat for shock.

Vaginitis

Vaginitis, an inflammation of the vagina, can be caused by 2 organisms.

- *Candida albicans* is a fungus that often causes vaginal yeast infections, which can lead to vaginitis as the pH increases (becomes more basic). The chances of getting vaginitis increase if the patient is taking oral contraceptives, or if she is menstruating, pregnant, or has unprotected intercourse. If *Candida* is the cause, the patient will complain of a burning and itchy feeling in the vagina, as well as pain and soreness during intercourse. She also may note a vaginal discharge that resembles cottage cheese.

- Bacterial vaginitis most often is caused by bacteria in the genus *Gardnerella*, which normally inhabits the vagina. Patients may get this after a recent course of antibiotics because the antibiotic can kill off the good bacteria of the vagina, allowing the *Gardnerella* to grow uninhibited. This can happen regardless of age and can happen in children for the same reasons; it is not exclusively tied to intercourse or sexual activity. If *Gardnerella* is the cause, the patient will complain of a fishy smelling vaginal discharge and an itching, burning sensation.

Treatment for both forms of vaginitis is beyond the scope of the paramedic. Routine transport to a physician would be recommended. There is seldom any emergency associated with these infections.

Sexually Transmitted Diseases (STDs)

While in most cases the paramedic will not diagnose or treat any STDs specifically, a general understanding could prove helpful. Infections that cause PID are most concerning to the paramedic and include chlamydia, gonorrhea, and bacterial vaginitis. Common sexually transmitted infections (STIs) include the following.

- **Chlamydia**, one of the most common STIs, can cause infections of the eye and urethra. It can be treated with antibiotics.

- **Herpes**, a viral infection, can affect different parts of the body. Genital herpes is characterized by sores and blisters in the area of the body that is infected—genitals, mouth, buttocks, or anus. Sores can come and go with outbreaks. Transmission is possible though much less likely in the absence of the sores when the virus is dormant (not active).

- **Gonorrhea**: These bacteria love to grow in warm, dark, moist places and, as a result, can cause an infection in the anus, vagina, and penis as well as the mouth, throat, and eyes. Women are generally asymptomatic until the infection spreads to other organs, particularly when it causes symptoms consistent with PID in addition to painful intercourse and urination. Painful vaginal burning and itching is accompanied by a yellow-green discharge that can sometimes be bloody.

- **Genital warts**, caused by the human papilloma virus (HPV), is **by far the most common STD**. A vaccine is now available for 4 of the known strains of virus; 2 of those strains are responsible for >70% of genital cancers in both men and women. HPV can be passed from the mother to the infant during birth.

- **Syphilis** is an infection with the bacterium *Treponema pallidum*, and while it can be spread in nonsexual ways it most often is spread during sexual activity. Syphilis can occur in stages.

  - Stage 1 is characterized by a chancre that is small, round, and typically painless, which goes away on its own within about 6 weeks.

  - Syphilis can be treated with a single injection of penicillin G at any time during the first 2 stages.

  - In Stage 3 (most chronic stage), the bacteria slowly attacks the heart, eyes, nerves, brain, blood vessels, liver, and bones with meaningful symptoms not becoming evident for years. Symptoms include paralysis, dementia, blindness, Parkinson style tremors, and death.

Toxic Shock Syndrome

Toxic shock syndrome is a form of septic shock that can affect both men and women; however; it is most common in women who use tampons during menses. The sepsis is associated with infection with either *Streptococcus pyogenes* or *Staphylococcus aureus*. Women were believed to get this more often because tampons would leave behind fibrous pieces in the vagina and invite infection. This problem has become much less common since tampon manufacturers improved their products to not leave fibers behind.

Patients will complain of a wide array of complaints, including syncope, fever, sore throat, vomiting, diarrhea, and headache. The patient's condition could quickly deteriorate to shock if antibacterial treatment is not initiated quickly. Kidney and liver failure and DIC are all possible courses for the untreated patient. The patient with toxic shock syndrome must be managed aggressively and treated for shock, including fluid resuscitation and treating any cardiac dysrhythmias that are present.

Ruptured Ovarian Cyst and Ovarian Torsion

Ovarian cysts are formed on a regular basis and house the developing oocyte before it is released during ovulation. Occasionally, these cysts do not rupture and release the ovum; these cysts disappear spontaneously and rarely cause an issue. Occasionally, however, after normal ovulation, the now empty cyst fills with blood and begins to stretch. This stretch will cause a dull achy pain on one side of the lower abdomen. As the cyst stretches, pressure builds up, leading to rupture. When an ovarian cyst ruptures, sudden, intense pain quickly follows. This pain starts in a lower abdominal quadrant and can radiate throughout the abdomen and to the back. It also may be accompanied by rebound tenderness from blood in the peritoneum as well as nausea and vomiting.

Ovarian torsion occurs when an ovary twists on the ligament to which it is attached. This can cause pain and symptoms similar to that of a ruptured ovarian cyst and is usually caused by an ovarian cyst that has not ruptured.

Treatment for each condition is primarily aimed at pain relief and making the patient comfortable. This often is described as the worst pain a woman has felt, so fentanyl or morphine are appropriate treatments. Initiate an intravenous line on the patient for medication administration, but fluids are not likely to be needed. Because nausea and vomiting are common symptoms with both conditions, 4 mg ondansetron can be administered. The patient should be transported in a position of comfort if one can be found.

Prolapsed Uterus

A **prolapsed uterus** is not a particularly common condition, but it occurs when the uterus drops from its normal position and sometimes becomes visible outside the body. Women who have had multiple vaginal births are at risk for this condition. Women age 65 and older are at risk for this condition regardless of birthing history because the ligaments that hold the uterus suspended in the abdomen weaken over time.

The patient may complain of feeling as if something is bulging in her vagina or may complain of lower abdominal pressure, particularly upon standing. A visual genital examination (a rare occurrence for a paramedic) should be performed; evaluate the vaginal opening for anything protruding from it. If there is tissue present, do not attempt to replace it or push it back into the vagina. Instead, lightly cover the tissue with moist sterile dressings and transport the patient to the hospital. If the patient is in severe pain, contact medical control for orders on administering analgesia.

Sexual Assault

Sexual assault can occur to any person, not just a woman, of any age at any time. The most common type of assault is rape. Children and older adults represent some of the most common targets. Sexual assault can involve more than just penetration of the patient's body and often involves injuries to the rest of the body beyond just the genitalia.

Assessment

Sexual assault is a crime; consequently, the patient is essentially a crime scene. Questioning of the patient should be done only as the patient allows. Very often, the patient will not want to recount what just happened. Focus the assessment on what hurts and what the patient needs treated. As in any gynecologic emergency, professionalism, support, and empathy are of the utmost importance. From initial contact, ask if the patient prefers a male or female provider in the back of the ambulance; the patient may not feel comfortable with a person of the same sex as the assailant. Make every effort to make this happen. In addition, it is recommended that more than one person who is not associated with the patient accompany the patient in the back of the ambulance. This precaution is to establish more than one independent observer to what happens there and to avoid implicating EMS or police in the assault.

For multiple reasons, the physical assessment of the genitals is not recommended. First, any examination may remove valuable evidence from the perpetrator. Second, this is generally a sensitive spot for any assessment to take place, and the assault only compounds that fact. Third, there often is nothing different that the paramedic will do after assessing this area. Only in cases of impaled objects and life-threatening bleeding should this area be evaluated on any patient, male or female. The remainder of the assessment should be completed as time allows and should be thorough so that other medical or traumatic findings are not missed.

Treatment for the patient who has been assaulted centers on providing comfort and addressing pain and anxiety. Deciding to treat pain and anxiety should be left to the discretion of the medical control physician because these medications can possibly alter the patient's ability to recall events accurately in the near term when the investigation is in the most critical stage.

Crime Scene Preservation

In a sexual assault, as with any assault, stabbing, or gunshot wounds, victims of a crime and the scenes in which they are found need to be preserved and documented. This way, law enforcement can still do their important investigation while EMS provides care to the victims. With this in mind, EMS providers should always follow the direction of law enforcement, even if it makes on scene care more difficult. The goal on any crime scene is to carefully gather the patient and get off the scene as swiftly as possible. This goal will help prevent the providers from leaving something behind or inadvertently having evidence cling to them as they move about the scene.

The patient's body is essentially a crime scene and should be treated that way. Employ the following measures to help preserve evidence for collection at the hospital.

- Prevent the patient from washing their hands or any part of the body because this can eliminate evidence.
- Remove any clothing cautiously and deliberately. If clothes need to be removed as part of the normal course of critical patient treatment, avoid cutting through any holes, especially those that could have resulted from a bullet or a knife. Avoid cutting or contacting blood or semen stains. Try to stay near a normal seam.
- Any clothing that is removed should be placed in paper bags and held for evidence. Plastic bags should not be used because these will allow mold to grow and possibly destroy trace physical evidence.
- Place the patient's hands into paper bags and secure them with tape to the wrists. This may be done by police prior to EMS arrival but should be done before the patient has the opportunity to touch other objects and lose evidence.

Documentation

Document anything that is observed or experienced on the scene or with the patient. The EMS providers will likely be called to provide testimonial evidence during a trial if it occurs. **Testimonial evidence** is evidence that witnesses provide from oral documentation or facts. It is helpful to incorporate such evidence into the patient care chart clearly and factually, free from embellishment or opinion. Anything the patient tells you during the transport should be documented; use quotes whenever possible and avoid paraphrasing.

Any treatment conducted on the patient needs to be clearly documented, especially intravenous attempts, intramuscular or subcutaneous medication administration, and any medication given. Any missed and successful intravenous location should be documented clearly because, if this patient does not survive, the coroner may mistake the hole the paramedic put in the patient as a place where an assailant injected a medication to facilitate the assault. Any medication you give should be accurately documented as well, especially sedatives and narcotics, because a perpetrator can use these on their victims to make them easier targets. It is for this reason that a medical control physician is not likely to order these types of medications to be given until blood can be legally drawn to test for drugs in the patient's system prior to arrival at the hospital.

OBSTETRICS

This section will cover everything related to birth. It begins with a discussion on conception and fetal development, including fetal circulation. Maternal changes during pregnancy will be discussed along with medical issues that can go along with these changes. Next will be preterm emergencies associated with pregnancy. This section will then conclude with a review of the stages of labor during normal deliveries. Since the APGAR Score is determined before the conclusion of the third stage of labor, it is included in this section as part of the continuum of perinatal care.

Pregnancy Anatomy and Physiology

As the ovum passes through the fallopian tubes, if it encounters sperm within approximately 24 hours of ovulation, fertilization may occur. Fertilization of the ovum usually occurs in a fallopian tube. After fertilization, the fertilized ovum, now called a **zygote**, continues to travel down the fallopian tube and implants in the endometrial lining somewhere within the uterus where it will grow and develop into an embryo and then into a fetus. Implantation happens about a week after fertilization.

By the time of implantation, the zygote has undergone multiple rounds of cellular division and is now called a **blastocyst**. What was once a single cell, by the time of implantation has features that will become the fetus, placenta, and amniotic sac. Implantation can cause some spotty painless bleeding that may be alarming to the mother who does not yet know she is pregnant or dismissed easily as early, light menstruation.

Implantation causes a cascade of changes in the mother as well. Shortly after implantation, the union of the blastocyst with the endometrial lining signals the lining to begin to release hCG, which stimulates the corpus luteum in the ovary to continue to release progesterone. Progesterone is responsible for maintaining the endometrial lining throughout pregnancy. Within 10 days from implantation (<3 weeks after conception), the embryo has developed a placenta, an umbilical cord, and an amniotic sac, and the rudiments of a heart have already begun to beat rhythmically.

By the end of the third week of pregnancy, the circulatory system is complete with some vasculature, a heart, and red blood cells. The neurological system is beginning to develop, and distinct areas of the brain can be differentiated. By the end of the fourth week, extensive folding of a previously basically flat embryo has given rise to the cranial vault, spinal cord, and the chest and abdominal cavities. The digestive tract also begins to develop, oriented by the location of the brain. The brain is essentially complete with all the distinct features it will have in simply smaller versions; growth will continue in the brain to enlarge itself for several weeks to come. Limb buds also begin to appear once the spinal cord is complete.

Over the next several weeks, development will continue at a rapid rate. The digestive system with all the accessory organs is visible and essentially complete by the end of the sixth week. The eyes have begun to take shape and orient themselves near the brain. The kidneys will be completely formed and functioning by the end of the 6th week, and glucagon is being produced by the fetal pancreas. From about the eighth week on, the structures critical to life outside the womb have developed, and the musculoskeletal system continues to develop bone, cartilage, tendons, and muscles. The fetus will not be capable of survival outside the womb for about another 4 months, however, because it is still too small. After the 28th week of gestation, the fetus is said to be viable if it is born prematurely, although it still requires extensive care.

The infant floats in a watery fluid called **amniotic fluid** or **amnion,** which is contained within the **amniotic sac** and serves to provide an essentially weightless environment in which the infant will develop. Later on, the fetus will consume the amnion and pass wastes into the fluid, so it also serves an excretory function.

The umbilical cord and placenta connect the fetus to the mother. The fetus gets all its O_2 and nourishment from the mother via these structures. Nearly everything the mother consumes can pass across the placental barrier, including sugar, protein, water, alcohol, and most illicit and prescription drugs. Though drugs of any kind are a concern throughout pregnancy, they are most dangerous during the rapid development that occurs between the third and eighth weeks. During these weeks in particular, drugs can interfere with proper formation of the circulatory and nervous systems in particular but also the digestive and endocrine systems.

Fetal Circulation

The fetal circulation is different from that of the independent person. The veins carry oxygenated blood away from the placenta and toward the fetus, whereas the arteries carry deoxygenated blood toward the placenta and away from the fetus. A way to remember this is that the **A**rteries carry blood **A**way from the fetus and therefore are **A**noxic (without O_2).

Within the fetus, circulatory differences also are present. Because the lungs of the fetus are not responsible for oxygenation of the blood until after birth, it is energetically favorable to the newborn to largely bypass the pulmonary circuit. Blood that enters the right atrium of the heart has already been oxygenated from the placenta and can pass as expected into the right ventricle, but it also can pass through the **foramen ovale** directly into the left atrium. The blood that goes directly into the left atrium is then eventually pumped to the rest of the body through the aorta as normal.

The blood that entered the right ventricle also has 2 options: some blood will go to the lungs to nourish the cells of the lungs themselves, but some blood will pass from the pulmonary artery directly into the aorta through the **ductus arteriosus**. This bypasses the pulmonary circuit and helps deliver the most blood to the body as possible with each beat.

Within 30 minutes after the neonate takes its first breath after delivery, the ductus arteriosus and foramen ovale will close, establishing adult circulatory pathways. Pay particular attention to the areas that blood has a choice of direction.

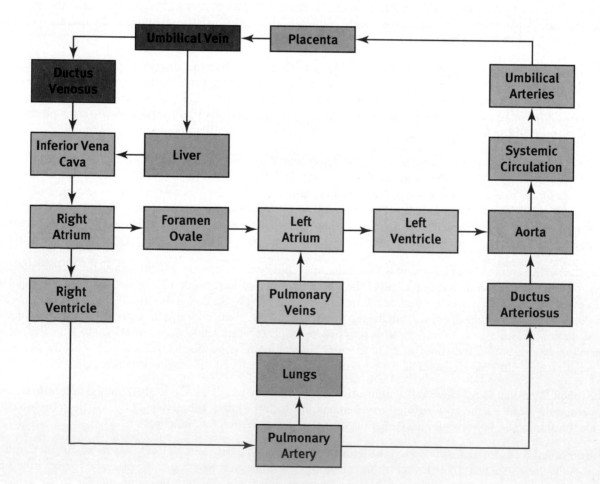

Figure 7-4. Chart of Fetal Circulation

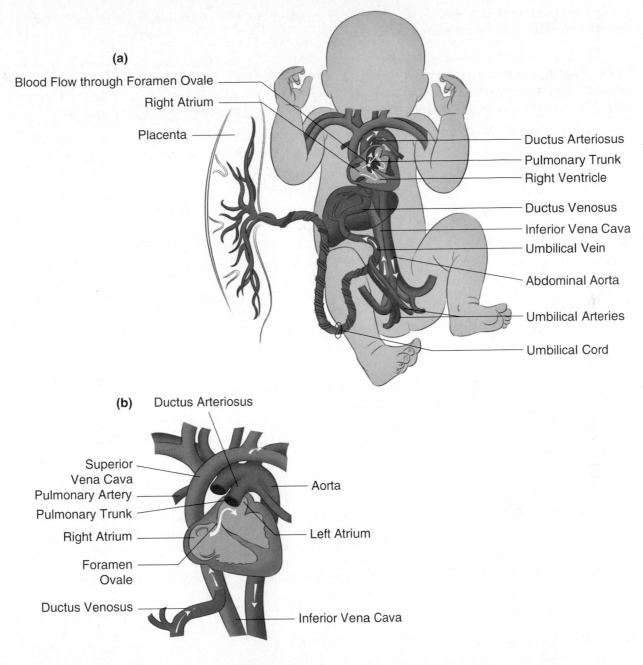

(a)

Blood Flow through Foramen Ovale

Right Atrium

Placenta

Ductus Arteriosus

Pulmonary Trunk

Right Ventricle

Ductus Venosus

Inferior Vena Cava

Umbilical Vein

Abdominal Aorta

Umbilical Arteries

Umbilical Cord

(b) Ductus Arteriosus

Superior Vena Cava

Pulmonary Artery

Pulmonary Trunk

Right Atrium

Foramen Ovale

Ductus Venosus

Aorta

Left Atrium

Inferior Vena Cava

Figure 7-5. Fetal Circulation
(a) Systemic fetal circulation. (b) Enlarged view of fetal circulation highlighting the 3 fetal shunts.

Maternal Changes During Pregnancy

The gravid female also experiences many physiologic and anatomic changes during pregnancy to be able to carry and metabolically support the growing fetus. Changes occur in the circulatory system, the urinary system, and the digestive system.

Circulatory Changes

Blood volume increases by approximately 50% during the course of pregnancy, increasing the volume from about 4.5 L to approximately 7 L. This increase is necessary to meet the perfusion needs of the fetus as well as maintain the perfusion of all maternal organs, particularly the kidneys. Furthermore, this prepares the mother for delivery, where the mother can lose in excess of 500 mL of blood during a normal spontaneous vaginal delivery (NSVD) and sometimes as much as 1,000 mL during a cesarean section. This excess volume allows for an autotransfusion of blood from the uterus as it contracts back to maternal circulation.

Red and white blood cell counts increase during pregnancy. The red blood cell count increases by nearly 35%, which is why most women take prenatal vitamins or, more recently, simply an iron-containing multivitamin. The increased rate of erythropoiesis makes an iron supplement essential; without it, pregnant women can suffer from pregnancy-related iron-deficiency anemia. White blood cell counts typically triple during the course of the pregnancy.

The maternal heart actually increases in size to be able to handle the polycythemia and increased circulating volume by anywhere from 10% to 15%. This increases overall cardiac output about 40% from about the 22nd week of pregnancy through the end. Helping increase the cardiac output, the heart rate also increases to a new normal resting rate about 20 beats per minute higher than before the mother was pregnant.

Respiratory Changes

The respiratory system experiences stress as well and for a variety of reasons. First, a lot more blood is circulating that needs to be oxygenated. Second, the mother's overall O_2 demand has increased to meet her increased metabolism as well as the fat metabolism of the developing fetus. Third, as the fetus develops and the uterine fundus pushes superiorly, it will push the abdominal contents against the diaphragm. This is initially compensated, limiting the ability of the mother to expand her chest cavity. This results in an overall decrease to the tidal volume in late stages; however, early on, the tidal volume and minute volume increase, each by as much as 50%.

Urinary System Changes

The kidneys increase in size by up to 30%, and the ureters can actually increase in diameter to accommodate the increase in urinary output. Consequently, the mother increases the amount of urinary output volume, therefore increasing the frequency of urination. Complicating the increased urine volume produced is a marked decrease in the volume of the urinary bladder. This is why pregnant women feel as if they are constantly urinating!

GI and Metabolic Changes

The GI system experiences decreased motility because of increased progesterone levels, which can lead to heartburn and belching. It also can exacerbate vomiting if food stays in the stomach for too long. The weight of the fundus on the lower intestines, coupled with decreased overall motility, can lead to constipation. The combined metabolism of the mother to accommodate the weight gain and structural changes as well as provide for the fetus's metabolic needs often can lead to an increase in carbohydrate intake. Women can develop diabetes during pregnancy, called **gestational diabetes**, as a combined result of increased carbohydrate intake and cellular decline in insulin sensitivity despite an increase in insulin production in the pancreas.

General Assessment of the Pregnant Patient

First, let's clarify some pregnancy-specific terminology.

- **Gravidity.** The number of times a person has been pregnant, regardless of outcome of the pregnancies. If a patient is pregnant with multiple fetuses, she is still pregnant only once.
- **Parity.** The number of births the patient has had (including stillbirths).
- **Abortions.** The number of spontaneous or elective abortions a patient has had. Spontaneous abortions are any fetal deaths that occur at <20 weeks of gestation; elective abortions can occur at any gestational age.
- **Living.** The number of live children the mother has born. This is strictly an infant who had any pulse or respiratory activity. It does not change if the infant was not able to survive. The number increases only if the infant was born after 20 weeks.

Using this GPAL shorthand method, a patient who was currently pregnant with one child and had viable twins from a previous pregnancy with no prior elective abortions would be G:2, P:2, A:0, L:2. Once this hypothetical mother has the child from her current pregnancy, the numbers would change to G:2, P:3, A:0, L:3. Some physicians may break down the parity number further to clarify term and preterm. Preterm would be any infant born prior to 36 weeks of gestation.

- **Nulligravida.** A female who has never been pregnant.
- **Nulliparous.** A female who has not given birth.
- **Primigravida.** A female who is pregnant for the first time.
- **Multigravida.** A female who has been pregnant more than once, regardless of outcome.
- **Multiparity.** Having given birth multiple times.
- **Grand multiparity.** A female who has given birth more than 5 times.

The history of the pregnant patient is not materially different from that of any other adult patient. As with any other patient, investigate the chief complaint, independent of the pregnancy, while keeping in mind how this may all be affecting the fetus. Keep in mind during the assessment of any female of childbearing age that she may be pregnant.

Once it is confirmed that the patient is pregnant, specific pregnancy questions should be asked. First find the GPAL values for the patient and document any history of abortion of any kind. Higher numbers of pregnancies that concluded with vaginal deliveries could result in a precipitous delivery, meaning the infant could deliver remarkably fast. Determine how the previous pregnancies ended, paying particular attention to any cesarean section history, especially if vaginal delivery is imminent. Vaginal birth after cesarean can be complicated and carries an increased risk of uterine rupture. In addition, determine if the patient has had prenatal care of any kind and if the physician has any concerns about the pregnancy or delivery.

Antepartum Complications Related to Pregnancy

Many problems are unique to the pregnant population. This section will look at the conditions that a woman could face exclusively because she is pregnant. This will include any problem related to pregnancy, not problems related to delivery. Each section will contain pathophysiology and assessment points to identify the problem, using both interrogation and the physical examination, and treatment options for the paramedic to consider.

Supine Hypotension Syndrome

Because of the increasing size and weight of the fundus, the expanded uterus, patients who are in their third trimester should not lie on their back. This can cause **supine hypotension syndrome**, which results from the fundus lying on and compressing the inferior vena cava and possibly also the aorta. This can materially interfere with blood returning to the heart from the lower extremities and abdomen, possibly leading the patient to pass out after about 5–7 minutes if left uncorrected. Maternal hypotension means the placenta, and by extension the fetus, will be hypoperfused. Extended hypoperfusion of the fetus could result in fetal demise.

Patients will start to show early signs of shock before they pass out, including anxiety, nausea, dizziness, and tachycardia. If the patient is supine, such as if she has to be confined to a backboard, suspect this as a cause. The condition can be remedied if the backboard is tilted toward the patient's left, or if the patient is allowed to lie in the left lateral recumbent position. If patient condition does not improve after these maneuvers, consider fluid resuscitation.

Hyperemesis Gravidarum

Hyperemesis gravidarum is a condition where the patient has excessive vomiting episodes, often more than 4x daily. The cause is unknown but seems to be related to particularly high hCG concentrations in the blood. Patients with this condition often are sensitive to smells that can trigger vomiting. This can be so bad as to affect electrolyte balances and pH and water balance in the body. Patients often are hypovolemic and may be hypoglycemic as well.

The assessment of these patients is a general assessment that should include orthostatic vital signs if the patient is capable. Assess the skin and mucous membranes for evidence of dehydration. In addition to preparing for more vomiting during patient contact—which could be projectile vomiting—transport the patient in a position of comfort and initiate ECG monitoring and an intravenous line of NSS. If the patient is hypotensive or tachycardic, consider administering 500 mL NSS. Check the blood glucose level and administer 25 g D50 if <60 mg/dL. To help control vomiting, administer 4 mg ondansetron intravenously and 50 mg diphenhydramine intravenously or intramuscularly if medical control permits.

Hypertensive Disorders

Hypertension in the pregnant patient is a significant cause for concern, particularly if it began during the pregnancy.

- Hypertension that began before the pregnancy is not necessarily an immediate threat.
- Pregnancy-induced hypertension, by contrast, is often a sign of preeclampsia, a group of early warning signs that the patient may have eclampsia. Symptoms of **preeclampsia** include edema (usually of the face, hands, ankles); protein in the urine; and hypertension, all of which began or worsened after the 20th week of pregnancy. Preexisting renal problems, diabetes, and the African American race predispose a patient to preeclampsia. A patient who has a seizure in addition to these symptoms is diagnosed with **eclampsia**. Treatment for preeclampsia in the prehospital environment includes high-flow O_2, especially if the systolic blood pressure (SBP) is >160 or the diastolic blood pressure (DBP) is >105. Transport comfortably but quickly, preferably to the hospital of choice, possibly for emergent delivery.
- First-line treatment of seizures from eclampsia is 4–6 g magnesium sulfate administered over approximately 15 minutes. Seizing will usually stop with just the loading dose. For extended transport times, a maintenance infusion of magnesium should be initiated at 1–2 g/hr and should be slowed if the patient shows a declining mental status. Although magnesium will likely control the seizure, if it persists, 4 mg lorazepam is the next line drug of choice. Blood pressure should be monitored and not treated prehospital because it needs to be slowly lowered to avoid fetal compromise. However, medical control may order 20–40 mg of labetalol every 15 minutes, or 5–10 mg of hydralazine every 10 minutes as needed to maintain SBP 140–160 mmHg and DBP 90–110 mmHg.

Gestational Diabetes Mellitus

As mentioned earlier in this section, the patient may develop diabetes as a result of being pregnant. The patient may present similar to any patient who is diagnosed with diabetes and is not pregnant and may have high or low blood sugar levels. This can be assessed and managed as previously discussed.

Toxoplasmosis

Toxoplasmosis is a parasitic infection that women can get, most commonly from handling cat litter or ingesting food contaminated with the parasite. Pregnant women are encouraged to eat only thoroughly cooked meat and to not change cat litter boxes. This disease does not have any symptoms and is detectable only with a blood test. Newborns also do not show any specific symptoms, but they may develop learning, visual, and hearing difficulties later in life.

Vaginal Bleeding During Pregnancy

This chapter has already discussed one of the major reasons for bleeding in the pregnant patient: the ectopic pregnancy. But several other conditions unique to the pregnant patient can involve spontaneous vaginal bleeding.

Abortion

Abortion is the expulsion and death of a fetus prior to being viable outside the uterus. (Depending on the text, this can be at any time prior to 20 or 28 weeks of gestation.) For consistency, this text will use **20 weeks as the cutoff**. What follows is an explanation of the degrees of abortion the paramedic may encounter in the field.

In **spontaneous abortion,** the body ends the pregnancy without warning. This can be caused by chromosomal abnormalities in the fetus, from a failed implantation, or from failed maintenance of progesterone from either the corpus luteum or the placenta. Illicit drug use increases the possibility of spontaneous abortion. In most cases, no definite cause can be identified. Treatment is limited to emotional support and prevention of shock. If the patient has not already done so prior to EMS arrival on the scene, apply a pad to the vagina but do not pack the vagina.

Elective abortion is a type of abortion that is a conscious decision on the part of the mother to end the pregnancy. If carried out in a doctor's office, hospital, or clinic, there are not nearly as many complications as when the mother takes it upon herself to elicit the abortion. Toxic herbal and chemical preparations can be taken that make the blood toxic to the fetus, which also may have negative effects on the mother. A person desperate to end a pregnancy may insert various instruments into the uterus in an attempt to forcibly detach the placenta from the endometrium, which can lead to profuse and life-threatening bleeding. When facing a patient who has had or attempted to perform an elective abortion, remember to be professional and reserve judgment.

In a threatened abortion, conditions that threaten the survival of the pregnant person (e.g., dehydration, malnutrition) bring that patient close to having a spontaneous abortion. Reversal of the causative problem often can halt the abortion, and the mother can carry to term or closer to it. Alternatively, a threatened abortion may proceed all the way to a complete abortion or become an incomplete abortion. Patients who have experienced a threatened abortion and still have a viable pregnancy (fetal heart tones are present, and the fetus is moving as before) are usually placed on near total bed rest to prevent such symptoms from happening again. In a threatened abortion, although the fetus's viability is threatened, it remains alive, the cervix remains closed (this is not assessed by paramedics), and fetal and placental tissue has not been passed. Treatment is aimed at supportive care for any presenting symptoms and should include emotional sensitivity and professionalism on the part of the responders.

In an **inevitable abortion**, the cervix has dilated; vaginal bleeding often is profuse and contains clots and may contain endometrial, placental, or fetal tissue. In this case, the abortion is not yet complete but cannot be stopped or reversed. Treatment should include emotional support whenever possible, but aggressive fluid resuscitation and treatment of shock are priorities.

If a threatened abortion is not successfully treated, it may proceed to become an **incomplete abortion**, in which only a portion of the products of conception—fetus, placenta, and amnion—are expelled while some remain in the uterus. An inevitable abortion may conclude as an incomplete abortion and require medical care to become a complete abortion. A complete abortion is where none of the products of conception remain in the uterus. Treatment for an incomplete abortion cannot be done in the field, and a paramedic's care is limited to emotional support and treatment of any other secondary symptoms, such as septic or hypovolemic shock.

On rare occasions, the fetus may die, but the body does not expel it. This is a **missed abortion**. Treatment for a missed abortion is dilation of the cervix and curettage, which is scraping of the endometrial lining.

Abruptio Placenta

Abruptio placenta occurs when the placenta begins to detach from the uterine wall prematurely, often long before the infant has actually been delivered. There are many causes for this condition, including drug and alcohol abuse and smoking, but the most common reason is maternal hypertension. External blunt trauma is the next most common reason. Abruptio placenta may result in slight, moderate, or profuse vaginal bleeding and should be considered in cases of vaginal bleeding in late-term pregnancies. It is possible for the patient to lose a lot of blood to the point of being hypotensive yet show no or minimal external bleeding. The placenta or amniotic sac can prevent the blood from actually escaping the vagina. Therefore, placental abruption should be considered whenever the pregnant patient in the 3rd trimester appears to be in shock.

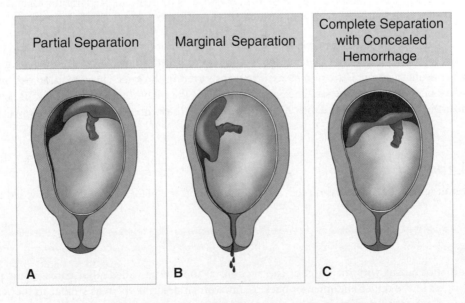

Figure 7-6. Abruptio Placenta Presentations

Treatment for placental abruption is supportive and should include high-flow O$_2$, intravenous fluid infused at a rate to maintain a SBP >100 mmHg, and rapid transport to a hospital capable of handling emergency deliveries.

Placenta Previa

Placenta previa occurs when implantation has occurred low in the uterus and the placenta develops over the cervical os, or opening. Placenta previa can be described as marginal, partial, or complete, depending on its relationship with the os. In a marginal placenta previa, the placental edge lies extremely close to the os and could impact NSVD. In partial placenta previa, the placenta does obstruct the os to a measurable degree. The placenta completely covers the os in complete placenta previa.

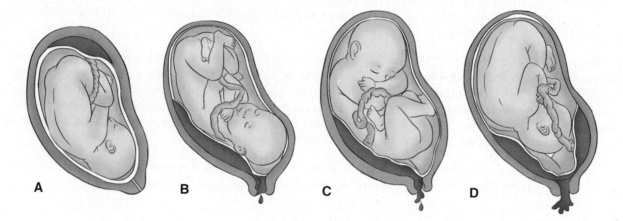

Figure 7-7. Types of Placenta Previa
(A) Normal placenta. (B) Marginal placenta previa. (C) Partial placenta previa. (D) Total or complete placenta previa.

This condition can be completely unknown to the mother who has not received any prenatal care and does not present a problem to either the fetus or the mother until delivery. In the patient who has had prenatal care, the mother will be scheduled for a cesarean section at about the 38th week of gestation to minimize the possibility of the body initiating natural childbirth. There is only one way out of the uterus naturally for the infant, and in the case of placenta previa, it is through its own blood supply. As the cervix starts to dilate in preparation for natural childbirth, vaginal bleeding will begin and remain constant or increase over time.

Treatment for the patient with placenta previa is the same as for abruption placenta: prepare for and treat for shock. In placenta previa, the paramedic should encourage the patient to breathe slowly and deeply through contractions to help the mother avoid pushing. Patients also may be transported in the knee-chest position, where the mother's knees and chest are in contact with the stretcher, and her pelvis is the highest part of her body. This will temporarily help minimize the pressure of the infant on the placenta and "buy time" to get to the hospital without more bleeding.

Stages of Labor

Labor is the overall term for the process of delivering the fetus and the placenta and can be divided into 3 distinct phases.

Stage 1 of Labor

The first stage of labor begins with the onset of contractions of the uterus, called labor pains. These pains begin as an achy feeling, often in the upper abdomen or back. Many women describe them as similar to that crampy feeling that a person would get with diarrhea. Initially, the contractions may be as far apart as about 15 minutes, but they tend to get closer together as labor progresses. The timing of these contractions is typically measured from the beginning of a contraction to the beginning of the next, and the duration of a contraction is how long the pain lasts before fully subsiding. It is important as part of the assessment of the pregnant patient with contractions to measure and report both how long they last and the time in between each.

As the uterus contracts, the infant is forced into the cervix and eventually the vagina. As this happens, 3 major changes happen to the cervix. First, the cervix shortens and becomes thinner (called **effacement**). As this is happening, the os of the cervix begins to dilate and gets larger in diameter, eventually achieving a diameter of about 10 cm. Neither of these measurements and assessment points are something the paramedic will measure because these measurements are internal and require extensive training; however, it may be reported to the paramedic during an interfacility transport. Delivery is imminent when the patient is fully dilated and 100% effaced. A fully dilated cervix signals the end of the first stage of labor and the beginning of the second. It often is at a point prior to the presentation of the head that the bag of waters (i.e., amniotic sac) ruptures (breaks), releasing a gush of amniotic fluid.

Stage 2 of Labor

The second stage of labor begins when the head of the infant is visible with simple inspection of the vulva, essentially simultaneous with full dilation of the cervix. The presentation of the head is called **crowning**. Although any part of the infant can present, the head is by far the most common, with the buttocks presentation (**breach**) being the second most common. If the head presents, it will generally be face down and flexed with the chin in contact with the chest. At this point, contractions are typically <3 minutes apart, the strongest they have been thus far during labor, and often last a full minute, making them seem nearly constant to the mother.

As the head begins to present, it is incumbent on the paramedic to remain calm and appear in control, while assisting in a completely natural process. It often is difficult to decide whether to transport the patient who presents with contractions or stay on scene and await delivery. Some factors to consider in making this decision are as follows:

- The number of previous births the patient has had
- The duration of the contractions
- The interval of the contractions
- The mother feeling as if she needs to have a bowel movement
- Presentation of the head
- Whether the mother has had prenatal care
- If the patient is considered a high-risk pregnancy

Contractions of a frequent interval and long duration signal an imminent birth. If a mother has had multiple births prior to the current pending delivery, this delivery often will be much faster—on the order of minutes rather than a couple of hours that is typical of nulliparous patients. If the patient says that she needs to have a bowel movement, do not allow her because this reflex is caused by the infant pressing on the rectum similar to feces preceding a bowel movement. If the patient is considered at high risk or has not had meaningful prenatal care, unless delivery is imminent, it may be worth attempting to get to a hospital capable of high-risk deliveries rather than stay on scene.

If any of these are present, it is highly recommended to stay at scene and perform an emergency delivery. Establish a clean, preferably sterile, area around the patient but particularly under the mother's buttocks and between her legs and prepare the OB kit every ambulance should have.

The following are the steps and events that occur during the second stage of labor:

1. Position the mother in a semifowlers position with her knees drawn up to her chest. Have other personnel assist with this and prop her back up against something firm or have her partner or spouse support her. In addition, it is worth having another ambulance crew on scene with you because once the child is delivered, there will be two patients. If there is time, don gloves, mask, eye shield or goggles, and a gown. This will not be a clean event.

2. Once the infant has crowned, apply gentle pressure on the newborn's head during any contraction and attempt the mother makes to push. The goal here is to prevent an explosive delivery, which could lead to

vaginal tears. During the intermission between contractions, encourage the mother to rest and catch her breath. During this time, keep the labia moist.

3. As the head begins to emerge, it will naturally turn, typically toward the mother's left. Support the head as it comes out and do not resist this turn. If the bag of waters has not ruptured by this time, carefully tear it with your fingers or with the forceps or the scalpel from the OB kit to allow the amniotic fluid to drain.

4. After the head is completely out of the vagina, slip a finger alongside the neck to check for a **nuchal cord**— the umbilical cord wrapped around the neck—and loosen it or attempt to loop it over the infant's head. Another option would be to clamp the cord in two places and cut in between the clamps, being careful to not cut the infant or mother, if you are unable to loop the cord over the head.

5. Still with only the head of the infant out, and using the bulb syringe in the OB kit, suction the infant's mouth then nose, making sure to get in the pockets of the cheeks when suctioning the mouth. Always suction them in alphabetical order: mouth then nose. Accomplish this by squeezing the bulb outside the infant and then insert the tip with the bulb compressed. After the tip is in the desired location, let go of the bulb, allowing it to reinflate and suck up the mucus and amnion in the mouth and nose.

6. On the next contraction, guide the infant's top shoulder out of the mother by applying gentle traction downward, being careful to not push too hard on the infant's head, which could cause nerve damage to the infant. Once that shoulder is free from its likely hang-up on the pubic bone, lift up on the infant's head, still during the contraction. This should free the lower shoulder from the perineum.

7. Once the shoulders are free, the torso, pelvis, and legs will deliver quite rapidly. Be prepared to hold the infant as it emerges. Remember, it is very slippery and wet. Set the newborn down on the area between the patient's legs. It is essential to keep it at the same level or lower than the vagina until the cord is cut.

8. If the paramedic is comfortable and it has not already been done, now is the time to clamp the cord and cut it between the clamps once it has stopped pulsing. One clamp should be placed at about 7 inches from the neonate and the other about 10 inches from the neonate whenever possible. If the paramedic is not comfortable cutting the cord, leave the newborn at this level to prevent flow of blood out of the infant and into the placenta.

9. Suction the mouth and nose again if needed. Dry the infant and wrap them in a dry blanket to preserve body heat. Place the neonate on the mother's belly if she is able to hold the newborn.

10. Assess an Apgar score and record the time of birth for the patient care report and the legal time of birth.

11. Proceed with newborn resuscitation guidelines from later in this chapter if needed.

The delivery of the child concludes the second stage of labor.

Stage 3 of Labor

The third stage of labor begins once the neonate is fully delivered and concludes with the delivery of the placenta. The placenta will be approximately the size of a dessert plate. Do not tug on the remainder of the umbilical cord in an attempt to accelerate this process. Within about 30 minutes, the placenta should deliver with a few more contractions. If after an hour the placenta has not yet delivered, transport the patient to the hospital because this may indicate a problem. Place the placenta in a plastic bag and bring it to the hospital; the physician will check it to ensure that the entire placenta has been expelled. Placenta retained in the uterus can lead to a lethal postpartum hemorrhage.

APGAR Scoring

The **Apgar score** is an assessment tool that assigns a numerical value to each assessment point. The score is calculated officially at 1 and 5 minutes of life, although the tool can be used at any time to evaluate the vitality of the newborn. For each section, assign the best score for the neonate from 0 to 2 and total the score for the 5 sections. Normal infants score 7 and higher.

Table 7-1. The Apgar Score

Letter	Meaning	Score	Description
A	Appearance/ skin color	2	Completely pink
		1	Peripheral cyanosis (hands and feet)
		0	Central cyanosis
P	Pulse	2	>100
		1	Present but <100
		0	Absent
G	Grimace: irritability	2	Avoids noxious stimulus
		1	Weak avoidance of stimulus
		0	None
A	Activity: muscle tone	2	Actively resists extension of extremities
		1	Weakly resists extension of extremities
		0	None/limp
R	Respiratory rate	2	Forceful cry
		1	Slow respiratory rate or gasping
		0	None
0–3 Severely depressed, critically ill newborn			
4–6 Moderately depressed, monitor closely, transport rapidly			
7–10 Normal			

PERINATAL COMPLICATIONS OF LABOR

Some issues may come up during the process of labor that the paramedic needs to be able to recognize and treat. These issues often are not predicted through ultrasounds available with prenatal care and can crop up in any patient.

Premature Rupture of Membranes

Premature membrane rupture occurs when the bag of waters ruptures more than an hour prior to the onset of labor. There are several possible outcomes to this condition. First, it may heal, and the pregnancy will continue as if nothing happened. Second, this could lead to infection if labor cannot proceed, which could later result in loss of the pregnancy. Finally, and most commonly, labor will either begin naturally or through medicinal induction within about 48 hours. This is not something that will affect the delivery overall; the paramedic should be aware that rupture of membranes does not, by itself, predict delivery.

Meconium Staining

Meconium is the infant's first bowel movement. This ordinarily happens after birth; however, when the infant is under duress, it will pass this stool into the amnion as part of its panic. Ordinarily, the amniotic fluid is clear to a slight pale yellow. Meconium-stained amniotic fluid that represents fetal distress is foul smelling, sticky, and greenish black. Fetal distress can be caused by any number of conditions, including nuchal cord, fetal developmental problems, trauma, hypoxia, and abruptio placenta.

The infant, for the entire time it is in the uterus, inhales the amnion, and this will include the meconium-stained amnion. If the mother has passed meconium-stained amniotic fluid, the paramedic must prepare for the potential delivery of a very sick infant. The infant may not be breathing or may be breathing ineffectively and require extensive support to survive. More will be covered on the topic of newborn resuscitation later.

Uterine Rupture

Uterine rupture may occur during delivery, particularly if the patient has any kind of scar tissue in the uterus, such as what may occur from a previous cesarean section. This could prove to be lethal to both the infant and the mother because of the inability to expel the infant and extensive bleeding from the uterus and possibly the placenta. If this happens while in the paramedic's care, the patient may be able to relate that she once had strong contractions, but recent contractions have felt weaker. This is proceeding in the wrong direction; contractions should get stronger as they progress toward delivery. Patients also will appear in shock with pale, sweaty skin. All patients presenting with imminent delivery should get an intravenous fluid infusion, and it is even more important for this patient to receive.

Preterm Labor

Preterm labor is any labor that begins after 20 weeks of gestation and before the start of the 37th week of gestation. If the due date is still remote, the hospital course may be to try and curtail the contractions and preserve the pregnancy. Neonates are not viable outside the uterus until about the 20th week, and most physicians consider viability to be after the 28th week of gestation, although some intrepid neonates have survived births earlier than 28 weeks.

Precipitous Labor

Precipitous labor begins and ends with delivery in <3 hours. This may happen most commonly in multigravida and multipara mothers. In this situation, the contractions are stronger and more effective, increasing the chances that the patient tears as a result of a fast birth. It is important that the paramedic coach the mother through the delivery and encourage her to breathe through some contractions if needed.

Postterm Pregnancy and Labor

A normal term for a pregnancy is 40 weeks, so any pregnancy that lasts beyond 42 weeks is considered postterm. Although there is no direct threat to the mother for carrying beyond 40 weeks, the placenta may not be able to transfer enough nutrients and O_2 to a child who has grown much beyond this time. Because fetuses may be larger than normal in this condition, there is an increased risk of delivery problems, including cephalopelvic disproportion and shoulder dystocia. Causes for retention of the fetus beyond 40 weeks are not well outlined.

Fetal Macrosomia

Fetal macrosomia represents an infant weighing >4,000 g (or 8 lb 13 oz) at birth, regardless of gestational age. Genetics and ethnicity play a significant role in predisposing a fetus to a high birth weight, with Hispanic patients being more likely to have a macrosomic child. Diabetes as a baseline or gestational diabetes also is a risk factor for a large infant. Male children also typically weigh more than female children, so they are disproportionately more likely to be macrosomic at birth.

Cephalopelvic Disproportion

Cephalopelvic disproportion is a situation where the size of the infant's head exceeds that of the opening of the pelvis. Frequently, the mother knows this is a problem ahead of time if she has had sufficient prenatal care. It is not possible to deliver this child through normal vaginal delivery, and attempting to do so may cause massive uterine bleeding and life-threatening problems to the mother and infant.

Intrauterine Fetal Death

Intrauterine fetal death differs from an abortion of any kind because it happens after the 20-week threshold. Its causes often are difficult to determine and can vary from intrauterine umbilical cord strangulation to a complication of diabetes or eclampsia to intrauterine infection. Labor may not even occur naturally, and if it does, labor may not start for weeks after the fetus' death. Upon expulsion from the uterus, the fetus may have blisters on the skin or skin actually sloughing off. It also may have already begun to putrefy and have dark discolorations depending on the degree of decomposition. The mother may or may not know that this has happened, and very little can prepare the mother or family for what the fetus will look or smell like. As a paramedic, try not to pass judgment and ensure professional behavior at all times. There is no need to attempt to resuscitate an obviously dead fetus.

COMPLICATIONS OF DELIVERY

Although a vast majority of deliveries are completely normal and free of complications, paramedics must be prepared for delivery complications. This section will discuss the complications of delivery and the best treatment for each.

Prolapsed Cord

For fetuses with a **prolapsed cord**, the child is not yet visible, and crowning has not yet happened; however, the umbilical cord is visible, being looped outside the vagina. In most cases, though, the delivery process will continue to progress as if nothing is wrong. Yet this could prove problematic for the fetus as it will likely pinch off the umbilical cord too early, cutting off its own blood supply as it descends further and further into the pelvis. This presentation cannot be vaginally delivered in the field—or in the hospital, for that matter—and should not be attempted; this presentation will require cesarean section.

Transport the patient in the knee-chest position, where the woman's pelvis is the highest part of her, to have gravity help keep the child in the uterus. One paramedic should hold the cord for the duration of patient contact and ensure that it continues to have a palpable pulse. If the pulse should disappear, the fetus is likely beginning to press on it. Insert a gloved hand into the patient and gently but firmly push or lift the part of the fetus compressing the cord off it. This paramedic will then be committed to this patient in this position until a crash cesarean section can be accomplished and the fetus is delivered.

Multiple Gestations

Twins are not terribly complicated, typically. Twins often are smaller than single gestation infants born during the same week of gestational age. This low birth weight may predispose the neonate to needing some degree of resuscitative care after birth. The 2nd and any sequential neonates will be born about half an hour apart.

The procedure for birthing twins is not any different from single births; it just gets repeated. For twins, there will always be one umbilical cord for each neonate. The number of placentas may vary. If there are two umbilical cords attached to one placenta, then the twins are said to be identical. Conversely, fraternal twins each have their own placenta. As they are born, write the time and some kind of identifier on a piece of tape and wrap it like a bracelet around the ankle. Do not just apply the tape to the infant.

Cephalic Presentation

In normal, headfirst deliveries, the crown or vertex of the head presents when the fetus's head is flexed, with the chin touching its chest. Occasionally, the head can hyperextend, resulting in a face-first presentation. Even more rare is when the head presents, parietal area first, called the military presentation. Although field deliverable, it is one of the hardest cephalic presentations for the mother to deliver and can result in an arrested delivery or extreme pain for the mother.

Shoulder Dystocia

Shoulder dystocia occurs when the fetus's shoulders are too broad to deliver and is a common complication of fetal macrosomia. It is diagnosed after the head delivers and the upper shoulder gets stuck on the pubic bone. The first sign of shoulder dystocia is what is called the turtle sign, which is where the fetus's head pushes out during a contraction and pulls back into the mother somewhat, analogous to a turtle retracting its head. This often is an unexpected complication, even in the hospital, and becomes a threat to the survival of the fetus for two reasons. First, the cord often is compressed between the fetus and the woman's vaginal wall. Second, the birth canal compresses the entire chest, reducing or eliminating the fetus's ability to breathe.

The delivery needs to be completed most likely before transport to the hospital, so being familiar with maneuvers designed to relieve shoulder dystocia is necessary. The mnemonic for remembering the order of the maneuvers is, appropriately, HELPERR:

- **Help.** Call for additional help.
- **Episiotomy.** The paramedic cannot do this.
- **Legs.** Flex the legs at the hip as far as they can possibly go, essentially almost putting the knees in the armpits. This is called the **McRobert maneuver**.
- **Pressure.** Exert suprapubic pressure straight down on the fetus's anterior shoulder while the patient is being held in the McRobert maneuver. The goal is to disimpact the anterior shoulder.
- **Entry Maneuvers.** This first involves an attempt at internal rotation of the fetus to dislodge either the anterior or posterior shoulder.
- **Remove Posterior Arm.** In this maneuver, the paramedic attempts to identify the posterior forearm and hand, gently pulling it free of the birth canal.
- **Roll the Patient.** Place the patient on all fours to try and straighten the spine and dislodge the posterior arm of the fetus.

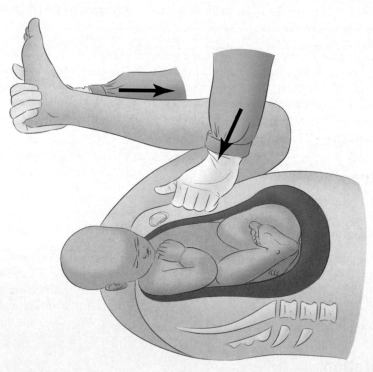

Figure 7-8. McRobert Maneuver and Suprapubic Pressure

If shoulder dystocia is encountered, call medical control as soon as possible and have the doctor on the phone help guide the processes. Make the decision to transport the mother in the knee-chest position.

Nuchal Cord

A nuchal cord is a cord that has been wrapped around the fetus's neck as a result of their normal movements in utero. As discussed in the normal birth outline, as soon as the neonate delivers in a headfirst delivery, slip a finger in between the cheek and shoulder of the neonate after it rotates into the side-facing position. If pulsing is felt, or the cord can be seen, attempt to loop the cord back over the head of the neonate if there is enough slack. If there is not enough slack, loosen enough cord to be able to clamp it in two places and then cut the cord between the clamps. This must happen so that the delivery can be completed, and the neonate does not die of strangulation.

Breech Presentation

Breech presentations occur when the buttocks is the presenting part and are more common in premature births. These presentations can be delivered in the field; however, they are not ideal. It is not uncommon for breech births to be harder deliveries for the mother and last longer. There also is the very real possibility for the infant's head to become stuck in the birth canal despite the rest of the body successfully delivering. If the infant's head gets stuck and the rest of the body has delivered, first attempt to free the child by carefully lifting the child's ankles upward in a circle toward the abdomen. This maneuver should free the head. If it does not and the head remains stuck, the child is in serious danger of asphyxiation. In this case, gently but quickly slide two fingers between the vaginal wall and the infant's face and push up on the infant's cheeks with one finger on each cheek. This will create a small gap through which the infant should be able to breathe. The paramedic who does this will be committed in this position until the infant's head is freed from the mother at the hospital. At no point in time should anyone forcibly yank on the infant to try to extricate the child.

Limb Presentation

On rare occasions, and for not clearly understood reasons, a limb of the infant may be the presenting part. This can be any of the four limbs, but most commonly it is a leg, although the infant may be lying transverse in utero, thus presenting an arm. This presentation is not field deliverable, and the patient will need a cesarean section. Transport this patient in the knee-chest position with the pelvis as the highest part of the mother, so that gravity can aid in keeping the child in. If both legs are the presenting part, the infant may be deliverable in the field in the same manner and with the same considerations as a breech presentation.

POSTPARTUM COMPLICATIONS

As previously discussed, pregnancy alone can be hard on the mother's body. Birth can come with its own set of problems, as well. After giving birth, the mother is still not fully in the clear. Problems associated with having given birth can present anywhere from hours to weeks after birth. As the uterus returns to its normal position in the pelvis and hormone levels return to prepregnancy levels, several problems can arise for the new mother after giving birth.

Pulmonary Embolism

A PE is by far one of the most serious complications of childbirth and is the most common cause of maternal cardiac arrest during the perinatal time frame. Air, thrombus, amniotic fluid, or water (after a water birth) may enter maternal circulation and lodge in the lungs. This will result in the sudden onset of chest pain and shortness of breath, tachycardia, and all the other PE symptoms described in chapter 4. Be prepared to aggressively manage this patient's airway and provide 100% O_2.

Uterine Inversion

Uterine inversions occur for unknown reasons and are therefore unpredictable, although they are believed to happen most frequently when there is strong traction (pulling tension) on the umbilical cord with a placenta that is attached to the uterine fundus (superior portion). It is fortunately relatively rare and is lethal in about 15% of patients who experience it. Uterine inversions are classified by the degree of inversion.

- A uterine inversion where the uterus inverts and stays within the uterine cavity and does not extend beyond the cervical os is called an **incomplete inversion.**

- A **complete uterine inversion** occurs when the fundus of the uterus extends beyond the os but remains within the body.

- A **prolapsed inversion** occurs when any portion of the uterus is visible beyond the vaginal opening.

Treatment for uterine inversion is supportive care and includes the provision of 100% O_2 and at least one intravenous line with fluid delivery titrated to maintain blood pressure; fluid boluses may be required to maintain the pressure, especially in the presence of a postpartum hemorrhage (PPH). Oxytocin should be stopped and withheld once inversion is recognized. Magnesium sulfate or terbutaline can be administered on order from the medical control physician if needed.

Postpartum Hemorrhage

PPH is defined as any bleeding in excess of 500 mL during the first 24 hours after vaginal delivery or 1,000 mL after cesarean section. Early PPH occurs within the first 24 hours. Late PPH occurs within the first 6 weeks after delivery. Causes for PPH include the following:

- Retained placenta (A piece of the placenta remains in the uterus.)
- Placenta accreta (Blood vessels from the placenta burrow into the myometrium instead of remaining within the endometrial layer.)
- Lacerations
- Instrumental delivery
- Fetal macrosomia
- Uterine atony (a lack of muscle tone in part or all the uterus)
- Hypertensive disorders
- Induction of labor and augmentation of labor with oxytocin

Treatment in the field is rather limited. But take the following steps to treatment while rapidly transporting the patient to the hospital.

1. Perform fundal massage. This is not gentle therapeutic massage that a person might get at a spa. This is more like kneading dense bread. Knead the uterus in circles.
2. Encourage the mother to breastfeed, particularly if it is within 24 hours.
3. Add 10 units of oxytocin, if available, to 1,000 mL NSS and infuse at about 20–30 mL/min.
4. Initiate 2 large-bore intravenous lines and run crystalloid solutions wide open.
5. Do not pack, internally examine, or insert anything into the vagina.

Trauma and the Pregnant Patient

This section will focus on both considerations in traumatic events that are unique to the pregnant patient because of both changes in mother's physiology and the fundus itself. Motor vehicle accidents and domestic violence are the primary causes of trauma in the pregnant patient. The focus then will be on the trauma with which the paramedic should be concerned during each trimester.

During the first trimester, the uterine fundus is still well within the pelvic girdle and therefore protected. The abdominal contents have not yet begun to shift, and circulation of the patient has not materially changed. Injuries and sequelae from abdominal trauma are largely unchanged from that of the nonpregnant patient.

During the second trimester, rapid growth of the fundus occurs, often leading to balance issues for the pregnant female and increased falls. The uterus itself is protected early on, but during the course of the trimester, abdominal organs are pushed upward and backward while the abdomen protrudes. The urinary bladder is now more superior and anterior, meaning that it is more susceptible to rupture in blunt or penetrating trauma. The mother's circulating volume has increased by nearly 50% by the end of the trimester. Consequently, it may take more bleeding to show typical signs of shock, and the mother's body will sacrifice the baby to save itself during times of severe hemorrhage. Blunt trauma and deceleration injuries increase the chances of abruptio placenta and spontaneous initiation of delivery. All these concerns continue through the third trimester as well.

The fetus through all this is rather well protected. It has the amnion to cushion it and slow its overall movements during rapid decelerations, such as what may happen during falls or motor vehicle accidents. Beyond that, layers of muscle, fat, and other connective tissue provide an added barrier. During penetrating trauma, such as gunshots and stabbings, the mother may actually fare a bit better because of the presence of the fetus. In such attacks, the fetus often bears the brunt of the injuries. During assessment, ask the mother if she has noted any fetal movement since the traumatic event. Ask her if there is any possibility of having ruptured her water or if there is any vaginal bleeding.

Treatment of the fetus is accomplished with excellent treatment of the mother. In trauma patients where the abdomen could have been involved, supplemental O_2 is always recommended. O_2 is a first-line treatment in all cases of potential fetal distress, abruptio placenta, maternal hypovolemia, or hemorrhage. If the patient's condition requires a backboard, tilt the backboard to the patient's left to minimize the chances of supine hypotension syndrome. The pregnant trauma patient can benefit from intravenous fluids, even if hemorrhage is not directly observed. If ventilations are required, breathing slightly faster and closely monitoring $EtCO_2$ is recommended because of the pregnant patient's normally increased respiratory rate and volume.

NEWBORN RESUSCITATION

In the previous sections, the normal birth of a newborn was presented, including initial care routines of suctioning, drying and stimulating the infant, keeping it warm, and positioning it on the mother's belly whenever possible. Abnormal births and presentations also were presented, as well as risks for fetal distress. This section will focus on describing what to do if the neonate is not born vigorous and crying, as more than 90% of children are. The section concludes by discussing common problems and treatments of the infant during the first month of life.

Assessment

Infants who are not crying forcefully or who are not moving actively after birth will need to be resuscitated, to varying degrees. Meconium staining, perinatal vaginal bleeding, maternal trauma, premature membrane rupture, and any other problem identified during prenatal care all increase the chances of the newborn needing some resuscitation. Within 30 seconds of birth, even before the first Apgar score is obtained, the infant needs to be quickly assessed for the ABCs. The inverted triangle will help guide the paramedic's stepwise planning to newborn resuscitation.

Inverted Triangle

The inverted triangle is a means of remembering the steps to newborn resuscitation. It is designed to indicate, at the top, the treatments and interventions every infant will receive. Descending down to the tip of the triangle illustrates the interventions that very few infants require to survive. Progression through the inverted triangle will be based on the infant's response to each higher level. Children are incredibly resilient when it comes to treatments, but this is especially true of newborns. With this in mind, movement from one level to the next should be rapid, roughly every 30 seconds or so.

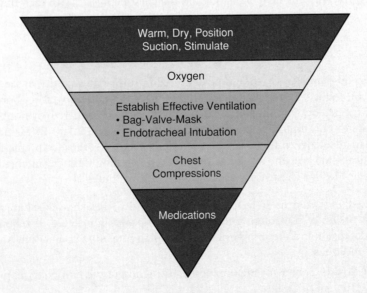

Figure 7-9. The Inverted Triangle of Newborn Resuscitation

Warm, Dry, Position, Suction, Stimulate

As mentioned in the previous section, upon delivery, every infant will receive these steps. Maintaining the body temperature of the infant is essential. In the back of the ambulance, if it is comfortable for the EMS crew, it is frigid for the newborn. The infant should be dried off from the blood and amnion covering them as best as possible. During these treatments, the infant should be positioned on their back. After each intervention is completed and the child is breathing and becoming increasingly pink, place the infant on the belly of the mother to aid in delivery of the placenta and minimize blood loss. Suction the mouth first and then the nose. Although this is done immediately after the head presents and rotates, it should be done again after full delivery to ensure that nothing was missed. Deeper suctioning should be performed if the amnion was meconium stained (more on this later). Stimulation most often is accomplished simply during the drying process. However, if this has not worked sufficiently, flick the soles of the feet or rub the child's back. If, after all of this is completed or 30 seconds has passed and the infant is not yet lively and vigorous, move down the triangle to the next level: oxygenation.

Oxygenation

Hypoxia is the most likely cause for any respiratory or cardiac depression found in the newborn. Transient hypoxia occurs in every newborn because of compression of the umbilical cord between the vaginal wall and the infant during a normal delivery; therefore, addressing this hypoxia is of highest importance. The assessment here needs to focus on respiratory and heart rates. The rates should be >30 (with the infant having a strong cry) and >100. Cyanosis of the hands and feet under these conditions is considered normal, and the infant does not require any further treatment; simply monitor the child and be alert for an unlikely decline in status.

Central cyanosis when the heart rate is still >100, however, requires blow-by O_2 because there may be another reason for the continuing cyanosis of the trunk or mucous membranes. O_2 can be delivered with O_2 tubing blowing a stream of air across the infant's face or with a simple non-rebreathing mask. In most cases, the infant will "pink-up" after just a few minutes of supplemental O_2. If O_2 is used for more than a few minutes, it should be humidified. O_2 should be discontinued if cyanosis of the trunk and mucous membranes resolves because excessive O_2 administration to a newborn can be harmful to the eyes.

Ventilation

If the infant is apneic for a period of 20 seconds or more at any point in time after birth, or the pulse rate is found to be <100 beats per minute, positive pressure ventilation should be initiated immediately. This should be continued until the heart rate improves to >100 beats per minute. Other signs that indicate the likely need for **positive pressure ventilation** include nasal flaring, grunting, and retractions. The retractions may be intercostal, subcostal, or supraclavicular. In **see-saw respirations**, the belly puffs out and the chest depresses with each inhalation, then vice versa during exhalation.

Bag-Valve-Mask

Because infant chests vary in diameter, O_2 should be delivered in sufficient quantity to see the chest rise, typically about 3–6 mL/kg of O_2 or about 1/10 the volume of an infant BVM. Ventilating a newborn may take more force than may otherwise be expected because the lungs have not fully inflated or there may not be enough surfactant in the lungs for them to inflate easily and fully. Blow-off valves often found on infant BVMs may release at a pressure lower than that required to adequately inflate a newborn's lungs, particularly those of premature newborns. After the first few breaths after delivery, the pressure needed to obtain chest rise should lessen, and breaths should continue to be delivered to a volume needed for chest rise at a rate of 40–60 per minute.

Oral airways are rarely used on newborns. In fact, if they can be avoided, they should be because the hard plastic may cause trauma to the soft tissues of the palate if the airway is improperly inserted. If required, airways should be inserted using a tongue depressor and slid into position rather than rotated as in an adult. An oral airway can be life saving in the following conditions:

- **Bilateral Choanal Atresia.** A bony or membranous obstruction in the nasopharynx prevents airflow through the nose. This can be fatal.

- **Pierre Robin Sequence.** This sequence is a series of developmental anomalies that result in a small chin and a tongue positioned more posterior than normal. These often result in airway obstruction that an airway will definitely alleviate. Less invasively, placing the infant prone also may alleviate this condition.

- **Bradycardia.** Children respond to periods of hypoxia by first becoming bradycardic. Whether the hypoxia is a direct result of a long delivery, respiratory distress after delivery, or periods of apnea, bradycardia is frequently present. In most cases, the bradycardia responds to ventilation and oxygenation. If bradycardia does not respond to ventilation, consider other possible causes, including acidosis and hypothyroidism. Vagal stimulation from suctioning; intubation; or motion of a placed orogastric tube, nasogastric tube, or ETT against the hypopharynx is possible. More will be discussed on the pharmacologic interventions for bradycardia later.

If, after about 30 seconds of BVM use, the heart rate or the respiratory rate of the child has not increased, move to the next stage of resuscitation: intubation.

Intubation

Most newborns are resuscitated to full activity and respiratory and heart rates with O_2 or a few minutes of ventilation with a BVM. If ventilation takes more than a few minutes, intubation should be considered because it will protect the airway from aspiration and minimize the chances of gastric insufflation from aggressive ventilation. Intubation should be considered any time it is expected that positive pressure ventilation will be used for an extended time. Intubation is specifically indicated when there is meconium staining or congenital diaphragmatic hernia.

Meconium staining signals possible meconium aspiration in the neonate. As noted previously, the fetus is consistently inhaling the amniotic fluid. If there is meconium in it, the fetus could inhale that as well. If the fetus then gets this into the lungs, it will likely result in severe respiratory depression and infection, which are associated with a high morbidity. This leads to atelectasis and hypoxia. It also will prevent the newborn from inhaling and inflating their lungs, resulting in a condition known as persistent pulmonary hypertension of the newborn and continued shunting of the blood in the heart through the foramen ovale and ductus arteriosus.

Ordinarily, after delivery, the infant is dried, warmed, and stimulated, but these procedures are not recommended in the meconium-stained infant, especially if the amnion was black and particulate. Instead, when the amniotic fluid contains meconium, aggressive suctioning beyond what would normally be done for any other normal newborn should be performed first, before drying, warming, and so on. To adequately clear meconium cleared from the lower airways, suctioning is performed using an ETT as a suction catheter attached to a meconium aspirator, which is then attached to the suction tubing. Next, using a laryngoscope and the usual intubation technique, suction deep into the trachea until there is nothing left to suction. Remember to suction out the cheek pockets as well. Discard the ETT. If deep suctioning yielded meconium in the lower airways, intubate and ventilate at a rate of 40–60 per minute with sufficient volume to see the chest rise. This is warranted in most meconium-staining cases.

A **congenital diaphragmatic hernia** is where the infant is born with its abdominal organs within the chest cavity. The stomach and perhaps some intestines have herniated through either the esophageal hiatus or another abnormal opening of the diaphragm, causing the mediastinum to shift to the opposite side of the hernia. This can be diagnosed on prenatal ultrasound, so the mother may be able to relay this information to the paramedic during the birth, allowing time for the paramedic to prepare. If there was no prenatal care, such a condition would not be known; however, assessment of the newborn can reveal clues. Instead of being round, the abdomen would be flat or even sunken because of the lack of abdominal organs. There may be bowel sounds in the chest cavity in addition to severe respiratory distress.

For any newborn who has severe diaphragmatic hernia, early intubation is recommended because BVM places the patient at unnecessary risk for gastric insufflation. Because the stomach is in the chest, gastric insufflation will only further diminish available lung capacity. Ventilating these newborns is something of a balancing act as far as the pressures needed to generate lung inflation are concerned. Such infants tend to have underdeveloped lungs as a result of ongoing pressure from the abdominal organs during gestation, making them more susceptible to barotrauma. On the other hand, higher pressures may be needed to get any air into the lungs for the same reason. If available, the newborn should receive an orogastric tube to relieve gastric distension. Rapid transport to a facility capable of emergency surgery on a newborn is recommended.

Positive pressure ventilation whether via BVM or intubation can cause a **pneumothorax** in a newborn. The pneumothorax also may be caused by damage to the lung from meconium aspiration. Relieve the pneumothorax in the same way as an adult, only with a smaller 22-gauge over-the-needle intravenous catheter inserted in the 2nd intercostal space just above the 3rd rib to avoid the vascular and nerve bundle that lies inferior to the 2nd rib. A newborn with a pneumothorax should be intubated to secure the airway and help monitor increasing airway pressure after initial relief of the pneumothorax.

Compressions

Chest compressions should be initiated in any child who is pulseless or has a heart rate of 60 or less after 30 seconds of effective positive pressure ventilation. In most cases, there also should have been 30 seconds of ventilation through a properly placed ETT or LMA as well as prior to beginning compressions. Compressions should be continued until the heart rate improves to >60 beats per minute. Compressions can be performed in one of two ways as recommended by the American Heart Association.

Compressing the sternum with both thumbs, with the hands encircling the chest so the fingers support the spine is the ideal way to compress the chest. But this can be done only if there are two paramedics: one paramedic performs the compressions, and one paramedic ventilates the child. The thumbs should be over the lower third of the sternum. The person performing the compressions is located at the head of the patient, whereas the person doing the ventilating is located to the side. This will allow yet another paramedic to cannulate the umbilical vein to acquire vascular access (more on this later). A 3:1 ratio of compressions to ventilations should be performed, and each set of 3:1 should be complete in about 0.5 seconds. This will ensure about 90 compressions per minute and 30 breaths per minute. Pulse or ECG rhythm checks should be performed only after about every minute of compressions and ventilations.

The alternative method should be done by placing 2 fingertips on the sternum and the second hand behind the infant's shoulders to support the spine. Ventilations are then delivered by a second paramedic. Compressions and ventilations should be delivered at the same rate as above. Check the pulse after 60 seconds of well-coordinated compressions and ventilations.

Traditional **vascular access in a newborn** is difficult and can be very time consuming. Cannulation of the umbilical vein provides an ideal site for fluid resuscitation and medication administration. Ideally, this is accomplished with an umbilical catheter; however, any intravenous catheter can be used as long as it is <4 cm in length and the diameter can fit the umbilical vein. The steps for umbilical catheterization are as follows:

1. Clean the length of the umbilical cord from the infant to about 3 cm away from the skin with alcohol or, preferably, povidone-iodine. Keep the area as sterile as possible, ideally draping the area with sterile drapes and using sterile gloves.

2. Attach a 3–5 mL prefilled syringe to a 3-way stopcock that is also attached to a 3.5–5 Fr umbilical catheter and flush saline through the catheter.

3. Cut the cord between the infant and the first cord clamp about 1–2 cm from the infant while pinching it shut with a cord tie proximally.

4. Insert the umbilical catheter into the umbilical vein. The umbilical vein will be the larger diameter vessel of the three options and will have a thinner wall compared with the other two arteries. This often is referred to as putting the catheter "in the mouth and not the eyes."

5. Advance the catheter about 2–4 cm into the vein until blood can be aspirated into the syringe. Do not advance beyond about 5 cm; further advancement could cause liver and heart cannulation.

6. Flush the catheter and tape into place.

Medications

Medications are at the tip of the inverted triangle because they are rarely required for newborn resuscitation. In most cases of the obtunded newborn, they can be resuscitated with effective ventilatory support. Medications in the pediatric population are generally weight based, so an estimated weight will be needed. Full-term infants are generally between 3 and 4 kg, with 3 kg considered the weight used for full-term newborns. Preterm infants can weigh <1 kg. This section will focus on conditions primarily treated with medications.

Bradycardia

Continuing from the discussion earlier in this section, although bradycardia most often is remedied with effective ventilation and oxygenation, there are some occasions where medications may need to be given. The medication of choice in a newborn is 0.01–0.03 mg/kg epinephrine 1:10,000 IV followed by a flush to get the medication into central circulation. Higher doses are not recommended because of profound and counterproductive hypertension of the newborn. Administration of the epinephrine via the ETT should be given at 10 times the intravenous dose or 0.1 mg/kg. Pulses should be checked about 1 minute after intravenous administration and about 3 minutes after ET administration.

Narcotics

Other sources of bradycardia may include the infant's response to narcotics. If the mother was a chronic narcotic user, administration of naloxone is not recommended for respiratory depression or bradycardia in the infant because of the increased possibility of fatal seizures the sudden withdrawal can induce. Instead, the infant should be weaned off the narcotic during the first few days or weeks of life. Conversely, if the respiratory depression could be from perinatal short term, acute narcotic use, then 0.1 mg/kg naloxone to a maximum of 2 mg is recommended.

Hypoglycemia

Hypoglycemia in the newborn is defined as any blood glucose reading <45 mg/dL, although many infants do not show symptoms until the readings are <20 mg/dL for a significant amount of time. Most term newborns will have sufficient glycogen stores to survive 8–12 hours without becoming significantly hypoglycemic because they have spent much of the 3rd trimester storing glycogen in their heart, liver, lungs, and skeletal muscle. Premature infants, on the other hand, have not had the opportunity to create these stores, so they are more likely to become hypoglycemic after birth. Stressed newborns also are more likely to present or become hypoglycemic.

Because symptoms often are vague, including irritability, limpness, eye rolling, tremors, twitching, or seizures, evaluate the blood sugar level of every infant behaving unusually. Unlike in the adult or even the older child, perform a heel stick on the newborn instead of a finger stick. This will be less painful for the child and can more easily be milked for the adequate amount of blood. If the blood sugar level is <45 mg/dL, administer 2 mL/kg of a 10% dextrose solution intravenously or intraosseously. Maintain the temperature of the newborn because hypothermia places an added stress on the child.

Pro-Tip

A 10% dextrose solution may need to be made because it often is not carried on an ambulance. This can be accomplished by taking D50 and discarding 40 mL from the prefilled syringe. Then refill the syringe with NSS to a total of 50 mL. This will result in 5 g in 50 mL or a 10% solution.

Acidosis

Despite adequate ventilation, oxygenation, and chest compressions, bradycardia may be a result of acidosis. The treatment of choice in adults is sodium bicarbonate, but this is associated with increased morbidity of the newborn and should be avoided. Treatment instead focuses on volume expansion as if the patient is hypovolemic. This will help in clearing metabolic acids.

Hypovolemia

Hypovolemia is difficult to detect in newborns because newborns react to just about every event with bradycardia, including hypovolemia. In persistent bradycardia, especially with cofactors including abruptio placenta, sepsis, or multiple births, hypovolemia should be considered. Treatment for this is 10 mL/kg NSS or Lactated Ringer's (LR) intravenous or intraosseous that can be repeated up to 3 times before switching to blood is recommended.

OTHER CONDITIONS REQUIRING ACUTE INTERVENTIONS IN THE NEWBORN

Until now, the assessment and treatment of problems that may present during birth or immediately after birth were addressed, specifically those relating to the newborn who is obtunded and distressed. This section will discuss those issues not directly related to the pregnancy or the act of delivery. This group of issues a newborn may face may not present for a few days to weeks after delivery.

Seizures

Seizures in an infant often are related to a significant underlying issue, although they may be difficult to discern from other activities of the newborn. The causes of seizures in newborns are listed. Seizures that occur within the first three days of birth are most likely caused by one of the first three on the list, whereas the rest of the list may begin three days after birth.

- Hypoxic ischemic encephalopathy
- Hypoglycemia
- Other metabolic disturbances
- Meningitis or abscess
- Epilepsy
- Intracranial bleeding
- Congenital brain malformations and encephalopathy
- Drug withdrawal

Hypoxic events during or around birth can lead to **hypoxic ischemic encephalopathy** and are the single most common reason for seizures in the newborn, often with the fastest onset after birth, with the first seizure occurring as soon as 12 hours after birth. Seizures from this cause frequently start off subtly and worsen during the first few days of life. The newborn seizure should be differentiated from jitteriness. This is easily accomplished by gently applying pressure to a limb or passively moving one or more extremities. This will halt jitteriness, but it will not have any impact on a seizure. Jitteriness is not associated with eye deviations.

Hypoglycemia is noted separately from "other metabolic disturbances" because it is by far the most common metabolic disturbance to lead to seizures. The other metabolic disturbances include the following:

- Electrolyte imbalances, especially hypocalcemia, hyponatremia (sodium), and hypomagnesemia
- Abnormalities of proteins and amino acids
- Increased ammonia levels from liver problems
- Toxins

Assessment of the newborn would be incomplete without asking the mother about the situation surrounding birth, including normal versus cesarean, meconium staining, a nuchal cord, or any other prenatal complications. Hypoglycemia should always be assessed and treated as noted in the hypoglycemia section. Phenobarbital and benzodiazepines should be administered only under the advice of a physician.

Vomiting

Anyone who has ever been around newborns knows all too well that they vomit. Often. It is seldom a cause for concern. It becomes worrisome if the vomiting interferes with weight gain, causes weight loss or dehydration, or appears bloody or bilious. Any of these may indicate a pathologic problem that needs to be addressed relatively quickly. As with vomiting at any age, aspiration is always a concern; it is especially concerning in newborns because they are not able to adjust to empty their mouths or avoid it when lying on their backs.

The causes of vomiting include the following:

- **Esophageal Atresia.** Atresia is the failure of the esophagus to properly develop and connect to the stomach. It may or may not be associated with a fistula, or unnatural connection, between the upper esophagus and trachea. Frothing after birth, and vomiting and choking with feeding, likely indicate this issue.

- **Infantile Hypertrophic Pyloric Stenosis (IHPS).** In this condition, the pyloric sphincter at the distal end of the stomach has thickened, and the stomach is unable to empty normally into the small intestine. Consequently, the stomach contracts forcefully to try and force the chyme (stomach contents) through it. Instead, this often manifests as projectile vomiting. Infants with this often also appear malnourished and dehydrated, and they possibly have hypoglycemia or other electrolyte imbalances.

- **Intestinal Atresia or Stenosis.** Atresia here refers to a malformation of the bowel; stenosis is a narrowing of the bowel. If this occurs in the upper portion of the gut that is proximal to the ileum, the patient may present with bile-stained projectile vomiting, which helps differentiate it from IHPS (the vomit is not bile stained). If it occurs in the ileum or the large intestine, the infant will avoid feeding, have a distended and often hard abdomen, and possibly have a reduced amount of bowel movements.

- **Malrotation.** In this condition, the intestines fail to coil properly during gestation, resulting in a 270° rotation of the intestines around the superior mesenteric artery, the major artery branch off the aorta that services the gut. This results in the small intestine being crowded into the right side of the abdomen, and the ascending colon ends up being in the epigastric region. The child often will have bilious, sometimes bloody, vomit. If it is significant, the vomit may even smell like feces. It can be found prior to birth, although it can be diagnosed at any age. Surgical procedures can correct it.

- **Meningitis.** The child will present with projectile vomiting in addition to a fever and nuchal stiffness. Because the plates of the skull are not yet fused, the child also may appear to have an oversized head.

- **Drug Withdrawal.** Vomiting can be a symptom of drug withdrawal (if the mother was a narcotic user).

- **Meconium Plug.** The failure of the last segment of the large intestine to relax and allow the meconium to pass results in a mechanical obstruction. This can cause abdominal distension and feeding avoidance similar to intestinal atresia.

Treatment for vomiting in the newborn will ultimately be related to the cause. Initially, manage the ABCs and attempt to establish intravenous access. Check the blood glucose level and treat if needed. Be prepared for further vomiting episodes and the need to suction or manage the airway. Dehydration may be indicated by sunken fontanels or skin tenting if the vomiting has been going on for more than 24 hours. A fluid bolus of 10 mL/kg is indicated in that case and can be repeated up to 3 times with the goal of a more active child. Antiemetics are not indicated in newborns.

Premature and Low Birth Weight Infants

Any infant born before the completion of the 37th week is considered premature or preterm. Often, there is no discernible reason for the child to have been born preterm; however, the following are some causes that may lead to prematurity:

- Maternal dehydration
- Infection
- Placental insufficiency
- Polyhydramnios (too much amniotic fluid)
- Preeclampsia
- Cervical incompetence (cervix opens too early)
- Abruptio placenta
- Multiple births
- Trauma

Premature children face a difficult battle to simply survive outside the mother, especially the more remote the actual due date. They may fight through such issues as respiratory distress, respiratory suppression, and possibly apnea because of surfactant deficiency. Without surfactant, the lungs cannot slide smoothly, and the mechanics of breathing become immeasurably more labored. Preterm infants also are predisposed to infections and sepsis because of a poorly functioning immune system. Nervous system compromise is common with intraventricular hemorrhage and periventricular leukomalacia (a form of cerebral palsy). Nervous system disorders can be caused by extended periods of perinatal hypoxia or the administration of hypertonic solutions.

Preterm infants are not necessarily born with a low birth weight; however, it is the most common reason for a newborn to be of low birth weight. Low birth weight is any newborn of any gestational age weighing <2,500 g or 5.5 lb. An infant weighing <500 g is unlikely to survive overall, but the infant stands the best chance in a hospital with a neonatal intensive care unit.

The best treatment for any child born either preterm or low birth weight is to keep the child warm and provide respiratory support as needed during rapid transport to a hospital that is capable of taking care of high-risk infants. Respiratory support and oxygenation should be given only to ensure adequate breathing and heart rate and should not be provided simply as a matter of course. Although long-term O_2 exposure can cause retinopathy of prematurity, which is abnormal development of the vasculature of the retinas, O_2 should not be withheld from the infant who is hypoxic. This could essentially be sacrificing the brain to care for the eyes because the brain is much more sensitive to periods of diminished O_2 supply.

Neonatal Jaundice

Infants often are born with a yellowish tint to their skin called jaundice. In the adult, jaundice can be caused by hepatitis or liver failure; however, in the infant, jaundice is the result of the liver being unable to conjugate bilirubin during the first week of life. Infants have a higher mass of red blood cells, and it is believed that the increased rate of erythrocyte destruction and metabolism exceeds the liver's ability to conjugate the resulting bilirubin. Generally, this is not a cause for concern, and it is almost a rite of passage for the newborn because it is seen to some degree in so many newborns. That said, bilirubin is neurotoxic, so high levels of bilirubin need to be addressed. The paramedic will not be able to address or meaningfully treat neonatal jaundice except to know that it will likely be the reason for altered mental status in a newborn with yellowish skin. The paramedic can start an intravenous line on the infant to temporarily dilute the bilirubin and to help minimize long-term effects; however, transport to the hospital is ideal.

Thermoregulation in the Newborn

The newborn's thermoregulation system is immature and does not respond as in older children or adults. Newborns do not sweat to release heat; they are not able to shiver to generate heat when they are cold. As a result, newborns can become overheated when bundled in a heated car or in direct sunlight or may even become cold when they are in an otherwise comfortably heated house. Newborns have a higher volume-to-surface-area ratio, which means that even under normal circumstances they will lose body heat faster, even in warmer temperatures.

Fevers in newborns are relatively rare and often are not the presenting feature of an infection. Newborns can actually become hypothermic during an infection and are at higher risk for hypoglycemia and metabolic acidosis because of the immune response. Neonates with illnesses often become somnolent, have a reduced appetite, and wet fewer diapers.

Hypothermic newborns are a cause for concern because this is more likely the presenting sign of illness. Hypothermia also leads to increased metabolic activity to try and generate heat because they cannot shiver, leading to hypoglycemia and possibly metabolic acidosis. As hypothermia progresses, they may slow their respirations or become irritable. They also may have **acrocyanosis** (cyanosis of the hands and feet) or become bradycardic. To rewarm the neonate, skin-to-skin contact is the best and can be used after drying the infant and placing the infant on the mother. Avoid using heated water bottles or heating pads, which can cause burns or hyperthermia.

Congenital Heart Diseases

A variety of congenital heart diseases (CHDs) are listed here, and the paramedic should have at least a working knowledge of them. Aside from the supportive measures mentioned throughout this chapter, EMS will not be able to do much for the infant with these conditions. Fortunately, many are not immediately life threatening upon birth;

however, most will require surgery, often within 6 months or so after birth. The conditions and the most common signs or symptoms are presented.

- **Ventricular Septal Defect (VSD).** VSD often is a malformation of the septum between the ventricles, which results in a net movement of blood from the left ventricle to the right because of the significantly higher pumping pressure the left ventricle generates. This leads to pulmonary hypertension as a result of the increased flow and also may result in a decreased systemic blood pressure.

- **Pulmonary Stenosis.** The pulmonary valve is damaged and often no longer opens fully. This causes an outflow problem from the right ventricle. Consequently, the right ventricle hypertrophies because of higher pressures needed to move blood out, so blood flow to the lungs decreases. Patients often present with JVD and cyanosis, especially during feeding.

- **Tetralogy of Fallot.** This combines four (hence tetralogy) conditions into one comprehensive CHD. The conditions are pulmonary stenosis, right ventricular hypertrophy, VSD, and an overriding aorta. The first three were described previously. An overriding aorta is caused by the position of the VSD in relation to the aorta. Because of this malformation, the aorta will receive some deoxygenated blood from the right ventricle. The degree to which the aorta is connected to the right ventricle will determine its degree of "override." These result in a child who is often cyanotic throughout the day but especially when crying, eating, or active at all. Infants will have "tet spells," where they become centrally blue and may even pass out as a result of working too hard to breathe and an overall lack of O_2.

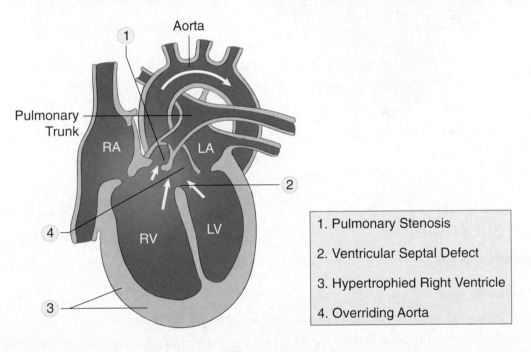

Figure 7-10. Tetralogy of Fallot

- **Atrial Septal Defect.** This results from the failure of the foramen ovale to close, so blood is able to shift between the atria. This causes mixing of the blood and can cause the patient to be cyanotic.

- **Patent Ductus Arteriosus.** This is failure of the ductus arteriosus to close as it normally does after birth. As it does prenatally, this shunts blood away from the lungs, resulting in low oxygenation systemically. If O_2 is administered to a child and the pulse oximetry does not increase, patent ductus arteriosus may be the cause. It can lead to CHF in the infant.

- **Truncus Arteriosus.** A condition where the pulmonary artery and the aorta are a single vessel. These patients often have CHF caused by the massive increase of blood flow to the lungs. Surgery divides the trunk into vessels.

- **Tricuspid Atresia.** This is a frequently fatal condition in which the infant lacks a tricuspid valve that, in turn, results in an undersized or absent right ventricle. Patients will have significantly decreased or absent blood flow to the lungs. The **Fontan procedure** redirects the vena cava and the hepatic portal veins directly into the pulmonary arteries. The result is a dual-chambered heart with one ventricle and one atrium—the left in both cases—to pump blood systemically and to the lungs.

- **Transposition of the Great Arteries.** This condition results in the pulmonary artery being connected to the left ventricle and the aorta being connected to the right ventricle. This results in blood returning from the body going right back out to the body without ever being oxygenated, and blood returning from the lungs heads right back to the lungs. Often, the systemic hypoxia can cause the foramen ovale and the ductus arteriosus to remain patent, allowing some oxygenated blood to reach systemic circulation. A VSD also may be present in patients with transposition of the great vessels.

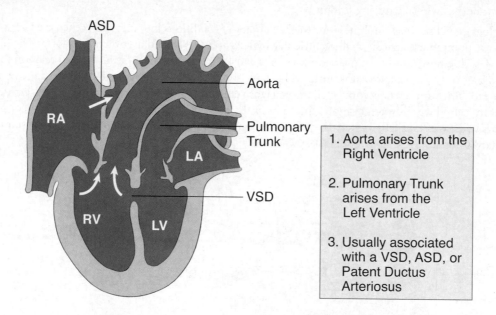

1. Aorta arises from the Right Ventricle

2. Pulmonary Trunk arises from the Left Ventricle

3. Usually associated with a VSD, ASD, or Patent Ductus Arteriosus

Figure 7-11. Transposition of the Great Vessels

REVIEW QUESTIONS

Select the ONE best answer.

1. Which of the following best describes the role of hCG during pregnancy?

    A. Causes an increase in the production of FSH and LH.

    B. Maintains the corpus luteum, which stimulates the production of estrogen and progesterone.

    C. Turns the ruptured follicle into the corpus luteum after ovulation.

    D. Stimulates the development, production, and release of milk from the mammary glands.

2. A sexually active, 35-year-old female presents with a 2-day history of increasing RLQ pain. She states that she has a history of tubal ligation reversal 4 months ago and has been actively trying to get pregnant with her new husband. She has not taken a pregnancy test and denies fever. Assessment reveals rebound tenderness and spotting vaginal bleeding. All of the following could cause the patient's symptoms EXCEPT:

    A. Ectopic pregnancy.

    B. Ovarian torsion.

    C. Ruptured appendix.

    D. Ruptured ovarian cyst.

3. A 27-year-old female complains of diffuse lower abdominal pain. She complains of an associated fever and chills and this morning noted that the pain worsened when she walked. She takes birth control pills and rarely uses condoms despite having multiple partners. She is conscious and alert. Which option indicates the most likely cause of the patient's symptoms?

    A. Endometriosis

    B. Uterine pregnancy

    C. Toxic shock syndrome

    D. PID

4. In fetal circulation, most of the blood bypasses the lungs of the fetus by going through which of the following?

    A. Foramen ovale

    B. Ductus venosus

    C. Hepatic portal system

    D. Ventricular septal foramen

5. A 37-year-old female who is 36 weeks pregnant calls the ambulance because she has an intense headache and is dizzy. She also notes blurred vision in her right eye. Vital signs are HR: 110, BP: 158/92, RR: 18, and SpO_2: 97%. You suspect:

    A. CVA

    B. Eclampsia

    C. Preeclampsia

    D. Migraine

6. The following are all true regarding abruptio placenta EXCEPT:

    A. External, visible bleeding can be profuse.

    B. Commonly caused by external blunt trauma.

    C. The placenta covers or partially covers the cervical os.

    D. Should be suspected with a late-term pregnancy in a person with hypotension.

7. Which of the following events takes place during the 2nd stage of labor?

    A. The infant is born.

    B. The placenta is delivered.

    C. The bag of waters breaks.

    D. The head of the fetus is visible at the vaginal opening.

8. After a newborn has been dried, warmed, and suctioned, which of the following is the next step for a child with a heart rate of 80 who is weakly crying and pulling back into the fetal position?

    A. Begin CPR.

    B. Administer blow-by O_2.

    C. Ventilate with a BVM.

    D. Suction again with a meconium aspirator.

9. The most immediate and effective treatment a paramedic can perform for the patient with postpartum hemorrhage is:

   A. Fundal massage.

   B. Administer oxytocin.

   C. Infuse up to 2 L crystalloid wide open.

   D. Administer 2 g magnesium sulfate slowly over 10 minutes.

10. Use the following scenario to answer questions 10 and 11.

    You just helped deliver a newborn who the mother estimated at 34 weeks gestational age. The amniotic fluid was stained with greenish-black meconium, and particulate matter was present. The cord was wrapped around the infant's neck twice. The newborn is limp, is blue centrally and peripherally, has only agonal respirations at a rate of 5, has a heart rate in the 30s, and exhibits no response to pain.

    What is this infant's Apgar score?

    A. 0

    B. 1

    C. 2

    D. 3

11. I.   Dry, warm, position, stimulate.

    II.   Suction mouth then nose.

    III. Suction hypopharynx with meconium aspirator.

    IV. Ventilate with BVM.

    V.   Chest compressions.

    Place the above steps in the correct order for the meconium-stained infant in the scenario.

    A. I, II, III, IV, V

    B. I, II, IV, V, III

    C. III, II, I, IV, V

    D. III, II, IV, V, I

ANSWERS AND EXPLANATIONS

1. **The correct answer is (B).** hCG stimulates the corpus luteum to continue to produce estrogen and progesterone, which maintains the uterine lining through early pregnancy until the placenta can produce its own estrogen and progesterone. (A) is the function of GnRH. (C) is the function of LH. (D) combines the functions of 2 hormones: prolactin (production of milk) and oxytocin (let-down or release of milk).

2. **The correct answer is (B).** Of the options listed, ovarian torsion (B) is least likely to cause rebound tenderness. Rebound tenderness is caused when the patient's peritoneum is irritated, most often from blood or infection. Ectopic pregnancy (A) is the most likely cause of those listed because of the history of increasing pain. As the zygote grows, the pain will increase and lead to bleeding. Ovarian cysts (D) most often result in a sudden onset of severe pain and rarely present slowly over days. A ruptured appendix (C) is a possibility; however, since this is caused by an infection, it will likely be accompanied by a fever as well as nausea and vomiting, and it has a longer time of onset.

3. **The correct answer is (D).** PID is caused by any of a variety of organisms that can be transmitted sexually, including chlamydia, candidiasis, gonorrhea, and bacterial vaginitis. Endometriosis (A) is a condition where the endometrial lining grows on the internal organs outside the uterus. This may cause diffuse lower abdominal pain, but rarely is it associated with a fever. Uterine pregnancy also could cause some mild midline or even diffuse lower quadrant pain, particularly during implantation; however, fevers and urinary pain are not associated symptoms. Toxic shock syndrome (C) can produce all these symptoms; however, it is strongly correlated with tampon use, not sexual activity or organisms associated with an STI.

4. **The correct answer is (A).** The foramen ovale is a hole in the septum between the right and left atria. Blood that passes through this from right to left will bypass the pulmonary circuit. The ductus venosus (B) bypasses the liver and does not affect systemic or pulmonary circulation. The hepatic portal system (C) is the circulation of the liver. A ventricular septal foramen (D) does not normally exist. If there is a hole between the ventricles of the fetus, it is called a VSD and will be repaired surgically.

5. **The correct answer is (C).** This patient is exhibiting common signs of preeclampsia. Some additional symptoms a patient may complain of include swelling of the hands, feet, and face; syncope; and protein in the urine. The patient will have eclampsia (B) only when she has a seizure resulting from the hypertension and fluid retention. CVA (A) and migraine (D) are not likely.

6. **The correct answer is (C).** This describes placenta previa.

7. **The correct answer is (A).** The 2nd stage of labor begins after crowning and continues through completion of the delivery of the infant. (C) and (D) each occur during the first stage of labor, which begins with the onset of contractions and ends with crowning. During this stage, the bag of waters most commonly breaks. The third stage of labor is when the placenta is delivered (B).

8. **The correct answer is (B).** A newborn who has a heart rate <100 but >60 should receive blow-by O_2 for approximately 30 seconds to a minute. If the infant still does not improve with O_2, positive pressure ventilations with a BVM (C) would be appropriate. If the heart rate is <60, CPR should be administered (A). Deep suctioning, such as with a meconium aspirator (D), would not likely be necessary.

9. **The correct answer is (A).** Immediately when recognizing a postpartum hemorrhage situation, fundal massage can be started immediately without any equipment. (B) and (C) are appropriate next steps to complete while the fundus is being massaged. Magnesium sulfate (D) is not indicated in postpartum hemorrhage.

10. **The correct answer is (C).** The score is as follows:

    - Activity: Flaccid = 0
    - Pulse: Present, slow = 1
    - Grimace: None = 0
    - Appearance: Blue centrally and peripherally = 0
    - Respiratory effort: Present, slow = 1
    - Total: 2

11. **The correct answer is (D).** The infant needs to be thoroughly suctioned first with a meconium aspiration device, including the hypopharynx and trachea with the aid of direct laryngoscopy. As soon as the suctioning is complete and both the mouth and nose are reasonably free of meconium, ventilations should be initiated because the respiratory rate is agonal at a rate of 5. Finally, chest compressions can be initiated immediately because the heart rate is <60.

Trauma 8

Learning Objectives

- ❏ Describe anatomy, physiology, and physics associated with traumatic injuries.
- ❏ Assess and treat hemorrhage; soft-tissue injuries; and thermal, chemical, electrical, and radiation burns.
- ❏ Assess and treat musculoskeletal injuries, including fractures, dislocations, sprains, and strains.
- ❏ Differentiate, assess, and treat various head injuries, neurological injuries, and spinal cord injuries.
- ❏ Differentiate, assess, and treat thoracic injuries to the heart, lungs, and great vessels.

Trauma involves injury to the person by any outside force. Injuries the body can sustain and overcome are widely varied and often depend on how long it takes a person to get definitive care at the hospital. EMS plays a very important role in this aspect of trauma care. As the paramedic, it is your responsibility to rapidly triage, treat, and transport a patient to a facility capable of continuing treatment. In many cases, surgical procedures are required to alleviate injuries, repair internal lacerations to organs, or set broken bones. Getting the patient to such a facility capable of emergency operations is the overarching goal of paramedicine for the trauma patient.

Throughout this chapter, there will be references to the **index of suspicion**. The index of suspicion is that nagging feeling that something more than can be seen or otherwise experienced is wrong with the patient. It also is anticipating that something more is wrong and potentially life threatening. For example, keep a high index of suspicion that your patient has a developing pneumothorax when you find crepitus and a rib fracture, despite not having notably diminished lung sounds of JVD. It may turn out not to be true, but a high index of suspicion will lead the paramedic to treat aggressively, possibly leading to saving time and ultimately a life.

PHYSICS OF TRAUMA

Trauma results when the amount of energy that is transmitted into the human body exceeds the body's ability to cushion itself or dissipate the transmitted energy. Think about it this way: If a person were to punch another person in the shoulder, the victim would likely not even sustain a bruise from it. In this case, the body of the person who was punched successfully dissipated the energy the punch delivered to it, and trauma from the event is minimized. If this same person would instead have been hit with a baseball bat in the same shoulder swung by a professional major league baseball player, the victim would likely come away with a few broken bones. In this case, the body did not successfully dissipate the energy, and a traumatic event occurred. Warning: Do not attempt this thought experiment in real life!

Energy

Various kinds of energy can cause injury to patients.

Mechanical energy is the energy of an object, generally an object in motion. Mechanical energy in physics has two distinct components: kinetic energy and potential energy. **Potential energy** is energy that an object possesses based on the virtue of its position and, therefore, its potential to release energy. For example, a ball sitting on the ledge of a tall building has potential energy, but no energy that will hurt anyone anytime soon, until it falls off the ledge. Once it does fall off the edge, it now possesses **kinetic energy** (**KE**), which is the energy of motion. Cars in motion, things falling, or airborne bullets all possess KE. If they impact a person, the person may sustain injuries.

Chemical energy is released whenever existing chemical bonds are broken. When these bonds are broken, they release heat. If the heat is high enough, it can produce burns. Chemical energy is released in dramatic fashion whenever something burns or explodes, but it also can be more insidious, such as when an acid gets on skin.

Electrical energy is a special form of chemical energy and can be found in electrical lines or lightning strikes.

Pressure, although not technically an energy, is a force. If this force is applied in high enough quantity, it can cause injury. Think back to the information on changes in pressure during diving.

Kinetics and Force

The mechanism of injury is something that every paramedic should evaluate in a trauma patient. This helps determine how much energy was transferred to the patient and predict what injuries the patient may have sustained. Evaluating the mechanism involved may not always be obvious. The quantity and direction of the force and energy play an important role as well as the duration of time the force is exerted.

The KE an object possesses is exclusively dependent on two factors: mass and velocity. The **mass** of an object is essentially its weight, and **velocity** is the distance the object travels per unit of time. Velocity, by definition, also specifies a direction. According to the equation, the velocity of the object impacts the overall KE significantly more than the mass of the same object. This means that a light object traveling at a high rate of speed could potentially carry more KE than a large object moving slowly.

$$KE = \frac{1}{2}mv^2$$

The KE of a falling object, on the other hand, is entirely dependent on the height from which the fall started and the mass of the object falling. During the fall, the potential energy an object possesses before it begins to fall is completely converted to KE just before it impacts the earth. With this in mind, the potential energy of the object is based on the height of the object, the mass of the object, and the acceleration due to gravity. The acceleration due to gravity is always 9.8 m/s^2 within a reasonable distance from sea level on Earth. Unlike in the kinetic energy equation, the values that can change in this scenario are height (h) and mass (m). Neither impacts the overall energy of the falling object more than the other.

$$\text{potential energy} = mgh$$

The variable in this equation that will affect injuries suffered by a patient most, however, is height. For this reason, paramedics focus on the height of the fall far more critically than the mass of the patient falling.

Aside from these finite values that have a measurable effect on the patient, other factors include the position of the patient during the impact, the object the patient impacted, the duration of time the force or the energy is applied, and the overall resistance of the body area impacted. These factors are not completely independent of each other.

The position of the patient at the time of impact can have wide-ranging effects on the degree of trauma sustained. For example, a person who fell out of a tree stand and landed on their buttocks or feet will have a completely different prognosis and set of injures than the person who landed headfirst. The child who is hit by a car while attempting to run out of its way will sustain different injuries than the child who turns and faces the car. Finally, the person who is sitting sideways in the passenger seat of a car, perhaps talking to passengers in the backseat will have different injuries during a head-on collision than the person who is seated properly. Although it is not necessarily possible to say which of the patients in these pairs of examples would fare worse in most cases, it is understandable that they would have different injuries.

The object on which the falling patient lands or against which the patient in a vehicle impacts plays a significant role in the patient's injuries. This often has to do with extending the period of time the force is applied. To put this into perspective, think of the stunt person who falls from a building. When landing, no injury occurs because the person impacts a large, air-filled pillow that slowly brings the body to a stop. The stunt person does not collide with the pavement, which would instantly bring the person to a stop and result in untold injuries.

Consider the less dramatic fall down the stairs: a person who falls down an iron fire escape likely will suffer more injuries than a person who falls down the same number of thick carpeted steps. In the case of the stunt person's pillow or the patient who fell down the carpeted steps, what each person landed on spread out the area of the impact and lengthened the time of the impact, lessening the injuries. It also is the concept behind vehicular airbags, which extend the time over which a person decelerates.

Finally, the impact resistance of body parts has to do with the likelihood that injuries will be sustained as a result of some impact. The younger person playing impact sports is less likely to sustain injury than an older adult because of a flexible rib cage, for example. Certain body parts are also more resilient to damage as well. The solid organs of the body are much less compressible and are therefore more likely to rupture when compressed. Air-filled organs, on the other hand, can dissipate the impact more successfully, similar to the stunt person's pillow.

Scientific laws rule over what happens during any collision. The **law of conservation of energy** states that energy can neither be created nor destroyed, but it can be converted from one form to another. This is illustrated in a car crash when a car collides with an immovable object: the car bends, windows break, and the sound of the impact all release the KE the car possessed just before the impact. The energy also is converted into heat because of the friction of the car against the object.

Newton's **First Law of Motion** states that an object at rest will remain at rest until acted on by an outside force; an object in motion will remain in motion and traveling in a straight line unless acted on by an outside force. This also is seen in motor vehicle crashes. After the car comes to a complete stop, the person inside will continue moving forward at the same velocity as immediately before the impact, until the seat belt tenses or the person collides with the steering wheel or airbag.

Newton's **Second Law of Motion** states that the force an object will exert on another object is equal to the product of the mass of the object and the acceleration of that object. This is a little bit more difficult to experience. Acceleration is the change in velocity over a specific period of time. Let's consider a car that collides with the immovable object and say that the 1,000 kg car is moving at 20 m/s (meters per second or approximately 45 mph). An accident of this type brings the car completely to rest in about 0.5 second. This makes the acceleration (or in this case, deceleration) of the car during the accident 40 m/s^2 (20/0.5 = 40). Multiplying these values together, the force exerted on the car—and by extension the occupants—is 40,000 N. (The unit of force is the Newton.) In the equation, F represents the force, m is the mass of the object in question, and a is the acceleration of the object. Note also that a represents the change in velocity (v) divided by time (t).

$$F = ma$$

$$a = \frac{\Delta v}{t}$$

Blunt Trauma

Injuries resulting from compression or nonpenetrating forces are called blunt trauma. Motor vehicle accidents and falls account for the majority of causes of blunt trauma and also are known as **deceleration injuries**. Earlier, it was noted that at the time of a vehicle crash, although the car stops, the occupant continues to move at the same speed as prior to the collision until the person encounters the steering wheel or some other object in the car. As the patient makes contact with this object, the person's exterior begins to slow down, but the interior organs continue to travel at the same speed. As the body wall undergoes impact, the person begins to compress, resulting in injury, especially to the solid organs. Based on the point of impact on the patient's body and the factors noted prior, injury patterns can be predicted.

Some common injury patterns in motor vehicle crashes are as follows:

Front-End Impacts. This impact occurs when the deceleration force is directly opposite the initial direction of travel. The occupant will slow down at the same rate as the rest of the car and will sustain injuries of the anterior part of the body. Unrestrained occupants will travel either the down-and-under route or the up-and-over route. The down-and-under route will result in lower body injuries predominantly as the knees impact the underside of the dashboard, whereas the up-and-over route could result in the patient's head colliding with the roof or windshield, and the chest and abdomen colliding with the steering wheel. Ejection is possible if the velocity of the patient is too great for the windshield to stop it.

Lateral or T-Bone Impacts. These collisions place the brunt of the force on the passenger compartment door panel at about the midpoint of the car. The occupants on the same side of the impact will suffer the greatest injuries as their seating area becomes compressed and they are essentially squeezed between the colliding object and the center console (if present) or by the other occupant if the overall width of the car changes that drastically. In this kind of collision, the head will snap violently downward and toward the direction of the impact resulting in whiplash injuries and possibly brain injuries. The chest and hips are directly impacted, and fractures or a pneumothorax are possible, if not likely.

Rollovers. If the lateral impact is below the center of gravity of the vehicle, the impact may cause the car to roll over. This has the potential to cause myriad injuries, especially if the patient is unrestrained. Unrestrained patients in a rollover accident could be ejected from the vehicle or end up in another location within the vehicle from where they started. Maintain a high index of suspicion with these unrestrained patients because wherever they come to rest, they did not arrive there in a friendly way.

Rear-End Impacts. The collision often is from a car traveling faster and colliding with slower moving traffic. In an isolated impact, this is usually the most survivable crash with the fewest major injuries. Whiplash injuries are most common as the head moves backward relative to the body during the impact but then snaps forward as the car slows down again. This may be the worst of the issues. However, if during the collision the car is pushed into another car or into oncoming or cross traffic, injuries are no longer predictable and could very well be life threatening.

Rotational or Quarter Panel Impacts. Often occurring at an intersection, one vehicle impacts another at the area of the tire, rather than the middle of the vehicle as in a T-bone. Because the impact is away from the center of mass of the vehicle, it will rotate to dissipate the energy from the impact. Injuries are widely varied and depend largely on the point of impact relative to the passenger and whether the passenger was restrained or not.

Pro-Tip

On any crash scene, take a moment away from patient care and evaluate the damage to the vehicle. Note deformity in inches from where the exterior of the car was before the impact to where it is now, keeping in mind that most modern cars are designed to crumple around the passenger compartment, transmitting energy around the passenger compartment rather than through it. Note intrusion into the passenger compartment; anything more than a foot is considered a significant mechanism. Note if any airbags deployed and if the seatbelt was used. Note whether the surrounding windows are intact. Finally, note any damage to the interior of the passenger compartment, dashboard, steering wheel, or center console. All of this is part of a comprehensive patient assessment and should be relayed to the receiving facility and documented in the patient care report after the call.

Restraints

Seatbelts and airbags have saved countless motorists' lives because they prevent ejections, minimize passengers impacting the inside of the vehicle, and expand the time of impact of the patient and spread the forces of the impact over a greater area. Seatbelts can cause injuries of the chest, including bruising and possibly fractured ribs or clavicle, but these injuries likely pale in comparison from what could have happened without the seatbelt. The airbag relies on rapidly expanding hot gases to inflate faster than the forward movement of the patient. Consequently, minor burns from the powder and gases of the airbag often are reported. Abrasions to the chest and face also are complications of airbag deployment. Children in the front seat can be killed by the airbag expansion.

Motorcycle Crashes

Motorcycle crashes can happen in the same way as with cars, except that the riders do not have any meaningful protection. Ejection from the motorcycle is highly likely, and injuries are not predictable. There are several types of motorcycle impacts.

Head-on Impact. This stops the motorcycle's forward movement. In this type of collision, the rider is usually ejected up and over the handle bars. This motion could result in one or both of the rider's legs becoming caught on the pegs while simultaneously contacting the handlebars. This type of collision often results in bilateral femur fractures or possibly tibia or fibula fractures.

Angular Impact. This is close to a sideswipe impact but often results in one of the rider's legs becoming temporarily trapped between the bike and the car. This can result in extensive orthopedic damage to that leg.

Laying the Bike Down. This is an option the driver may take to avoid a worse collision. This allows the rider to deliberately separate from the bike. If the rider has worn proper protective equipment, including lower body leather or Kevlar, this should minimize long-term injuries and even may eliminate road rash. If the biker is not able to separate from the bike, however, the results could be devastating.

Motorcycle helmets are no longer required in many states, although more safety-oriented riders still opt to use them. If a helmet was worn at the time of the accident, the paramedic should evaluate it for abrasions or cracks and take it along to the hospital with the person who was wearing it. Any damage found on the helmet should be assumed to have been transmitted to the rider's head and neck until proven otherwise at the hospital. If the rider is still wearing it when EMS arrives, it should be removed carefully to allow for better access to the airway and proper in-line immobilization.

Pedestrian Accidents

In a pedestrian accident, there are three impacts, each of which can cause injuries. First, a car or truck collides with the individual, leading to injuries of the lower extremities, often ripping feet out of tightly laced shoes. Second, the torso, upper extremities, and head collide with the hood, causing injuries to those areas. Finally, the force of the impact provides sudden acceleration to the pedestrian and throws the patient. The third impact is when the person finally hits the ground and comes to rest. Adult pedestrians are more likely to be hit on their side as they walk or run to get out of the way, whereas children tend to turn and face the oncoming vehicle, resulting in more facial trauma caused not only by facing the vehicle but also their shorter stature.

Falls

As mentioned earlier, the severity of injury is primarily a result of the height from which the patient has fallen. Remember also that the acceleration due to gravity is 9.8 m/s^2, which means a person falling for just 2 seconds will hit the ground at nearly 45 mph! The duration of the fall can be impacted only by the height from which the person falls. Falls from heights of 3 times the height of the person are generally considered a significant mechanism of injury, and falls of about 50 feet (5 stories) or more are not likely survivable.

Extending the amount of time for deceleration increases the likelihood that a person will survive the fall. This can be accomplished with a large inflatable pillow for the stunt person; for shorter falls, it can simply include falling onto softer ground rather than cement. Consequently, what a person lands on plays a great role in severity of injury. In addition, it is worth noting that water at high speeds or falls from great height offer little in the way of a softer landing place and can be as hard on the body as concrete in a fall. Finally, take a moment to evaluate what the patient may have collided with on the way down. A straight fall without hitting any obstructions is generally less significant than one that struck many obstructions on the way down because each obstruction will be a narrow, rather than broad, point of impact on the body. It also may cause the body to rotate, further complicating the injuries sustained.

The physical condition of the patient could impact the severity of injuries that a patient sustains. Remember that the older adult with brittle bones will become more easily injured than a younger child under the same conditions. Furthermore, the medications the patient takes and their comorbid conditions, such as cardiac or lung disease or diabetes, may significantly impact the recovery time from any injury—regardless of severity.

Finally, the part of the body that sustains the initial impact during a fall also can affect the severity of the injury. Children frequently fall headfirst simply because of the disproportionate amount of mass concentrated in their upper bodies. Landing with legs outstretched and knees locked can transmit the impact all the way up into the pelvis and spine, which can lead to acetabular fractures and compression fractures of the vertebrae.

Blast Injuries

During an explosion, 5 types of injury can occur: primary, secondary, tertiary, quaternary, and quinary. **Primary blast injuries** are caused entirely by the pressure wave generated by the blast itself. **Secondary blast injuries** result from shrapnel, rocks, or anything in the vicinity of the blast becoming airborne and striking the patient. The pieces of material can travel in excess of 2,000 mph and can impale the victim. **Tertiary blast injuries** are caused by a person being hurled into the air and into another object, such as a wall, or knocked over onto the ground. These occur as a result of the pressure wave. **Quaternary blast injuries** are caused by other events surrounding the blast, such as burns from hot gases or flames or respiratory conditions resulting from the inhalation of toxins. Finally, **quinary blast injuries** are found in the so-called dirty bomb. This releases contaminants, such as fertilizer, VX gas, deadly bacteria, or radioactive materials, into the surrounding area during the explosion.

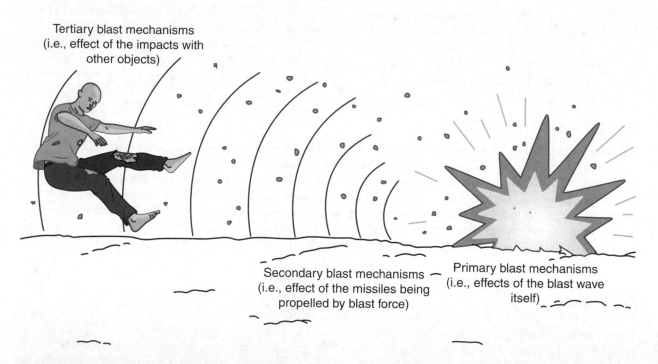

Figure 8-1. Primary, Secondary, and Tertiary Blast Injuries

Treatment of blast injuries requires a high index of suspicion and means being prepared to treat life-threatening injuries. The injuries can be as wide ranging as ruptured tympanic membranes, lungs, and other gas-filled structures as a result of the pressure wave and other blunt trauma to burns, lacerations, and fractures. It is possible to spend extensive amounts of time in projecting possible injuries resulting from any one of the above levels of blast injuries, but it is best to conduct a thorough head-to-toe assessment, aggressively treating any derangements of the ABCs found.

Penetrating Trauma

Penetrating trauma includes any type of puncture to the skin at least, but it usually involves underlying structures. Penetrating trauma is classified as low, medium, and high velocity. Low-velocity penetrating trauma encompasses stab wounds and penetrations sustained from falls or countless other ways of puncturing the skin. The severity of a stab wound is determined by the following factors:

- Damage to structures underlying the area of the skin penetrated.
- Is the knife waved around inside the body or just plunged into it? Moving it around can have the effect of broadening out the area of the stab wound.
- What is the depth of the penetration?
- Was the penetrating object removed and reinserted? If the knife or other object is plunged in and allowed to remain, the knife or penetrating object's presence may be enough to tamponade any bleeding, making the injury less significant than it may otherwise have been.

Medium- and high-velocity penetrating wounds are generally from a firearm or other projectile. Firearms, listed here in decreasing order from high velocity to medium velocity, include rifles, shotguns, and handguns. Rifles produce the highest muzzle velocity of weapons and fire a single, comparatively large bullet that follows a straight path.

The shotgun is still considered high velocity; however, the initial velocity is slower than that of a rifle and higher than that of a handgun. The shotgun, in contrast to rifles and handguns, fires a shell that is loaded with smaller pellets. The pellets vary in size but tend to scatter upon ejection from the muzzle. At distances less than about 30 feet, the shotgun blast can be devastating: the unevenly shaped pellets cause widespread injury, tearing and shredding through the tissue, carrying clothing, hair, and other material into the wounds they create.

The handgun fires a single bullet at a time with reasonable accuracy—more than the shotgun but less than the rifle— because of both the shorter barrel and sight radius. Bullet diameters for the handgun can vary anywhere from less than a quarter inch to nearly half an inch. The larger the bullet diameter, the more likely it is to travel in a straight line and the more difficult it is to be deflected off a straight pattern. Smaller bullets can ricochet off organs of differing densities or bone, whereas larger ones are more likely to tumble in a straight line. Tumbling increases the amount of damage done along the travel pathway. Furthermore, the cavitation wave the bullet produces, similar to the wake a fast-moving boat leaves in water but in all directions, can cause even more damage and bruising to surrounding tissues.

Much discussion often is given to entrance and exit wounds and how to distinguish each type. As a paramedic, the wounds should not be labeled "entrance" or "exit"; rather, an objective description of each should be given clearly in the patient care report. Although it is true that entrance wounds often are small, roughly approximating the size of the bullet that entered, and exit wounds often are large and appear as if an explosion happened just below the skin caused by the cavitation wave, this is not an absolute rule. Instead, document the appearance and location of any wounds found.

GENERAL ASSESSMENT, TRAUMA CRITERIA, AND TRANSPORT DECISIONS

Genuine multisystem trauma calls can be extremely stressful for the paramedic. A whole lot went wrong all at once, resulting in difficult scenes and multiple patients with widely varying complaints. The scenes more often than not are a chaotic hub of activity, sometimes involving multiple agencies and levels of training, occasionally with conflicting priorities. The extrication of the patient may require hours of time and specialized equipment, and the coordination of efforts to free a patient is complicated. Finally, patient injuries are sometimes occult and need to be found through diligence of a systematic assessment.

General Assessment

The assessment of the multisystem trauma patient should follow a systematic and consistent pattern to minimize the possibility of missing something. **Multisystem trauma** refers to a traumatic event that involves more than one of the body's systems. For example, a patient who fell and sustained a pneumothorax and fractured ribs has sustained damage to the respiratory and musculoskeletal systems. This is always more significant than an isolated injury, such as an eye injury or a fractured ankle. The body can more readily deal with the isolated injury, rather than multiple and widespread problems all at once.

The assessment should begin by assessing the airway, breathing, circulation, disability, and exposure.

- **Airway.** Focus on determining the patency of the airway during respirations and assess for the patient's ability to maintain a patent airway going forward. If the patient is not likely to be able to maintain their airway, consider intubation or the placement of an alternative airway.

- **Breathing.** Focus on the quality and effectiveness of breathing; initially, a rate is not required. If breathing has adequate tidal volume and appropriate minute volume, provide supplemental O_2. If breathing is deemed inadequate or ineffective, provide positive pressure ventilations with a BVM and consider intubation as soon as feasible if the patient is not combative, clenched, or seizing.

- **Circulation.** Assess all of the following: (1) observe for any massive bleeding, (2) assess for skin color and temperature, and (3) assess for the presence and quality of a pulse. Here again, pulse rate is not specifically needed—fast, slow, or normal is sufficient during this rapid assessment. At this point in the assessment, control any major external bleeding and begin to plan for prevention of and treatment for shock.

- **Disability.** Once the ABCs have been addressed, assess the neurological status of the patient. This is done generally with AVPU and then more specifically by obtaining a GCS reading. Assess for loss of consciousness and overall level of consciousness.

- **Exposure.** In multisystem trauma, it is not possible to fully assess the patient who is still clothed. The patient should be stripped completely naked, except, under most circumstances, their underwear. It is rarely necessary to assess genitalia or breasts in the trauma patient. If it should be necessary, expose the area for assessment and treatment and then cover the area back up as soon as treatment allows. Maintenance of dignity is important unless it interferes with treating a potentially life-threatening injury. Whenever possible, perform this step in the confines of the ambulance, not in the view of the general public.

Vital signs should always be obtained as soon as possible and every 5 minutes or so throughout contact. The patient who has sustained multisystem trauma should be placed on a cardiac monitor, and intravenous access should be obtained with fluids running to maintain an SBP of >100. Minor bleeding should be bandaged at this point, and extremities suspected of having a fracture or dislocation can be splinted. It is worth keeping in mind, however, in massive trauma, that the paramedic may never get to any meaningful assessment or treatment beyond managing ABCDE.

Trauma Criteria

The paramedic will need to decide if the patient needs to go to an accredited trauma facility or can be treated at a regional or community hospital. In many cases, when multisystem trauma is present, a trauma facility is recommended. The American College of Surgeons has made recommendations on which patients need a trauma center. A patient who meets any of the following criteria should be transported to a trauma center via the most efficient means possible.

- **Physiological Criteria**
  - GCS ≤13 at any point during patient contact
  - SPB ≤90 at any point during patient contact (<110 in patient >65 years)
  - Respiratory rate outside the range of 10–30 per minute or on ventilatory support

- **Anatomic Criteria**
  - Any penetrating trauma to head, neck, torso, or proximal extremities
  - Chest trauma, including fractures
  - Two or more proximal long bone fractures
  - Crush injury to any extremity
  - Degloving injury
  - Pulseless extremity
  - Amputation proximal to the wrist or ankle
  - Pelvic instability
  - Open or depressed skull fracture
  - Paralysis

- **Mechanism of Injury Criteria**
  - Fall >3× the body height (children) or 20 ft (adult)
  - Car versus pedestrian or bicyclist where the person is thrown, run over, or struck at speeds >20 mph
  - Motorcycle crash at speeds >20 mph

- Car crash involving any of the following:
  - ° Intrusion into passenger compartment >12 in.
  - ° Ejection from the vehicle
  - ° Death of another occupant in the same vehicle
- **Special Considerations**
  - Patient age >55 years
  - Patient is pregnant
  - Burns of any kind with other trauma present
  - Patient takes anticoagulants or has a bleeding disorder
  - EMS provider judgment

Mode of Transport

If any of the aforementioned criteria are met, the patient must be taken to a trauma center. The paramedic must make the decision on how to get the patient to the hospital. There are two options: ground or air. The paramedic should consider the following criteria before electing to fly the patient:

- Can the trauma center be reached within about 20 minutes by ground? If the transport time is less than about 20 minutes, factoring in weather and traffic, then the patient should be transported by ground. Outside that range, aeromedical flight should be considered.
- Is there difficulty in accessing the patient? This can be caused by rough or remote terrain, such as forest trails or extensive off-road travel needed, or entrapment and the need for complicated, time-consuming extrication. If the rescue company predicts that the patient will take long enough to extricate and that a helicopter could have landed by the time the patient is freed from the vehicle or extricated from the rough terrain, and injuries meet the previous criteria, then flight is recommended.
- Does the patient require medical care beyond that of the resources available on the scene? Flight nurses and paramedics generally have a broader scope of practice and can provide more extensive care than ground crews. This can include the administration of paralytics to aid in intubating a combative patient or the patient whose jaw is clenched as a result of a head injury. If this level of care is needed and not available on the ground transport unit, aeromedical transport is preferred.
- Is this a **multiple casualty incident** (**MCI**)? If multiple patients are at an event, it is advisable to send the most critically injured by air so that the ground resources are not stripped from a certain area. With that in mind, it is not recommended to send any of the patients from an MCI by air if the patients do not meet criteria. Aeromedical transport is exorbitantly expensive and rarely covered by any insurance.
- If the region requires without exception that ambulance patients be brought to the nearest facility, then sending the patient by air will alleviate this requirement. Going to the nearest facility should be only under extreme circumstances, such as weather conditions that make it unsafe to fly, unavailability of helicopters, or ground transport to a trauma center that would exceed 20 minutes.

INCIDENT MANAGEMENT AND TRIAGE

Incident management and triage often are the paramedic's responsibility. On a scene with multiple patients, or the potential for multiple patients, the paramedic must employ a system of response, treatment, and transport to maximize the greatest number of casualties surviving the incident with the least long-term deficits. This can be accomplished by using the **National Incident Management System** (**NIMS**) to help guide responses and effective, rapid triage on scene to help identify the most life-threatening conditions among the casualties.

Incident Command System

NIMS provides a structure for the effective running of a situation. If all responders are familiar with the system and the guidelines for operating within it, the casualties will suffer the least long-lasting ill effects, and the providers will be able to operate in a safe environment. The **incident command system** has the following components:

- Command structure
- Preparedness
- Resource management
- Communications and information management and dissemination

Incident Commander

The incident commander (IC) will be the person in charge of the overall operation of the scene. In many cases, this is the local fire chief, fire marshal, or other designated officer. (Rarely is it a person from EMS.) The IC is responsible for scaling up (or down) the operation as needed, and for assigning roles to arriving personnel. Any roles not assigned are inherently retained within the role of the IC.

There are 2 types of command systems:

- **Unified Command System:** joint command structure (each agency knows the role it would play in the event of an actual incident)
  - Often major incidents that are planned well ahead of time across agencies that will be involved with primary wave of response, e.g., a nuclear power plant 'practice run' for a meltdown situation
  - Triage and evacuation procedures, among others, are practiced across the teams
- **Single Command System:** single person command structure;
  - Often medium-to large-scale incidents that cannot be anticipated, e.g., a multiple vehicle crash or a natural disaster
  - IC should be well-identified by both the uniform and location from which operation is led

Finance Sector Chief

The finance sector chief will be responsible for all costs associated with a large-scale incident. This is particularly essential when multiple agencies are responding. The finance sector chief often is part of a unified command structure, and the expenses are tallied well in advance of the event.

Logistics Sector Chief

Logistics is planning, so the logistics sector chief is responsible for procuring and distributing supplies to be delivered directly to a scene. The supplies include not only medical supplies but also food, water, fuel, and lodging for the providers on scene. This person does not have any direct responsibility for the transport destinations of patients.

Operations Sector Chief

The operations sector chief is responsible for the operation of the scene and all tactical operations. This includes all branches related to patient care. The branch leaders report to the operations sector chief. Usually there is only one operations sector chief, but multiple officers may report to the operations sector chief.

The tactical operations branch officers who report to the operations sector chief are as follows:

- **Triage Officer:** Responsible for the team of personnel triaging each patient from the scene or area that they have been tasked by the operations sector chief
- **Treatment Officer:** Responsible for the care delivered in the triage area; has several providers assigned to each triage area to provide care and remain accountable for the patients in that area; also responsible for ensuring that any patients who refuse care or transportation are documented on paper, so that those involved in the incident are accounted for

- **Transport Officer:** Responsible for assigning patients from triage/treatment area to ambulances, buses, or wheelchair-accessible vans for transport to the hospital or other temporary housing; should keep track of where the patients are sent so they may be reunited with loved ones at a later date; also responsible for keeping track of any patients who cannot be resuscitated
- **Staging Officer:** Responsible for maintaining an ongoing list of available transport-capable units as they arrive to the scene and as they are called away by the transport officer (these units include not only ambulances but also buses and wheelchair-accessible vans for noncritical transport from the scene)
- **Extrication Officer:** Responsible for overseeing rescue operations (often bridges EMS and fire operations on a scene because of the responsibility to extricate patients (fire) and to get patients to the triage sector [EMS]); usually functions under EMS branch but often (ideally) is cross-trained in both extrication and EMS knowledge
- **Rehabilitation Officer:** Responsible for the care and well-being of the providers on scene, including fire and EMS branches; has the authority to remove a provider from the operation for medical reasons or to ensure adequate sleep; usually functions under the EMS branch

Planning Sector Chief

The planning sector chief is responsible for solving issues as they arise during an operation that are unrelated to treatment or transportation. This individual, for example, may be tasked with finding temporary housing for displaced individuals who are not otherwise hurt and not in need of medical care, or they may need to work on getting supplies to the scene. Ultimately, this person works closely with the logistics sector chief and the IC to ensure smooth operation of the scene.

Command Staff

The IC may need to rely on several individuals to work with the public, media, and other sector officers on especially large-scale incidents, such as natural disasters.

- **Safety Officer:** Responsible for the provision and maintenance of safety throughout the operation for any condition that may become a problem for providers; has the authority to stop an entire operation if a threat to providers is identified, and restart only once problem is resolved
- **Public Information Officer:** Responsible for relaying information to media outlets about the state of the ongoing operation (under the direction of the IC); assigned later in the operation and is positioned well away from the operation, both to keep the members of the public and media safe and to minimize distractions on the scene
- **Liaison Officer:** Responsible for disseminating information across the command structure, to ensure all providers are up-to-date on the latest information and status of the operation

Triage

Triage is a system of sorting patients at an MCI in a manner that ensures that the patients with the most life-threatening conditions receive the fastest care. This system allows a small team of rescuers to do the greatest good for the vast majority of patients.

Primary triage takes place as soon as the patient arrives at the triage sector. This is the first and arguably cursory evaluation of the patient. Often performed by the triage officer or a designee, once triaged, the patient is assigned an initial triage category. This category often is of a higher priority than the patient's condition may warrant after a more detailed assessment.

When the patient arrives at their primary triage area as assigned during primary triage, the patient is reevaluated during the **secondary triage** process. This better reflects where the patient should be and, by extension, the priority with which the patient can be transported. The patient is assigned **Green**, Yellow, **Red**, or **Black** colors that designate the severity and priority of the patient's condition.

- **Green.** Low priority, non-life-threatening injuries. These patients will remain on scene longer in most cases and may receive transport to a hospital by a means other than an ambulance.

- Yellow. Delayed transport, moderate injuries not likely to be life threatening. Patients in this category may have visible fractures of distal extremities or spinal injuries with or without paralysis. These patients will not have severe impairments to respiratory or cardiovascular systems. In addition, they will not have a known apparent change in mental status.

- **Red.** Immediate transport, life-threatening or potentially life-threatening condition. These patients have known and apparent changes in mental status or derangement in respiratory or cardiovascular systems. This can include patients with chest pain and respiratory distress independent of the injury. Patients who regain spontaneous respirations with an airway adjustment or adjunct or who have spontaneous respirations after being given 5 rescue breaths are tagged **red**; if these fail, they are tagged **black**. Patients experiencing a severe psychiatric emergency, whether directly related to the incident or not, may be given a **red** tag so that they are removed from scene more quickly, thus minimizing their impact to the scene. Injured rescuers should be transported immediately off scene to minimize the morale impact on the remaining rescuers.

- **Black.** Deceased or unsalvageable patients. Patients garner a **black** tag when they have signs inconsistent with life, such as cardiac arrest or severe chest or head injuries. Patients in respiratory arrest with a pulse get a **black** tag if manual adjustment of the airway (head tilt/chin lift or an oral pharyngeal airway) does not result in spontaneous, life-sustaining respiratory effort on the part of the patient.

START Triage

START triage is the recommended primary triage guidelines for a disaster response. Following this 6-step approach will allow the triage officer or a designee to rapidly evaluate all accessible patients on a scene and direct them to the treatment areas.

The first step is to get all the walking wounded off the immediate area of the scene. These will all be tagged **green** and sent to the treatment area.

The next steps involve an evaluation of breathing for each patient remaining on the scene. If the patient is not breathing, reposition the airway and reevaluate. Use the **red** tag if with repositioning the patient begins to breathe spontaneously; use the **black** tag if the patient fails to begin breathing.

If the patient is breathing, is the *estimated* respiratory rate between 10 and 30? If outside this range, the patient is tagged **red** and sent to that treatment area for secondary triage. If the patient is breathing, move to the next evaluation point, circulation.

Does the patient have a strong *radial* pulse? If so, move to the next evaluation step of mental status. If the patient does not have a strong radial pulse, and it is found to be either weak, irregular, or absent, the patient is tagged **red** and sent to that treatment area.

If the paramedic makes it this far in the triage process on any patient, the patient is essentially hemodynamically stable, and the final evaluation point is the patient's mental status. If the patient is able to follow commands, the patient is tagged yellow and sent to that treatment area. If the patient is unable to follow commands, the patient is tagged **red** and sent to that treatment area.

This process can be completed in less than 30 seconds for every patient, and it is cohesive if more than one person is completing the primary triage of each patient. Obviously, it is likely that a lot of patients will be triaged to the red category, many of whom will be overtriaged. Once to the red treatment area, the personnel there can do a more in-depth assessment of the patient and choose to either keep the patient in that category or reduce the patient's priority to yellow or green if appropriate.

Table 8-1. START Triage Principles

Step	Assessment Question	Outcome	Next step	
1	Capable of walking?	Yes	→	
		No	→	Go to Step 2
2	Breathing?	Yes	→	Go to Step 3
		No	→	Go to Step 4
3	RR between 10 and 30?	Yes	→	Go to Step 5
		No	→	
4	Reposition, now breathing?	Yes	→	
		No	→	
5	Pulse present?	Yes	→	Go to Step 6
		No/weak	→	
6	Follows clear commands?	Yes	→	
		No	→	

Special Triage Considerations

Certain patients should be triaged higher than their conditions may otherwise indicate. Injured or ill rescuers should be transported immediately. Individuals on scene who are exhibiting signs of psychiatric illness, including hysteria and aggression, should be removed as soon as possible (this kind of behavior is contagious and could cause the situation to get out of control quickly). Additionally,

- **Lightning strike** will require a significant alteration to these triage guidelines. Patients in cardiac arrest due to a lightning strike need to be triaged in "*reverse triage*," i.e., they will receive a **red** tag (not black) in all triage situations (the reason being that such patients will likely recover from the event with rapid appropriate treatment, while most other trauma patients in cardiac arrest will not).

- **Contamination with hazardous materials**—chemical or biological—will require patients to be decontaminated before going to the triage sector. This is to prevent contamination of the triage area, treatment area providers, ambulances, and equipment. Once decontaminated, these patients can be triaged as usual.

SOFT-TISSUE INJURIES AND BLEEDING

The skin, also known as the **integument**, is the largest organ in the body and is composed of two distinct layers: the epidermis (outermost layer) and the dermis (inner layer). The integument serves several important functions.

Structure and Function of Skin

The skin serves four functions:

- **Protection.** The skin minimizes trauma from mechanical forces that would otherwise be caused by the simple act of walking or bumping into things. It prevents microorganisms and toxic chemicals from entering the body.

- **Sensory.** The skin contains nerve endings for pain and pressure plus hot and cold. This helps keep the rest of the body informed about the external environment.

- **Temperature Regulation.** The capillaries near the skin, lying within the dermis and subcutaneous layers, can be dilated to release excess heat or constricted to conserve heat. The arrector pili muscles attached to hair follicles can raise hair off the skin, which has the effect of trapping heat near the skin in an alternate method of temperature regulation.

- **Water Balance.** The skin helps the body maintain water balance by not allowing water to evaporate from the body through the skin. This also helps maintain the body's internal environment.

Epidermis

The **epidermis** is primarily responsible for preventing water loss and protecting the body from the external environment and mechanical forces. The innermost portion of this layer is made of living cells that begin at the base of the layer and push outward toward the surface. As these cells move outward, they become filled with a protein called keratin and die. They are then known as the stratum corneum, which makes up the tough, outer layer of skin. The epidermis also contains sporadically placed melanocytes that are responsible for the production of melanin. A person with more melanocytes will have a darker skin.

Dermis

The **dermis** lies immediately underneath the epidermis and is made up of tough elastic fibers called **collagen** and **elastin**. These work together to make the skin resistant to tearing and distortion. Also within the dermis lie the capillaries responsible for thermoregulation. White blood cells called macrophages and lymphocytes are located throughout the dermis as well and serve as a first-line defense against any pathogens that may get across the skin or as a result of cuts or abrasions. The following structures also lie within the dermis:

- Nerve endings (sensory fibers for pressure, pain, and temperature)
- Sweat glands
- Hair roots
- Sebaceous glands

Subcutaneous Tissues

A layer largely consisting of fat (adipose) cells that provides insulation and cushioning, **subcutaneous tissue** underlies the dermis and is superficial to the major muscle groups. The subcutaneous tissue also is highly vascular.

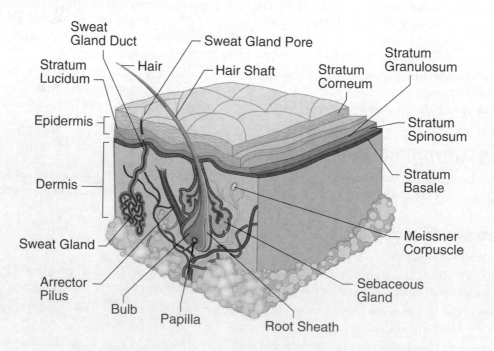

Figure 8-2. Anatomy of the Skin and Subcutaneous Tissue

Hemorrhage

Hemorrhage can be internal or external, but either one can be severe enough to lead to hypovolemic, specifically hemorrhagic, shock. Humans contain 65-70 mL/kg of circulating blood at any time, which correlates to approximately 5 L of blood in an average-sized adult. The loss of just 1 L of blood in an adult, whether internally or externally, will lead to vital sign changes and the onset of signs of shock. To broaden this number, the body cannot tolerate a loss of more than 20% of the circulating volume. The type of vessel lacerated will determine how quickly the body will lose blood and what the bleeding looks like if the bleeding is external.

- **Arterial Bleeding.** Often spurting initially, arterial bleeding can slow to a continuous flow if the loss is significant enough. If the vessel is cut perpendicularly, the vessel can clamp down and minimize bleeding; if the vessel is cut along its axis, it will actually open further and continue to bleed. Neither laceration type is likely to clot because of the pressure of the pulse wave.
- **Venous Bleeding.** This is slower and a darker red than arterial bleeding. Lacerations to larger veins can lead to significant blood loss, and the end of the vein that is closest to the heart may draw in air, leading to an air embolism. Remember to cover both ends of the vein when controlling bleeding.
- **Capillary Ooze.** Capillaries are under very little pressure and, therefore, tend to seep or ooze. Breaks in capillaries are the most likely to clot and stop bleeding on their own.

Under normal circumstances, minor bleeding will clot off and stop in about 10 minutes. The following conditions or situations will interfere with normal clotting processes.

- **Medications.** Beta-blockers may prevent the vessel from constricting, thereby allowing further bleeding. Anticoagulants such as aspirin, clopidogrel, warfarin, or enoxaparin will delay or inhibit clotting.
- **Hemophilia.** Genetic condition where the patient lacks the ability to clot. This patient will not clot, and a simple laceration could become life threatening.
- **Extensive Damage to the Vessel.** This will prevent normal clotting from happening because the clot cannot close all the areas of bleeding.
- **Hypothermia.** Cold will inhibit the necessary enzyme reactions from occurring, and, therefore, the clotting cascade will not occur.

Closed Wounds and Internal Hemorrhage

Closed wounds are widely varied in severity and can lead to life-threatening blood loss. The following are examples of closed wounds or internal hemorrhages, complete with symptoms and prehospital treatment.

Contusions. Commonly known as bruises, contusions involve breaks in the capillary vessels underneath the skin, without actually breaking the skin. These generally are not life threatening, and little prehospital treatment is required.

Hematomas. Larger subcutaneous vessels and sometimes arteries can be ruptured and bleed more heavily than the capillary vessels in contusions. This results in a raised, blood-filled area resembling a large blister. This bleeding can continue to the point where pressure builds up and underlying tissues are deprived of blood and therefore O_2. This can result in necrosis to the area. Although not life threatening, untreated hematomas can lead to significant tissue damage. The paramedic should apply ice or a cold pack to the area if possible. Also, mark the edges with a pen so that later assessments will clearly reveal whether the hematoma is still growing. Definitive treatment is sterile drainage at the hospital.

Compartment Syndrome

Within all 4 limbs, individual muscle groups are surrounded by a tough covering called **fascia**, which confines the muscles to a finite compartment. Bleeding or swelling that occurs within this compartment raises the pressure within the compartment. Compartment syndrome results when the pressure within the compartment rises too high and circulation to the muscle within the compartment is compromised. If this is allowed to continue for an extended period of time, irreversible tissue death (necrosis) can set in. This can happen with soft-tissue injuries or fractures to the limb.

Symptoms of compartment syndrome include the **6 Ps**:
- Pain (generalized in the area of the compartment)
- Paralysis
- Paresthesia (numbness or burning sensation in the area)
- Passive stretch pain (stretching or extending the muscle within the compartment will induce more pain)
- Pressure
- Pulselessness (distal to the injury)

Prehospital treatment for compartment syndrome is limited to rapid transport and delivery of the patient to the emergency department before the extremity is pulseless. Narcotic pain relief may be attempted, but it is usually unsuccessful at relieving pain. Splinting the extremity to prevent further injury is recommended; however, it is critically important to make sure that there are pulses after splinting if they existed before splinting. Applying the splint too tight can increase the possibility of compartment syndrome. The administration of high-flow O_2 will maximize the amount of O_2 the tissue is receiving. Providing intravenous crystalloid fluid also will maximize the flushing of toxins resulting from rhabdomyolysis.

Internal Hemorrhage

Internal bleeding from injury to internal organs can be difficult to find or assess. If the patient has sustained abdominal or chest injuries, presume that there is internal bleeding. This maintains a high index of suspicion so that the patient will receive a higher level of care. If the abdomen is firm to palpation or if there is any bruising over either flank (the Grey Turner sign) or around the umbilicus (the Cullen sign), there may be internal bleeding. Rebound tenderness is a sign of peritoneal irritation, which could be from blood in the perineum or other toxins from ruptured bowels.

Hemorrhage should be suspected and transport initiated to a trauma center for emergency surgery. Initiate cardiac monitoring and an intravenous line. Consider a 200–500 mL bolus or run the intravenous line wide open if the patient is already showing signs of shock.

Open Wounds and External Hemorrhage

Open wounds bleed externally, so the amount of blood lost often is visible. This means that it is much more likely to accurately estimate the amount of blood lost, making it easier to anticipate the onset of shock. Open wounds have a greater capacity to bleed than internal wounds, which often can be self-limiting because of the confined space in which to bleed.

With open wounds, however, there is a greater likelihood of contamination of the wound with bacteria and other debris. Although this does not necessarily pose an acute threat to the patient, in an isolated open wound, such as an abrasion sustained from a low-speed fall from a pedal bicycle, the wound should be irrigated with sterile water before placing the bandage. Deeper wounds and burns may require more aggressive debridement at the hospital.

Abrasions

Abrasions are very shallow wounds that occur when the skin is dragged across a rough surface. This will essentially remove parts of the epidermis, exposing the nerve endings found in the dermis to air. This is what causes the most pain. Rinsing the abrasion may cause the patient more pain in the short term, but it may be better for the patient to help minimize the chances of infection. Cover lightly with a bandage.

Amputation

An **amputation** is the partial or complete separation of a digit or limb from the patient. In **partial amputations**, the limb remains attached to the person only via an isthmus of skin. In **complete amputations**, the limb is completely detached. Bleeding in an amputation often is less than anticipated because the vessels are able to constrict.

The paramedic should be cautious about jagged, exposed bone ends that could catch on something or cause a laceration to the rescuers.

A unique amputation is the degloving injury. In this injury pattern, the bones are usually left intact, with only the skin removed from the body—the way one would remove a glove or a sock. Often times, the skin is removed overall intact, but the appearance is particularly gruesome. This, and any shredding or tearing full amputation, often will have excessive bleeding because the vessels were not cut cleanly transverse.

Treatment for an amputation begins with cleaning the remaining part of any debris. Wrap the stump with sterile roller gauze. In the unlikely event that the bleeding is profuse, immediately consider a tourniquet placed on the proximal limb. For the amputated part, rinse it with saline and wrap loosely with gauze soaked in sterile water or saline. Place the part in a plastic bag and seal the bag. Place the bag inside a cooler with cold packs or ice but do not let the part or any portion of the part freeze. The part should not be submerged in water and should not be in direct contact with the ice. Transport the patient immediately, whether or not the part can be located.

Avulsion

An **avulsion** occurs when a flap of skin is torn loose, either partially or completely. In a **partial avulsion**, the skin flap is still attached to the patient; in a **complete avulsion**, the chunk of skin is completely removed, almost like removing a piece of cheese from a block of cheese with a cheese slicer.

Bleeding with an avulsion is dependent on its location. An avulsion of the scalp or facial skin may bleed profusely, whereas an avulsion of the back or dorsal forearm, for example, may ooze only. Begin treatment for an avulsion by washing the area where the flap was removed with sterile water. Return the flap to its original anatomic position. If it was a complete avulsion, give the best approximation of its original location. Cover the wound with a dry sterile dressing. If available, apply a cold pack to extend the time that the flap of skin will remain viable.

Bites

Human and animal bites, though often minor soft-tissue injuries, expose the patient to a wide variety of infections. The human mouth contains far more strains of bacteria that can cause infection than either the dog or cat. Wild animals can have any number of bacteria in their mouths and also may have the virus that causes rabies. Any bite, especially human, where the skin is broken should be seen at a hospital.

Treatment for bites with broken skin should include the following:

- Calm the patient who is anxious about being bitten.
- Irrigate the wound with sterile water or saline.
- If the bite involved tearing, such as if a dog bites a person and the person yanks their arm free, try to replace the tissue to where it came from as in an avulsion.
- Control bleeding with a dry sterile dressing.
- Transport to the hospital for suturing, antibiotics, and possible surgical resection.

Crush Syndrome

When an extremity is crushed under a considerable weight, such as a car that fell off a jack or during a building collapse, extensive damage to the body can occur the longer the body is under the weight. The crush weight alone can splinter bones and rupture muscles. A person can recover from these injuries if the weight can be removed relatively quickly. **Crush syndrome** can develop in any person trapped for any period of time. It is especially likely to happen after four hours or more under the crushing item, or when arterial blood flow is compromised.

Primarily, crush syndrome results in tissue necrosis to the area under or distal to the crushing object. This results in rhabdomyolysis in all the muscles in this region because of the lack of circulation. Rhabdomyolysis is the breakdown of skeletal muscle, which releases myoglobin into the bloodstream. The myoglobin can cause acute renal failure if not treated aggressively. In addition to rhabdomyolysis, all cells, including the muscle cells in the area, release into the bloodstream waste products of metabolism. These waste products include acids from anaerobic respiration, CO_2, urea, and potassium from both cellular death and metabolism. This combines for an isolated area of metabolic acidosis. Clots also can form throughout the extremity because of hemostasis.

As a result of all this developing while the crushing object is in place, the level of toxins in the crushed extremities can reach lethal quantities in 4 hours depending on the extent of the area crushed. Therefore, removal of the object without first initiating medical treatment could result in almost immediate patient death from cardiac arrest. After ensuring scene safety and accessing the patient, conduct as much of the primary survey as possible and address any threats of the ABCs. At this point, it is important to monitor the patient while coordinating efforts to remove the crushing object from the patient. Take the following steps just prior to removal of the crushing object.

1. Place the patient on the cardiac monitor and monitor continuously for ECG changes consistent with hyperkalemia.

2. Establish intravenous or intraosseous access in any accessible, unaffected extremity or the external jugular vein and infuse normal saline, not lactated Ringer solution, which contains potassium.

3. Once the team is ready to remove the crushing object, administer 1 mEq/kg sodium bicarbonate intravenously or intraosseously.

4. Infuse up to 1 L normal saline solution. Continue infusing at least another liter as the object is being removed.

5. If the cardiac monitor is showing signs of hyperkalemia, including peaked or tented T waves or a P wave with decreased amplitude, give 1 g calcium chloride or calcium gluconate.

Mannitol can be used to accelerate diuresis. Lasix should not be used because it can add to the acid present in the blood. If medications are not an option, apply a tourniquet proximal to the crush if possible. Consult medical command before readministering of the medications and for assistance in establishing the intravenous fluid flow rate.

Lacerations

Lacerations are cuts that often extend deep into the dermis and sometimes beyond. The severity of the laceration will depend on the structures that were damaged from the laceration. An **incision** is a special kind of laceration, where the edges are very precise and the cut was made intentionally, generally with a surgeon's scalpel. Apply direct pressure and elevation and move quickly to a tourniquet if arterial bleeding is noted or if the bleeding does not stop with direct pressure and elevation.

Puncture Wounds

Any instrument that penetrates the skin and underlying structures is a puncture wound. This can be from a knife, a nail, or a shard of wood kicked up by a saw blade. With puncture wounds, always assume that it is deeper than can be assessed and that more than just skin and subcutaneous tissue are involved. The penetrating objects also can deliver bacteria and debris deep into the body, so infection is a common complication. Shock can develop quickly, from blood loss or damage to fluid-filled, hollow organs, such as a bladder or the GI tract.

If the penetrating object has been removed prior to EMS arrival, treatment is much the same as that for a laceration: Clean with sterile water or saline and bandage.

A more unique situation presents when the penetrating object has been left in the patient. This is now called an impaled object and should not be removed; the object may be tamponading internal bleeding. The only reasons to manipulate an impaled object would be if its presence is too cumbersome to get the patient into the ambulance or if the object is attached to something else, such as a fencepost or car antenna. At any rate, motion of the object itself or of the patient around the object should be limited to minimize the chances of causing or worsening internal bleeding.

Treatment of the impaled object is more complicated than a laceration or an open puncture wound. First, minimize movement of the soft tissues immediately surrounding the impaled object because this could further damage those structures. Apply bulky padding around the impaled object so that its motion is limited. Bulky dressings can include rolls of gauze or blankets and towels, depending on the size of the impaled object. The only time an impaled object should be removed is if it interferes with the airway or the performance of CPR. Removal of an object impaled through the facial cheek is acceptable because it may interfere with the airway, and the paramedic can provide direct pressure to both sides of the wound, minimizing bleeding.

General Treatment Guidelines

Managing External Hemorrhage

1. Maintain body substance isolation.
2. Protect the airway and manage the C-spine if necessary.
3. Apply direct pressure to the wound.
4. If the wound continues to bleed, apply a tourniquet proximal to the injury and proximal to the elbow or knee.
5. Tighten the tourniquet until distal bleeding stops and a distal pulse is no longer palpable.
6. Secure the tourniquet in place.
7. Write "TK" and the exact time the tourniquet was applied on a piece of tape and apply the tape to the patient's forehead. If tape isn't available, write it directly on the patient's forehead.
8. Transport rapidly to a trauma center or helicopter. If the patient is showing signs of shock, or to treat for shock prophylactically, conduct steps 9–12:
9. Position the patient supine or in Trendelenburg position if there is no head injury.
10. Administer high concentration O_2.
11. Cover the patient in warmed blankets and maintain body heat.
12. Initiate at least one intravenous or intraosseous line and administer up to 1 L fluid to maintain a blood pressure.

Hemostatic agents are chemicals that are introduced into a wound that has bleeding that is not able to be stopped with direct pressure and is usually in an area where a tourniquet cannot be placed. They come as a powder or embedded in specialized dressings. The chemicals absorb the water from the blood and activate the clotting cascade. These were designed for the military and are not typically recommended in areas where transport times are short.

Internal Bleeding

The only definitive care for internal bleeding is generally surgery. The best treatment a paramedic can do for a patient in the field is to recognize that the patient is, in fact, bleeding internally or maintain a high index of suspicion that the patient could have internal injuries and rapidly transport the patient to the hospital. During transport, the patient should receive at least one, preferably two, large-bore intravenous lines with fluids running wide open. Although this will maintain blood pressure, it will not replace the O_2-carrying power of blood, so even this will eventually become insufficient.

BURNS

Burns are soft-tissue injuries resulting from the sudden and violent release of energy. Burns can occur from a release of heat in the form of fire, energy from chemical reactions, or radiation released from radioactive substances. Damage to the skin in such a profound way also affects body systems other than just the skin; there may be airway burns compromising the respiratory system, fluid shifts can lead to hypovolemia and cardiovascular compromise, and destruction to the skin will open the person up to the risk of a massive infection that overtaxes the immune system. This section will discuss all these issues from all 3 major burn sources.

Temperature is a quantitative measure of how much energy an object possesses. As an object gains or absorbs energy, its temperature will rise a predictable amount. Conversely, if an object releases energy, its temperature will drop a predictable amount.

Practical Point

When baking cookies, you may notice that the cookie sheet itself cools off considerably faster than the cookie itself. That is because of the predictable nature of the 2 different materials. The water in the cookie releases a tremendous amount of energy as it cools, so it takes longer to release that energy than the cookie sheet, even though they were the same temperature when they came out of the oven. It is the process of releasing this energy—by transferring it to another object, in this case human tissues—that is the root cause for all burns.

Thermal Burns

Thermal burns occur when the heat source a body comes in contact with exceeds the body's ability to dissipate that heat. Thermal burns are dependent on the following:

- Length of time the body is exposed to the heat source
- Temperature of the heat source
- Amount of energy the heat source releases when it comes in contact with the body
- Type of heat source

The longer the body is exposed to the heat source, whether it is a flame, a hot stove, or water from a shower, the more significant the burn. This is because the body has more time to absorb the energy being released. The burn will likely involve deeper layers and a broader area, perhaps even beyond the local area of contact. The hotter the source, the more energy it has to release, resulting in a more significant burn.

The amount of energy an object possesses at any given temperature will vary based on the type of material that comprises it. Pull a beach towel off a metal fence on a hot sunny day, no problem; touch the hot fence for a long enough period of time, and a person may get a burn. Water, whether liquid or steam, will release more energy per gram than any other household substance. (For those curious, ammonia will release more energy; however, most people do not have vats of hot ammonia sitting around their houses.) Remember, there does not need to be a flame for a person to receive a burn.

Types of Thermal Burns

Thermal burns can be classified as follows:

- **Contact Burns.** Burns caused by coming in direct contact with a hot object. Reflexes often limit the damage done as a result of contact burns. These can be more severe if a patient is restrained or impaired by alcohol or a medical condition. A contact burn also can be a sign of abuse in adults age 65 and older and the very young, especially if there is a pattern to the burn.
- **Flame Burns.** Caused by open flame, these often are the deepest burn, especially if the patient's clothes are on fire.
- **Flash Burns.** These burns are caused by sudden heat from an explosion or being near a lightning strike. These are usually minor in nature, although sometimes they can have a lasting effect on the eyes.
- **Scald Burns.** This type of burn can be seen in any age patient, but it is most commonly found in children and handicapped, especially as a result of cooking. Scald burns can result from hot liquids being spilled off the stove by children reaching up or even from the showerhead if the hot water heater is set too high. Scald

burns can cover a broad area, particularly if they soak into clothing because the burn will continue to deepen until the energy of the water is used up or the clothing can be removed. If it gets into the diaper of a child (or an adult), it can be especially destructive to the genitals.

- **Steam Burns.** When steam comes in contact with any surface, it will condense back into liquid water. This change releases a colossal amount of energy—in fact, more than 6 times the highest defibrillation setting per gram of water. This steam can not only burn the skin of the hands and face but also cause serious burns of the airway if it is inhaled.

- **Inhalation Burns.** In a fire, inhalation of superheated air can cause airway burns. In an airway burn, the airway lining swells, sometimes to the point that it closes off the airway completely. The superior structures, including the epiglottis, larynx, and pharynx, are often the worst burned because they are the first to dissipate the heat energy. The patient with upper airway burns will require fast, aggressive airway management before it closes off entirely.

Smoke Inhalation

CO is the predominant chemical in smoke and is largely responsible for deaths associated with smoke inhalation. CO poisoning and its treatment were discussed in chapter 6. However, it is worth mentioning that the pulse oximetry in a person with smoke inhalation may be 100%. Despite this, always provide high-flow O_2 either via a non-rebreathing mask or positive pressure ventilation.

During a fire, the most lethal part of a fire is the smoke, not the flames or the intense heat. The smoke, along with the superheated air surrounding it, is so hot that it contributes to airway damage. This can contribute to swelling of the airways and should be considered whenever a patient has soot around the mouth and nose or singing to the facial hair or nose hairs. Smoke also contains a wide array of toxic chemicals.

Other chemicals in structure fire smoke include cyanide and hydrochloric acid. Cyanide is a poison that will shut down the electron transport chain in cellular respiration, and hydrochloric acid is a strong acid that can destroy living tissue. These chemicals can cause problems but are usually not in a concentration high enough to be a concern.

Burn Severity

- **Superficial burns** (formerly "*first-degree burns*") are a typical sunburn. Only the epidermis is affected. The skin will be red, hot to the touch, and often swollen and painful. When touched, the skin will blanch and return to the red color. The patient is extremely sensitive to touch because of damaged nerve endings.

- **Partial-thickness burns** involve the epidermis and can be subdivided further:

  - *Moderate partial-thickness burns* typically involve only the superficial dermis, and the hair follicles remain intact. The skin will be red with fluid-filled blisters. The redness will blanch when touched and return to the color.

  - *Deep partial-thickness burns* also will have blisters and damage deeper into the dermis. The hair follicles, sweat, and sebaceous glands are damaged. Such a burn also may be deep enough to destroy pain receptors in the dermis. The burn will not be painful in some areas.

- **Full-thickness burns** involve the entirety of the epidermis and the dermis, burning all the way down to the basement membrane where the skin anchors to the fascia and new skin cells are generated. The skin will appear white and waxy and charred or leathery. This is called **eschar** (pronounced "ESS-car") and is dry, hard, and tighter than regular skin. The eschar can tighten to the point that it acts as a tourniquet on extremities or greatly hampers chest excursion during breathing. All nerve endings are destroyed, so patient feels no pain (except perhaps on the edges where partial and superficial burns may exist).

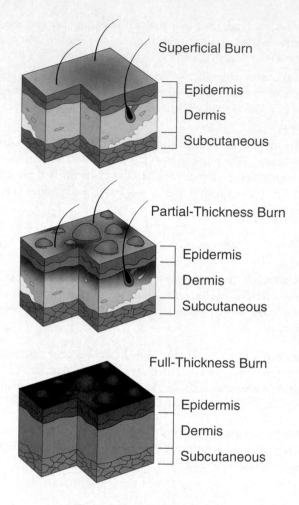

Superficial Burn

Epidermis

Dermis

Subcutaneous

Partial-Thickness Burn

Epidermis

Dermis

Subcutaneous

Full-Thickness Burn

Epidermis

Dermis

Subcutaneous

Figure 8-3. Burn Severity

Thermal Burn Assessment and Treatment

By now, it should go without saying that scene safety is the first thing to assess on any call.

- Assessing the scene is of paramount importance.
- Unless you are trained as a firefighter and equipped with the proper gear (including the self-contained breathing apparatus), never enter a building that is (or was recently) on fire.
- Leave it up to the firefighters to bring any patients to the ambulance or triage area. When they do, ask them about the thickness of the smoke, the area in which they found each patient relative to the location of the fire or the drift of the smoke, and how long it took them to get each patient out from the time the alarm was sounded. These questions will provide valuable information about the scene.

Body substance isolation for the burn patient should, whenever possible, include gloves and a gown. Skin can come off in sheets after a burn, so protection may be warranted beyond just gloves. Once the patient arrives, ensure that the burning process has stopped and that the patient is, in fact, no longer on fire; it is possible that the clothes are still smoldering or still hot enough to intensify burns. Wet the patient down and remove all clothing as soon as the patient can be touched. This is essential because polyester will turn to solid plastic when heated, holding more heat against the patient and worsening the burn.

Only now is it possible to begin the primary assessment. During the airway and breathing portion, note any signs and symptoms that may signal smoke or heated air inhalation:

- Facial burns
- Singed facial and/or nose hair
- Cough
- Black sputum, lips, nasal lining (carbon)
- Hoarseness
- Wheezing (bad)
- Stridor (worse)

If the patient has any of these signs and symptoms, suspend the remainder of the assessment and prepare to aggressively manage the airway. Early recognition will invariably lead to early intervention, which will be life saving in the patient with the above conditions. Begin first with nebulized saline. This will help the patient with the conditions noted above who is currently breathing. It also may help lubricate the airway and accelerate the removal of contaminants in the lungs and airways. If this does not work, or respiratory distress is increasing or stridor or wheezing is present, field intubation may be necessary.

Only the most experienced paramedic should attempt an intubation of this patient because there may be only one opportunity for successful intubation. As the upper airways swell, any irritation to them will make them swell faster, quickly eliminating the opportunity for airway maintenance.

Intubation may also be attempted on a person who is conscious, agitated, anxious, or otherwise uncooperative (due to the pain from the burn or other trauma). If the patient is able to understand the need for the intubation, explain it thoroughly, with ongoing communication throughout and after the process. Take the following steps:

1. Prepare all equipment necessary for the intubation, including a smaller tube than would otherwise be used. Consider starting with a 6 or 5.5 cuffed tube in an adult to enhance chances of success. It is also worth having a couple of different sizes prepared at the same time to facilitate switching between sizes quicker.
2. Place a stylette in the selected tube and conform the tube to the preferred shape.
3. Lubricate the external part of the ETT liberally with water soluble lubricant.
4. If available, spray the patient's mouth with lidocaine spray. It will already be painful from the burn; the laryngoscope will only exacerbate this and make the patient more resistant to the procedure.
5. Ideally, the patient should receive rapid sequence intubation (RSI) for this. Sedate with 2 mg Versed, 1.5 mg/kg lidocaine, and 0.1 mcg/kg fentanyl. Administer 20 mg etomidate for induction followed with 1.5 mg/kg succinylcholine chloride for paralysis.
6. Introduce the ETT and secure with a commercial tube holder. Evaluate placement with lung sounds and $EtCO_2$.

If these steps do not work or intubation is no longer possible, a tracheotomy may be required.

Once the airway is secure and patent, evaluate circulation. Assess peripheral pulses at any of the usual places, with preference to those that are not under burned areas if possible.

- Assessing blood pressure may be challenging if the extremities are burned. If possible, avoid taking a blood pressure over a burned area. If the patient has any partial- or full-thickness burns on the body, it is safe to presume that the patient will be hypovolemic eventually, and begin to treat for such a case.
- Establish at least one peripheral intravenous as soon as possible for fluid resuscitation and pain management.

Practical Point

Severe burns will result in a fluid shift out of the vasculature and into the interstitial space, resulting in profound and potentially lethal hypovolemia.

As long as circulation is intact, evaluate the total body surface area (BSA) burned and the degree to which the patient has been burned to determine the burn severity. BSA is determined as a percentage of the total body surface, using one of two common methods:

- **Rule of 9s** (more commonly used) assigns regions of the body percentages in multiples of 9 across the entire body for the adult. (This changes slightly in infants about 1-year-old who lose 9% from their legs and gain it back in their head.) Approximations are all that is needed for this step because the paramedic will not be able to accurately determine the exact amount in the chaos of initial care and the scene.

- **Rule of palms** states that the percentage of BSA burned can be estimated using the patient's palm as a reference. The patient's palm—including fingers—is approximated as 1% BSA; therefore any area the palm can cover equates to approximately 1%.

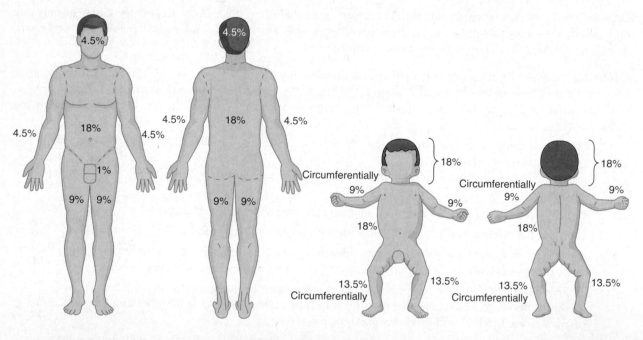

Figure 8-4. Rule of 9s
(A) Adult. (B) Infant.

Table 8-2. Adult Burns

Severity	Burn Thickness or Area	Criteria
Critical	Full-Thickness	Burns involving hands, feet, face or genitalia
		Circumferential burns of torso, arms or legs
		>10% BSA
	Partial-Thickness	>30% BSA
	Any Thickness	Airway or respiratory involvement
		Other trauma such as fractures
		Patient age <5 or >55 with any "moderate" burn
Moderate	Full-Thickness	2% – 10% BSA with 0% in hands, feet, face or genitals
	Partial-Thickness	15% – 30% BSA
	Superficial	>50% BSA
Minor	Full-Thickness	<2% BSA with 0% in hands, feet, face or genitals
	Partial-Thickness	<15% BSA
	Superficial	<50% BSA

Once the BSA burned has been estimated, fluid resuscitation can be fully planned. The **Parkland formula** is used to determine the amount of fluid in milliliters the patient will need within the first 24 hours after the incident. Half of this amount is to be administered in the first 8 hours, with the remaining half given over the remaining 16 hours. The Parkland formula is 4 times the BSA times the patient weight in kilograms.

$$\%BSA \times weight\ (kg) \times 4 = mL\ fluid$$

Normal saline is preferred to lactated Ringer solution because it contains potassium. Because of the extent of cellular damage that has already occurred, potassium levels in the blood may already be elevated. Mortality in burn patients increases the longer the patient goes without intravenous fluid resuscitation. The paramedic's goal should be to establish at least one large-bore peripheral intravenous line and begin running fluids. This process should not delay the transport of the patient to the helicopter or the hospital.

Pain Management

For burn patients, pain management is an essential part of the care plan. The pain the burn patient experiences is extraordinary and often requires multiple doses of pain medication to achieve a reduction in pain level because the patient's metabolism has increased from the burn process and the anxiety. In addition, absorption is altered because of fluid shifts, so intravenous or intraosseous administration is required. Begin with 0.1 mcg/kg fentanyl or up to 10 mg morphine sulfate and consult medical control for further orders.

Electrical Burns

Electrical burns are a difficult burn to assess because much of the damage is internal. For an electrical burn to happen, the electricity must complete a circuit by entering the body and then flowing into another wire or the ground. When the circuit is completed, the electricity flows into the body from the point of contact with the live electrical source until it exits the body. High-voltage electrical current, such as that from outdoor electrical supply lines will follow the shortest path to the nearest conductor or the ground. Lower voltage sources under 1,000 V, such as household interior wiring, will usually take the path of least resistance to electrical flow, which is usually nerves and blood vessels.

Between the entry and exit wounds, electricity produces immense heat from the natural resistance of human tissue to electricity. The electricity also will cause skeletal muscle tetany, freezing a person in position connected to the electricity source if the current is high enough. Skeletal muscle tetany can be powerful enough to cause fractures during the spasm. As the current increases beyond 20 mA, respiratory muscle paralysis sets in if the current flows through these muscles. Finally, VT may be induced with as little as 50–100 mA if the current flows through the heart. Although skeletal muscle tetany and respiratory muscle paralysis will subside when the electrical current stops, VT will not spontaneously convert to normal rhythm.

There are 3 types of electrical injury:

- **True electrical burns** (most common) occur when electricity flows directly into the body from a source and into another conductor or the ground.
- **Arc burns** often come from extremely high-voltage wires. Electricity essentially "leaps through the air" and into the body of a person close enough to the source to become a suitable conductor. Temperatures of the arc, because of the very high resistance of air, can reach well in excess of >9,000°F (5,000°C). If the arc initially contacts the person through a tool, for example, a screwdriver, the tool is vaporized.
- **Flame burns** occur when electricity flows through clothing and sets it on fire.

Before assessment can begin, ensure that the scene is safe and that the electricity has been turned off if the patient is still near the source of injury. Supply lines can spontaneously turn back on if they are programmed to do so to prevent long term black-outs. Once ensured of security from the electricity, proceed with assessment of the ABCs in the usual fashion; however, open the airway with the modified jaw thrust if needed; muscle spasms may have caused a neck injury. Ventilate as needed if not breathing or breathing inadequately; otherwise provide high-flow O_2. Initiate CPR if needed and defibrillate VF as soon as possible. Treat other cardiac dysrhythmias as needed.

During the secondary assessment, try to evaluate the likely path of the electricity through the body. Areas that have been affected will tend to be extremely hard as a result of the damage. Essentially, the tissues in this area have been cooked. Because the electricity will cauterize any bleeding it may have caused, external or internal bleeding is highly unlikely. Appropriately splint any fractures or dislocations found and document the presence of distal pulses.

Lightning Burns

Lightning differs from electricity in that the current from lightning is a direct current, which means it travels in only one direction, whereas electrical current in wires is typically alternating current. In addition, it lasts for only milliseconds, rather than exposing the patient until the current is turned off. Consequently, it more resembles a blast injury than what may be expected from a high-voltage electrical burn. It also is similar to arc burns, where a large, onetime discharge of electricity travels from a body—the cloud—to another body—a person or persons on the ground.

A person does not need to be struck directly to sustain the damaging effects from lightning. Often, the person receives a splash burn, which results from a lightning strike nearby and electricity traveling through the air from that point to the person. As the electricity spreads in the ground after striking the ground, the person also can sustain injuries from the ground current.

Treatment for the patient who was struck by lightning is very similar to that of the electrocuted patient. Unless there is still lightning activity in the area, and the patient is outside near a tall object, the likelihood that lightning will hit the same spot again is remote, so the scene is typically safe. The patient who is not breathing or is in cardiac arrest is the highest priority when there is more than one patient. Because lightning is direct current, it will act as a defibrillator, depolarizing the entire heart at the same time. As often as not, the heart will begin beating immediately after the lightning is done. Other times, it will restart after a defibrillation or 2 minutes of CPR initiated immediately after the strike.

Chemical Burns

Chemical burns result when certain types of chemicals come in direct contact with a patient's skin. The burn severity depends on conditions similar to those of a flame burn:

- **Chemical state.** No amount of gaseous O_2 will hurt a person in the near term. However, liquid O_2, such as what may be found in concentrators for home O_2 therapy, could cause significant burns if the tank were to rupture.

- **Concentration.** Concentration plays a big role in how long the patient needs to be exposed to the agent for the burn to occur. Some very dilute chemicals no longer pose a hazard, whereas for other chemicals, dilution slows or limits the damage done. Pure ammonia, for example, is a very strong base and can cause significant burns; however, when diluted, it works as a very effective household cleaner that can be used without a mask or gloves.

- **Depth of penetration.** Certain chemicals can burn deeper into layers of the skin, causing more damage.

- **Duration of exposure.** In most cases, the longer the patient has been exposed to the chemical, the worse the burn is. That said, some chemicals will do their damage in mere seconds, regardless of the concentration.

The type of chemical the patient was exposed to impacts the damage the patient will experience.

- **Acids.** Acids release hydrogen ions, which are responsible for the burning effect. As they react with the skin, a tough callus is formed, which limits damage to the skin. This is called **coagulative necrosis**.

- **Bases.** Bases release hydroxide ions into solution and essentially liquefy the skin. Fat deposits react with strong bases and essentially turn into soap (a process called **saponification**). Because cellular structures have a relatively large component of lipids as part of the cell membranes, the cells will liquefy and dissolve. Therefore, until all the hydroxide has reacted with fat in the area of contact, cellular destruction will continue to occur.

- **Oxidizers.** These help other items burn. Therefore, when they come in contact with skin, they can cause such a powerful reaction that the skin or clothing will actually catch on fire.

In many cases, treatment for chemical burns is related to removing the patient from contact with the chemical. This should largely be left up to the fire department for decontamination prior to arriving at the ambulance for treatment. Provided the chemical to which the patient was exposed is not violently reactive with water, the patient should be thoroughly washed off with excess water for at least 10 minutes if their overall condition permits. For treatment recommendations for each chemical, consult the Emergency Response Guidebook and Chemtrec for information on specific treatments.

Special consideration must be given to chemical burns of the eye. Any of the previously mentioned chemical types can cause burns in the eye. Because of the presence of tears in the eyes, even dry, water-soluble chemicals become more of a concern than they would be if they just got onto clothing or the skin. If chemicals get into the eyes, the eyes should be flushed for at least minutes with clean water. Never use antidotes in the eyes to try and counter the effects of the chemical because this can worsen the burn because of the heat released during the reaction or purely the chemical activity of the new chemical being introduced.

When flushing with water, remember to flush away from the other eye and minimize splashing. Hold the eyelids open and ensure that the water makes its way under each eyelid. Have the patient roll their eyes as well so that the water can more easily wash all areas of the eye. If contact lenses are present, remove them as quickly as possible because they can hold the chemical against the cornea, worsening the burn.

Radiation Burns

Although rare, radioactive materials are commonly found in industry and are sometimes associated with terrorist attacks and bombings. Response to such incidents should be limited to people who are specially trained and equipped to work in latent dangerous environments. Simply being in the area of a radiation exposure does not immediately make a person contaminated or able to expose others. However, being at an area where there was an explosion and having radioactive debris on the person does make the person contaminated and capable of contaminating the ambulance, the providers, and the emergency department.

Three kinds of radiation are released from radioactive material. What kind of radiation is purely dependent on the material in question:

- **Alpha Particles (lowest energy).** The alpha particles can easily be stopped by skin or clothing. Alpha radiation is a cause for concern only if the source is embedded in the patient, such as shrapnel, or ingested.

- **Beta Particles (higher energy).** The beta particles are stopped by aluminum and glass, so the ambulance will provide adequate protection from beta radiation, assuming it is not allowed on the patient. Beta particles are capable of causing damage to DNA, cancers, and other problems.

- **Gamma Radiation (high-energy with extensive penetrating power).** Gamma radiation can be stopped only by thick concrete, lead, or thick steel. The smaller the wavelength, the more energy the gamma ray possesses. As a result, it has more penetrating power. This also is dependent on the source.

Radiation is measured in **radiation absorbed dose** (**rad**) or **radiation equivalent in man** (**rem**). One hundred rad is equal to 1 Gray (Gy). People are exposed to radiation every day in small doses. This small dose is called **background radiation** and is about 0.36 rad per year. Major radiation exposures are measured on the Gray scale, which translates into about 1,000 times the amount of background radiation.

Acute radiation sickness is dependent on the dose of radiation received and duration of time for which it was received. Radiation sickness involves 3 presentations:

- **Hematopoietic,** a drastic drop in both red and white blood cells; can lead to profound infections
- **GI,** seen when the GI system receives the radiation dose; causes extensive vomiting and diarrhea
- **Neurovascular,** seen when the brain is involved in receiving the radiation dose; causes neurological symptoms, including confusion, dizziness, and headache

Mild radiation sickness begins from 1 to 2 Gy, is completely recoverable, and rarely results in long-term problems. Exposure to 2–5 Gy will result in moderate radiation sickness, and people at this level may experience long-term problems. Mortality rates exceed 50% of those exposed. Exposure to greater than 5 Gy, particularly with involvement of the GI system, is fatal within 1 week. If vomiting presents within 1–2 hours, death is assured. Exposure to greater than 8 Gy is fatal within 48 hours regardless of the area of the body primarily exposed.

Assessment is largely related to the onset of vomiting. Those who vomit outside of 1 hour of exposure have a greater than 95% survival rate from the exposure. If vomiting occurs within an hour, mortality rates exceed 80%. And, finally, if vomiting occurs within the first 10 minutes, death is guaranteed.

Radiation contact burns may occur when a patient handles or otherwise comes in direct contact with a radiation source. This may happen in certain places of employment or during the detonation of a dirty bomb. The appearance in the area of the exposure may resemble a localized chemical burn or sunburn. Radiation burns, in contrast to regular chemical burns, tend to appear hours or days after contact.

Treatment for radiation exposures involves determining the level of exposure and, first and foremost, the need to protect the EMS crew from harm. Once the providers are safe, assessment of the vomiting time frame is essential. Although radiation exposure–related vomiting is not treated the way other sources of vomiting can be, it is helpful to know the survivability of the exposure. Long-term treatment in the hospital will involve treating for the widespread infection and neutropenia (low neutrophil count) that results from exposure.

MUSCULOSKELETAL INJURIES

Fractures, sprains, and strains are common reasons for a patient to need an ambulance. Often, these are in the context of more serious, multisystem trauma. This section will discuss the musculoskeletal system and assessment and treatment of musculoskeletal injuries, focusing on those of the appendicular skeleton.

Muscles

Skeletal muscles are under voluntary control, which means that the patient controls all aspects of muscle movement. These muscles also are referred to as striated because under a microscope, they appear to have stripes. Skeletal muscle includes all the muscles attached to the skeleton, and they provide much of the bulk surrounding the skeleton.

Skeletal muscle is responsible for moving bones that are capable of movement, but skeletal muscle also is responsible for facial expressions, blinking, tongue movement, maintenance of posture, and swallowing. Skeletal muscle has a high metabolic rate and requires a constant flow of O_2. Consequently, skeletal muscles have a rich blood supply and often bleed profusely when injured.

Skeletal muscles that are attached to 2 bones have an insertion and an origin. The insertion is the end of the muscle attached to the bone that moves the most during contraction. The origin is the end of the muscle attached to the bone that moves the least during contraction. For example, the origin of the biceps muscle in the upper arm is the scapula, and the insertion is located on the radius in the forearm. When the biceps contracts, the forearm is flexed upward.

Skeletal Structure

The components of our skeletal system are divided into axial and appendicular skeletons. The **axial skeleton** consists of the skull, the vertebral column, the rib cage, and the hyoid bone (a small bone in the anterior neck used for swallowing); it provides the basic central framework for the body. The **appendicular skeleton** consists of the bones of the limbs (humerus, radius and ulna, carpals, metacarpals, and phalanges in the upper limb; and femur, tibia and fibula, tarsals, metatarsals, and phalanges in the lower limb), the pectoral girdle (scapula and clavicle), and the pelvis. Both skeleton types are covered by other structures (muscle, connective tissue, and vasculature).

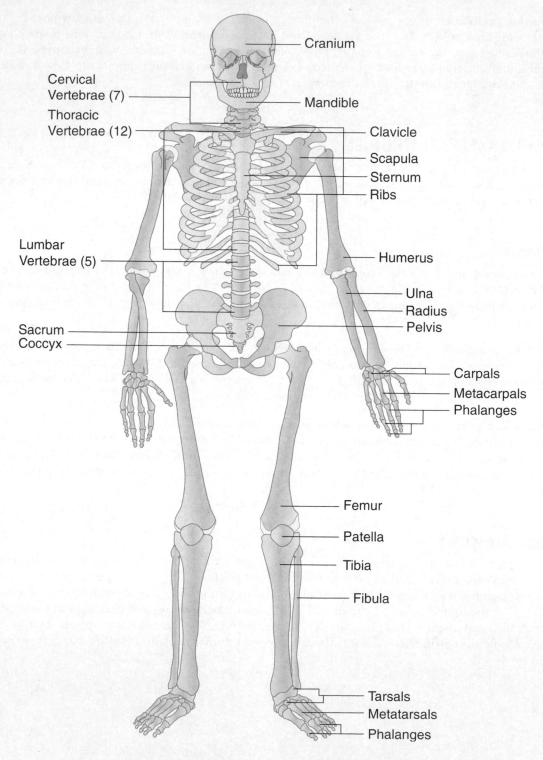

Figure 8-5. Anatomy of the Human Skeleton

The skeleton is created from 2 major components: bone and cartilage.

Skeletal Composition

Bone is a connective tissue derived from embryonic mesoderm. Bone is much harder than cartilage, but it is relatively lightweight.

Macroscopic Bone Structure

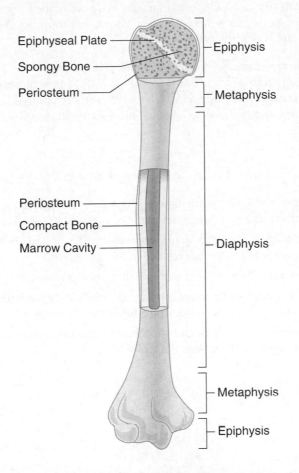

Epiphyseal Plate —
Spongy Bone —
Periosteum —

— Epiphysis

— Metaphysis

Periosteum —
Compact Bone —
Marrow Cavity —

— Diaphysis

— Metaphysis

— Epiphysis

Figure 8-6. Anatomy of a Long Bone (Humerus)

Bone's characteristic strength comes specifically from **compact bone**. It lives up to its name because it is both dense and strong. The other type of bone structure is **spongy** or **cancellous** bone. The lattice structure of spongy bone is visible under microscopy and consists of bony spicules (points) known as **trabeculae**. The cavities between trabeculae are filled with **bone marrow**, which may be either red or yellow. **Red marrow** is filled with hematopoietic stem cells, which are responsible for generating all the cells in our blood; **yellow marrow** is composed primarily of fat and is relatively inactive.

Bones in the appendicular skeleton are typically **long bones**, which are characterized by cylindrical shafts called **diaphyses** that swell at each end to form **metaphyses** and terminate in **epiphyses**. The outermost portions of bone are composed of compact bone, whereas the internal core is composed of spongy bone. Long-bone diaphyses and metaphyses are full of bone marrow. The epiphyses, on the other hand, use their spongy cores for more effective dispersion of force and pressure at the joints. At the internal edge of the epiphysis is an **epiphyseal (growth) plate**, which is a cartilaginous structure and the site of longitudinal growth. Prior to adulthood, the epiphyseal plate is filled with mitotic cells that contribute to growth; during puberty, these epiphyseal plates close, halting vertical growth. Finally, a fibrous sheath called the **periosteum** surrounds the long bone to protect it as well as serve as a site for muscle attachment. Some periosteum cells are capable of differentiating into bone-forming cells; a healthy periosteum is necessary for bone growth and repair.

Structures in the musculoskeletal system are held together with dense connective tissue. **Tendons** attach muscle to bone, and **ligaments** hold bones together at joints.

Cartilage

Cartilage is softer and more flexible than bone. Cartilage consists of a firm but elastic matrix called **chondrin** that is secreted by cells called **chondrocytes**. Fetal skeletons are mostly composed of cartilage. This is advantageous because fetuses must grow and develop in a confined environment and then must traverse the birth canal. Adults have cartilage only in body parts that need a little extra flexibility or cushioning (external ear, nose, walls of the larynx and trachea, intervertebral discs, and joints). Cartilage also differs from bone in that it is avascular (without blood and lymphatic vessels) and is not innervated.

Most of the bones of the body are created by the hardening of cartilage into bone. This process is known as **endochondral ossification** and is responsible for the formation of most of the long bones of the body. Bones also may be formed through **intramembranous ossification**, in which undifferentiated embryonic connective tissue (**mesenchymal tissue**) is transformed into—and replaced by—bone. This occurs in bones of the skull.

Joints and Movement

Like bone and cartilage, **joints** are made of connective tissue and come in 2 major varieties.

- **Immovable joints** consist of bones that are fused together to form **sutures** or similar fibrous joints. These joints are found primarily in the head, where they anchor bones of the skull together.
- **Movable joints** include hinge joints (such as the elbow or knee), ball-and-socket joints (like the shoulder or hip), and others. They permit bones to shift relative to one another.
  - Strengthened by **ligaments**, pieces of fibrous tissue that connect bones to each another
  - Consist of a **synovial capsule**, which encloses the actual **joint cavity** (**articular cavity**); a layer of soft tissue called the **synovium** secretes **synovial fluid**, which lubricates the movement of structures in the joint space
  - **Articular cartilage** contributes to the joint by coating the articular surfaces of the bones so that impact is restricted to lubricated joint cartilage (and not to the bones)

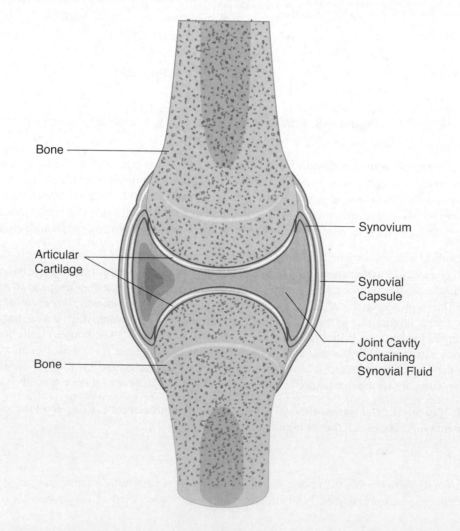

Figure 8-7. Structures in a Movable Joint

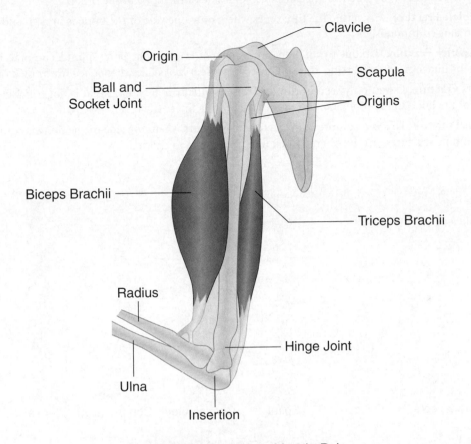

Figure 8-8. Antagonistic Muscle Pairs
The biceps brachii and triceps brachii are an example of a muscle pair that works antagonistically; the contraction of one causes the other to elongate.

Types of Fractures

A fracture is a break or crack anywhere in the bone. The break does not have to be completely through the bone. Fractures can be classified as follows:

- **Comminuted Fracture.** A single bone is broken in 2 or more places. Common in crush injuries but can occur in any fracture. When the bone is broken in 2 or more places, and the pieces of the bone are clearly defined, it also may be referred to as a segmental fracture.

- **Compression Fracture.** A fracture resulting from overloading of the bone. Often seen in falls from height. Common in vertebral body fractures.

- **Linear Fracture.** The fracture line is parallel to the shaft of the bone. May or may not be completely through.

- **Oblique Fracture.** The fracture line is at an angle to the shaft of the bone and completely through.

- **Spiral Fracture.** The break line twists around the shaft of the bone. Common in twisting injuries such as when a ski stays planted in the snow and the person spins on that leg as while falling.

- **Transverse Fracture.** The fracture line is perpendicular to the shaft of the bone and completely through.

Fractures can be defined based on completeness:

- **Complete Fracture.** The fracture line goes from one side of the bone to the other.
- **Incomplete Fracture.** Any of the fracture types where only one side of the bone is broken and the opposite side remains continuous.
  - **Greenstick Fracture.** Unique to children, in this type of fracture, the bone splinters on one side and remains intact on the other side. It is so named because it looks like when a healthy branch of a tree breaks.
  - **Stress Fracture.** Commonly seen in runners, it is essentially bone failure that is not completely from one side of the bone to the other. Often synonymous with a linear fracture.
  - **Torus Fracture.** This is a compression fracture that occurs when one side of the bone is compressed, causing minute fractures. A type of greenstick fracture unique to children.

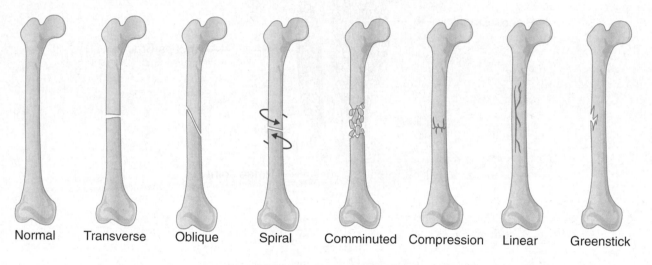

Normal | Transverse | Oblique | Spiral | Comminuted | Compression | Linear | Greenstick

Figure 8-9. Types of Fractures

Defining Fractures on Displacement

Nondisplaced fractures remain in alignment at the fracture site. This is most common in linear fractures but can happen during any fracture if the extremity is replaced into a neutral position. In a displaced fracture, the bone ends no longer align. These are the following types of displaced fractures:

- **Angulated Fracture.** The fracture site causes a bend in the shaft of the bone.
- **Avulsion Fracture.** During a sudden contraction of a muscle, such as during a seizure or during a sports game, the insertion point of the muscle peels off a portion of the bone.
- **Depressed Fracture.** Most commonly associated with the skull, this fracture occurs when there is partial penetration into the skull causing it to break, leaving a dent behind.
- **Overriding.** After a fracture, the strength of the contraction of the surrounding musculature pulls on the bone ends, and they end up sliding past one another.

Open Versus Closed

One final way to classify fractures is by whether they are open or closed. In **closed fractures**, the skin over the fracture area is intact. In **open fractures**, the skin over the fracture site is lacerated, from either external trauma or the bone ends lacerating the skin from inside. Open fractures also carry with them the added considerations of increased incidence of infection and increased bleeding. Any time the skin is broken, the likelihood of infection increases. Bleeding will increase markedly, however, because when the bone ends are exposed, the tamponading effect of a closed fracture is lost. Bones often are highly vascularized, especially in the marrow. With that in mind, when bone ends protrude through the skin, bleeding worsens.

Signs and Symptoms of Fractures

Pain often is localized to the fracture site. In fact, pain often can be pinpointed to that area, not throughout the limb.

Deformity often will occur as an unnatural bend in the area of the fracture. If the fracture remains aligned, this may not be seen.

If the fracture becomes an overriding fracture and the muscles surrounding the fracture contract, **shortening** may occur, in which the affected limb may appear shorter than the other limb, if a comparison can be made. This is commonly seen in femur fractures.

Localized bleeding and tissue damage will result in **swelling** in the area of the fracture. Compartment syndrome is a concern when swelling is present. Bruising also may become apparent.

Crepitus is the feeling of the bone ends rubbing together. Sometimes it can even be heard. This should not be deliberately generated once it is found because it can cause more injury.

Patients with an extremity fracture often will not be able to move the limb **distal** to the injury, which can be caused by muscle entrapment in the fracture, lacerations to the muscle in the area of the fracture, or motor nerve damage. Frequently, pain with motion is enough to prevent deliberate movement. There also is the possibility of distal numbness if there is damage or entrapment of the sensory nerve in the area of the fracture. Distal pulses may not be palpable because of blood vessel entrapment, a laceration at the fracture site, or swelling that pinches off the vessel.

Assessment and Treatment

Treatment for any musculoskeletal injury begins with ensuring that the patient's ABCs are intact. Consider cervical spine immobilization if the patient could possibly have sustained a spinal injury as well. Orthopedic injuries and the pain they cause can be distracting injuries; this means that the patient may not even notice that they have neck or back pain because the pain from the fracture or dislocation is so severe. Any other life-threatening injuries or the presence of shock should, in most cases, be treated before any focus is placed on the orthopedic injury. For the purposes of this section, let's assume that there is an isolated injury to an extremity.

Evaluate the injured extremity for pain, deformity, discoloration, and swelling. If there is swelling, carefully mark the edges of the swollen area if they are well defined so that later when the area is assessed in the hospital, doctors and nurses are able to see if the swelling has worsened during the time that EMS was with the patient.

Next, check for pulse, motor, and sensation distal to the injury:

- **Pulse.** For arm fractures or dislocations, assess for the presence of a radial pulse; for leg fractures or dislocations, assess for a dorsal pedal pulse or a posterior tibial pulse. At this point, the primary concern is purely the presence or absence of the pulse on the affected side. When there is the opportunity, compare the strength of pulses from one side to the other. If the pulse is absent, attempt to realign the extremity prior to splinting as described below. If a pulse does not return after realigning the extremity, this is a true emergency because the area distal to the injury may be lost.
- **Motor.** Have the patient wiggle the toes or fingers on the affected side. Even if it is painful, one slight movement is enough to know that motor impulses are getting through.
- **Sensation.** Assess for sensation distal to the injury. Two nerve branches service the hands; therefore, both must be assessed to be thorough. This can be accomplished by having the patient close their eyes (no cheating!) while you brush the index finger and pinky. Sensation in the index finger means that the radial nerve branch is intact, and sensation in the pinky indicates that the ulnar nerve branch is intact. The case is similar in the feet where the big toe and the pinky toe can be assessed for sensation.

Pelvic and Hip Fractures

Pelvic fractures require a significant amount of force and are consequently fairly rare. They also are associated with a high mortality rate because of the concurrent damage to the structures underlying the pelvic bones. In addition, the pelvis can hold a lot of blood, which is difficult to assess. For these reasons, a pelvic fracture requires the paramedic to maintain a high index of suspicion for greater problems than just the orthopedic injury.

Types of Pelvic Fractures

Lateral and AP Compression

Pelvic fractures can result from lateral compression from falls or T-bone type accidents or from anterior-posterior (AP) compression from a head-on motor vehicle collision or a fall landing on the buttocks. In a **lateral fracture**, the ring of the pelvis tends to be compressed, reducing the overall diameter of the pelvis. Although this usually causes significant internal trauma, the bleeding gets tamponaded more quickly because of the reduced volume in the pelvis. In an **AP compression fracture**, often called an **open book fracture**, the pelvis widens, worsening any bleeding that may be occurring within the pelvis. It is called an open book fracture because in this type of fracture, the symphysis pubis spreads open like a book might when it is set on its spine. Remember also that because the pelvis is a ring, if the pelvic ring is broken in one location, it must be broken in a second location as well.

Vertical Shear and Straddle Injuries

Both vertical shear and straddle injuries involve an upward force directly on the pelvis. **Vertical shear injuries** result when a person lands on their feet with locked knees, transmitting the force of the fall all the way up through the legs to the pelvis. This can result in tearing of the ligaments of the pelvis and essentially splits the pelvis apart in the area of the symphysis pubis anteriorly and the sacrum posteriorly. **Straddle injuries** to the pelvis occur when a person lands almost exclusively on the perineum. The most common fracture that results is to the rami of the ischium. Injuries of this type usually result in more significant injuries to the perineum and the genitourinary system. Bleeding from this area can be substantial.

Hip Fractures

A **hip fracture** actually involves fractures of the proximal femur. The fracture can be an **intertrochanteric fracture**, which is a fracture of the proximal end of the shaft of the femur, or, more commonly, it will be a fracture of the neck of the femur, which is the area of the femur which articulates with the acetabulum of the pelvis. Both of these fractures can occur in patients of any age but are a much more common result of a fall in adults age 65 and older, especially those with osteoporosis. A **femoral neck fracture** is one of the most common sites of a pathologic fracture in the patient with osteoporosis. Pathologic fractures occur as a result of normal activity, not from any discernible traumatic event. In the case of a femoral neck fracture in a patient with osteoporosis, simply standing and adding weight to the femur again can be enough to break it.

Patients with a hip fracture will have the leg of the affected side shorter than the other. That leg will be rotated externally (laterally) as well. This shortening and rotation is a hallmark sign of a displaced hip fracture. Nondisplaced hip fractures are less common and may not show the classic shortening and rotation. Assess the extremity for distal pulse, motor, and sensation as previously noted. Splint the fracture with either a board splint long enough to immobilize the entire leg all the way up to the armpit or simply place the patient on a long backboard. After immobilizing the patient with either option, reassess the extremity for distal pulse motor and sensation. Blood loss is usually minimal; however, initiating an intravenous line and providing pain management is appropriate.

Treatment for Hip and Pelvic Fractures

Because of the high likelihood of internal injuries with pelvic fractures, the primary focus is to anticipate and treat for shock. Remove the patient's clothing and immobilize the patient on a long backboard. Initiate cardiac monitoring and at least one large-bore intravenous line with fluid running to maintain a systolic blood pressure >90. Once the patient has been immobilized and shock prevention measures have been initiated, attention should focus on stabilizing the pelvis. Although the long backboard itself can be a sufficient splint for most situations, the application of a pelvic binder is recommended.

A **pelvic binder** is a specialized splint that wraps around the pelvis. When properly secured, it will squeeze the open book fracture closed. It provides uniform circumferential pressure to stabilize the pelvis. This type of splint is far superior to a board splint or the backboard alone. This will reduce pain for the patient as well as possibly reduce the bleeding associated with the fracture.

Femur Fractures

Femur fractures often result from a high-speed impact directly to the upper leg, such as during a motorcycle accident, a motor vehicle accident, or a sports injury. Femur fractures can be associated with severe bleeding, which often is exclusively internal and can be up to 1,500 mL of blood lost into the thigh. The leg will most likely shorten as the muscles spasm and contract, generating extreme pain. Application of a traction splint to the affected leg, provided there are no other injuries in that leg, provides both pain relief and immobilization of the leg. Other treatment should include establishment of at least one large-bore intravenous line to treat or prevent shock. Analgesics are recommended especially if the traction splint has not fully addressed the pain.

Joint Injuries

Types of Joint Injuries

A **dislocation** is any displacement of the articulating surfaces of a joint. A dislocation may or may not be associated with a fracture in the same extremity. A dislocation often involves damage to the tendons surrounding the joint as well. The dislocated bone will lock into the new position because of the stretch and spasm of the muscles. Dislocations of the knee cap, elbow, and shoulder are among the more common. Dislocations to the hip joint are very common after an operation for a total hip replacement because the tendons have been manipulated during the operation.

A **subluxation** is a partial dislocation. In a subluxation, the articulating surfaces are no longer properly aligned. Because some of the tendons and ligaments are still intact in the joint and the joint is not locked into place as it is in a dislocation, the patient may have some capability of movement in that joint.

A **sprain** occurs when ligaments are stretched or torn. This can result from the joint being unnaturally twisted or a transient dislocation or subluxation that spontaneously resolves. Sprains commonly occur in the knee, ankle, and wrist.

When a muscle or tendon is stretched beyond its normal length, a **strain** is the result. This can occur during periods of excessive use or when the muscle is put into use in a violent manner, such as when a basketball player cuts from running in one direction to the other suddenly. Muscle strains are usually described as aches that worsen with use of the injured muscle.

Signs and Symptoms of Joint Injuries

Sudden swelling immediately following a sudden burst of pain, called **edema**, is common, particularly in sprains. This is often located directly superficial to the injured ligaments. The swelling can be significant to occlude blood flow distal to the injury. Always check for a distal pulse, motor, and sensation and document any deficits.

Pain for both sprains and dislocations is usually severe and in many cases worse than that of fractures. With an isolated closed fracture, pain is usually related to the amount of soft-tissue injury; in a dislocation or sprain, muscle spasms in the area contribute to ongoing, often worsening pain.

More common with sprains, discoloration and bruising often appear within 24 hours or so of the injury.

Assessment and Treatment of Muskuloskeletal Injuries

Response to any musculoskeletal injury begins with assessment of the patient's ABCs. The presence of any life-threatening injury or shock should, in most cases, be treated first—even if the patient's focus is on an orthopedic injury. Orthopedic injuries can be amazingly distracting. The pain from a fracture or dislocation may be so severe that the patient does not even notice neck or back pain. Consider cervical spine immobilization if the patient could possibly have sustained a spinal injury as well as the orthopedic injury. For the purposes of this section, we will assume that there is an isolated injury to an extremity.

Evaluate the injured extremity for pain, deformity, discoloration, and swelling. If there is swelling, carefully mark the edges of the swollen area if they are well defined; this will allow comparison later. At the hospital, doctors and nurses who assess the area will be able to see if the swelling has worsened since EMS was with the patient.

Next, check for pulse, motor, and sensation (PMS) distal to the injury:

- **Pulse.** For arm fractures or dislocations, assess for the presence of a radial pulse; for leg fractures or dislocations, assess for a dorsal pedal pulse or a posterior tibial pulse. If the pulse is absent, attempt to realign the extremity prior to splinting as described below. If a pulse does not return after the extremity is realigned, this is a true emergency because the area distal to the injury may be lost. (At this point, the primary concern is purely the presence or absence of the pulse on the affected side. When there is the opportunity, compare the strength of pulses from one side to the other.)
- **Motor.** Have the patient wiggle the toes or fingers on the affected side. Even if it is painful, one slight movement is enough to demonstrate that motor impulses are getting through.
- **Sensation.** Assess for sensation distal to the injury. Two nerve branches service the hands; both must be assessed. This can be accomplished by having the patient close their eyes (no cheating!) as you brush the index finger and pinky. Sensation in the index finger means that the radial nerve branch is intact, and sensation in the pinky indicates that the ulnar nerve branch is intact. The case is similar in the feet, where the big toe and the pinky toe can be assessed for sensation.

Practical Point

In the trauma assessment station and in any oral station involving trauma, be sure to mention checking distal pulses, motor, and sensation (distal PMS) at these points in the sequence:

- Before initiating any movement or treatment (crucial)
- After splinting a fracture or dislocation (crucial)
- After moving the patient, e.g., from ground to stretcher (recommended)

General Management Guidelines for Musculoskeletal Injuries

It is not practical to describe treatment of every possible fracture or dislocation a patient may sustain, but the useful mnemonic RICE outlines the basics. RICE stands for the following:

- **Rest.** Stop using the painful extremity. (This usually takes care of itself.)
- **Immobilization.** Apply a splint.
- **Cold.** Apply a cold pack.
- **Elevation.** Prop the extremity to the level of the heart or higher to minimize pain from swelling.

Splinting and Immobilization

Once the PMS assessment is complete, fractures and dislocations need to be immobilized using a splint. Adequate splinting of a fracture means immobilizing the joint above and below the fracture. Thorough splinting of a dislocation means immobilizing the bones above and below the dislocated joint. The splint can be a pillow, a padded board, a vacuum splint, or any other object that limits the motion of the fracture or dislocation. Splinting should not supersede treatment of life-threatening injuries.

The following steps outline the proper splinting procedure:

1. Remove clothing to expose the area above and below the injury.

2. Apply a dressing to any wounds in the area before applying the splint. If this is an open fracture, do not push the bone ends back into the body or manipulate the extremity such that the bone ends recede into the body.

3. If the extremity is angulated, EMS has only one opportunity to return it to a neutral position. Tell the patient that you are going to try to align the injured limb. Grasp the extremity distal to the injury and gently return the extremity to the neutral, in-line position while also gently pulling along the axis of the extremity. This step must be attempted if the limb does lacks a pulse distal to the injury. Note: If you encounter severe resistance or the patient experiences extreme pain (some pain is to be expected), abort the attempt to realign the extremity and splint it in the most comfortable position achievable. Failure to regain pulses after a failed alignment attempt constitutes a genuine emergency threatening the limb.

4. Once the extremity lies in a neutral position (or if it is being splinted in the position found), apply a splint that is long enough to immobilize the bones or joints that need to be immobilized. The long backboard can be a sufficient splint for any fractured extremity.

5. Secure the splint tightly to the extremity, but not so tight as to cut off circulation.

6. Reassess distal PMS and monitor throughout transport. If the patient loses pulses in the extremity, consider loosening the splint. If that does not help, expedite transport to the hospital.

Injuries to the upper extremity and certain types of shoulder dislocations are best splinted with a **sling and swath**. The sling can be made from a triangular bandage. It should support the entire forearm from elbow to wrist, with the ends tied around the neck of the patient and the knot padded to minimize pressure on the soft tissues of the neck area. The swath is a band made from another triangular bandage tied around the body of the patient; its purpose is to prevent movement of the extremity in the sling and provide added support. Both should be tied such that they provide support and position the arm away from the body, but they should not impede breathing.

A **traction splint** is applied to the lower extremity when an isolated mid-shaft femur fracture is suspected. The traction pulls the contracted upper leg muscles into a neutral position. Often, this splinting is enough to relieve the pain from the femur fracture. It also can help minimize bleeding in the area of the fracture. Traction splints should *not* be employed if there is any other suspected fracture or dislocation to the same leg, either proximal or distal to the femur.

Once the extremity is splinted, applying a cold pack over the injury can be beneficial. It can help limit pain and control localized inflammation. It also can reduce swelling over time. Hot packs should be avoided for most injuries, particularly in the acute phase; after the first 48 hours of an injury, however, heat may be helpful.

Pain Management

Proper immobilization of a musculoskeletal injury often provides significant pain relief for the patient, in some cases even eliminating the need for pharmacological intervention. Proper splinting also includes raising the injured area above the heart in the absence of contraindicating factors (such as a head injury with a lower extremity fracture). In addition to splinting, application of cold packs or ice to the injured area can bring relief. Cold slows the transmission of pain signals to the brain and can also help limit swelling, another source of pain in an injury.

In cases where pain from a musculoskeletal injury cannot be mitigated with splinting, immobilization, or application of cold, the paramedic has several medication options to control a patient's pain. The National Registry recognizes the following narcotic and nonnarcotic pain relievers for musculoskeletal pain management: morphine, fentanyl, nitrous oxide, ketorolac, and ketamine. (Refer to the Appendix for information on common EMS dosages and routes for these medications.)

Other Musculoskeletal Problems

Most of these disorders are more chronic in nature rather than acute and are seldom seen in the field. In addition, they may not require aggressive treatment from the paramedic. Unless otherwise indicated, treatment for patients with the following ailments includes ruling out acute trauma and making the patient comfortable for transport to the hospital of their choice.

Arthritis

Strictly speaking, **arthritis** is an inflammation of any joint, which, over time, will result in destruction to the joint. This will cause significant chronic pain for the patient. **Osteoarthritis** is believed to be from general wear and tear of the joint that occurs with aging. **Rheumatoid arthritis** is an autoimmune disease where the body's defenses attack the joints, leading to swelling and damage. Rheumatoid arthritis can occur at any age. Finally, **gout** is a form of arthritis that results from the body's inability to eliminate uric acid. Uric acid salts crystallize in the joints, which can cause chronic pain that increases across time. Patients with gout will be on a medication called allopurinol, which is commonly used as a diuretic to help the kidneys remove uric acid more efficiently.

Spinal Stenosis

Spinal stenosis is a narrowing of the spinal canal. It is a chronic condition that worsens over time. Eventually, it will cause back pain that leads to numbness inferior to the level of the stenosis. The stenosis is not typically throughout the spine but rather at one or only a couple of locations.

Overuse Syndromes

Long-term repetitive motions will lead to inflammation and pain in the affected area. **Tendinitis** results when one or more of the tendons in a joint become inflamed. **Bursitis** is inflammation of the bursa sac present in the joint that cushions the joint. Inflammation of the carpal tendon in the hand leads to the most common form of overuse syndrome, called **carpal tunnel syndrome**. The inflammation of the tendon located at the proximal portion of the palm of the hand causes compression of the underlying median nerve and blood vessels. A patient with carpal tunnel syndrome will present with numbness and tingling of the lateral hand, the thumb, and the index and middle fingers.

HEAD, NECK, AND SPINE INJURIES

This section will focus on injuries involving the face and sensory organs as well as neurological trauma of the head, brain, and spinal cord. Injuries to the sensory organs can make oral assessment and history taking more difficult for the provider. Injuries possibly involving the spine need to be treated cautiously because rough handling of the patient during extrication or transportation could result in a worsened injury. Head injuries can be difficult to care for because the patient can be combative, have seizures, or be resistant to treatment. The section starts by looking at the anatomy and physiology of each region, along with injuries and treatment for any injuries that may occur within that region.

Anatomy of Face and Sensory Organs

Bones of Face

The face and skull are made up of several bones held together at immovable joints, often called **suture lines**. The following lists the major bones of the face and the cranium. "Paired" noted in the definition indicates that the bones exist as separate bones on the right and left side of the face.

- **Frontal Bone.** Makes up the forehead.
- **Nasal Bones.** Paired; make up the bridge of the nose.
- **Maxilla Bones.** Paired; make up the anterior portion of the hard palate in the mouth, which is the bone into which the upper teeth are anchored and is the upper jaw. Also makes up a portion of the medial portion of the orbit, along with the lacrimal bones.
- **Lacrimal Bones.** Paired; forms the lateral wall of the orbit.
- **Palatine Bones.** Paired; make up the posterior third of the hard palate of the roof of the mouth.
- **Zygoma or Zygomatic Bones.** Paired; make up the inferior orbit and lateral cheek on each side. The zygomatic process makes the anterior portion of the zygomatic arch.

- **Temporal Bones.** Paired; comprise the side of the face anterior and superior to the ears. The posterior portion of the zygomatic arch is part of the temporal bone. The mastoid process posterior to the ear on both sides is part of this bone as well.
- **Mandible.** The entirety of the lower jaw.

Bones of Skull

In addition to the temporal bone and the frontal bone, these bones comprise the **cranial vault**. "Paired" noted in the definition indicates that the bones exist as separate bones on the right and left side of the skull.

- **Sphenoid Bones.** Paired; located between the temporal and frontal bones, deep to the zygomatic arch. The sphenoid also makes up the anterior portion of the base of the skull and the posterior orbit.
- **Parietal Bones.** Paired; located posterior to the frontal bone, make up the top of the head.
- **Occiput or Occipital Bone.** Makes up the posterior part of the skull.
- **Vomer.** Makes up the posterior nose and a small portion of the midline base of the skull.

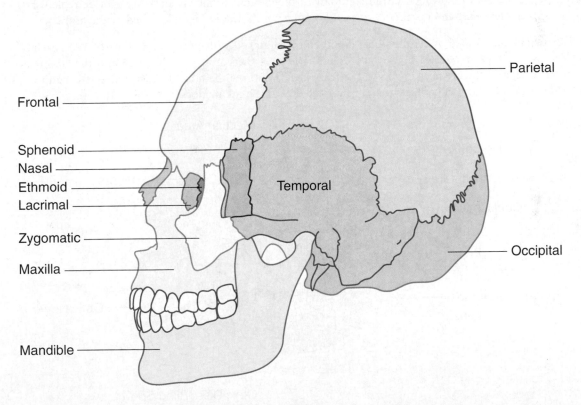

Figure 8-10. Bones of the Skull, Lateral View

Eye

The **eye** is a complex sensory organ. As noted in the neurological section earlier in the book, several different nerves are responsible for the sense of vision (optic nerve, CN II) and the motion of the eyeball itself (oculomotor nerve, CN III; trochlear nerve, CN IV; and abducens nerve, CN VI). The extraocular muscles of the eye are responsible for movement of the eye and looking in different directions.

The **cornea** is a thin layer of colorless cells that covers the anterior portion of the eye over the pupil. This is a very delicate layer, and it does not take much to cause a corneal abrasion.

The **pupil** is a hole in the iris through which light passes.

The **iris** is the colored part of the eye that dilates and constricts to control the amount of light entering the pupil.

Located just behind the pupil and iris, the **lens** focuses light on the retina to form an image. The thickness of the lens is controlled by the ciliary muscles, which attach to the lens on all edges of the lens.

The **retina** is a photosensitive layer of specialized cells that receive light entering the eye and convert the light into an electrical signal. The area of the retina with the most light-sensitive cells is called the **fovea**. This area of the retina allows for the clearest vision; other areas of the retina are less sensitive and therefore produce the less detailed image of the peripheral vision.

Once the retina converts the image to an electrical signal, it travels to the **optic nerve** and eventually to the visual cortex in the posterior region of the brain for interpretation. The **optic disk** is an area of the retina that does not contain any light-sensitive cells and is often called the **blind spot**.

Most of the globe of the eyeball is composed of a tough fibrous tissue that is white in color, called the **sclera**.

The lens and supporting ciliary muscles divide the globe of the eyeball into a large posterior chamber and a much smaller anterior chamber. The anterior chamber is filled with a fluid called the **aqueous humor**. The posterior chamber is filled with a clear fluid called **vitreous humor**. If the vitreous humor is lost, it cannot be replenished by the body, and the patient may end up blind. Aqueous humor, conversely, can be replenished by the body.

The **lacrimal gland**, located under the upper eyelid on the lateral edge, drips tears into the eye. With each blink, the tears drift across the eye and wash away any debris. The tears then drain from the eye into the lacrimal duct on the medial corner of the eye near the nose. The tears then drain into the nose. Tears also keep the **conjunctiva**, the underside of each eyelid that contacts the eye, lubricated so that blinking does not scratch the eye.

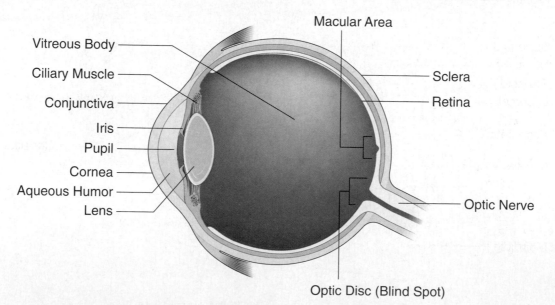

Figure 8-11. Structures of the Eye, Lateral View

Ears

The **ears** are responsible for hearing; however, they also are responsible for maintaining a person's balance and orientation in space. The vestibulocochlear nerve (CN VIII) is responsible for both of these senses and has 2 branches: the auditory branch and the vestibular branch. First, the sound will be followed along its progression; then the vestibular system will be discussed.

The ear has three subdivisions conveniently named the outer, middle, and inner ear. Sound first contacts the **pinna**, which is the outermost structure of the external ear. The sound is then funneled into the ear canal, where it contacts a thin membrane called the **tympanic membrane** or **eardrum**. The tympanic membrane is the division between the outer and middle ear.

The eardrum vibrates and transmits the sound through three bones collectively called the ossicles: the **malleus**, the **incus**, and the **stapes**. The bones conduct the sound in that order to the oval window in the vestibule, and with that, the sound enters the inner ear. The **eustachian tube** connects the inner ear with the posterior pharynx, allowing the inner ear pressure to remain equal to atmospheric pressure.

The structure of the inner ear is the **cochlea**. As sound travels through this snail-shaped organ, the vibrations reach the **organ of Corti** that has specialized hairs that are sensitive to particular frequencies. Each hair then stimulates a nerve fiber of the auditory branch of the vestibulocochlear nerve. This electrical impulse is interpreted in the auditory centers in the temporal lobe of the brain.

Also within the inner ear, unrelated to the sense of hearing, are the semicircular canals, known as the **vestibular system**. Three semicircular canals arranged in perpendicular axes send signals to the brain to alert it to the body's orientation in space and its relative speeds in each direction—side to side, front to back, and vertically.

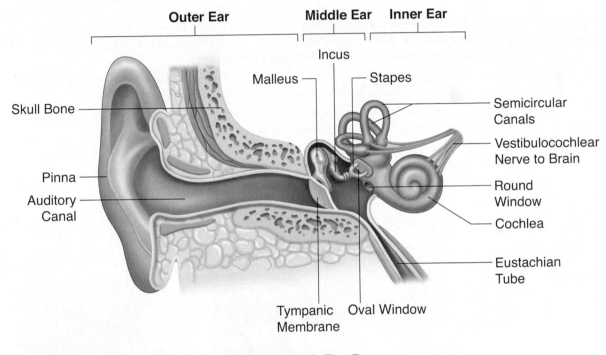

Figure 8-12. The Ear

Injuries of Face and Sensory Organs

Facial Fractures

Fractures of the bones of the face occur as a result of blunt trauma, such as the case of an unrestrained driver or passenger who collides face first with the dashboard or the windshield. A patient with facial fractures has sustained forces between 30 g (nose) and 100 g (maxillae and orbit), which is more force than astronauts experience during takeoff (about 3 g). As a result, although a facial fracture may be visually stunning, it is more likely that the patient has a significant—often lethal—brain injury.

Facial fractures can present in a variety of ways depending on the bone that was fractured; however, all of them will present with bruising at the very least and likely nearby lacerations. Facial fractures that result in a fracture to the bones of the base of the cranial vault may cause CSF to leak out. If this happens, CSF can be seen mixed with blood coming from the ears and/or the nose. To assess this, perform the halo test: Dab a little blood coming from the ear or nose on a 4 × 4 bandage. If there appears to be a pale yellow ring around the red blood, this indicates CSF.

In addition to likely brain injury, the patient may present with significant airway compromise caused by bleeding into the airway, swelling of the airways, and possibly foreign bodies lodged in the airway (teeth). Airway compromise is the primary concern in nasal and mandibular fractures because they are directly involved in the airway.

Mandibular fractures, in addition to the aforementioned airway compromise and bleeding, also may present with **malocclusion**. Malocclusion is a change in the articulation of a patient's teeth. The patient also may complain about pain on biting. Patients may not be able to talk in cases of fracture or dislocation of the temporomandibular joint because they are no longer able to close their upper and lower jaws.

Orbital fractures are most likely to occur on the inferior or lateral portion of the orbit and significantly less likely to happen in the superior edge of the orbit, which is the frontal bone. Any fracture, but particularly inferior orbital fractures to the orbit, carries with it the possibility of entrapment of or damage to facial nerves, resulting in numbness to the face. Extraocular muscles also may become entrapped or lacerated by the fractures. This will result in the patient's eye not being able to follow the provider's finger.

Zygoma fractures, also called cheek fractures, result in apparent asymmetry of the face with the affected side flatter than the other. Numbness and paralysis often result in that cheek, upper lip, and teeth. Eye movement can be inhibited as well.

Maxillary fractures are perhaps the most dramatic of any facial fracture and require the most force to occur. They will present with instability of much of the face and malocclusion as a possible symptom caused by shifting of the upper jaw. Fractures involving the maxillae are referred to as **LeFort fractures**.

- **LeFort I.** The fracture line is located across the inferior portion of the nose and results in a floating palate. Essentially, the entire upper jaw has been freed from the rest of the skull.
- **LeFort II.** The fracture line begins in the bridge of the nose and in a lateral and inferior direction, more or less following the natural maxillae suture line inferior to the orbits.
- **LeFort III.** A completely free-floating face. The fracture line is across the bridge of the nose and through the posterior orbit. This fracture often is referred to as **craniofacial dissociation**.

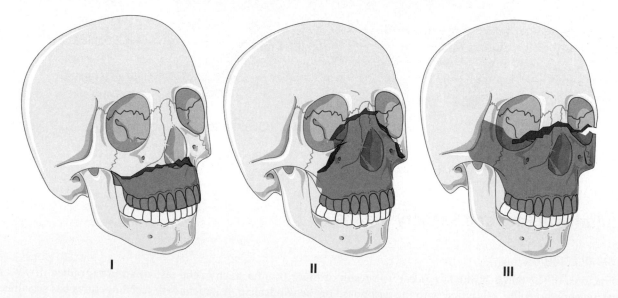

Figure 8-13. LeFort Fractures

Treatment of facial fractures often involves an extended focus on establishing and maintaining a patent airway. Manually open the airway, using only the modified jaw thrust to protect the cervical spine. An ETT is highly recommended if the patient requires positive pressure ventilation because the instability of the facial structures will make obtaining a seal for BVM unlikely. Suction should be liberally used before and during intubation attempts to clear the airway of blood, vomit, and any dislodged teeth. Because of the increased likelihood of fractures to the base of the skull with facial fractures, inserting anything into the nose is contraindicated. This includes nasopharyngeal airways, nasogastric tubes, and blind nasotracheal intubation. Application of a cervical collar in this patient, either before or after intubation, may help stabilize the jaw and support facial structures. Rarely, needle cricothyrotomy may be required to establish an airway; however, if needed, it should be employed early and quickly.

Eye Injuries

Eye injuries are concerning because they often result in some degree of vision loss, even if only temporarily. As a result of the temporary vision disturbance and the patient's contemplation of permanent visual loss, the patient often has a high degree of anxiety with an eye injury. Eyes, like any other part of the body, can be subjected to blunt and penetrating trauma and are particularly sensitive to chemicals, heat, and irritants.

For a laceration or impaled object to the eye or eyelid, do not apply direct pressure to the eye. The application of pressure to the eye can be extremely harmful to the patient. First, pressure to the eye can stimulate a vagus response leading to bradycardia. Second, if the globe is lacerated or punctured, pressure can force aqueous or vitreous humor out of the eye, and, in extreme cases, the lens, iris, or even retina can be forced out of the eye as well. Any of these can lead to permanent blindness. Although the eyelid may bleed heavily, the eye does not often bleed much.

If the impaled object is still present in the eye, the goal is stabilization of the object to prevent further injury. Placing a cup or bulky dressings around the object and covering both the patient's eyes is recommended. Covering both the patient's eyes causes the patient to minimize eye movement, thereby providing protection against more damage from the impaled object. When applying the dressing and covering either eye, be sure to not apply pressure to the globe of either eye. In addition, this will effectively make the patient blind, so treat the patient as if they are:

- Tell them what will happen before starting the procedure. While with the patient, the paramedic should narrate as much of their activities as possible to help allay the patient's anxieties.
- Make every effort to maintain gentle contact with the patient. This allows the patient to know where the provider is at all times so that the patient does not get startled.

Objects on the eye surface can be more than just a nuisance. They can cause corneal abrasions or lacerations. Chemicals can lead to conjunctivitis or inflammation of the conjunctiva. Flush the affected eye with water away from the unaffected eye. Do not allow the patient to rub their eyes.

Because the eye is somewhat recessed within the socket (orbit), blunt eye injuries are relatively uncommon. Blunt trauma can result in rupture of the globe or **hyphema**, bleeding into the anterior chamber of the eye. The retina also can detach from the sclera as a result of blunt trauma. Blunt trauma in the area of the eye can cause the eye to protrude from the orbit. If the globe is exposed, place a moist sterile dressing directly in contact with the avulsed eye and cover with a dry sterile bandage that includes both eyes.

Ear Injuries

External ear injuries are generally limited to the pinna and are the same as any other area of the body. Soft-tissue injuries to the external ear often heal poorly because of the poor blood supply. The result is often a deformed pinna called **cauliflower ear**.

Blunt injuries to the ear typically do not result in meaningful external injury; however, it is possible that the eardrum will rupture. This is especially likely when a person is slapped in the ear, such as might happen during an assault. It also may occur if the patient is close to an explosion. Bleeding is possible, though typically it is light. If there is bleeding from the ears, never pack the canal. Instead, loosely bandage the ear to allow the blood to drain. If there is bleeding from the ear, perform a halo test to evaluate for CSF.

Head Injuries

Head injuries can result from blunt and penetrating trauma to the skull. Head injuries can occur from falls, assaults, sports-related injuries, motor vehicle collisions, or gunshot wounds. They often can involve neurological deficits that can range from short-term anterograde amnesia to unconsciousness, brainstem herniation, and eventual death. In the previous section, it was noted that facial injuries can transmit energy to the brain, leading to injuries there as well. The types of skull fractures will be presented first; the implications on the brain will be discussed a bit later.

Basal skull fractures are fractures to the base of the skull and can result from impacts on any area of the head; however, large forces are usually required to cause basal skull fractures. Signs and symptoms of a basal skull fracture often include blood and CSF leaking from the ears, nose, or both. This can be found by performing the halo test described previously. Patients with basal skull fractures also may have periorbital ecchymosis, known as raccoon's eyes, or ecchymosis in the area of the mastoid process called the Battle sign. Both of these take a while to form and are considered late signs not usually seen immediately following the traumatic event.

Linear skull fractures are a closed, nondisplaced fracture of the skull that often results from blunt trauma. If the underlying brain is not injured, then the fracture itself is not typically anything to worry about.

Depressed skull fractures are fractures that result from blunt trauma to the skull, resulting in multiple fractured pieces of skull in one area. The result is a dent or a depression of the skull. Such fractures can cause shards of skull to become embedded in the brain tissue, leading to profound neurological deficits. Concurrent basal skull fractures are possible when this much force has been imparted to the skull.

Head injuries can be open or closed. In an **open head injury**, brain tissue is exposed as a result of skull fracture. In a **closed head injury**, brain tissue has still been injured regardless of whether the skull has been fractured. But brain tissue is not exposed. Remember, with every fracture listed here, if the scalp over the top of the fracture is broken, it is considered an open fracture. This is not the same as an open head injury.

Traumatic Brain Injury

Traumatic brain injury is any injury to the brain that results in transient or permanent cognitive, intellectual, or emotional changes. A **primary brain injury** is the actual injury to the brain as a direct result of the insult. This injury can be through penetrating trauma such as a gunshot wound; however, it is much more likely the result of blunt trauma to the head and brain. After the head is impacted, say by the concrete sidewalk during a fall, the brain will continue to move within the cranium until it collides with the inner wall of the cranium. At this point, the brain is injured in the same area of the initial impact. This is called a **coup injury**. If the force was great enough, the brain may then bounce off the cranial wall and into the other side of the cranium, thus injuring the side of the brain directly opposite the point of impact. This is called a **contrecoup** injury.

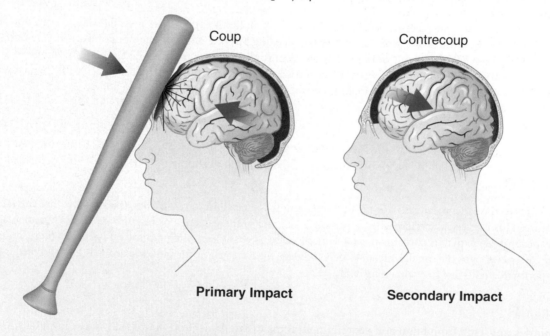

Figure 8-14. Coup and Contrecoup Injuries
The coup injury is caused by the initial impact; the contrecoup injury is caused by the brain bouncing backward and colliding with the other side of the skull, opposite the impact.

Secondary brain injuries happen after the brain has been directly injured. These injuries include the damage to the brain tissue that results from bleeding into the brain and swelling of the brain. This also can include any infections and abscesses that can occur with open head injuries. Finally, cerebral ischemia, hypoxia, and infarct can happen when blood flow to a particular area of the brain is compromised for even just a short period of time.

Secondary brain injuries can lead to a worsened patient outcome because the skull is not capable of expanding to make room for the swelling brain after an injury. Because swelling will occur whether or not the brain has a place to go, it will first move into the potential spaces within the cranium. These include the small volume initially occupied with CSF. Once that space has been occupied, it starts to occlude the blood vessels within the cranial vault. Throughout this process, the pressures within the head are increasing. This is referred to as increasing ICP.

As this pressure increases, the brain recognizes that it is getting hypoxic as a result of the pressures building up, so, as a matter of self-preservation, it orders an increase in blood pressure. Blood pressure increases. However, not knowing what is happening in the brain, the carotid sinuses, which measure pressure, recognize an increase in pressure that they did not call for and order the heart rate to slow down. So, the heart rate slows down. This cycle of increasing blood pressure and decreasing heart rate will continue and worsen as the pressure in the skull continues to rise.

The brain does this to maintain cerebral perfusion pressure (CPP). The minimum CPP required to perfuse the brain under normal circumstances is 60 mmHg and can be calculated by subtracting the ICP (which cannot be measured in the field) from the mean arterial pressure (MAP). MAP is shown on automatic blood pressure cuffs as a number in parentheses but can be calculated by doubling the diastolic number, adding to it the systolic number, and dividing by 3.

$$MAP = \frac{2(\text{Diastolic}) + \text{Systolic}}{3}$$

$$CPP = MAP - ICP$$

Normally, ICP is less than 15 mmHg and can be 0. Therefore, it is essential that the MAP of any patient, especially the patient with a head injury, be kept above 60 mmHg by maintaining blood pressure and providing fluids.

As the brain continues to swell, after occluding the blood vessels, now kept open only with the markedly increased blood pressure, the only other option for the brain in a closed head injury is to herniate out of the foramen magnum at the base of the skull through which the spinal column passes. To do this, it must first push out the medulla and midbrain, which includes the respiratory centers of the brain. Pressure and damage to the respiratory center result in an ataxic respiratory rate, which tends to be fast, shallow, and irregular. This type of respiration will not be effective in maintaining oxygenation or removing CO_2 and will lead to a respiratory acidosis that can possibly cause the cerebral arteries to dilate, further worsening the ICP. Ataxic respiration, combined with bradycardia and hypertension, is called the Cushing triad or the Cushing reflex. This is a hallmark sign of a potentially lethal brain injury.

Signs and symptoms to look for when assessing a patient with a head injury include the Cushing triad but also include evaluation of pupil equality. As the brain swells, it will exert pressure on the oculomotor nerve, causing one pupil to be dilated and sluggish to react or completely unreactive to light. The patient may vomit without a previous complaint of nausea. The patient may have an altered mental status or have had a transient loss of consciousness prior to EMS arrival.

Specific Types of Brain Injuries

Concussion

Concussion is a diffuse brain injury that can occur with any blow to the brain. Concussions are most common in deceleration injuries, such as those that result from sports injuries, motor vehicle crashes, and falls. A concussion is not associated with long-term debilitation. Loss of consciousness is not necessary for a person to have sustained a concussion. Patients may be amnestic to the events that caused the injury and may show either anterograde or retrograde amnesia, but a patient may not have either.

Diffuse Axonal Injury

A **diffuse axonal injury** is characterized only once in the hospital. These injuries are differentiated from a concussion because the brain has sustained more extensive damage to the axons of the neurons, resulting in interrupted transmission of nerve signals. Axons can be sheared or torn off the nerve bodies, which is often not survivable or results in permanent deficits. Stretching of the axons, instead of shearing them, is survivable but may result in some long-term impairments depending on the area of the brain affected.

Intracranial Bleeds

Cerebral Contusion

Cerebral contusions are a bruise within the cerebrum in a local area. This is worse than a concussion because this actually results in structural damage to the brain and a loss of the blood-brain barrier, resulting in a longer period of neurological deficits than with concussion.

Epidural Hematoma

An **epidural hematoma** is located outside the dura mater between the meninges and the skull. Epidural hematomas are most commonly caused by blunt trauma and linear fracture to the temporal bone and a laceration to the middle meningeal artery that underlies it. The trauma to the head that leads to the epidural hematoma usually first causes the patient to lose consciousness. The patient will then regain consciousness and have a "lucid interval" before losing consciousness again after the ICP has critically increased. Often, the patient also will display unequal pupils.

Subdural Hematoma

A **subdural hematoma** results when one or more of the veins that lie between the dura and the brain are torn during a traumatic event. This is very common in falls and motor vehicle accidents sustained by adults age 65 and older because the distance between the brain and dura mater expands as a result of atrophy of the cerebral tissue. Here, blood accumulates beneath the dura but still outside the brain tissue. It has the capacity to increase ICP; however, it takes a much longer time to develop than an epidural hematoma; sometimes it is not clinically apparent for days or weeks after the injury.

Intracerebral Hematoma

An **intracerebral hematoma** is worse than a cerebral contusion because the bleeding is heavier and affects a larger area of the cerebrum. Although the blood can be surgically removed from within the brain tissue, there is still a very high likelihood of death with this type of injury.

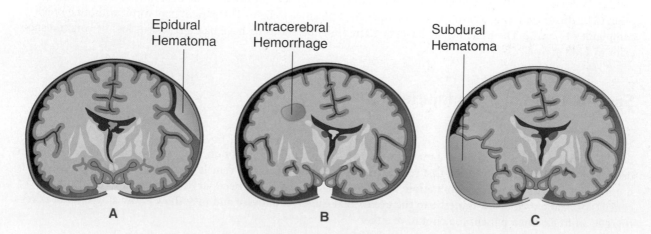

Figure 8-15. Intracranial Hemorrhages
(A) Epidural hematoma, (B) intracerebral hemorrhage, and (C) subdural hematoma.

Subarachnoid Hemorrhage

Bleeding into the subarachnoid space where the CSF circulates leads to a significant headache as a result of meningeal irritation. A **subarachnoid hemorrhage** is associated with a high mortality rate; those who survive often have significant clinical deficits. Signs and symptoms include those associated with closed head injury.

Neck and Spine Injuries

Anatomy of Neck

The anterior neck has several relatively superficial structures of concern when assessing neck trauma. First, along the midline is the trachea, and located superficial to the thyroid cartilage of the trachea is the highly vascular thyroid gland. Immediately lateral to the trachea lie each of the carotid arteries. They are reasonably protected with overlying muscles. Moving further laterally are the jugular veins. Also within the neck, in the area of the carotid arteries, are several cranial nerve bundles, including the vagus nerve among others.

Neck Injuries

Penetrations and lacerations to the anterior neck can be immediately life threatening. The trachea is particularly vulnerable to lacerations because of its prominent location. Lacerations to the trachea will result in heavy bleeding and difficulty breathing. Treat a lacerated trachea similar to a dislodged tracheostomy tube. Place an ETT directly through the hole in the anterior trachea, inflate the cuff, and either allow the patient to breathe unaided through the tube or ventilate as needed.

If the great vessels—either the carotids or the jugulars—are lacerated, bleeding will be massive. Controlling the bleeding can be tricky because the application of pressure to the bleeding site can stimulate a vagus response. A failure to occlude both sides of the lacerated vessel can result in a massive air embolus directly into the brain if the laceration is on the superior side of the carotid or directed into the heart if the lacerated vessel is one of the jugulars. In addition to the massive bleeding, patients could present with neurological deficits as a result of a possible air embolus or simply the lack of cerebral blood flow. Apply an occlusive dressing to lacerations of the great vessels of the neck and apply enough pressure to control bleeding.

Blunt injuries to the neck most commonly will result in tracheal fractures. If the cartilaginous rings are broken, then the trachea is no longer able to remain open when the patient takes a breath. This will cause severe—possibly fatal—difficulty in breathing because the trachea collapses with each inhalation. Rapidly providing positive pressure ventilation is essential for this patient. If the tissue of the trachea also is ruptured, air may escape into the mediastinum and cause additional problems as the pressure builds up.

Anatomy of Spine

Thirty-three vertebrae make up the spinal column. The vertebrae surround and protect the bundle of nerves that is the spinal cord. Each vertebra is connected to a vertebra above and below it with multiple ligaments and cushioned from each with a cartilaginous pad located between the vertebral bodies. All vertebrae have the following features:

- **Vertebral Body.** The bony mass that makes up most of the body. It articulates with the cartilage between each vertebra.
- **Pedicle.** The area between the transverse process and the body. This is a smooth area above and below which spinal nerves exit the spinal column. This notch is called the **intervertebral foramen.**
- **Transverse Process.** Forms points of attachment for ligaments and projects posteriorly and laterally from the vertebra.
- **Spinous Process.** Projects posteriorly from the vertebra. In lumbar vertebrae, they project inferiorly as well. They are sites for muscle and ligament attachment.
- **Vertebral Foramen.** The space through which the spinal cord passes.

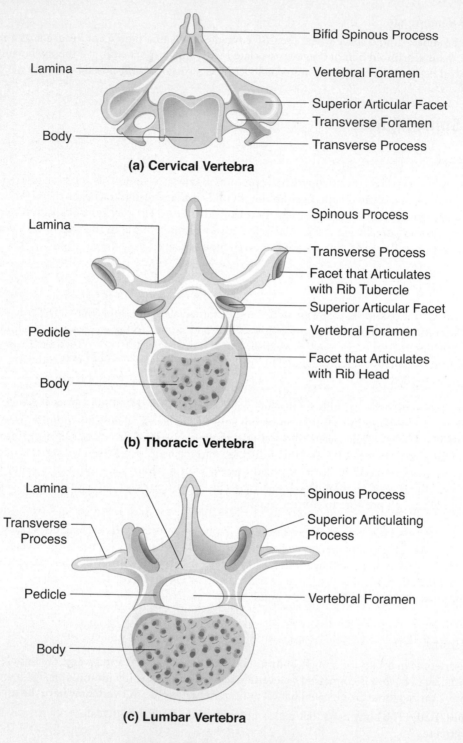

(a) Cervical Vertebra

Labels: Lamina, Body, Bifid Spinous Process, Vertebral Foramen, Superior Articular Facet, Transverse Foramen, Transverse Process

(b) Thoracic Vertebra

Labels: Lamina, Pedicle, Body, Spinous Process, Transverse Process, Facet that Articulates with Rib Tubercle, Superior Articular Facet, Vertebral Foramen, Facet that Articulates with Rib Head

(c) Lumbar Vertebra

Labels: Lamina, Transverse Process, Pedicle, Body, Spinous Process, Superior Articulating Process, Vertebral Foramen

Figure 8-16. Types of Vertebrae

The vertebral column is divided into five different sections. The vertebrae are identified based on their location and number, working superior to inferior. For example, the first thoracic vertebra is named T-1.

The Cervical Vertebrae (7). Each of the other cervical vertebrae differs from the remainder of the column in that they all have a foramen on the lateral sides through which passes the vertebral arteries. They are the only vertebrae that have this feature. C-1 and C-2 differ from each of the other 5 in this section and have specific names: atlas and axis, respectively. The axis (C-2) provides the axis on which the atlas (C-1) spins when the head turns from side to side.

The Thoracic Vertebrae (12). Each thoracic vertebra is associated with a pair of ribs that articulates on the lateral facets. The spinous processes are slightly more pronounced because they have more muscle and ligaments attached than other vertebrae.

Lumbar Vertebrae (5). Lumbar vertebrae have the largest and thickest vertebral bodies because they support the weight of much of the body superior to it.

Sacrum (5). These vertebrae are fused together within the ring of the pelvis.

Coccyx (4). The vestiges of our tail, injuries to the coccyx are usually insignificant, despite being extremely painful.

Spinal Cord

The spinal cord transmits messages from the brain to the PNS and from the PNS to the brain. Sensory signals travel on the afferent (ascending to the brain) tracks, whereas motor signals travel on the efferent (exiting the brain) tracks to the muscles of the body. Spinal nerves exit the spinal column in between every vertebra and are named according to the vertebra above it. Inferior to L2, the spinal cord the nerve roots take on the appearance of a horse's tail. This region is aptly referred to as the **cauda equina** and services the lower extremities.

Spinal Column Injuries

The neck is the only area of the spine that allows for a comparatively wide range of motion. So injuries are caused by flexion, rotation with flexion, and hyperextension. Each injury type can result in different presentations.

Flexion injuries result from any incident where the head can whip forward suddenly. They can result in fractures to the atlas and axis or dislocation of these joints. Each of these can be described as either stable or unstable. Unstable injuries are more significant and can result in stretching or tearing of the spinal cord. Flexion when combined with rotation of the head, such as what may happen during a lateral impact during a motor vehicle accident or an assault or tackle in a football game, can result in even worse injuries to the C-1 and C-2 area.

Hyperextension injuries can occur anywhere in the spine, but mostly occur in the cervical spine. Hyperextension of the cervical spine can result in a **hangman's fracture**. A hangman's fracture is a fracture to C-2 that results in bilateral fracture to both pedicles. This is an unstable fracture but does not typically result in a cord injury.

Compression injuries can result from vertical compression of the spine, also known as axial loading. This often results in **burst fractures** of the vertebral body anywhere along the spine. It is most commonly found in the cervical and lumbar vertebrae because the cervical vertebral bodies are the smallest of all, and the lumbar already support the most weight, so any more load can result in fracture. The compression force can come from above, such as hitting the crown of the head on the roof of a car during a collision or from below as might happen when jumping from a height and landing on the feet with locked knees. Most of these fractures are stable relative to causing cord injury; however, continued movement of the fractured vertebra could force a piece of bone into the cord, lacerating it.

Spinal Cord Injuries

Primary Cord Injuries

A **primary cord injury** is any cord injury resulting directly from the traumatic event. This can include complete or partial transection from penetrating trauma. Primary injury from blunt trauma is more varied. Transection of the cord can still occur with blunt trauma after the ligaments that hold the vertebrae together are torn. This leads to an unstable dislocation of the vertebrae in that area, which could lead to one sliding off the other and cutting the spinal cord. Fractures to the vertebra can force a piece of bone shrapnel into the cord, leading to partial loss of neurological function on the affected side. Injuries such as these result in permanent deficits.

Hemorrhage into the spinal canal and contusions to the spinal cord itself can lead to temporary or permanent deficits. **Spinal distraction**, or the stretching of the spinal cord resulting from the vertebrae being pulled apart can cause small tears in the neurons or acute swelling. Each of these may result in normal radiology studies and may be referred to as **SCIWORA**, which stands for "spinal cord injury without radiological abnormality".

Secondary Cord Injuries

Like any other tissue in the body, the cord can swell as a result of trauma leading to a temporary loss of neurological function distal to the injury. It is not uncommon for a patient to have normal feeling and motor function after an incident but later have paresthesias or movement problems distal to a traumatic spine injury. What follows is a list of secondary cord injury syndromes with their symptoms and prognoses.

Anterior cord syndrome results from disruption of the anterior region of the cord often caused by flexion injuries. The patient will present with motor and sensory loss to the area inferior to the injury.

Central cord syndrome is associated with hyperextension injuries of the cervical spine. Patients with this type of injury will have a loss of function of the upper extremities, whereas motor function of the lower extremities tends to remain intact. Patients may have acute bowel and bladder dysfunction with this and also may have variable changes in their sensation to pain and temperature of the upper extremities. This injury is common in older adults, particularly those with arthritis of the spine or spinal stenosis. Recovery from this often is complete but with bilateral hand weakness sometimes persisting.

Posterior cord syndrome is likely with extension injuries, though much less common. Patients with this syndrome will have a decreased sensation to light touch and proprioception. **Proprioception** is the person's ability to perceive position in space without having to look at the limb.

Cauda equina syndrome is caused by lesions in the L-1 and L-2 area, including hemorrhage, transection, and penetrating injuries. In addition to low back pain, it can lead to paresthesias to the lower extremities, particularly those areas that would contact a saddle. Patients also will present with decreased rectal tone and have bowel or bladder dysfunction.

Brown-Sequard syndrome can be thought of as lateral cord syndrome, though it is never referred to this way. It results from damage to one side of the cord from either distraction, transection, or a penetrating injury. Damage to all nerve tracts on one side of the spinal cord leads to loss of motor and light touch and vibration on the side of and inferior to the injury. This also will lead to the loss of pain and temperature sensation on the side opposite the injury.

Neurogenic shock can result from any of the above injuries. It causes widespread dilation of vessels inferior to the spinal cord lesion. This, in turn, leads to hypovolemia relative to the size of the container. Patients will present pale and diaphoretic superior to the injury and flushed and dry inferior to it.

The assessment of suspected spinal cord injuries should involve careful palpation of the entire spinal column. Encountering a step-off, or an area where the spine is no longer a continuous line, indicates a possible transection of the cord or a distraction injury at least. As with extremity fractures, assess distal pulse, motor, and sensation, particularly in the lower extremities and document findings. Anytime the patient has or is suspected of having a spinal cord injury (SCI), the patient should be carefully transferred to a backboard and fully immobilized with a cervical collar and head immobilization devices. Anytime the patient is transferred or moved in any way, reevaluate pulse, motor, and sensation of the extremities.

Treatment of SCIs has two major goals. Minimizing the progression of secondary spinal injuries should be the primary goal. This is accomplished by employing spinal motion restriction devices, such as the short spine board if the patient is found seated, and securing the patient to a long backboard as well, regardless of position found. Second, the patient should be treated for shock, and steps should be taken to prevent the onset of shock. Often, an SCI is not the only issue facing the patient, so completing a full secondary assessment and the treatment of any life-threatening conditions found should not be ignored.

CHEST INJURIES

With the relatively flexible rib cage surrounding the vital structures of the heart and lungs, the paramedic needs to maintain a high index of suspicion when presented with any trauma involving the chest. An intact rib cage does not always mean that the heart and lungs have avoided injury. Chest injuries can lead to profound respiratory and cardiovascular compromise. This section will discuss the injuries to the chest and treatments the paramedic will need to initiate.

Chest Anatomy

The chest is surrounded and protected by the rib cage and sternum. The 12 pairs of ribs can be classified as either true ribs, false ribs, or floating ribs. All ribs articulate posteriorly with a thoracic vertebra. The **true ribs** are the first 7 pairs of ribs and connect to the sternum anteriorly. **False ribs** consist of the lower 5 pairs of ribs and have no direct connection to the sternum. They either connect through merging with other ribs or do not connect at all. The lowest 2 pairs of ribs have no anterior connection to the sternum and are called **floating ribs**. The area of the ribs closest to the sternum is made of cartilage in younger populations to allow for greater flexibility and resiliency.

The area between each rib is called the intercostal space and is numbered based on the number of the rib superior to it. Within this space are the intercostal muscles, which are responsible for raising and lowering the rib cage during respiration. Just to the inferior side of each rib is the neurovascular bundle, which contains the artery, vein, and nerves for that area.

The **sternum** or breastbone can be divided into three regions. The superior portion is called the **manubrium**. The center portion is known as the body of the sternum. The manubrium connects to the body of the sternum at an angle known as the **angle of Louis**. Finally, the most inferior part is called the xiphoid process.

The posterior chest also has ribs, but has the thoracic vertebrae at the midline. The **scapula** is located over the upper third of the posterior back and makes up the posterior point of articulation of the humerus in the shoulder. The clavicle joins here as well to make up the **acromioclavicular joint**.

Within the rib cage lie the heart, lungs, esophagus, and great vessels. The **mediastinum** lies on the midline and contains the esophagus, trachea and bronchi, and heart and great vessels.

Lateral to the mediastinum are the lungs, three lobes on the right and two on the left. The lungs are surrounded by two layers of tough connective tissue called **pleura**. The layer closest to the lung is called the **visceral pleura**, and the layer closest to the chest wall is called the **parietal pleura**. In between the layers is a serous fluid that lubricates the pleura, allowing the lungs to slide smoothly during inhalation and exhalation.

Two layers of fibrous tissue surround the heart as well. The inner layer is called the **epicardium**, and the outer layer is the parietal layer and is called the **pericardial sac**. Its purpose is to protect itself and the surrounding structures from the constant motion of the heart.

The inferior border of the thorax is the **diaphragm**, which can be as high as the 5th rib during exhalation. It can then descend to cause inhalation and recede well inferior to the xiphoid.

Chest Wall Injuries

Patients do not often suffer just a single injury to the chest when they are injured. If a patient has a rib fracture, there is also the possibility of a pneumothorax underlying the fracture. Chest bruising can lead to a cardiac contusion or a pulmonary contusion. For purposes of this text, isolated injuries will be described; however, the paramedic needs to know that more injuries than just those that can be seen or felt may exist. A thorough assessment of the chest will be necessary to effectively treat all the injuries the patient may have. It was mentioned at the opening to this section and is reiterated here: Maintain a high index of suspicion with any patient who has sustained a chest injury or has sustained a significant mechanism of injury.

Rib and Sternal Fractures

Rib fractures are the result of blunt trauma to the chest. Occasionally, people have been known to fracture ribs during a particularly forceful cough or sneeze. Rib fractures are extremely painful for the patient, even when there are no underlying injuries. Patients with a rib fracture will often self-splint to minimize the movement of the fractured bone ends against each other. They will complain of sharp, constant pain that came on suddenly and does not radiate. The pain also will worsen during inspiration or movement. Crepitus may be palpated in the area of the fracture as a result of the pressure exerted during palpation and from the act of breathing.

Sternal fractures require a much more significant amount of force. Consequently, this fracture is associated with a high incidence of underlying injuries. The heart or lungs often are bruised in addition to the fracture. If they are still conscious, patients will complain of excruciating midline chest pain as a result of the traumatic event. Patients also will have bruising and crepitus in the area of the fracture.

Treatment of rib and sternal fractures is similar and primarily directed at splinting the fracture. The best way to accomplish this is with a pillow held in place with a couple of triangular bandages. This will minimize the movement of the bone ends, thereby alleviating pain. Because the pain often leads to reduced tidal volume on the part of the patient, administer O_2 to help the patient breathe easier and prepare to treat for shock. With these injuries, be alert for the possibility of more insidious life-threatening conditions, including a cardiac contusion, cardiac tamponade, a pulmonary contusion, and pneumothorax.

Flail Chest

A **flail chest** occurs when two or more consecutive ribs are broken in two or more places. This is a significant injury and very often is complicated by an underlying pneumothorax or a pulmonary contusion. It is possible to have an entire side of the rib cage flail or have the sternum flail as well.

Because the flail segment now moves independent of the rest of the rib cage, the physics of breathing is materially impacted. Remember that normal ventilation is caused by the ribs and diaphragm being able to create a negative pressure within the thorax, thus allowing atmospheric air to rush in. Similarly, during exhalation, the diaphragm relaxes, creating a higher pressure in the chest cavity than outside the body, allowing air to be pushed out. During inhalation, the flail segment also moves into the chest cavity and pushes out during exhalation. This is called **paradoxical motion**. This increases the amount of pain the patient is experiencing and increases the risk for a punctured lung and resulting pneumothorax, if one was not already there.

To go along with the paradoxical motion, a patient will obviously complain of shortness of breath and chest pain. There may be bruising over the flail segment. A finding of diminished or absent breath sounds on the side of the flail segment is suggestive of a pneumothorax. Be alert for other signs of pneumothorax.

Treatment for the flail segment begins by stabilizing and splinting the segment in a similar manner as for rib fractures. The patient will need supplemental O_2 and may benefit from positive pressure ventilation. Intubation should be considered, especially if the patient lacks a gag reflex and is unable to protect their airway. If present, treat the pneumothorax. The patient also should have at least a large-bore intravenous line initiated and run wide. Monitor the heart rhythm throughout contact and treat any dysrhythmias as they present.

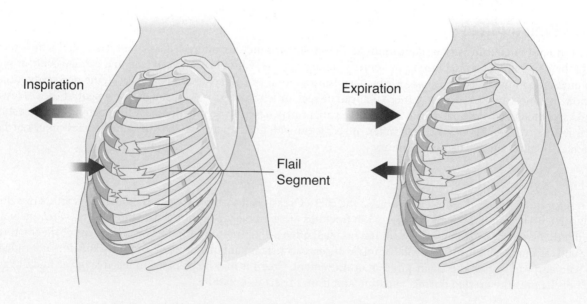

Figure 8-17. Flail Segment Demonstrating Paradoxical Motion

Lung Injuries

Pneumothorax

A **pneumothorax** results from a punctured lung that allows air to escape into the potential space between the visceral and parietal pleura. In a simple pneumothorax, air accumulates in this space but does not develop enough pressure or flow out of the lung fast enough to build pressure and become a tension pneumothorax. In a **tension pneumothorax**, the pressure in the pleural space builds to the point that the injured lung becomes compressed or collapses. As the lung collapses and air pressure and volume increase on the affected side, the pressure can force the mediastinum and its contents toward the unaffected side.

A pneumothorax also may develop as a result of a penetrating wound to the chest wall. This new hole in the chest wall will allow air in on inhalation and may or may not allow the air out on exhalation. This is known as a **sucking chest wound**. If this new hole is greater than 2/3 the area of the trachea, air will preferentially enter the chest wall hole over the trachea. The larger this hole, the more quickly the lung will collapse and the more rapid the decline of the patient's status. Even though air may exit the hole on exhalation, some will remain in and build up over time with each successive breath.

The following findings are suggestive of a pneumothorax:

- **Chest Trauma.** Blunt or penetrating trauma to the chest can result in a pneumothorax. Often, a person will take a deep breath and hold it while seeing an impending accident. This action makes lung trauma more likely. Rib fractures or a flail chest concurrent with the pneumothorax is also possible.

- **Diminished or Absent Breath Sounds.** This finding in an otherwise healthy person is an early finding in pneumothorax, sometimes even before the patient complains of shortness of breath.

- **Subcutaneous Emphysema.** This is air that has escaped the lungs and become trapped in the skin. Palpating this area will feel like there is popping under the skin. The skin may even feel inflated.

- **Hyperresonant to Percussion.** This means that tapping over the affected side sounds hollow and echoes. To percuss a patient, place the nondominant hand over the area to be percussed and tap the middle finger of that hand with a finger or two of the other hand.

- **JVD.** JVD results when there is a backup of blood that is draining from the head. It is clinically significant when the patient's head is raised >45°. It presents in pneumothorax when the pressure has built up to the point that it begins to inhibit the venous return of blood to the heart, the ejection of the blood from the right side of the heart, or both.

- **Tracheal Deviation.** As the pressure builds up and the mediastinum is displaced, the trachea deviates from its normal position in the midline and gets pushed toward the unaffected side. Because it takes some amount of time for the pressure to build up, this is considered a late sign.

- **Pulse Oximetry Decreased and Not Improving with Supplemental O_2.** As the lung collapses, the alveoli collapse as well (atelectasis). This results in an area of the lung, and therefore blood in capillaries, that do not receive O_2. Providing O_2 will not resolve this, so pulse oximetry does not improve despite high-flow O_2.

Treatment for a pneumothorax begins with cardiac monitoring, the establishment of at least one large-bore intravenous line, and the provision of high-flow supplemental O_2. If the patient is not breathing or is breathing inadequately, positive pressure ventilation should be initiated. Intubation should be considered if it is expected that the patient will require extended periods of ventilation. Definitive treatment for a pneumothorax is placement of a chest tube in the hospital, but for EMS, interim definitive treatment is needle thoracostomy. A needle thoracostomy allows the air to escape from the intrapleural space giving the lung a chance to re-expand. This often immediately relieves difficulty breathing in the spontaneously breathing patient or makes positive pressure ventilation easier.

Needle Thoracostomy

If the patient presents with most of the signs and symptoms listed above, follow these steps to perform a needle thoracostomy. Although this procedure is not usually necessary for a simple pneumothorax, it may need to be performed on a person with an open pneumothorax.

1. Identify the landmarks for needle placement.

    - Second intercostal space, midclavicular line, just above the third rib to avoid the neurovascular bundle that lies just inferior to the rib above. This can be easily found by identifying the angle of Louis and sliding laterally into the second intercostal space.

    - Fifth intercostal space, midaxillary line, just above the sixth rib. This location, in many cases, should be the second choice.

2. Cleanse the chosen location with alcohol or povidone iodine.

3. Insert the large-bore (>16 gauge) intravenous catheter at a 90° angle to the skin and push it all the way to the hub.

4. Remove the needle from the catheter and leave the catheter in place. Air, blood, or both may be quickly released through the catheter.

Some texts recommend using a makeshift flutter valve. They suggest cutting the finger off a medical glove and inserting the catheter through the fingertip of the glove before inserting the needle into the chest. Other texts identify that in the short period of time this will be in place, it is not likely to provide much added benefit when weighed against the benefit provided by getting the needle into the chest in a more timely fashion. Follow local protocols.

Hemothorax

The presence of blood in the intrapleural space can have the same effect as air, given enough time to accumulate, and blood flow. The sign and symptoms of a **hemothorax** are similar to those of a pneumothorax but with a couple of exceptions. Instead of being hyperresonant to percussion, a hemothorax is said to be dull to percussion. Also, JVD may or may not be present depending on how much blood has been lost to the pleural cavity. Finally, the patient will present with worsened tachycardia and hypotension as a result of the blood loss. Treatment is the same overall for the patient with the hemothorax, with added emphasis on fluid resuscitation. The patient should receive at least a liter of fluid during transport, and efforts should be taken to maintain the blood pressure after the needle thoracostomy is performed.

Rarely is it just one or the other—blood or air—present in the pleural space after chest trauma. Often both are present simultaneously. This is called a **hemopneumothorax**. It is treated the same way as either a hemothorax or a pneumothorax.

Pulmonary Contusion

A **pulmonary contusion** is a bruise to the lung tissue. Within the first 24 hours or so, patients may not have any complaints related to the bruising of their lung, and the biggest sign may be a ventilation perfusion mismatch and some mild chest pain that worsens with inhalation. A **ventilation perfusion mismatch** is essentially where it appears that the patient is breathing adequately. In other words, tidal volume is appropriate, and the mechanics of breathing are within normal limits. However, the pulse oximetry reading is lower than would otherwise be expected given a normal ventilatory status. An area of the lung is no longer able to transfer O_2 into the blood because of broken capillaries. Over time, this area also swells, leading to atelectasis, which can further complicate the respiratory status.

Treatment for a pulmonary contusion is largely related to increasing the FiO_2. Administer high-flow O_2 to the patient. Positive pressure ventilation is recommended if the patient's respiratory status is declining. Establish an intravenous line for access, but fluid administration should be limited because it may worsen the pulmonary edema already beginning. Fluid should be administered to maintain cardiac output and improve a falling blood pressure.

Cardiovascular Injuries

Cardiac Tamponade

Also known as pericardial tamponade, **cardiac tamponade** is a condition where fluid or blood accumulates within the pericardial sac surrounding the heart. Similar to what a pneumothorax does to a lung, as pressure builds up from blood in the sac, the heart begins to get compressed. Blood can accumulate slowly or rapidly depending on the source of the bleeding. As compression of the heart begins, the following signs and symptoms will become apparent.

- **Distant Heart Sounds.** Heart sounds in a person with cardiac tamponade are described as distant or muffled.
- **JVD.** The thinnest and most pliable structures within the pericardium are the atria and veins and are therefore the first to be compressed as pressure builds. Once the pressure on the external wall of the atria exceeds that of the pressure inside the atria, blood begins to back up in the vena cava, which is seen as JVD. This also has the effect of reducing preload.
- **Hypotension.** Because of both the reduction of preload and the inability of the heart to expand against the pressure outside, the blood pressure falls.
- **Narrowing Pulse Pressure.** The pulse pressure is the difference between the systolic and the diastolic numbers of the blood pressure. This value will decrease as the pressure builds.
- **Electrical Alternans.** This is seen on the ECG as a changing appearance of the electrical cycle on the printout, which is caused by the compressed heart swishing around in the blood surrounding it. The oscillation has the effect of changing the axis that the ECG is seeing from beat to beat. Although bigeminy should be ruled out, electrical alternans is a classic finding in pericardial tamponade.

The presence of hypotension, JVD, and muffled heart tones is collectively referred to as the Beck triad.

Treatment for cardiac tamponade includes monitoring the cardiac rhythm and treating any dysrhythmias found. Prepare for cardiac arrest, with the most likely presenting rhythm being some form of pulseless electrical activity. Initiate at least one large-bore intravenous line and run fluid wide to try and increase preload. Definitive care for pericardial tamponade is a procedure called **pericardiocentesis**, which EMS cannot perform. In pericardiocentesis, a needle is inserted into the pericardium, and the blood is drawn off, allowing the heart to expand and beat normally. Rapid transport to a trauma facility capable of rapid surgical intervention is necessary.

Myocardial Contusion

A bruise to the heart muscle can occur as a result of the rapid deceleration of the chest wall leading the heart to collide with the chest wall. This results in hemorrhage and swelling of the myocardium and can lead to electrical dysrhythmias. Anytime the cells of the heart become irritated, whether from hypoxia or structural damage—both of which are possible in a myocardial contusion—electrical disturbances are to be expected. The disturbance can be as mild as occasional ectopic beats or as lethal as VT or VF. It is essential to diligently monitor the cardiac rhythm and perform serial 12-lead ECGs on a person with this condition.

As a result of the bruising and the swelling in an area of the heart, the mechanics of the heart may be affected as well. Bleeding and edema will interfere with the full contraction of the myocytes in the area of the bruise, which can lead to decreased cardiac output. Hypotension can result from myocardial contusion.

Treatment for this condition, in addition to careful monitoring of the electrical activity of the heart includes establishing an intravenous line and providing enough fluid to maintain blood pressure. Excessive fluid may negatively impact cardiac output because the heart is not able to squeeze as hard as under normal conditions. This also can lead to pulmonary edema.

Myocardial Rupture

Medically, **myocardial rupture** is seen in a person who has had a heart attack that results in a large area of necrotic heart muscle. Such a person likely has had poorly controlled high blood pressure. The result is the necrotic area fails, and the structure of the heart is lost. Death almost always follows. The extreme forces and pressures that can occur during a traumatic event may lead to myocardial rupture, where the wall of the heart fails. Most patients do not survive, but those who do require rapid transport to the nearest trauma center. Treatment for the patient with myocardial rupture is supportive and includes cardiac monitoring, at least one intravenous line, supplemental O_2, ventilation, and CPR as needed.

Commotio Cordis

Recall from chapter 5 that the T wave of the ECG has absolute and relative refractory periods. This means that during the absolute refractory period, no energetic impulse can cause the ventricles to depolarize. During the relative refractory period, represented on the ECG as the downslope of the T wave, at least one myocyte has been fully repolarized and is capable of depolarizing again and either starting or propagating another heartbeat. If that myocyte receives a sufficiently energetic impulse, it will be depolarized, causing a new wave of depolarization to be spread to the surrounding cells.

Now the heart is in an electrically confused state, where some of the cells are depolarized or actively depolarizing and others are still becoming repolarized. This results in chaotic and disorganized electrical activity in the ventricles, which often will lead to VF or VT and sudden cardiac arrest.

In **commotio cordis**, a direct blow to the chest, perhaps by a struck baseball or a well-timed punch, can provide this sufficiently energetic impulse. This is most likely to happen in children and teenagers because their chest wall is still pliable, which leads to the energy being easily transmitted to the heart. Electrical disturbances are likely, even in the conscious patient. Electrical defibrillation is the definitive treatment for the unconscious patient in VF or VT and should be performed as quickly as possible. Continue treatment for patients in cardiac arrest as per normal. Early CPR and early defibrillation represent the best chance of survival for this patient.

Traumatic Aortic Disruption

Traumatic aortic disruption is arguably the most severe of all the deceleration injuries described here. In this situation, the body stops moving suddenly from a relatively high speed, such as might be achieved during highway driving. After the body stops moving, however, the heart continues its forward momentum and swings on the aorta, which is securely attached to the posterior chest wall. With sufficient speed, the aorta wall fails and tears. With a large enough tear, the patient will bleed out into the chest cavity within 1 or 2 minutes of the collision.

Treatment for this patient is largely supportive. Only very few patients with this condition survive until EMS arrives and even fewer survive to arrive at the hospital. Maintenance of blood pressure, provision of an airway and O_2, and CPR if needed are the mainstays of treatment for this patient.

Other Chest Injuries

Diaphragmatic Rupture

Diaphragmatic rupture can occur as a result of penetrating trauma that lacerates the diaphragm or as a result of a sudden and massive increase of intra-abdominal pressure, such as might occur in a person who gets run over by a car or who has something heavy fall on top of them. This condition can be complicated when the abdominal contents herniate into the chest cavity. If the abdominal contents herniate into the chest, bowel sounds may be present in the chest. Patients may complain of difficulty breathing as a result of becoming reliant on the intercostal muscles for all respirations. With the diaphragm ruptured, it can no longer contract in a coordinated way to allow for normal breathing physiology. Patients also may have considerable injuries to the abdominal contents, particularly the spleen, liver, and stomach, because these organs lie just inferior to the diaphragm.

Treatment for diaphragmatic rupture begins with assisting the patient's breathing as needed and providing supplemental O_2. Because the lungs rest on the diaphragm posteriorly, remain alert for the development of a pneumothorax and, if found, treat accordingly. Patients with this injury also are likely to be profoundly hypotensive that may result from bleeding from the liver and spleen. Establish one or two large-bore intravenous lines and run fluid wide to treat for shock. Control any external bleeding that may be present but do not pack any stab or gunshot wounds.

Tracheobronchial Injuries

Tracheobronchial injuries are rare and can be caused most commonly by penetrating trauma but also secondary to rib fractures or CPR. These injuries carry a high likelihood of death because of airway obstructions, bleeding into the lower airways, and the patient's inability to ventilate the alveoli. Air will escape the laceration and can lead to a pneumothorax if it is located in one of the bronchi. It also could lead to a **pneumomediastinum** if the laceration is in the proximal bronchi or trachea.

The location of the injury plays a big role in the mortality of the patient. If the injury is located in the superior portion of the trachea, an ETT may be able to be placed past the laceration, allowing the patient to possibly breathe on their own or be able to be successfully ventilated. If the laceration is in the bronchi or distal trachea where an ETT cannot bypass it, positive pressure ventilation can be disastrous, resulting in inflation of the entire mediastinum all the way into the face. In this case, if the patient is breathing, positive pressure ventilation should be avoided.

Traumatic Asphyxia

Traumatic asphyxia results when the patient's chest is compressed between two objects. The compression forces blood in the chest into the nearby veins and arteries of the head, neck, liver, and kidneys, causing them to rupture. This also can cause ocular and subconjunctival hemorrhage and **exophthalmos** (protrusion of the eyeballs). This often is a fatal injury. However, in the event that the patient survives the compressive force, assess and treat any life-threatening conditions found, including cardiac rhythm disturbances, pneumothoraces, and other injuries. Anticipate hypotension if not already present. Treatment should include large-bore intravenous lines, supplemental O_2, and positive pressure ventilation. Intubation often is required.

ABDOMINAL INJURIES

Abdominal injuries can be caused by penetrating and blunt trauma. For the paramedic, determining the exact structures injured is not as essential as being able to recognize that an abdominal injury has occurred. This section will talk very broadly about the abdominal examination and presentations of certain injuries. Finally, certain injuries that require treatment beyond just intravenous fluids and cardiac monitoring will be discussed. In addition, the abdominal anatomy is discussed in chapter 6 in the section titled Gastrointestinal Emergencies.

The abdomen is particularly susceptible to blunt and penetrating trauma. It is not protected with bone like the chest and pelvis to help mitigate some of the forces involved in either type of trauma. It is highly vascular, so bleeding can occur from just about anywhere in the abdomen in meaningful amounts to quickly lead to shock. Laceration of any hollow organ in the abdomen—the stomach, intestines, or bladders—can lead to not only massive hemorrhage but also sepsis if the contents leak out.

Abdominal injuries should, therefore, be treated as a potentially lethal and true emergency. At this time, nothing can be done in the prehospital world for an abdominal injury. These injuries require surgical intervention to repair the laceration or remove the organ in its entirety, such as might occur from a lacerated spleen.

Unlike pain from other trauma, abdominal pain often is diffuse throughout the abdominal cavity, making it difficult to confidently isolate the source of the injury. Furthermore, because so much is going on in any of the 4 quadrants, even if the pain can be narrowed down to 1 quadrant, it could still be from any of several organs. For example, in the URQ, pain could be from liver lacerations, kidney lacerations, a gall bladder rupture, large or small intestine trauma, or lacerations to the head of the pancreas. Any of these could result in significant hemodynamic instability from internal bleeding.

Assessment of the patient with the closed abdominal injury begins by exposing the area and evaluating for any bruising. Periumbilical bruising (the Cullen sign) or bruising to either or both flanks (the Grey Turner sign) are strong indicators of internal bleeding. They are somewhat late signs, however, and, if present, the person has either been bleeding for a while or is bleeding heavily.

Next, each of the four quadrants should be palpated firmly, compressing the abdomen 2–3 inches using the entire area of the fingers, not just the tips. The quadrant furthest from the painful quadrant should be palpated first, while the quadrant the patient identified as painful should be saved for last. This is done because if the painful quadrant is palpated first, it may hinder the patient's ability to tell if the other quadrants are pain free during palpation. During palpation also note if the abdomen is rigid. This can be from blood in that area or muscular guarding of the area. Either of these are good indicators of an injury to that quadrant.

Management of the patient with a closed abdominal injury should largely be supportive, with an eye toward prophylactic shock prevention. Administer high-flow O_2 as with any multisystem trauma patient. Initiate at least one large-bore intravenous line as soon as possible without delaying transport to the hospital; initiate a second if time permits. Initiate continuous cardiac monitoring and treat any dysrhythmia found. Treat any external wounds.

An **evisceration** is a deep laceration to the abdominal cavity that results in the abdominal contents spilling outside. Needless to say, this is a very serious injury that requires rapid transport to the nearest trauma center. Do not palpate over the eviscerated abdomen or the contents. Do not attempt to push the contents back into the abdomen. Instead, cover all the exposed contents with a moist sterile dressing and then cover the entire area with another bandage to keep warm. Initiate at least one intravenous line and treat for shock.

REVIEW QUESTIONS

Select the ONE best answer.

1. Which of the following patients—all of the same weight, gender, and age—are likely to sustain the worst injuries?

   A. A fall from a height of 25 ft (~8 m) onto grass

   B. A fall from a height of 25 ft (~8 m) onto cement

   C. An unrestrained patient involved in a motor vehicle crash at 25 mph (~10 m/s) with airbag deployment

   D. An unrestrained patient involved in a motor vehicle crash at 25 mph (~10 m/s) with no airbag deployment

2. Recent advances in the manufacture of automobiles have significantly reduced the injuries a driver sustains during a crash. Heavy damage to the front of the vehicle alone is not considered a significant mechanism of injury anymore. Which of the following still represents a mechanism of injury capable of resulting in significant injury to the restrained driver?

   A. Ejection from a motor vehicle

   B. Lateral or T-bone type crash on the right side

   C. Quarter panel collision with rotation

   D. Side-over-side rollover

3. Which of the following is NOT found in the dermis layer of the skin?

   A. Melanocytes

   B. Nerve endings

   C. Peripheral vasculature

   D. Sweat glands

4. Use this information for questions 4 and 5.

   A patient has been trapped under debris during a structure collapse for approximately 8 hours before you are able to access the person. The person's left leg is crushed with a steel support beam. The person is conscious, alert, and oriented, complaining of pain and dizziness. The patient's vital signs are HR: 100, BP: 96/56, RR: 24, and SpO_2: 96%. You have initiated a peripheral intravenous line and placed the patient on a cardiac monitor. You observe this 12-lead ECG result:

   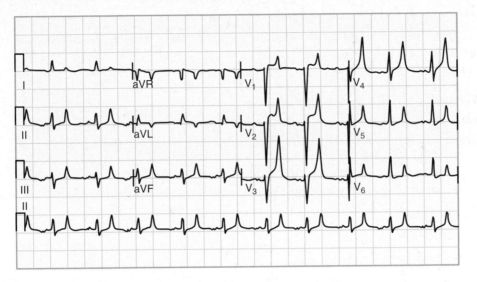

   What is the most appropriate next treatment for this patient and rhythm?

   A. 1 L lactated Ringer solution

   B. 1 mEq/kg sodium bicarbonate

   C. 1 g calcium chloride or calcium gluconate

   D. 150 mg amiodarone, slow over 10 minutes

5. Impaled objects may be removed from a patient in all the following instances EXCEPT:

   A. The object is impaled in the patient's facial cheek.

   B. The object interferes with effective patient transport.

   C. The object interferes with the performance of CPR.

   D. The object interferes with airway maintenance.

6. Use the following information to answer questions 6–8.

   You arrive on the scene of a fire, and the firefighters bring you a patient who was trapped inside the house. The patient has sustained partial- and full-thickness burns over the anterior abdomen, anterior upper legs, and circumferential lower legs below the knees. The person's genitals were spared injury. The person weighs approximately 265 lb, is conscious and alert, and is maintaining their own airway with the following vital signs: HR: 118, RR: 24, BP: 108/54; SpO_2: 100%.

   What is the approximate BSA burned?

   A. 27%

   B. 31.5%

   C. 36%

   D. 45%

7. Approximately how much fluid should the patient receive in the first 8 hours after the incident?

   A. 5,800 mL

   B. 8,700 mL

   C. 17,345 mL

   D. 19,000 mL

8. Which color triage tag should be provided during the primary triage if the patient was part of a larger incident?

   A. Red

   B. Yellow

   C. Green

   D. Black

9. Exposure to which of the following forms of radiation is potentially the most lethal?

   A. Alpha particles

   B. Beta particles

   C. Gamma radiation

   D. Ultraviolet radiation

10. All of the following are true of splinting EXCEPT:

   A. Splint both ends of the fractured bone.

   B. Check distal pulse, motor, and sensation before and after splinting.

   C. Pad over any bony areas.

   D. Place the fractured extremity in a neutral position prior to splinting.

11. Epidural hematomas are most commonly caused by which of the following?

   A. Aneurysms

   B. Dural lacerations

   C. Lacerations to meningeal veins

   D. Lacerations to meningeal arteries

12. You have been called to an indoor rock-climbing gym, where a patient fell off the top of the rock climbing wall after a rope failed. The patient is conscious and alert, answering questions appropriately. The patient is complaining of mid-back pain, numbness and paralysis to the right leg, and loss of pain sensation in the left leg. You suspect which spinal cord injury?

   A. Anterior cord syndrome

   B. Brown-Sequard syndrome

   C. Cauda equina syndrome

   D. Posterior cord syndrome

13. Your patient was struck in the chest with a baseball bat during a street brawl. He is complaining of severe chest pain that gets worse when he coughs and shortness of breath. The patient has a large bruise in the center of his chest with no crepitus noted. Lung sounds are clear bilaterally. The patient's vital signs over 15 minutes are listed. What condition does your patient most likely have?

Initial: HR: 118, BP: 126/84, RR: 24, SpO_2: 98% on room air
10 min: HR: 124, BP: 116/80, RR: 24, SpO_2: 98% on room air
15 min: HR: 130, BP: 104/88, RR: 24, SpO_2: 98% on room air

A. Cardiac contusion
B. Cardiac tamponade
C. Pulmonary contusion
D. Pneumomediastinum

ANSWERS AND EXPLANATIONS

1. **The correct answer is (B).** Of all those listed, the fall from a height of 25 ft unleashes the greatest amount of energy on the patient. More energy means the patient will experience a greater force when hitting the ground. Option (B) also has the highest impulse—the force is spread out over a shorter amount of time—because the patient hits cement rather than grass (A). The grass is softer, so, like an airbag, it extends the time the body takes to slow down. The patient possesses substantially less energy, and, therefore, less force is imparted onto the patient in either motor vehicle crash option compared to the falls.

2. **The correct answer is (A).** Ejection from a motor vehicle during a crash remains a significant mechanism of injury because of the multiple number of impacts the patient will receive. The remaining impacts are still capable of causing injury; however, most will be less severe than those in a person who was ejected.

3. **The correct answer is (A).** Melanocytes are pigmented cells located in the epidermis.

4. **The correct answer is (C).** This patient needs to receive calcium chloride or calcium gluconate, even before removing the steel support beam. This ECG shows peaked T waves, flattened P waves, and a widened QRS, which are highly indicative of hyperkalemia. Releasing the crushing element would release even more potassium into circulation for this patient, so calcium ahead of that would be most appropriate. (B) is appropriate; however, it will not also treat the rhythm as calcium would. Sodium bicarbonate is used to primarily neutralize the metabolic acids produced during anaerobic respiration. Lactated Ringer solution (A) contains potassium and could serve to only worsen the situation. Amiodarone (D) may be necessary but should not be the 1st-line treatment in an anticipated hyperkalemic situation.

5. **The correct answer is (B).** If the object interferes with effective patient transport because it is too large or bulky, it must be trimmed. This is the only reason an object should be trimmed. The remaining options are all reasons an object can be removed from a patient.

6. **The correct answer is (C).** The approximations to arrive at this answer are as follows: The abdomen is approximately 9%; the entire anterior of each leg is 9% each; and because the lower legs were both circumferentially burned, it is 4.5% for each. This adds to 36%.

7. **The correct answer is (B).** The Parkland formula is as follows: BSA burned times 4 times the weight in kilograms. So, the total amount of fluid needed in the first 24 hours is $36 \times 4 \times 120.5$ kg = 17,345 mL, which is answer (C). The question asks for the fluid in the first 8 hours, which is half the total amount, or approximately 8,700 mL.

8. **The correct answer is (B).** The patient's respiratory rate is between 10 and 30; the patient has a palpable pulse, is alert, and is able to follow simple commands. This patient may be upgraded to red (A) during secondary triage; however, the initial triage places the patient as a yellow. This patient's condition is not minor in nature and should never be a green (C). Black (D) is reserved for the deceased and those anticipated to die, and this patient is not likely to die in the near term.

9. **The correct answer is (C).** Gamma radiation, even in small doses, can be lethal in a high enough concentration. Alpha (A) and beta (B) particles would potentially be lethal in high doses only if the particles get internal. Ultraviolet radiation (D) can be lethal but only after long-term exposure leads to melanoma. Wear sunscreen!

10. **The correct answer is (A).** If a bone is fractured, it should be placed in a neutral position (D) with padding over bony areas (C), and the bone and the 2 adjacent joints should all be immobilized. After the splint is applied, check the distal pulse, motor, and sensation.

11. **The correct answer is (D).** Epidural hematomas are caused when cerebral arteries are lacerated. The middle meningeal artery is the most commonly lacerated. Aneurysms (A) rarely lead to epidural hematomas and are more likely to lead to intracerebral hemorrhage. Dural lacerations (B) are not directly associated with either epidural or subdural hemorrhages. Subdural hemorrhages are caused by venous lacerations (C).

12. **The correct answer is (B).** These symptoms describe Brown-Sequard syndrome. Anterior cord syndrome (A) presents with motor and sensory loss to both lower extremities. Cauda equina syndrome (C) will result in numbness to those areas that would come in contact with a saddle as well as loss of rectal tone. Finally, posterior cord syndrome (D) would result in bilateral decreased sensation to light touch and proprioception.

13. **The correct answer is (B).** Based on the information given, the narrowing pulse pressure that can be seen in the serial vital signs most likely indicates a developing cardiac tamponade. A reassessment of the patient when this is noted would reveal muffled or distant heart sounds and JVD increasing. A cardiac contusion (A), though possible, would not be the 1st thought here because there is no mention of ECG changes, such as VF, VT, or ST changes. A pulmonary contusion (C) can be reasonably ruled out along with pneumothorax because the pulse oximetry reading remains constant and the lung sounds are clear and equal. Pneumomediastinum (D) also should be a consideration in such a chest injury; however, it is not the most likely option here. Pneumomediastinum would most likely present with subcutaneous emphysema, particularly in the area of the neck.

Life Span Development and Pediatrics

Learning Objectives

❑ Describe physical, behavioral, and intellectual developmental changes that occur across the life span.

❑ Differentiate, assess, and treat pediatric respiratory emergencies.

❑ Differentiate, assess, and treat causes of pediatric shock.

❑ Differentiate, assess, and treat causes of pediatric altered mental status and pediatric seizures.

A person's body from infancy to late adulthood goes through many changes. Patients who are very young or very old often have conditions not otherwise seen in the population between the ages of 8 and 55. Calls for pediatric patients often evoke feelings of fear and anxiety in EMS practitioners largely because of unfamiliarity with changes in medication dose, fear of a sudden decline in patient stability, or concern about a difficult assessment because the child cannot verbalize a complaint in the same manner an adult might.

This chapter will explore changes throughout the life span, beginning with the newborn infant and progressing through late adulthood. Then the differences between adult assessment and physical examination findings will be compared with the pediatric anatomy. Finally, pediatric emergencies and their treatments will be addressed.

VITAL SIGN CHANGES

Vital signs change the most over the life span between newborn and adolescence. Generally, the younger person will have a faster heart rate and respiratory rate than the adult ≥18 years. These will gradually slow down to what is familiar for adults. The younger person will have a lower blood pressure to begin with at birth that will gradually increase to adulthood.

Table 9-1. Normal Vital Sign Ranges Throughout the Life Span

Age	Pulse	SBP	Respirations
Newborn (0–1 month)	100–180	50–70	30–60
Infant (1–12 months)	100–160	70–90	25–50
Toddler (1–3 years)	90–150	80–100	20–40
Preschool (4–5 years)	80–120	80–100	20–30
School age (6–12 years)	70–120	80–110	15–25
Adolescent (13–17 years)	60–100	90–120	12–20
Adult (18+ years)	60–100	100–140	12–20

Infants, 1 Month to 1 Year Old

Infants go through many rapid changes throughout the first year of their lives, in addition to the change from fetal circulation to normal circulation. Infants will approximately triple their birth weight by their first birthday. The lungs also will rapidly expand and develop faster during their first year than at any time after.

The infant's respiratory system is different from an adult's in many ways. Infants breathe using their diaphragm primarily and are, therefore, referred to as belly breathers. Their intercostal muscles are weak and play nearly no role in breathing. Infants have a proportionally larger tongue than adults, meaning it takes up more space in their mouths than an adult's. The airway is much narrower and shorter than an adult's. The airway diameter roughly approximates the diameter of the child's pinky.

Infants have the following reflexes:

- **Moro Reflex.** Also known as the startle reflex, the Moro reflex causes the infant to extend their arms and spread the fingers as if to grab something.
- **Rooting Reflex.** Brushing an infant's cheek makes the infant turn in the direction of that cheek and look for, or root for, a nipple.
- **Sucking Reflex.** The infant will instinctively suck on anything placed in their mouth.
- **Palmar Reflex.** Touching the infant's palm causes the infant to grasp onto that item.

The fontanels are the soft spots located on the top of the infant's head. The anterior fontanel is located where the two parietal bones and the frontal bone meet, and the posterior fontanel is located at the vertex of the head at the intersection of the parietal bones and the occipital bone. Two others are located on the lateral skull; however, they are not easily palpable. The fontanels will close by the 18th month of life.

Toddlers and Preschoolers, 1–5 Years Old

During this age, children grow rapidly, expanding their musculoskeletal system and further developing alveoli and bronchioles in their ever-expanding lungs. Potty training occurs during this stage. Children also begin to explore their world because they have begun to walk early in this stage. Falls are common because even though they can walk, their ability to balance may not yet have caught up. They often will place things in their mouth as part of their exploration, so choking and poisoning are a concern in this age group.

During this age group, particularly for preschoolers, it is helpful to involve the children in their own care whenever possible. Although it is not advisable to give them an option regarding treatment between receiving or not, for example, "Should I start this intravenous line or not?" it will be helpful to ask, instead, "Should I start this intravenous line in your right or left arm?" This option will give children ownership over their care and, by extension, trust in the provider.

School-Age Children, 6–12 Years Old

Development in this age group slows to a steadier pace compared with that of earlier age groups. Later in this group, puberty will begin, along with all the changes it brings. Girls usually experience menarche (the beginning of menstruation) when they are this age.

As children get older, their reasoning methods change and develop.

- During **preconventional reasoning**, children make decisions either to get what they want or simply avoid punishment.
- **Conventional reasoning** follows, and is rooted in getting approval from peers and society.
- **Postconventional reasoning** follows as children begin to make decisions based on their beliefs and conscience.

Adolescents, 13–17 Years Old

During this time, teenagers experience a growth spurt, gaining height along with bone and muscle mass. The girl's growth spurt typically finishes before the boy's. Their body shape takes on that of an adult. If it has not happened yet, menarche will happen during this time.

Teenagers also increase their need for privacy and struggle for independence from their parents. They will prefer to have all medical questions directed to them and allow them to tell their story. The parents need to be involved in decision making because adolescents are still dependents to the parents and guardians. Adolescents may not share all information with EMS, especially if the information is sensitive in nature, such as involving drug or alcohol use or sexual activities. With this in mind, it may be helpful to have a member of the team interview the parents or guardians away from the child while another interviews the patient.

Adulthood, 18–60 Years Old

Over this time frame, chronic conditions become noticeable. The body that was performing at its optimal level at about 25 years old starts to lose muscle mass and develop more fatty deposits. Later in this stage, women begin menopause and can begin to develop menopause-related osteoporosis. If the person has had children, they will have already grown and likely moved out of the house by the later end of this life stage. During this time, those who are parents will now have to readjust to a home without children, often referred to as the empty nest syndrome.

Late Adulthood, >60 Years Old

Declines in functioning of nearly every system are noticeable in patients during this age range. Long-term cardiovascular atherosclerotic buildup starts elevating blood pressure and increases the risk for ACS and CVA. Chronic respiratory diseases increase, where even nonsmokers who have lived in urban areas can begin to show signs of COPD. Type 2 diabetes may be diagnosed and contribute to the risk factors for other disease processes.

During the decline, patients begin to no longer be able to do the things that they were once able to do. They also may start seeing friends and family members die. They may have continual aches and pains and become partially or completely dependent on pain medications. These—combined with feeling unneeded because they are now retired and their children are no longer at home—can all contribute to intense feelings of depression.

PEDIATRICS

Paramedics often say that pediatric calls are the call they fear most. Although it is true that children cannot be treated simply as small adults, they are not something to be feared. In this portion of the chapter, the goal is to allay that fear so that you can be more confident when you arrive to the side of a sick infant or toddler.

Major Anatomic and Physiological Differences

Allusions were made to a couple of specific anatomic and physiological differences earlier in this chapter because they appear in specific age groups. Here, the discussion will focus on the major differences between children and adults and include the impact of the difference on prehospital assessment and treatment. The differences will be listed in head-to-toe order, not necessarily the order in which they would be found during a physical examination and not necessarily in any particular order of importance.

- Children have a higher surface-area-to-volume ratio, which means they are at greater risk of hypothermia in any exposure. They generally have less fatty tissue to act as insulation, which serves to only increase the potential for hypothermia.
- A smaller absolute circulating blood volume means that blood loss becomes more significant at lower volumes. Children actually have more circulating blood per kilogram than adults (relative volume).

- Children's higher circulating blood volume per kilogram combined with their ability to more adequately constrict blood vessels means that they will be able to maintain blood pressure longer than an adult. This also means that they are in compensated shock for a longer period of time, resulting in a more sudden crash of the blood pressure as they enter decompensated shock.

- The fontanels remain open up to age 1 year: the posterior fontanel closes at 1.5–3 months, and the anterior fontanel closes at about 12–18 months. Until the fontanels close, they can be a great assessment tool for evaluating hydration status and ICP. If the fontanel is sunken, the infant is significantly dehydrated. If it is bulging out of the skull, the ICP is increased, possibly as the result of a head injury or hydrocephalus.

- The head of a child is much larger relative to the rest of the body. This can cause the child to often "lead with the head" during falls from any height, thus increasing the chances of sustaining significant head injuries even under less than significant mechanisms.

- The occiput of the head extends beyond the back of the child. This means that traditional immobilization methods may cause the child's neck to flex, potentially compromising the airway and the cervical spine. Padding under the shoulders will be necessary to relieve this.

- The airway is shorter and narrower than that in an adult. Also, the tongue takes up more space in the mouth.

- The airway is narrowest at the cricoid ring in children compared with the vocal cords in the adult.

- Infants are obligate nose breathers for the first few months of life. This means that any amount of mucus can dramatically affect their ability to breathe. Sometimes, suctioning the nares is all that is needed to alleviate the child's difficulty breathing.

- Children have a higher basal metabolic rate than adults, which means, by extension, that they have a greater O_2 demand. O_2 demand can exceed 7 mL/kg/min in newborns compared with approximately 3.5 mL/kg/min in adults. This increase in O_2 demand is achieved with a faster respiratory rate despite a tidal volume similar to that of an adult.

- The alveolar minute volume is increased in children as well, which results in a diminished functional reserve capacity. Therefore, lung infections and trauma can have a dramatic effect on oxygenation. Respiratory distress and shock can set in much more suddenly in such a child.

- The chest wall of a child is extremely pliable, even well into adolescence. This can lead to significant injuries to the organs underlying the ribs, even in the absence of rib fractures. Any bruising across the chest of a child should be considered significant until proven otherwise via x-ray at the hospital.

- The spine of a child is much more pliable than that of the adult because the tendons are not as taut. This can result in SCIWORA and a lack of assessment evidence that can indicate a spinal injury. Maintain a high index of suspicion with any significant mechanism of injury.

- Abdominal organs are more anterior and less protected by the rib cage. Therefore, abdominal trauma can be more significant in younger children, even with relatively minor mechanisms such as low-speed motor vehicle crashes in the presence of properly placed restraints.

Specific Pediatric Emergencies

Respiratory Problems and Hypoxia

Children's breathing problems are classified as respiratory distress, respiratory failure, or respiratory arrest.

Table 9-2. Respiratory Conditions and Treatment

Condition	Compensation	Signs and Symptoms	Treatment Options
Respiratory distress	Compensated	Retractions, nasal retractions, sniffing position, and tripoding in older children	High-flow O_2 and nebulized albuterol for wheezing
Respiratory failure	Decompensated	See-saw breathing in infants, altered mental status, head bobbing, cyanosis, bradycardia, and slowing respirations	High-flow O_2 and positive pressure ventilation
Respiratory arrest	None	No breathing, marked bradycardia, and cyanosis	Positive pressure ventilation, intubation, and CPR for HR <60

Pro-Tip

There is no hard and fast break point between respiratory distress and respiratory failure, so spending time classifying the patient is neither necessary nor helpful. Beginning more aggressive treatment earlier in the course of treatment, however, is always better than waiting until symptoms worsen.

Respiratory Emergencies

Please refer to chapter 4 for information on the following respiratory emergencies: asthma, anaphylaxis, croup, and epiglottitis.

Cystic fibrosis is a genetic disease that often is discovered early in life, usually by the second birthday. Its hallmark is excessive, thick secretions of mucus in the lower airways and a high salt content in sweat. Patients have a difficult time clearing these secretions and often are hospitalized for infections such as pneumonia and bronchiolitis. Treatment for a patient with cystic fibrosis is largely symptomatic and may include bronchodilators, humidified O_2, and possibly positive pressure ventilation.

Commonly known as whooping cough, **pertussis** is caused by an infection with bacteria and transmitted via respiratory droplets. Its symptoms are similar to the common cold, with a runny nose, sneezing, and coughing, but as the disease worsens with time, the cough will take on the characteristic "whoop" sound with inspiration. The coughing can become so severe that the patient presents with respiratory distress and cyanosis. If pertussis is suspected, take airborne precautions, including surgical mask and eye protection.

Bronchiolitis is a swelling of the lower airways similar in nature and presentation to asthma, but it results from a viral infection called respiratory syncytial virus. Because asthma is rare in children under 1 year old, the virus is most likely causing the symptoms. Regardless of the ultimate cause, the treatments are identical. Albuterol or nebulized racemic epinephrine should be administered; in severe cases, positive pressure ventilation may be needed as the patient moves from respiratory distress to failure.

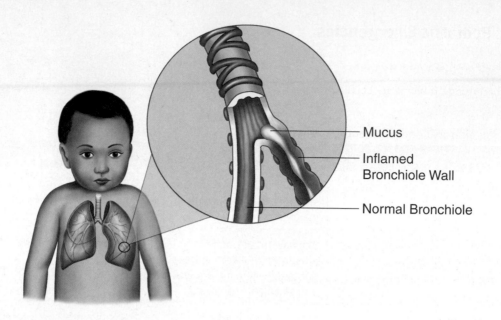

Mucus

Inflamed
Bronchiole Wall

Normal Bronchiole

Figure 9-1. Bronchiolitis

Treatment of Respiratory Emergencies

Children in respiratory distress often benefit from supplemental O_2. With their relatively low tidal volumes and high metabolic O_2 demand, any disease process that affects alveolar ventilation or respiration should receive high-flow supplemental O_2. A child who is still responsive may not tolerate a face mask despite needing that volume of O_2. In this case, blow-by O_2 across the nares can be similarly effective without stimulating anxiety in the child. The child's caregiver can be a resource in a situation such as this because the caregiver may be more successful at holding the tubing near the child's face.

Initiation of positive pressure ventilation should begin at the first sign of a decrease in respiratory effort or level of consciousness. Ensure that the proper size BVM is used for ventilation but avoid overinflation of the lungs. Children's lungs are more susceptible to barotrauma from forceful ventilation compared with an adult's lungs, and it is not uncommon for a rescuer to use an adult bag on the child. If this is the case, ensure that the ventilation volume is just enough to see the chest rise and that the person providing the positive pressure ventilation is focused on that critical job. According to **AHA 2020 updates** to CPR and ECC, the recommended rate for ventilation for a child is 1 breath every 2–3 seconds, or 20–30 breaths per minute. **This replaces prior recommendations based on new research.**

Intubation of children should be performed for any of the following reasons:

- Poor seal of the mask to the face
- The need for extended resuscitation times
- Cardiac or respiratory arrest
- Head or facial injury
- Inability to protect and maintain the airway (because patient is obtunded)

Selecting the size of the ETT can be difficult in a child. In children <8, the size of the airway at its narrowest point can be approximated by comparing the size of the ETT to the pinky of the child. The diameter also can be calculated by adding 16 to the patient's age in years and then dividing the result by 4.

$$\text{ETT size in mm} = \frac{16 + \text{age (in years)}}{4}$$

Pro-Tip

This equation will give you the anticipated size for an uncuffed tube. If you have only cuffed tubes, reduce the tube size by 0.5 mm. (An 8-year-old child would get a 6 uncuffed tube: $(16 + 8)/4 = 6$, but a 5.5 cuffed tube.)

Based on the **2020 AHA updated guidelines** for CPR and ECC, a cuffed tube is now recommended whenever possible to prevent air leaks.

When preparing to intubate, in addition to having suction and other ancillary equipment prepared, always have available a tube one size higher and one size smaller than the expected size tube.

If the benefit to the child outweighs the possible risks, then the child should be intubated. The risks, in many cases, can be anticipated ahead of time, with steps taken to mitigate them. The risks of intubation include the following:

- Damage to teeth and gums from using the upper teeth or gums as a fulcrum
- Trauma and swelling to the oropharynx, tongue, and epiglottis
- Worsened hypoxia from prolonged intubation attempts
- Unrecognized esophageal intubation
- Stimulation of an intact gag reflex and resultant vomiting
- Increased ICP
- Bradycardia from vagus nerve stimulation

The child who is intubated should be constantly reassessed specifically for tube displacement and the effects of barotrauma. Use the mnemonic **DOPE** to assess the child, especially when changes in ventilatory status present.

- **D: Displacement**
  - Check that the tube is still in the trachea with auscultation of the lungs and direct laryngoscopy.
  - Check that the tube has not been pushed deeper and is still at the same centimeter mark at which it was originally placed.
- **O: Obstruction**
  - Mucus, blood, vomit, or other secretions can obstruct the tube, preventing ventilation or exhalation.
  - Suction the tube using a soft-suction catheter.
- **P: Pneumothorax**
  - Increased difficulty ventilating the patient is indicative of a developing pneumothorax.
  - Assess for signs of a pneumothorax, including tracheal deviation, JVD, and absent or diminished lung sounds. These can be very difficult to evaluate in the infant who has a minimal neck that can hide JVD and tracheal deviation.
- **E: Equipment**
  - Ensure O_2 is flowing.
  - Evaluate tubing for crimping or kinks. This should include the ETT.
  - If using a mechanical ventilator, replace it with a BVM and manually ventilate for a few minutes.

Pro-Tip

DOPE is the mnemonic you will need to know for the test. However, it can sound rather crude if you were to say to your partner, "Check the DOPE," in the presence of the child's caregivers. Not only that, but the mnemonic places evaluation and treatment of a pneumothorax ahead of equipment failure. Instead, POET is an alternate mnemonic for evaluating a patient who is intubated. The letters stand for placement, obstruction, equipment, and tension pneumothorax, and it sounds a little friendlier to say, "Check the POET!"

Shock

Shock in any person regardless of age is the lack of perfusion to end organs. Children can experience the same types of shock as an adult. The major difference between children and adults is that children can remain in compensated shock for a longer period of time. However, when the time comes that the child can no longer maintain blood pressure, it is because the child has completely exhausted every compensatory mechanism available. The blood pressure drops alarmingly fast, often without warning; if the child is not already receiving aggressive pressure support therapy, irreversible shock is imminent.

Compensated shock is characterized by tachycardia in the child. Young children do not sweat nearly as readily as older children and adults. Pallor centrally and mottling of the skin peripherally should be concerning because both indicate shunting of blood from the peripheral circulation to the central circulation. Capillary shunting in children is more successful than in adults, so seeing this should alert the paramedic to begin treatment.

As the shock progresses and compensated shock becomes decompensated, the child becomes lethargic and can no longer respond to familiar surroundings. Children will no longer cry when they are taken away from their parents or regular caregivers. If they can still make a sound, it will be a weak whimper that is short lived after a painful stimulus. Peripheral pulses will no longer be palpable, and central pulses will remain strong before fading later. A child who is first encountered in this state should receive aggressive fluid resuscitation and pressor support as soon as possible with vascular access most likely started with an intraosseous line.

Hypotension will be profound as the child begins to decompensate. The minimum systolic blood pressure (SBP) in a child can be calculated by adding 70 to twice the child's age in years.

$$SBP = 70 + 2 \times age \text{ (in years)}$$

Anything approaching this value should be concerning because it will become significant shock. Anything below this value should be treated aggressively.

Treatment of Shock

The cornerstone of shock treatment in the child is fluid resuscitation. Therefore, vascular access in the child in shock is essential. The access may be intravenous or intraosseous, and fluid should be able to flow freely or with pressure added to the intravenous bag. For the child in symptomatic shock who is tachycardic with other signs such as pale cool mottled skin or altered mental status, fluid should be given as a bolus of 20 mL/kg. This dose may be repeated up to 3 times before blood or blood products are required.

Once the vascular access has been obtained and the fluids are being administered, treatment should be targeted to the cause or type of shock.

Anaphylactic Shock

- Epinephrine, 1:1,000 solution, 0.01 mg/kg up to a maximum dose of 0.3 mg intramuscularly
- Diphenhydramine, 0.5–1 mg/kg to a maximum of 50 mg
- Methylprednisolone, 0.5 mg/kg to a maximum of 60 mg

Neurogenic Shock

- Methylprednisolone, 0.5 mg/kg to a maximum of 60 mg

Septic Shock

- Aggressive fluid therapy is the most important treatment. Administration in excess of 60 mL/kg may be required.
- Treat hypoglycemia with 0.5–1 g/kg of a 25% dextrose solution to a maximum of 50 g. Hypoglycemia may not be initially present, but after the administration of fluids, the patient may become relatively hypoglycemic.

Cardiogenic Shock

- Fluid bolus should be administered slowly—and the patient reassessed frequently during the bolus—to ensure that the patient does not become fluid overloaded.
- Contact medical control for the preferred pressor medication and dose if needed. Often in children, the preferred pressor is epinephrine 0.1–1 mcg/kg/min as an intravenous or intraosseous infusion, titrated to the desired effect.

Altered Mental Status

Altered mental status in children can be caused by any of the same reasons that adults can experience AMS. The mnemonic AEIOU-TIPS lists the major reasons for a person present with an altered mental status.

Table 9-3. AEIOU-TIPS

A	Alcohol
E	Epilepsy and endocrine electrolytes
I	Insulin
O	Opiates
U	Uremia
T	Trauma temperature
I	Infection
P	Poisoning psychogenic
S	Shock and stroke

Treatment for any of these reasons is largely the same as in the adult population. Every patient with an altered mental status should be checked for low blood sugar even if there is no history of diabetes.

Overdoses and Poisonings

Overdoses and poisonings in children can vary widely, and can be accidental or intentional.

- Younger children are more likely to accidentally overdose on medications, thinking they are candy. These overdoses can be catastrophic and should be treated symptomatically with appropriate supportive care.
- Older children are more likely to intentionally overdose on prescription medications or street drugs. They may also do this with the intent of achieving a euphoric state or to execute a plan of suicide. Treat these situations symptomatically.

Seizures

Seizures in children can be caused by a number of factors. Hypovolemia, sepsis, underlying abnormalities, epilepsy, and fever are all common reasons for a child to seize. It may not be possible to determine the exact cause in the field. Febrile seizures are most common, but the child should be assessed to rule out other causes for seizures, including head injuries and stroke.

A febrile seizure occurs when a child's temperature rises very quickly, often as the result of an infection rather than environmental hyperthermia, although hyperthermia is possible as well. Febrile seizures occur in children between the ages of 6 months and 6 years. A child who has had a febrile seizure in the past is predisposed to having another febrile seizure.

Treatment for this type of seizure most often is supportive. This type of seizure seldom requires intervention because it typically lasts less than 5 minutes, and the child returns to normal within an hour of the event.

Anticonvulsants are not usually indicated for this reason. Rapid, active cooling often is contraindicated as well because the resulting rapid drop in core body temperature could precipitate another seizure. If the child is bundled up or under multiple blankets, removing the child from the blankets is all the cooling that would be recommended in this situation.

Children having an epileptic seizure, on the other hand, will require more aggressive interventions. These children should receive O_2 to maintain a pulse oximetry reading of >95%, and high-flow O_2 during ongoing seizures regardless of the pulse oximetry. Establishment of an intravenous line is recommended as soon as the seizure activity subsides. Anticonvulsant medications should be administered according to the patient's weight. It is best to use a length-based tape to determine the doses of the medications.

REVIEW QUESTIONS

Select the ONE best answer.

1. Which inborn reflex causes the infant to turn their head toward the side where someone or something is brushing their cheek?

    A. Moro reflex

    B. Palmar reflex

    C. Rooting reflex

    D. Sucking reflex

2. Which fontanel remains open longest and can provide a point of assessment into a child's hydration status?

    A. Anterior fontanel

    B. Mastoid fontanel

    C. Posterior fontanel

    D. Sphenoid fontanel

3. Which reasoning type is characterized by children whose actions are rooted in getting approval from peers and society?

    A. Common sense reasoning

    B. Conventional reasoning

    C. Preconventional reasoning

    D. Postconventional reasoning

4. You have a 16-year-old female complaining of abdominal pain. She tells you in confidence that she is pregnant and shows you the OTC pregnancy test with a positive reading. She asks you not to tell her parents because she does not want them to know. You believe the pain she is having is related to the pregnancy. Knowing this, are you able to discuss your care plan with her parents in most states?

    A. No, because she is pregnant and considered the individual according to consent and privacy laws.

    B. No, because she asked you not to, and you must always respect any patient's wishes.

    C. Yes, because she is a minor, and the parents are ultimately responsible for her care.

    D. Yes, because you did not witness the patient taking the test, therefore you cannot trust that it is hers.

5. Which of the following best explains why children are at greater risk for hypothermia than adults?

   A. The thinner chest wall allows heat to escape from the central circulation and the core at a faster rate.

   B. The higher basal metabolic rate means that more energy goes into cellular metabolism.

   C. The higher surface-area-to-volume ratio means that the child's core mass is closer to the ambient air than in an adult.

   D. The smaller absolute circulating blood volume leads to a more rapid loss of heat when blood is pumped to the extremities.

6. You have a 7-year-old male patient who presents with a 3-day history of fever and cough productive of a thick whitish brown sputum. The patient's lung sounds are rhonchi over the right lower lung field with scattered wheezing. Vital signs are HR: 142, RR: 28, BP: 98/56, T: 102.9, SpO_2: 94% on room air and 98% on 4 LPM O_2 via nasal cannula. The child is alert but sleepy and is sitting up and answering questions appropriately. You have the child on the O_2, and it is well tolerated. The next most appropriate treatment for this patient is:

   A. Continuous positive airway pressure (CPAP).

   B. 20 mL/kg bolus of 0.9% saline solution.

   C. 2.5 mg albuterol in 3 mL saline via a nebulizer.

   D. 0.5 mg ipratropium bromide via a nebulizer.

7. Use the following scenario for questions 7 and 8.

   You are called to a residence for a 23-month-old male who fell into a backyard pool and was found unresponsive. Rescue personnel have the child out of the pool and are providing CPR and ventilations with a child-sized BVM when you arrive. The ECG shows pulseless electrical activity and an agonal ventricular rhythm. A pulse is generated with compressions.

   You elect to intubate this child for the 15-minute ride to the hospital. What size tube would you anticipate is the most appropriate?

   A. 3.5, cuffed

   B. 4.0, cuffed

   C. 4.5, cuffed

   D. 5.0, cuffed

8. Shortly after beginning the transport, the child's O_2 saturation begins to drop. What should you do first?

   A. Increase the O_2 flow rate.

   B. Suction the ETT.

   C. Extubate and ventilate with just the BVM.

   D. Check the position of the ETT.

9. A child with altered mental status presents with rapid and deep respirations and a 3-day history of vomiting and excessive urination. Which of the following represents the most likely cause for these symptoms?

   A. Hypovolemia

   B. Hyperglycemia

   C. Drug overdose

   D. Respiratory acidosis

10. Treatment for a febrile seizure most often requires:

    A. 1 mg lorazepam.

    B. active cooling with cold packs.

    C. 0.2–0.5 mg/kg diazepam intravenously.

    D. Only monitoring and supportive measures.

ANSWERS AND EXPLANATIONS

1. **The correct answer is (C).** This describes the rooting reflex, in which the infant roots for food (nipple) in response to something touching the cheek. The Moro reflex (A) causes the infant to spread out their arms and legs in response to being startled. In the palmar reflex (B), the infant closes their hand when something touches the palm of the hand. The sucking reflex (D) happens whenever something is inserted into the infant's mouth.

2. **The correct answer is (A).** The anterior fontanel does not fully close until between 12–18 months of age. This fontanel is also the largest. The mastoid fontanel (B) generally closes between 6 and 12 months. The posterior fontanel (C) is generally the 1st to close between 1.5 and 3 months of age. The sphenoid fontanel (D) closes at about 6 months of age.

3. **The correct answer is (B).** Conventional reasoning is decision-making based on the child's desire for the approval of others. In preconventional reasoning (C), a child makes decisions and undertakes actions to get something desired or avoid punishment. In postconventional reasoning (D), the child makes decisions and undertakes actions according to their own internal moral compass. Common sense reasoning (A) is not a defined stage in the development of reasoning.

4. **The correct answer is (A).** The Health Insurance Portability and Accountability Act and other laws pertaining to the rights of privacy and confidentiality state that a minor is considered the individual, particularly when it comes to making decisions regarding pregnancy. Such decisions include testing for STDs, prescription contraceptives, and decisions regarding pregnancy-related care. Respecting the patient's wishes (B) is always a good idea whenever possible; however, when it comes to a plan of care for a minor, "just because she asks you not to" is not a strong enough reason, except in the aforementioned cases.

5. **The correct answer is (C).** This correctly describes why children, particularly infants, are at greater risk for hypothermia in all environments. A thinner chest wall (A) means that children are at greater risk for internal chest injuries. A higher basal metabolic rate (B) has a greater impact on O_2 and nutrient consumption and is more likely to help maintain a child's core temperature. A smaller circulating blood volume (D) means that a child needs to lose less fluid overall before showing signs of shock and has little direct impact on thermoregulation.

6. **The correct answer is (B).** This child is showing signs of compensated shock bordering on decompensation and is possibly septic from the infection. The SpO_2 indicates that the child is oxygenating effectively, so albuterol (C) and ipratropium bromide (D) are not indicated at this time. CPAP (A) is never an appropriate choice when pneumonia is suspected.

7. **The correct answer is (B).** Because this child is almost 2 years old, the equation becomes $(16 + 2)/4 = 4.5$. Because the answers all indicate cuffed tubes, the size should be reduced by 0.5. Therefore, the answer is 4.0. (C) would be correct if it said "uncuffed."

8. **The correct answer is (D).** This represents D in the DOPE mnemonic. It is possible during transferring the patient from the ground by the pool to the ambulance that the tube became dislodged or pushed deeper. Suctioning (B) represents the O in DOPE and should be done 2nd. Increasing the O_2 flow rate (A) likely would not produce better oxygenation. Extubation (C) should always be a last resort.

9. **The correct answer is (B).** Hyperglycemia would present with Kussmaul respirations, which are deep and rapid along with the other symptoms mentioned. The child is likely hypovolemic (A); however, this is not the cause of the symptoms but rather a symptom. Drug overdose (C) does not usually cause any of the listed symptoms. This patient is in acidosis; however, it is metabolic in nature, not respiratory. Respiratory acidosis (D) results from decreased ventilation, such as in respiratory arrest.

10. **The correct answer is (D).** Most febrile seizures are self-limiting and require little more than monitoring the patient. Starting an intravenous line is optional because rarely do febrile seizures follow one after each other. Lorazepam (A) is not recommended in the pediatric population. Active cooling (B) is not usually necessary and could result in causing another seizure if the child begins to shiver. Because it is usually over, diazepam (C) is rarely needed.

EMS Operations 10

Learning Objectives

❏ Describe requirements and regulations of EMS systems.

❏ Describe workforce safety and the well-being of the paramedic.

❏ Describe public health initiatives and the paramedic's role in public health.

❏ Describe concepts related to emergency vehicle operations.

❏ Describe aspects of emergency communications, including components of a radio report and patient handoffs.

❏ Describe components of EMS documentation and medical/legal concepts.

❏ Describe considerations for scene operations, including mass casualty and disaster incidents, the incident command system, the basics of vehicle and other specialty rescues, and situations involving hazardous materials.

❏ Define preservation of the crime scene.

The topic of EMS Operations, which comprises 10–15% of the NRP Exam, covers the fundamentals addressed early in paramedic course content: **medicolegal, communications/documentation, and special situations** (rescue, hazardous materials, crime scene preservation, etc.). This chapter briefly reviews that information, concentrating on the topics that are most likely to be seen on the NRP exam.

Practical Point

EMS Operations was likely a topic covered in your EMT classes. On the NRP exam, this content is tested in combination with other topics, e.g., the principles of hazardous materials would be tested in the context of a burn patient or asphyxiation.

EMS HISTORY, PUBLIC HEALTH, AND PROVIDER WELLNESS

Emergency medical services have changed dramatically since their first U.S. appearance in the 1860s. EMS has evolved from the mere provision of a ride to the hospital, with little or no medical care provided en route, to the mobile emergency room that is the modern ambulance. Today's EMS professionals have much more responsibility for patient care and public service than ever before, with more on the horizon.

EMS History and Regulation

EMS in the United States dates to the 1860s, when the first use of a vehicle staffed with personnel capable of providing medical care is documented. The first ambulance operated in Ohio in 1865, and soon afterward the first ambulance service in the United States began operating out of Bellevue Hospital in New York City. It was not until after World War II, however, that EMS began to resemble its current form.

Emergency physicians began to staff mobile intensive care units in the 1960s. As time went on, public support grew to establish a class of specially trained technicians to take the place of physicians in this context. This arose not only in the form of new regulations and publications, but also in mainstream popular culture. The table records some of the most influential of these in the second half of the 20th century.

Table 10-1. Major Forces that Advanced EMS Development

Year(s)	Event	Impact
1966	The white paper "Accidental Death and Disability: The Neglected Disease of Modern Society" is published.	Developed collaborative financial and public health strategies for accident prevention efforts and community-based EMS Developed the concept of medical direction Created the basis of the 911 emergency call system
1972	The series *Emergency*, focused on L.A. County paramedics, airs on television.	Promoted public awareness of and demand for local EMS agencies
1973	Congress passes the Emergency Medical Services Act (EMS Act).	Defined the 15 required components for an EMS system (including integration of health services, EMS research, and regulation of medical direction, communication, education, and quality improvement)
1980s–1990s	The National Highway Traffic and Safety Administration (NHTSA) expands.	Provided EMS programs and initiatives nationally, through the powers of a federal agency

States refer to paramedics variously as "licensed," "certified," or "credentialed." While these terms are nearly synonymous, there are differences in level of authority between them.

- *Licensed* providers generally have the greatest autonomy; physicians and nurses are licensed by the U.S. state (or states) in which they practice.
- *Certified* providers work under the authority of a licensed provider such as a physician; this is the situation for many paramedics.
- *Credentialed* providers possess specific education but are not licensed or certified, e.g., a layperson who holds a CPR card.

Regardless of the terminology used by a given state, legally paramedics must work under the license and oversight of a physician medical director. A physician medical director is an individual or team of physicians who authorize a paramedic to work in their service. Medical direction can come in various forms:

- **Service Medical Direction.** One or more licensed physicians authorize paramedics to work to their level of certification.
- **Offline Medical Direction.** Protocols, standing orders, or guidelines outline everything that a paramedic is authorized to do, either for a patient or in a given situation, without consulting a licensed physician.
- **Online Medical Direction.** A licensed physician remotely gives orders for treatment of a patient live (generally by radio or cell phone), while the paramedic is with that particular patient.

Public Health

Major principles of both the EMS Act of 1973 and the NHTSA are public health education and prevention of harm. EMS can play an important role in promoting these goals by identifying and remediating injury and illness in their own geographic regions.

Wellness and Safety of the Paramedic

The wellbeing and safety of a paramedic are of paramount importance. To treat patients safely—and to sustain a career working day in and day out in EMS—paramedics themselves must be well. In earlier chapters, we discussed at length the concept of scene safety and the importance of maintaining situational awareness on scene. Before returning to this topic later in the chapter, here we address the *physical and mental health of the paramedic*.

Physical Wellbeing

The very nature of EMS involves unpredictability, alternating periods of high stress with "hurry-up-and-wait." Paramedics spend much of a shift sitting—waiting for a call, writing a chart, and riding in the ambulance. They work long shifts, often in excess of 12 hours, with little guarantee of eating a complete meal. These challenges, common to many EMS systems, mean that paramedics are often unable to make consistently good food choices. Nutrition and weight control are 2 related topics that contribute to the wellbeing of the paramedic and, consequently, to the quality of care they can give their patients.

With ever-changing nutrition guidelines, here are some general points on eating for optimal nutrition. A 2,000-calorie diet is recommended in most active adults, although some people need less.

- **Fruits**. Eat a variety of whole fruits. Minimize intake of fruit juices (which are effectively liquid sugar), and avoid corn syrup whenever possible.
- **Vegetables**. Eat vegetables in a wide variety of colors. Focus on orange ones and dark leafy greens.
- **Grains**. Make whole grains at least half of your intake of grains; whole grains contain more fiber and protein.
- **Proteins**. Focus on low-fat, lean meats, or choose poultry or fish. Bake, boil, or grill; avoid frying.
- **Dairy**. Dairy can provide much of the supply of calcium needed daily. Consume these foods sparingly, however, as they also tend to be high in fat.
- **Oils**. Oils and fats that are liquid at room temperature (e.g., canola and other cooking oils) are better for you than those that are solid at room temperature (e.g., butter or lard).
- **Water**. Drink plenty of water every day.

Following these recommendations can help you succeed in your weight-control efforts. In addition to managing intake, increasing your physical activity promotes weight reduction and maintenance goals. For those looking to lose weight, exercise is crucial.

Exercise extends benefits well beyond weight management. It also has been shown to mitigate stress and to improve mental capacity, sleep, sex life and function, and long-term health generally. These benefits result from 30 minutes of "vigorous exercise"—meaning activity that raises heart rate to approximately 80% of its maximum age-based heart rate. To calculate this target heart rate, subtract your age from 220, then multiply the difference by 0.8. For example, a 40-year-old would have a target heart rate of about 144 beats per minute (220 − 40 = 180; 180 × 0.8 = 144).

Inadequate sleep, smoking/vaping, and poor lifting mechanics can erase benefits gained from healthy eating and exercise. Working long hours can lead to poor sleep and sleep deprivation. Signs of **sleep deprivation** include loss of coordination, inability to concentrate, poor diet, and even depression. Efforts to eat well, avoid caffeine, and maintain something close to a regular sleep schedule will help reduce the effects of sleep deprivation.

Use of tobacco is one of the biggest health problems worldwide. If you don't smoke or vape, don't start; if you do, work to quit. The nicotine in tobacco and vaping products causes potentially lifelong, life-threatening cardiovascular and pulmonary changes. Nicotine is also one of the most difficult drugs to quit. Seek guidance from professionals, and ask for support and encouragement from friends and colleagues.

Proper lifting mechanics can be the difference between a long career in EMS and an early departure due to a lingering back injury. The very nature of EMS involves lifting and moving many patients, often from difficult positions or locations not designed for carrying a person or equipment. Follow these recommendations to maximize your safety during lifts and moves of patients:

- Plan your moves to minimize the number of lifts.
- Do not carry what can be moved on wheels.
- Coordinate lifts with your partner or team to minimize uneven distribution of weight. Ask for assistance if needed.
- *Always lift with your legs.* Your legs have the most powerful muscles of the body. Set your feet shoulder width apart on flat ground, keep your back straight with your head up looking at your partner, and lift as a unit.

Mental and Emotional Wellbeing

In EMS we see a lot of depravity—injuries, abuse, rape, suicides, homicides, and death—and illnesses of all kinds. We spend long hours away from family and friends, working holidays and weekends and overnights when other, "normal" workers can be with loved ones. We have notoriously poor sleep, poor diet, and chronic excessive stress.

This difficult environment can easily generate poor mental health and depression. Paramedics need to be aware of the warning signs not only in ourselves, but also in our partners and colleagues. Warning signs include feelings of depression, anxiety, agitation, or hopelessness; withdrawing from enjoyable friendships and activities; and sleeplessness or substance abuse. Should you see these signs in yourself or others, speak up, either to the affected colleague or your supervisor.

National Suicide Prevention Hotline
800-273-8255

Time away from the job is vitally important to manage **chronic stress**. Do your best to avoid "shop talk" with friends in the business during your off time. Engage in activities involving people who are not in emergency services. Develop hobbies that take your mind off of the job. Overtime may be nice, but pay attention to when you need to pull back and work only the regular shift. Take a vacation. Try meditation, yoga, or other mindful activity to help dissipate stress and promotes recovery from a shift.

These techniques help to manage the chronic job stress of EMS, but **acute stress** is another matter. Life events combined with acute job stress can be overwhelming. Severe calls can provoke strong emotions and lingering effects (nightmares and lost sleep, anger, tension, and mentally replaying events) that can seriously impact quality of life.

In situations of acute stress, do not go it alone. Call upon counseling or a critical incident stress debriefing team to help dissipate the acute stress that the job delivers from time to time. Tend to your own needs first, so that you may be able to help others later.

Paramedic Safety

Proper body mechanics (discussed earlier) will help prevent on-the-job injury. But paramedics also need to protect themselves from the patients themselves, diseases, and the hazards of the scene. This section discusses the basics of protection from diseases and hostile patients, as well as some everyday scene considerations. (Scene considerations for rarer events, such as rescues and acts of terrorism, are discussed later in the chapter.)

The paramedic can encounter infectious diseases on virtually every call. (Refer to the Medical Emergencies chapter for more information on how communicable diseases can be passed from patient to provider.) On scene and in the ambulance, the paramedic should consider wearing personal protective equipment (PPE) to safeguard against any of a litany of diseases the patient may have. During every call, nitrile gloves are recommended as a primary means of minimizing disease transmission, in addition to post-call handwashing. Gloves can prevent transmission of blood or fluid-borne illnesses.

Airborne and droplet-borne diseases (such as the respiratory illnesses pneumonia and Covid-19) can be transmitted through the air. Thus it is highly recommended that you wear at least a surgical mask during close, confined contact; protection is even greater if the patient can also tolerate wearing a mask. For higher-level protection, you may choose to wear an N95 mask or P-100 respirator. During aerosolizing procedures (such as intubation, suctioning, or administering nebulized medications like albuterol), a face shield or goggles can provide additional protection.

After the call, sanitize your equipment, paying particular attention to high-touch areas and equipment within 6 feet of the patient:

- Medical items, e.g., blood pressure cuffs, cardiac monitors
- Equipment, e.g., ceiling handrails, stretcher handles, compartment doors, door handles
- Incidental items, e.g., the clipboard, your pen

Certain scene types require a heightened attention to safety. Two notable examples are scenes with a violent patient and traffic accidents.

Violent Patients. Dealing with emotionally disturbed or violent people often requires more than just the ambulance personnel.

- *Request police presence* to help defuse the situation or secure the patient, as needed. There is no heroism in going in first and getting hurt or becoming a hostage.
- Once police are present and there are sufficient personnel to subdue the patient if needed, *consider the use of physical or chemical restraints* for as long as the patient presents a threat to self or bystanders.

Traffic Accidents. Street or highway scenes can be extremely dangerous for the providers, even more so at night. Take every precaution to make yourself and the ambulance more visible.

- If needed, use the ambulance to block the scene.
- Wear a vest or jacket that is road-safety yellow with reflective striping when outside the ambulance.
- Do not venture into lanes that are being used as travel lanes, even if controlled, and use caution when moving toward travel lanes.

Regardless of how visible you have made yourself, maintain a high degree of situational awareness. Drivers are often more interested in seeing the crash than looking for providers in the roadway.

Practical Point

Whenever possible, a fire truck should be the unit that protects a street or highway scene from oncoming traffic. It is bigger, has more emergency and scene lighting, and can withstand a much bigger collision than an ambulance. The ambulance should be the protection from traffic only in scenes that do not require a fire response.

COMMUNICATIONS, DOCUMENTATION, LAWS, AND ETHICS

This section covers important aspects of the paramedic's duties that are not directly related to patient care. Knowledge of technical aspects of communication will help the paramedic to relay information effectively to dispatch, other responding units, and receiving physicians and facilities. Proper documentation techniques will help the paramedic and patient if any aspect of the call is later contested in court. Finally, medicolegal and ethical considerations are discussed to clarify the paramedic's responsibilities and protections.

Communications

EMS communications are varied. EMS providers must be able to communicate with dispatchers and other first responders and other healthcare professionals. EMS communications have been discussed throughout the book, particularly rapport-building and interview situations on tested topics. Here we also address communication equipment, communication modalities, and regulations of the Federal Communications Commission (FCC). Lastly, we discuss reports to medical command as well as the handoff to personnel once at the hospital.

Communications Equipment and Methods

Despite the ubiquity of Internet and cellular communications, radio continues to be the mainstay of communication between EMS units, personnel, and dispatch. The system relies on several different components to work continuously and without fail. These components, and some alternate options, are as follows.

- **Base Station.** This fixed location is the main desk of communications, whether at the local, county, or regional level. The base station houses the most powerful transmitter of the components listed, as well as a receiver and an antenna (or multiple antennae) to reach the outer limits of the EMS coverage area, and often well beyond. The power of the base station, which is determined by the FCC, is generally greater than 45 watts.
- **Mobile Transceivers.** These devices are mounted in vehicles. With 20–50 watts of power, mobile transceivers are better able to reach dispatch over moderately hilly terrain than portable transceivers.
- **Portable Transceivers.** These are handheld devices with up to about 10 watts of power. Portable transceivers have a very limited range, particularly when operated within a structure. In some systems, these radios are used in conjunction with a repeater system situated in the ambulance.
- **Repeaters.** These devices do just that—they repeat. Repeaters receive a signal on one frequency (usually a low-power portable radio) and send it out immediately on another, more powerful frequency. Repeaters increase the range of the portable radio effectively to that of the mobile radio without having to go to the unit to make the transmission.
- **Remote Consoles.** Usually located in the hospital or at a medical command station, remote consoles receive radio reports and possibly biotelemetry from incoming units. They need to be more powerful and, possibly, reach farther than mobile units. Remote consoles can themselves be paired with a repeater or a trunked system and may also be able to receive and transmit on multiple frequencies.
- **Biotelemetry/Telemetry.** This device enables the paramedic to transmit data, not voice, to the hospital. Telemetry is becoming increasingly important for physicians to make treatment decisions for patients with stroke symptoms, abnormal ECGs, or chest pain.
- **Trunked Systems.** Trunking is a way for multiple agencies to operate on one frequency when needed. You can think of it as a rewiring of the system to connect different entities that need to communicate by selecting certain input and output frequencies. Trunked systems allow entities that are not normally on the same frequency to communicate clearly, as may be required during a mass casualty incident.

Modes of Radio Operation

The most familiar mode of radio communication is the **duplex** system. In this type of communication, a radio transceiver can both send and receive at the same time. Phones are the best example of a duplex system. Most radios used throughout EMS communications, however, use the **simplex** system. In a simplex system, the radio can either transmit or receive, but cannot do both at once. This is why, when multiple units try to transmit at once, one unit "steps on" the other. An alternative is a **multiplex** system, which combines two or more signals (often voice and data) over one frequency. Once again, cell phones are capable of multiplexing, which is why you can talk on the phone and surf the Internet while sending a signal to a Bluetooth speaker all at the same time.

All radio communications are based on the frequency of the waves transmitted. Every radio wave is measured in 2 ways: **wavelength**, which is the distance between the waves, and **frequency**, which is how many waves pass a fixed spot in 1 second. Frequency is recorded in units of **Hertz**, and a prefix to *Hertz* indicates a multiplier. For example:

hertz (Hz) = 1 wave per second

kilohertz (kHz) = 1,000 waves per second

megahertz (MHz) = 1 million waves per second

gigahertz (GHz) = 1 billion waves per second

EMS radio frequencies can be found in both the very high frequency (VHF) range of 30–175 MHz and the ultrahigh frequency (UHF) range of 300–3,000 MHz. Most commonly, medical communications occur in the high band of the VHF range, usually 150–160 MHz. Communications within urban areas and communications with the hospital are often found in the 450–470 MHz range of the UHF. Trunked systems may run upwards of 800 MHz. The specific operating frequencies are assigned and regulated by the FCC.

Communication over any of these frequencies can be hindered by terrain or the presence of metal structures. Generally, the higher the frequency, the less likely the signal will be impacted by obstructions. The higher the frequency, however, the shorter the overall distance the signal can travel.

Clarity and Content

There are many formal rules for talking on the radio, as well as general etiquette. These are far beyond the scope of this text. Here, we highlight the most important, farthest-reaching rules and guidelines that are most likely to be evaluated on the NRP Exam.

The best rule of thumb for communication via radio is to keep it short, direct, in plain English (rather than coded language), and related to the situation at hand. Another important general rule is that patient-specific communication, such as name and other demographic information, should be limited to what is needed for the provision of care of the patient. Following are some other recommendations for radio communication.

- Key up the microphone about 1 second before beginning to speak; this ensures the air is open and the first words are not cut off.
- State the agency being hailed first, followed by your unit number.
- Speak slowly, clearly, and at a normal tone as free from emotion as possible, with your mouth about 3 inches away from the mic.
- Become familiar with the phonetic alphabet for when something needs to be spelled out.
- Provide complex numbers one digit at a time to prevent misunderstanding. For example, a blood pressure of 180/62 might be communicated by radio as "one-eight-zero over six-two."
- Avoid profanity on the radio. The FCC can issue monetary fines or imprisonment for use of profanity.
- When receiving orders from a physician, be sure to use closed loop communication practices and repeat back any orders; this ensures the message was properly received and nothing was missed.

Medical Radio Reports and Hospital Handoffs

The radio report into the hospital should be brief and should paint as detailed a picture of the patient as needed for the situation. To alert the staff of your arrival when orders for further treatment are not needed, the report can simply include the patient's age, gender, chief complaint, brief history of present illness (HPI), and estimated time of arrival (ETA) into the ED.

In medical command situations where you *are* asking for further treatment orders seeking specialty care (such as a trauma alert, MI alert, or stroke alert), a more detailed picture should be shared. The report should conclude with your medical command question or recommendations for treatment. Consider using the **SBAR** method of communication recommended by the **Agency for Healthcare Research and Quality (AHRQ)**. SBAR stands for Situation, Background, Assessment, and Recommendation.

- **Situation** includes patient age, gender, weight if needed for care, and the chief complaint or problem. It may also include an upfront request for the orders you would like to receive by the end of your report.

- **Background** includes the HPI along with any pertinent signs and symptoms, or pertinent negatives. The word *pertinent* is important here to help focus the report—to keep it brief and aimed at obtaining the treatment you believe is needed. For example, the nurse or physician receiving your report on a cardiac arrest patient would likely not need to know that the patient had normal bowel movements prior to the arrest, but this recipient should know that it is a dialysis patient.

- **Assessment** includes your physical assessment and patient vital signs, along with any treatment you have rendered or have in progress at the time of the command call. It should also include what you regard as the highest priority problem you are treating.

- **Recommendation** is what you are requesting again. Include here dosages and frequency of medications needed/desired for the patient condition. Also include your recommendation for any specialty service activation.

The SBAR method can be used not only during radio communications, but also during handoff at the hospital. Although it is unlikely you will be making a treatment recommendation at that time, the other portions of the SBAR are important. During the handoff is also when you might include further information that could be helpful—things not directly related to the medical situation that you found out during your ongoing assessment. It is also important at handoff to convey any patient changes or treatment conducted since the radio report was given. Communication during this transfer is crucial for patient safety and continuity of care.

Documentation

Documentation is arguably the most important part of an ambulance response; it is often said, "If it's not documented, you didn't do it." The documentation of a run is a legal record. Among other things, it can protect the paramedic accused of malpractice and be a source of evidence in cases of personal injury, homicide or assault, and other felonies and misdemeanors. Accurate, concise, descriptive, factual documentation allows the paramedic to remember the call years after it actually happened.

The Patient Care Report

The **Patient Care Report (PCR)** documents everything pertinent that was done, evaluated, considered, and stated during the call, from response through delivery of the patient to the receiving facility. It is a confidential legal record that serves many purposes beyond simply documenting the events of the call.

The PCR includes information about the patient, scene, care rendered, and the patient's response to that care. Thus it will contain information protected by the **Health Insurance Portability and Accountability Act (HIPAA)**. This law, enacted in 2016, establishes permissible uses for the information contained in any medical record and identifies specifically who may access that information. Patient care records had always been considered private; however, HIPPA established stiff penalties for both individuals and agencies that violate a patient's right to that privacy.

HIPAA states that a healthcare provider may not disclose information that could identify a patient or link a person to a specific incident or diagnosis. It further states that only those with a need to access the full chart may do so. For example, billing personnel may need information from the entire chart to complete their job, whereas a quality assurance evaluator likely would not need access to patient demographics to evaluate the treatment rendered.

HIPPA recognizes that protected health information may also be shared with those not directly involved in patient care in other specific circumstances, for example:

- Birth
- Death

- Certain diseases and public health concerns
- Instances of suspected abuse or neglect
- Law enforcement concerns such as homicide, assault, or rape (among others)

HIPAA does not prevent a paramedic from using the chart to conduct quality assurance or continuing quality improvement; likewise, discussing generalities of the case as a means to debrief the incident does not violate the act. HIPAA also does not prevent the paramedic from providing information to any person who is or will be directly involved in the continuity of care. However, it *does* explicitly forbid you to share information with the media and even family members of the patient.

Format and Content

The PCR is generally completed electronically, as paper forms are being phased out worldwide. While the overall format is dictated by the software, the minimum required content remains the same.

Demographics

Patient demographics are needed for every call. These should include name, address, cell or home phone number, date of birth, and medical insurance information. For automobile crashes, car insurance provider should also be collected.

NEMSIS Information

The National Emergency Medical Services Information System (NEMSIS) collects data from ambulance companies nationwide. It is used in several ways, including:

- Tracking regional trends
- Bolstering EMS funding and insurance reimbursements
- Research purposes

The information collected by NEMSIS includes bodily locations of complaints (head, chest, extremities, etc.) as well as specific information about falls, car crashes, stroke, cardiac arrest, and work-related complaints.

Patient Care Information

All of your information on assessment, treatment, response to treatment, and transfer of care gets recorded in the narrative section of the PCR. The **narrative** is the area that describes the call to the reader. It should begin with dispatch information and the response initiation location.

Most software has an area where the vital signs, level of consciousness, and ECG interpretation are recorded. For clarity and uniformity, it is recommended that the bulk of the narrative follow the form of a **SOAP note**. The abbreviation *SOAP* stands for:

- **S**ubjective
- **O**bjective
- **A**ssessment
- **P**lan

The **subjective** section should contain everything told to you by the patient, bystander, or family member—the subject or subjects. This includes the chief complaint, OPPQRST, symptoms reported, and any other information that is conveyed by someone on scene. Allergies, medications, and past medical history can be included here but are often found in their own sections. This area can also contain descriptions of the scene, damage to the vehicle, and the nature or cause of a traumatic injury.

The **objective** section should contain everything that you have personally observed and found during the physical exam. While this can include highlights of vital signs and ECG findings, this information is often found in a flow-chart that is recorded by time completed.

The **assessment** section highlights what you believe are the top diagnosis priorities for the patient's treatment. When done by a physician, this is referred to as the differential diagnosis; for EMS purposes it can be called the working diagnosis. You should list here anything you wish to treat in the order of likelihood of the diagnosis. For example, for a patient with a chief complaint of chest pain and shortness of breath that you are treating, you might indicate:

1. Acute MI
2. CHF
3. Pulmonary embolism

Finally, the **plan** section is where you would record the treatments initiated—your plan of care—as well as the out-comes of those treatments. In most software programs, this takes the form of a flowchart similar to the recording of vital signs. If that is the case, referring to this section in the narrative is all that would be needed here. (Consider using this area to document treatment that should have been completed but was not, along with the reason for not com-pleting it.) This section should also include a note about transfer care of the patient to the hospital; this documents continuity of care and minimizes the chance that the paramedic is later accused of abandoning the patient. Whenever possible, record the name of the person receiving the patient, their level of certification (RN, MD), and the patient's bed number.

Medicolegal and Ethics

HIPAA, discussed in the previous section, is one of many laws and regulations governing EMS. This section covers some of the regulations facing EMS and healthcare in general.

Ethics

Ethical considerations for the paramedic can be summed up in 2 distinct but related concepts: "First, do no harm," and "Act in the best interests of the patient." Another rule of thumb when it comes to medical ethics is: Render the care and treat the patient the way you would want a loved one to be cared for and treated.

These guiding principles will help keep paramedics out of harm's way and enable them to render the best possible care for the patient. As a paramedic, you will often be held accountable for your and your team's actions from an ethical standpoint; from a legal standpoint, you will always be held accountable.

Laws and Legal Considerations

The paramedic could face one or both of 2 possible types of lawsuits depending on the entity bringing suit. In civil law, the patient or the patient's family may file suit against you. In criminal law, the state or other governmental entity brings the lawsuit against you.

Civil law is invoked when a patient sues you for such matters as abandonment, negligence, malpractice, and breach of duty to act. Civil law can also involve the paramedic who is called to testify for or against an individual encoun-tered in the course of EMS duties. For example, suppose the paramedic responds to a motor vehicle crash involving a work vehicle, and the person who was injured on the job and now unable to work sues for disability and workers' compensation. The paramedic might be called to testify about the crash site and the person's injuries.

The goal of civil law is to assign blame or responsibility, legally called **liability**, for an injury or loss. Once liability has been established, **compensatory damages**, or compensation (usually in the form of fines), are assessed by the court. These damages are usually assigned to compensate the patient (or kin) with money for medical costs and for physical and mental suffering. **Punitive damages** in excess of medical costs may also be awarded; these are designed to punish the plaintiff if the wrongdoing is found to have been intentional, avoidable, or the result of recklessness.

A civil suit requires the agreement of 9 out of the 12 jurors and is based on only a preponderance of the evidence provided—not beyond the shadow of a reasonable doubt, as in a criminal case.

Criminal law is invoked when the state files suit against you for breaking a law or statute, and it is brought by the government. A criminal lawsuit may arise against the paramedic accused of falsifying documentation or diverting controlled substances. Where there is a victim, the paramedic may face a criminal lawsuit, most often arising from accusations of assault, battery, false imprisonment, or defamation. Definitions of these terms are as follows.

- **Assault.** Causing fear of imminent bodily harm or breach of bodily security.
- **Battery.** Touching anyone without their consent; this does not have to result in visible injury.
- **False Imprisonment.** Occurs when a person is unjustifiably held against their will; in the context of EMS, this occurs when a person is transported without their consent and the act of transporting the person cannot be justified.
- **Libel.** Defamation taking the form of the written word. In the context of EMS, this can arise from a PCR that includes the opinions of the EMS provider.
- **Slander.** Defamation in the form of spoken words. The paramedic could be liable for slander if they violate a person's privacy. This would also violate HIPAA.

Laws Governing EMS

Many laws govern EMS and EMS providers, ranging from federal laws all the way down to agency-specific rules. Here are a few laws and rules with which you should be familiar and a brief description of each.

Medical Practice Act

U.S. states regulate the practice of medicine, usually in a state statute called a medical practice act. This act defines the minimum requirements and qualifications of each level of provider as well as the scope of practice for each. **Scope of practice** is the range of actions a healthcare worker is allowed to perform based on their level of certification. For the paramedic, these actions can be further modified by the service medical director or state medical director. Typically, the service medical director does not authorize actions that are outside those defined for each level of provider in the medical practice act.

Emergency Medical Treatment and Active Labor Act (EMTALA)

EMTALA was created in 1986 to prevent hospitals from performing "economic triage," the practice of sending away patients without means of payment to other hospitals or discharging them without evaluation or treatment. EMTALA guarantees evaluation and stabilization of those seeking emergency medical treatment and prohibits discrimination of any kind. This requirement has allowed providers to focus purely on the needs of the patient and not their ability to pay for services. Ethics plays a role here as well: Treat your patient as you would want to be treated. A homeless patient who is complaining of shortness of breath should receive exactly the same treatment as a penthouse dweller with the same complaint.

EMTALA also addresses destination determination for the paramedic. In some systems, paramedics may transport only to the closest hospital; other systems may require a medical command consult to direct transport to the patient's preference of hospital. EMTALA is also unique in that it allows individuals to sue for violations of the act; it is nonetheless extremely unlikely that an ambulance service or paramedic would be sued under provisions of EMTALA.

EMTALA regulates interfacility transports as well. The paramedic should make sure that the in-transit care they provide falls within their scope of practice. Examples of violations include:

- A BLS provider takes a patient who requires cardiac monitoring.
- A paramedic administers an infusion to a patient when that is outside the paramedic's scope of practice.

The paramedic should also assess the patient before transport to confirm the patient is stable enough for a safe transfer. Finally, bear in mind that transferring an unstable patient to another hospital for a reason *other than* a higher level of specialized care could itself be a violation of EMTALA.

Emergency Vehicle Operations and Transportation Laws

"Due Regard." Emergency vehicle (EV) laws vary from state to state; however, all of those laws require the driver to operate the vehicle with "due regard" for the public and other drivers. While operating an EV with warning devices engaged (including both lights and sirens), the driver may be able to pass other vehicles in ordinary no-passing zones or proceed through a controlled intersection against a red light. In these and similar circumstances, the other drivers in the area must grant the operator right of way. But when EV operators fail to obtain the right of way from other drivers and cause a crash, they are often found legally at fault in civil cases. Worse, they may be found criminally liable (through negligence) in a suit brought by any of the drivers on the road or the patient in the back of the ambulance.

In-Vehicle Restraints. During patient transportation to the hospital, responsibility for the safe arrival of the patient rests on the shoulders of the EV operator. Therefore:

- Secure the patient with all available seatbelts.
- Secure pediatric patients in their own car seats whenever possible or in a commercially available emergency pediatric car seat.
- Engage shoulder harnesses for the patient whenever possible (required by many ambulance insurers).

Should the need arise to remove these restraints to provide adequate patient care, it is recommended that this need be documented.

The driver is also responsible for the safety of the provider in the patient compartment. The EMS provider is often in a less-than-secure position while actively providing patient care—seldom wearing a seatbelt or even able to brace for a collision. When not actively providing patient care, the provider should be secured with a lap belt and shoulder harness.

Destination Decision. In most cases, the patient has the right to decide where (within reason) they would like to be transported. When the patient is reasonably stable, the patient's choice should be honored whenever possible. If the patient is unstable, however, the patient should most likely be transported to the nearest "most appropriate facility." The most appropriate facility is one that is fully equipped to handle the severity of the patient's health needs and that also is within a reasonable driving distance beyond the actual nearest facility. For example, an unstable patient with an active MI should be transported to a facility capable of rapid interventions including angioplasty. Although protocols vary regarding the length of time beyond the nearest facility the ambulance should go to get to the specialty center, 20 minutes more is a good rule of thumb. In excess of that, transport to the nearest facility or aeromedical transport should be considered.

Refusal of Care. When a patient refuses care (be it treatment, transport, or both), the paramedic must be cautious. Refusals of care are among the most litigated areas of EMS and require special attention. For a refusal to be considered legally obtained and enforceable, the patient must meet several minimum standards, as follows.

- Patient must be conscious, alert, and oriented to person, place, and time.
- Vital signs should be within normal ranges for the age of the patient.
- The patient should not have sustained a head injury.
- Precautions should be taken to prevent relapse of whatever caused the original call. An example of this would be ensuring that a patient diagnosed with diabetes eats complex carbohydrates after experiencing an episode of low blood sugar.
- Patient is of legal independence (over 18, emancipated) or a parent or guardian is present to acknowledge the refusal and accept responsibility for the care of the minor.
- Patient must not be under the influence of drugs or alcohol.

If the patient does not meet these standards and is oriented to person, place, and time, or is capable of being cared for, medical command should be contacted.

The patient must be told all of the risks of not seeking an evaluation at a hospital and cautioned that the evaluation of the paramedic is not a substitute, regardless of the severity of illness or injury. The patient must also be encouraged to seek care on their own, from their own doctor or, if appropriate, by self-transport to the emergency department. Patient and provider should sign the refusal document, and it should be witnessed by a neutral party whenever possible.

Concepts Related to Consent

Consent is essentially permission to render care. Obtaining a patient's consent to render treatment minimizes the paramedic's risk of being accused of assault, battery, or unlawful touching. Consent can take either of 2 forms. In **informed consent**, the patient is told of the need for treatment and the means by which that treatment is to be performed, is permitted to make a decision about that treatment, and then agrees to accept the suggested treatment. **Implied consent** applies when a patient is unable to make a decision for any reason, e.g., unemancipated minor, altered mentation for any reason, mental incapacitation, unconsciousness, or under the influence of drugs or alcohol.

As mentioned earlier, treatment of most minors falls under implied consent, with a couple of notable exceptions. First, an adult other than the parent or legal guardian can make a decision on behalf of the minor patient; this is referred to as **in loco parentis**. Individuals who may make such a decision include day care personnel, school teachers, and the like. Second, **emancipated minors** are under the legal age of consent (usually 18) but hold legal documentation indicating that they are to be treated as adults. Emancipation is granted through the courts (most often), or due to marriage, military service, or current pregnancy. In the specific situation of a pregnant minor, the law generally regards the pregnant minor as emancipated and free to make all decisions for both herself and her unborn child—that is, *during pregnancy*. After delivery of the baby, minors who were previously emancipated while pregnant return to the status of legal minors with regard to decisions about themselves, but they retain legal decision-making authority with regard to their children.

Mandatory Reporting

As a paramedic, you may come across cases that are suspicious for child or elder abuse or neglect. If the situation is suspicious (i.e., the story does not match the injury or complaint), you are legally required to report that concern. If you fail to report something that you found suspicious during a call, you could be prohibited from practicing as a paramedic and face other serious consequences.

Bear in mind that merely reporting a case as suspicious does not establish the guilt of any party. Rather, it starts the process by which an investigation evaluates whether abuse or neglect exists. If that investigation concludes that there is not abuse or neglect, nothing happens to the individuals, nor do they ever find out who reported the suspicious case. Conversely, if it is determined that there is abuse or neglect, your report may have saved a life.

Negligence and Abandonment

In its everyday sense, *negligence* means a failure to act in a prudent manner. **Negligence** on the part of the paramedic, as a legal designation, requires 4 specific elements: duty to act, breach of that duty, proximate cause, and resultant harm. To win a civil suit for negligence against a paramedic, the plaintiff must prove all 4 elements.

- A **duty to act** is the responsibility to respond to a call or event, to render care, and to act within a generally accepted standard of care and to the level of certification. This responsibility exists any time you are "on duty." During this time, you have (presumably) full access to your equipment and are as capable of performing EMS actions as another equally equipped paramedic. When you are off duty, it may still be ethical to render aid. However, you will not legally be held to the same standard of provision of care, since you likely lack full access to equipment (e.g., you are in uniform but in a personal vehicle or in public). That said, if the care you do render is inappropriate or beyond the level your certification, liability may still exist.

- A **breach of that duty** exists if, for example, you fail to respond to a call in your area or you fail to render care that is within your certification's standard of care. The standard of care is established by comparing actions of the paramedic in question to the way a similarly trained paramedic from the same area would perform or react in a similar situation.

- **Proximate cause** means that any harm that resulted to the patient must be traceable to the actions taken by the paramedic. This burden of proof rests with the patient's legal team (or the legal team of the patient's proxy if the patient is incapable of acting on their own behalf or is deceased). Proximate cause is often the most difficult part of negligence to prove legally: A lot can happen after the paramedic treats the patient, making the origin of harm harder to pinpoint—and also, there was a reason the paramedic was called in the first place. Remember that lawsuits are most often about assigning blame, so being able to prove based on a preponderance of the evidence that the paramedic's actions were to blame for the harm is often clouded with other possible explanations for the harm. For example, suppose a patient sustained a head injury in an assault and was intubated and ventilated in the field. This patient recovers but sues the paramedic: Now the patient has headaches and weakness that, the patient's lawyer says, are the result of oxygen deprivation sustained during the intubation attempt. While that is a plausible explanation, documentation could refute it; furthermore, a traumatic brain injury could have these sequelae regardless of intubation attempts. Documentation is crucial to absolving or indicting the paramedic in such cases.

- **Resultant harm**, in this legal sense, can take a great range of forms including minor disability, loss of income, emotional distress, loss of aspects that existed prior to the incident, and death.

Under the law, **abandonment** is a specific type of negligence resulting from the failure to continue care once care has begun. This lack of continuation of care subsequently results in harm. Abandonment can occur if you begin treating a patient and leave them to treat another patient with more acute needs and fail to return to or hand over care of the first patient. It can also happen if you drop off a patient to any receiving facility and fail to notify appropriate personnel of the patient's arrival. Furthermore, the personnel notified at the hospital must be of a higher level of care (RN/NP/PA/MD); notifying a tech or support personnel is inadequate to ensure proper continuity of care.

End-of-Life Care and Decisions

End-of-life care, powers of attorney, and do-not-resuscitate (DNR) orders can be challenging for the paramedic. These are often complex, nuanced situations—which potentially means that each needs to be managed differently. When in doubt, check local protocols or contact medical command for situational guidance.

A patient may decide to make clear and legally binding how they would like their healthcare to be managed with an **advance directive**. These documents include living wills, DNR orders, and organ donor cards.

A person makes a **living will** while mentally intact and has it witnessed to put it into force (by an attorney or another person, depending on the state). Living wills spell out exactly what healthcare a person would like to receive in the event they are no longer capable of giving informed consent (e.g., persistent coma). The paramedic can often honor these requests but must contact medical command to be sure. Living wills also may designate a **healthcare power of attorney (healthcare POA)**; this is a person whom the patient has authorized to make healthcare decisions on the patient's behalf in the case of their own incapacitation. The healthcare POA may request and authorize treatment for the patient that the rest of the living will has specifically prohibited, causing confusion. The decision of the healthcare POA generally supersedes the rest of the living will. (Again, seek guidance from medical command.)

Do not resuscitate (DNR) orders express the patient's wishes regarding artificial ventilation, provision of CPR, and other lifesaving measures. The DNR must be signed by the patient and, in many states, a physician and/or lawyer. It is often difficult to know if EMS can follow these orders. If presented with a DNR, engage medical command for guidance. Online medical direction empowers EMS to stop any efforts that have already been initiated once a DNR is presented or to stop efforts if, in the course of allowed treatments, the patient goes into cardiac arrest.

SPECIAL RESPONSES: HAZARDOUS MATERIALS, TERRORISM, AND DISASTERS

Medical and trauma patients make up the overwhelming bulk of a paramedic's workload. In the course of a long career, however, you can expect to encounter situations that require special preparation. This section gives a high-level overview of responses to hazardous materials incidents, terrorism, and natural disasters, focusing on areas most likely to be tested in the National Registry Paramedic exam. (For information on triage and the National Incident Management System, see the Trauma chapter.)

Hazardous Materials

According to the Department of Transportation (DOT), a **hazardous material (hazmat)** is any substance capable of causing unreasonable risk to either human health and safety or the environment when commercially transported, incorrectly used, or improperly stored. The Occupational Safety and Health Administration (OSHA) and the Environmental Protection Agency (EPA) are the 2 federal agencies that are jointly responsible for developing and enforcing regulations related to hazmats in the United States.

OSHA and the EPA have outlined training levels for hazmat incident response in the Hazardous Waste Operations and Emergency Response (HAZWOPER) standards.

- Hazmat Awareness, the lowest level of hazmat understanding in the standards, is required for EMS responders.
- Higher training levels are required of personnel with greater responsibility for running hazmat operations: Operations, Technician, Specialist, Incident Commander.

As in poisonings, the severity of the incident depends on the hazardous material involved, its quantity or concentration at the point of exposure, and duration of exposure. When responding to a hazmat incident, you must identify the hazardous substance, determine how best to protect yourself and the public, establish the distance from the substance needed to isolate it, and determine what PPE is required to safely decontaminate and treat the patients.

Identifying the Hazmat

Vehicles that transport hazardous materials, including rail tank cars and shipping containers, are required to display a standardized placard for every substance in storage. These placards identify substances as flammable, poisonous, oxidizer, explosive, biohazardous, or radioactive. Hazmat shipping placards are regulated by the DOT. To find free, official placard examples and explanations from the DOT, search for "hazardous materials chart" on the DOT website: **www.fmcsa.dot.gov**

Hazmat placards typically bear a 4-digit number identifying a specific substance or class of substances. For example, a railcar displaying a placard with the number *1993* is carrying a combustible fluid (such as diesel fuel or home heating oil).

Every ambulance is required to carry the most up-to-date version of the *Emergency Response Guidebook* (*ERG*). In addition to identifying hazardous substances, this book provides the initial isolation zones, considerations for groundwater and sewer infiltration, and emergency medical treatment for various forms of exposure. *ERG* is a free publication of the DOT; you can download it from the DOT website or a smartphone app store.

Isolation and PPE

Once the substance (or class of substances) has been determined, it must be isolated. The first step in the response is to establish safety zones; this is done in coordination the fire department and hazmat experts. *ERG* will help determine the hot zone and the warm zone.

- The **hot zone** is the area immediately surrounding the location of the hazmat; only the highest level of hazmat-trained personnel should be here, wearing the appropriate level of PPE.
- The **warm zone** is the area where responders and victims are decontaminated; only personnel with high-level certification should be here, wearing appropriate hazmat PPE.
- The **cold zone** is farther from the incident; this is where EMS triage and transportation generally take place.

PPE for a hazmat response may be far more specialized than that used on a typical medical or trauma call, depending on the hazardous substance in question. Hazmat ensembles worn by various levels of responders are as follows:

- **Level A ensemble** (highest level of protection) includes a self-contained breathing apparatus (SCBA); these suits are gastight (completely unventilated), raising the concern of overheating.
- **Level B ensemble** includes an SCBA, giving a high level of respiratory protection; used when skin exposure to the substance poses low threat.
- **Level C ensemble** provides respiratory protection with a powered air-purifying respirator (PAPR) and minimal skin contact prevention.
- **Level D ensemble** (worn only by those in the cold zone) is little more than an N95 or P-100 mask; there is no protective suit.

Decontamination and Disposal

Everyone in the warm and hot zones of a hazmat incident must be decontaminated at the scene. Those who had direct exposure to the substance (**primary contamination**) are decontaminated first. Next come those who were exposed to the substance indirectly (**secondary contamination**), through contact with people or equipment that was directly exposed.

Decontamination is accomplished by one or more of the following methods.

- **Dilution** (most common decontamination method): Flowing water over the patient is generally the safest and most effective way to remove the contaminant. The effluent may be allowed to run into a sewer or captured if particularly hazardous to the environment.
- **Absorption**: Large pads or towels are used to absorb the contaminant.
- **Neutralization**: Changing the hazmat into something less harmful via a chemical reaction is rarely used on patients, because the chemical reaction generates a large amount of heat that can burn the patient.

Disposal of the products of decontamination is also a consideration. The water from a dilution process, the clothing of contaminant-exposed patients, and occasionally even the equipment used in the rescue must be discarded. When the loss of life is a real threat, controlling the effluent is secondary to decontaminating the patient and speeding their way to proper care. To the greatest extent possible, however, contaminated items should be kept to a minimum, managed with care, and disposed of appropriately as hazardous waste.

Terrorism and Natural Disasters

From the EMS perspective, terrorism and natural disasters have a lot in common. Both can result in multiple patients with myriad injuries, challenges to access all the patients who need emergency care, and disruption in normal communications.

Terrorism

While terrorism can manifest insidiously (e.g., cyber crimes and identity theft), the more overt and violent forms (e.g., use weapons or explosives) that result in physical harm are more relevant for the paramedic.

Unlike natural disasters, terrorist strikes tend to occur without warning. They are often volatile as well, especially early on. A variety of issues can complicate EMS response, for instance:

- Logistical chaos (compromised access, patients from various directions)
- Uncertainty about whether all hazards have been accounted for (structures rendered unstable, possibility of an invisible chemical or radiological agent)

Scene safety and security of the responders are of paramount importance. EMS responders to a terrorist strike—from the incident commander all the way through the paramedic rendering treatment—should maintain a high index of suspicion throughout the scene operations and should constantly be reassessing the situation. The paramedic should be deeply familiar with the Incident Management System (discussed in the Trauma chapter) and their role within the response.

Weapons of Mass Destruction

Explosives are perhaps the most common terrorist weapon; they cause extensive damage, potentially in the perpetrator's absence. Incendiary devices can be made from a variety of explosive and flammable materials (ammonium nitrate fertilizer, dynamite, propane, gasoline). This section introduces some other common weapons and concerns they raise for the paramedic.

Chemical Agents

Vesicants, or blistering agents, are chemicals that cause blisters on the skin after prolonged exposure. Agents of this type include mustard gas (sulfur mustard), lewisite, and phosgene oxime (CX gas).

- Skin symptoms include blistering, burning, redness, pain, and eye irritation and injury.
- Respiratory symptoms include stridor, hoarseness, cough, hemoptysis, and shortness of breath.

Treatment for vesicant exposure includes decontamination shower with copious amounts of water followed by pain control with any analgesic. Treat blisters as for any partial-thickness burn. Treat respiratory complications symptomatically and be prepared to ventilate or intubate as needed.

Choking agents such as chlorine and phosgene cause damage and swelling to the airways.

- Chlorine has a distinctive smell and rapidly causes symptoms of coughing and respiratory distress, consistent with pulmonary edema. However, CPAP and oxygen alone are unlikely to improve the patient's condition because air exchange has been compromised at the alveolar level, causing airway swelling and leakiness.
- Phosgene (not the same as phosgene oxime, mentioned earlier) smells like freshly cut grass. Symptoms are consistent with pulmonary edema (chest tightness, cough, and shortness of breath) and often manifest only hours later.

Treatment for both chlorine and phosgene begins with removal from the affected environment and decontamination of the patient. Aggressive treatment for respiratory conditions is also needed: oxygenation, intubation, and ventilatory support. Phosgene more than chlorine can result in excessive fluid production, so suctioning may also be necessary. All other treatment is supportive to the patient.

Pro-Tip

Always make sure that the patient has been thoroughly decontaminated. Insufficient decontamination is harmful not only to the patient, but also to the EMS provider through off-gassing: A contaminated patient could exhale enough of a damaging chemical agent to sicken the provider who inhales it. Likewise, off-gassing can occur when poison from the victim's clothing aerosolizes—again, making the EMS provider sick by breathing the contaminant. Nerve agents tend to be oily, so these chemicals may require more than flowing water alone to fully decontaminate the patient.

Nerve agents are notable for their power to kill a great number of people in a short time and with a small dose. Dozens of these agents exist, so identifying all of them here is not possible. The most common are sarin, soman, and VX. Most nerve agents are organophosphates, which cause the syndrome consistent with parasympathetic nervous system overstimulation. Bradycardia is one symptom. The acronym *SLUDGE* can help recall the other symptoms in this syndrome:

- Salivation
- Lacrimation
- Urination
- Defecation/diarrhea
- GI distress (vomiting)
- Eyes (miosis, or pinpoint pupils)

Treatment for nerve agent exposure includes parasympatholytics (e.g, atropine) and cholinesterase activators (e.g, pralidoxime chloride). Seizures should be treated as they occur with any benzodiazepine selected. Ventilatory support and CPR are often needed.

Cyanide is in a class all its own. It works by shutting down glucose metabolism at the cellular level, preventing the formation of sufficient ATP for cellular function—meaning death almost certainly follows. Treatment for cyanide exposure or ingestion is largely supportive. Cyanide poisoning is treated with hydroxocobalamin, sodium nitrite, and sodium thiosulfate. None of these medications are routinely carried on ambulances, so rapid transport with supportive measures (CPR, respiratory support) is recommended.

Biological Agents

Bacteria, viruses, and neurotoxins can be used as biologic weapons. The effects of these agents manifest only days or weeks after the initial exposure, potentially affecting responders as well as survivors of the attack. Treatment is supportive, with rapid transport to the hospital.

- Bacteria: anthrax, bubonic plague, pneumonic plague
- Viruses: smallpox, hemorrhagic fevers (Ebola)
- Neurotoxins: botulinum, ricin

Radioactive Devices

Certain chemicals give off radioactivity as they degrade. Radioactive decay can be rapid or slow and can produce effects that are beneficial (e.g., diagnostic x-rays) or catastrophic (e.g., nuclear reactor meltdown). Used in a weapon of terror, radioactivity can increase the geographic area of destruction, potentially rendering large areas no longer habitable by humans. See the Trauma chapter for information on radiation exposure and treatment.

Natural Disasters

Natural disaster responses can vary widely in scope, duration, and types of injuries generated. Earthquakes can quickly cause a lot of damage and injury but are generally over in minutes, while a hurricane can rage across an expansive area for weeks. Disasters that unfold relatively slowly (hurricanes, blizzards) tend to permit more EMS planning than a sudden event (volcanic eruption, earthquake).

Planning may involve bringing in extra resources from areas not predicted to be affected and housing them strategically in or beside the area expected to be hit. Identifying ingress and egress routes from the affected area is worthwhile (although the natural disaster could later obstruct those optimal routes). Planning can also identify where displaced persons might be sheltered (e.g., domed stadiums as used during Hurricane Katrina, churches, schools, and gymnasiums).

Other concerns that may be addressed during the planning stage include:

- Preparation and mobilization of disaster relief organizations
- Increased preparedness training for disasters likely to strike a specific region (e.g., earthquake response in California, hurricane response in Florida and the Gulf Coast)
- Internal and external communication contingencies
- Establishment of liaisons to communicate with media or other agencies

During the natural disaster, planning shifts to reacting. As damage reports start coming in, patterns of patient injury and illness become known, and responders start rescuing patients, the scope of the disaster dictates the deployment of resources. It may be necessary to break the incident down into multiple areas of operation.

The ICS implementation is far more complex than what most responders usually see. Triage, transport, and patient tracking are important not only for all the usual reasons, but also because they facilitate reunification of families. This saves a search—and avoids tying up precious resources—for "missing" persons whose whereabouts are known. It also assists in the IC's communication with hospitals, clarifying whether hospitals are full or can take more patients.

While patients are the immediate focus in any response, the responders also need consideration during extended operations. The IC should make sure that all personnel have regularly scheduled downtime, which should include sleep, food, and opportunity for exercise. Counselors should also be available at the crew staging and sleep areas to address responders' mental health needs.

SCENE CONSIDERATIONS

The paramedic will spend about half of every call on a scene. While general scene safety has been discussed earlier in the book, a few specific scenes merit further discussion. These are vehicle extrication, specialized rescue, and crime scene operations.

Practical Point

This discussion flags things to be aware of during various types of specialized rescues. In no way will it sufficiently prepare you for the "active rescue," but it will help you be more confident in thinking about ways to free your patient.

Vehicle Rescue

Vehicle rescue and technical rescue have similar procedures and considerations, so much of the discussion focuses on scenarios related to vehicle rescue, followed by some specific considerations for other rescue situations.

Steps of a Rescue

Steps of any rescue are largely parallel with those of a response to a medical emergency.

- **Preparation.** This includes education, training, and practice well ahead of any call.
- **Response.** This includes protocols for dispatching the rescue company and order of response of apparatus
- **Arrival and Scene Size-Up.** Before even exiting the unit, evaluate the extent of damage and consider what additional resources may be needed. Also consider the ingress and egress of additional units including ambulances. Identify potential hazards and identify a perimeter of control for situations that may require evacuation.

- **Stabilization of the Scene.** More on this to follow.
- **Accessing the Patient.** What tools or resources will be needed to gain access to the patient and extricate the patient? These can be simple, like cutting the window out of a vehicle or using leverage to lift a fallen tree limb off the patient. Or it may involve multiple hydraulic tools—for instance, to remove a car roof.
- **Disentanglement.** Planning the patient's removal from the wreckage may involve the paramedic when crush injuries are possible or partial amputations have been identified. Use caution when a patient is in close proximity to a tool being used.
- **Removal.** After disentanglement, the patient may be removed from the car. Removal may require more planning when the patient needs to be removed from a ravine, flowing river, or mountainous terrain.
- **Treatment and Transport.** Transport modality should be considered from the moment of contact. When the entrapment is particularly complicated and extrication will therefore be prolonged, consider air transport. Depending on the degree of entrapment and lack of access, it may be impossible to begin treatment in earnest until after the patient has been removed.

Scene Stabilization and Control Zones

Any scene needing a rescue may also need to be stabilized. The most obvious hazards should have already been considered. Other hazards may present themselves as you approach the scene and begin operations. During this time, also consider optimal ambulance ingress, parking, and egress. The first unit on scene considers these factors for itself at arrival; it should then expand consideration to all units en route as part of scene stabilization. Units should be parked to protect those operating on the scene (where appropriate) and out of the way of hazards (e.g., fumes, fluid runoff). Doing so also helps establish a perimeter of control.

While accountable to the IC or other specially trained personnel on scene, the paramedic must remain alert for and respond to specific hazards that may arise at any time, for instance:

- Visibility in operations on/near a roadway and/or at night
- Physical hazards to the rescuers requiring helmets and turnout gear

Control zones were addressed in the context of a hazardous materials response. The same concepts apply in a rescue, but with looser delineation between hot, warm, and cold zones. In vehicle rescues, it is common for the paramedic to be in the hot zone, actively involved in the rescue process and providing care to the patient. That is less common in more technical rescues (e.g., trench rescues, confined space rescues).

Special Rescue

Everyone on scene needs to have a shared mental model of the plan of rescue, including the patient(s) when appropriate. The paramedic may be in a position to provide guidance and direction to the rescue personnel based on an understanding of the situation or familiarity with the abilities of the rescue company. Often, however, the paramedic's role in a rescue is simply to wait until the patient has been removed.

As in hazardous materials response, there are training levels for technical rescue:

- **Awareness.** An introduction focused on scene safety and prevention of further injury
- **Operations.** Allows assistance in the rescue event
- **Technician.** Certified in the use of the equipment and management of the rescue scene

Confined Space

A confined space is an area that is surrounded by a structure and not intended for human occupancy. These can be grain silos, dumpsters, wells, or any area with limited entrance or exit space where a person could become stuck. Recall that asphyxiating gases that are heavier than air can accumulate in low areas. Thus the space may have insufficient oxygen or contain poisonous gases requiring the use of an SCBA. In any confined space rescue, assume that the atmosphere is hostile, and do not enter without proper training or a sufficient oxygen supply. Better yet, wait until the rescuers bring the patient out of the environment and possibly decontaminate them.

Trench Rescue

Trenches that are human-made (e.g., excavations for construction) should always be shored up as the excavation proceeds to prevent the sides from collapsing back in. Weight around the edges of an excavated area can increase the likelihood of collapse. Water saturation can worsen the severity of collapse. Upon collapse, the earth moved into the space can entrap a person and be heavy enough to cause crush injuries.

A paramedic should not enter a trench even to provide care for the trapped patient. The risk of further collapse is too great, potentially making the rescuer a second patient. Defer to those with understanding of the risks associated with a trench rescue. Until the patient is removed from the trench, create a wide perimeter and provide reassurance to the patient from a distance.

Water Rescue

Regardless of where you work, a water rescue is almost always a possibility. Besides pools, rivers, and ponds, local weather events like storm flooding or sudden snowmelt can create a water hazard. Swift-moving water is the most hazardous type of rescue for the rescuer—especially in areas that are not usually waterways, where submerged items pose an even greater hazard.

When you encounter someone in need of a water rescue, do not exceed your level of training. Talk to the person, assure them that more help is on the way, and encourage them not to panic. To remember the order of rescue efforts to attempt, use the mnemonic "Reach, throw, row, then go!"

1. **Reach.** Extend something sturdy that you can both grasp to pull the person to shore.
2. **Throw.** Toss a device (life ring on a rope, rope alone) that the person can grasp, allowing you to reel them into shore.
3. **Row.** Try to get to the person by rowboat or (in swift water) motorboat. A jet ski built for more than one may also work if the rescued person is capable of holding on.
4. **Go.** Get into the water yourself to attempt a rescue only if the other steps have failed.

Regardless of your familiarity with the terrain, you should always wear a personal flotation device (PFD) during a water rescue. A wetsuit or (for prolonged immersion in water) a drysuit may also be appropriate. In swift water, the rescuer is often tied to the shore/land with a rope to guard against being swept away upon entering the water. A water rescuer who loses footing should turn, feet first, in the direction of travel with the feet extended, so anything submerged first comes into contact with the legs. This approach also protects the head and allows the rescuer to see obstacles.

Eddies and boils pose distinct hazards for water rescuers.

- An **eddy**, like a whirlpool, is rotary movement of water along the water's surface.
- A **boil**, which churns perpendicular to the surface, could be powerful enough to hold a person under water.

Cold emergencies, including cold water rescues, require rewarming of the patient who has undergone the mammalian diving reflex: lowered heart and respiratory rates, and possibly unconsciousness. These physiological responses often permit a submerged person to survive longer in water that is less than 70°F (21°C) than in warm water.

Other Rescue Situations

In these "other" situations, let the experts secure the patient and bring them to your staging location. Maintain your own safety and ensure continuous communication or tracking with the IC and other team members. Following are a few thoughts to consider for each situation.

Search and Rescue

- Person of any age is lost somewhere
- Location varies widely (public park, cave system, city)
- Operations tend to take a long time (large area, many rescuers/agencies)
- Consider the elements faced (rain, snow, heat, cold) in your preparations for the patient
- Rescued and rescuers alike will need food and water

Structure Fires

- Approach the scene as a paramedic even if you are trained as a firefighter
- Expect fire rescuers to bring the patient to a safe zone for EMS care
- Use anything known ahead of time (e.g., entrapment, firefighter goes down) to anticipate patient needs and prepare ahead of time (e.g., laying out IV lines, airway options, supplies for a surgical airway)
- Consider what other resources may be needed, and set them in motion (e.g., helicopter, other ground units for transport so an ambulance always remains on scene)

Industrial Rescue

- Many agricultural and industrial machines have known pinch points, crush points, or pull-in points that can cause severe injury or death to the operator
- Prior to attempting any rescue, ensure that the machinery is turned off or disconnected
- If the patient is in an awkward position, use cribbing or other tools to support them
- Machine parts may need to be immobilized to secure the disentanglement process

Crime Scene Awareness

Crime scenes present unique challenges. To you, the person in your care is the patient; to law enforcement, the same person may be a victim, perpetrator, or witness. In addition to treating the patient with dignity and respect, the paramedic must mindfully preserve evidence from both the patient's person and the scene. Since anything the patient says could become part of the legal record, documentation is even more critical than usual. As ever, personal and crew safety comes first; then the paramedic can turn attention to the patients.

Preparation

EMS uniforms, body armor, and standard operating procedures or standard operating guidelines (SOP/SOG) should be considered in responses to a potential or known crime scene.

EMS uniforms often resemble those of law enforcement, sometimes even including a badge. Consequently, a perpetrator could mistake the paramedic for a police officer. Paramedics can also be the intentional target of a perpetrator who does not want a patient to survive. With this in mind, many services require paramedics to wear ballistic vests as a matter of routine protection.

Body armor, in addition to ballistic vests, is recommended for paramedics entering a known violent situation. Body armor can be bulletproof, stab proof, or spike proof. Remember that wearing a vest or armor is not a free pass to enter any scene; wait for law enforcement direction before entering and follow any available SOP/SOG established by your agency.

Potentially Violent Situations

Domestic Violence

Any residential scene is potentially the site of domestic violence, even if that is not the call you received. Maintain situational awareness throughout patient contact. Following are a few points to remember:

- Identify primary and secondary exits before you begin.
- Note the location of items that could become a weapon (e.g., kitchen knives) and everyone's proximity to them.
- Be aware of your body language and tone of voice (be assertive but not aggressive), and select your words and conversational topics with care.
- Take steps to establish a zone of calm, and separate the two parties as needed for your own safety and security.

Domestic violence scenes present a danger to the paramedic until the aggressor has been removed and law enforcement has stabilized the scene.

Gang Violence

Gang violence is surging across America, and not just in cities. When exposed to gang violence, maintain situational awareness and seek protection from law enforcement as needed. Keep in mind that a rival gang member may object to your tireless work to save the life of a person they just tried to kill. To limit exposure to the crime scene, it is recommended that you load the patient quickly and move out of the immediate area before working on patient care.

Active Shooter and Hostage Situations

All mass shootings are active shooter situations until proven otherwise—that is, until the shooter has been neutralized through surrender or death.

During an active shooter situation where there are already confirmed or suspected casualties, EMS no longer waits to enter the area until the law enforcement operation is complete. Instead, EMS is incorporated into the law enforcement operation, as follows:

- Mixed team: usually 4 armed police officers and 1 paramedic
- Team moves through scene, stops when a patient is found
- Paramedic initiates brief care (e.g., START triage, tourniquet)
- Team retreats, delivers patient to dedicated triage/treatment area

Paramedics can prepare further for such operations by training to become tactical medics.

While a hostage situation involves injured people, there is usually no opportunity to enter and get them out. These operations often last for hours, during which the police are in charge until the hostage-taker is neutralized. Maintain situational awareness. Do not become a hostage yourself.

Meth Labs

Any dwelling that a paramedic enters on the job could house a clandestine drug lab, where drugs like meth are "cooked" using household chemicals. This presents several areas of concern for the paramedic.

- Lab operators have an interest in keeping the lab secret; they could resort to violence against you or the law enforcement there to protect you.
- Owners have been known to booby trap clandestine labs to prevent accidental discovery.
- These "labs" may be chemically unstable, capable of exploding with enough force to level a home or a block.

Be alert for people acting suspiciously or studying your movements. It may not be a meth lab, but it may be something you are not supposed to see.

Preserving Evidence

The paramedic is responsible for preserving all types of evidence from actual and possible crime scenes. These include testimonial evidence and physical evidence.

Testimonial evidence is information communicated by the patient or other people on scene.

- Mainly captured through the run report
- Consists of observations on the scene and the patient, carefully and thoroughly captured by the paramedic
- Avoids the paramedic's opinions or judgment, which would cast doubt on its accuracy
- Includes actual quotes when possible

Physical evidence can include any tangible item but usually refers to blood or bodily fluids, body parts, and objects. The paramedic must not disturb evidence but, rather, must preserve it with as little manipulation as possible.

- Do not move a person who is obviously deceased until the police or coroner can properly document. The location and position of the body are physical evidence.
- Stay clear of walls and avoid repositioning furniture, which could interfere with physical evidence (e.g., obscuring a blood spray pattern on the wall).
- Leave any objects that may have captured blood or hair where they lie (e.g., shell casings).
- If something must be moved to care for the patient, document it in the run report.

Practical Point

If moving something to access or extricate the patient becomes necessary, ensure that it is documented in the run report.

Finally, the very patient you transport is "evidence" in some cases. Some important points to remember in such a case are as follows.

- **Penetrating injury (bullet wound, stab wound):** Be careful to not cut the clothing off through the point of entry.
- **Removed items:** Carefully place all items removed from the patient into a paper bag; seal and mark the names, including the name of the person who bagged the items.
- **Trace evidence:** A patient who struggled with an assailant may have trace evidence under the fingernails. To preserve it, wrap the patient's hands in paper bags secured to the wrists.
- **Sexual assault:** Prevent the victim from showering, douching, changing clothes, washing the hands, or urinating, since doing so may alter or wash away crucial evidence.

Document anything that you needed to remove from the patient, where it was left at the hospital, and with whom. Document all PPE you were wearing and whether you were wearing gloves (so your fingerprints are not mistaken for those of the perpetrator). Document clearly and thoroughly, including observations on scene or on the patient, without passing judgment.

REVIEW QUESTIONS

Select the ONE best answer.

1. Which of the following provides the greatest protection to the paramedic from a droplet-borne infection?

    A. N95 mask on the paramedic
    B. N95 mask on the patient
    C. Surgical mask on the paramedic
    D. Surgical mask on the patient

2. Which of the following communication equipment devices has the greatest range of transmission?

    A. Base station radio
    B. Handheld portable radio alone
    C. Handheld portable radio connected to a mobile repeater
    D. Mobile radio

3. Which of the following frequencies would be classified as ultrahigh frequency (UHF)?

    A. 155 MHz
    B. 155 GHz
    C. 375 Hz
    D. 375 MHz

4. Which of the following is NOT a component of the SBAR communication mnemonic?

    A. Scene
    B. Background
    C. Assessment
    D. Recommendation

5. A plaintiff files a lawsuit against a paramedic for neglect and is awarded $200,000 for loss, pain, and suffering. The legal term for this type of payment is which of the following?

    A. Accidental damages
    B. Compensatory damages
    C. Criminal damages
    D. Punitive damages

6. You are on scene with a 17-year-old female who fell down 2 steps at her high school. The patient is conscious, alert, and oriented to person place, time, and event. She states that she wishes to refuse transport to the hospital and that she is entitled to make her own healthcare decisions because she has a 6-month-old baby at home. Should you allow this patient to sign the refusal-of-care form? Why or why not?

   A. Yes. Once a female has been pregnant, she is legally an adult regardless of age.

   B. Yes. She is oriented to person place and time, so taking her to the hospital constitutes kidnapping and false imprisonment.

   C. No. She is under age 18 and not currently pregnant, so she is still the responsibility of her parents/guardians.

   D. No. She should be evaluated at the hospital to rule out head injuries and other occult injuries.

7. You are visiting a theme park with your family when someone waiting in line near you collapses. You identify yourself as a paramedic and begin chest compressions but do not administer breaths to the patient, who you believe is in cardiac arrest. The patient dies, and the family later sues you for negligence because as a paramedic you knew to provide breaths for the patient but did not. If the plaintiffs prove this allegation, will they win? Why or why not?

   A. Yes. Since the patient died under your care, there was clear and present resultant harm.

   B. Yes. Since you identified yourself as a paramedic, you had a duty to act at the level of a trained paramedic.

   C. No. Since you were not on duty at the time, there was not a breach of duty.

   D. No. Since you could not have provided ventilations safely, there was not proximate cause.

8. Which of the following is an example of an advance directive?

   A. Do not resuscitate order

   B. Living will

   C. Organ donor card

   D. All of the above

9. Which of these places the steps of a water rescue in the proper order?

   A. Reach, Throw, Go, Row

   B. Reach, Throw, Row, Go

   C. Throw, Reach, Row, Go

   D. Throw, Row, Reach, Go

10. You are on scene with a person who has been shot in the right chest. It is a sucking chest wound, and the patient is having difficulty breathing. You successfully establish an IV on the second attempt. You should include in the documentation for this patient all of the following EXCEPT:

   A. Caliber of bullet casing found on scene

   B. Furniture you moved during access or extrication

   C. Location of the missed IV attempt

   D. Location of wounds you suspect are from the bullet

ANSWERS AND EXPLANATIONS

1. **The correct answer is (A).** When treating a patient suspected of having a droplet-borne infection, the paramedic gains the greatest protection by wearing an N95 mask. If the patient can tolerate it, the patient can wear a surgical mask for even greater protection against transmission.

2. **The correct answer is (A).** Of the options presented, the base station radio has the most power and therefore would have the greatest range of signal transmission. A handheld portable radio (B) by itself has the smallest range of the options presented. A portable radio connected to a mobile repeater within a vehicle (C) and a mobile radio mounted to the vehicle (D) have ranges of transmission that are approximately equal to each other but substantially less than that of a base station.

3. **The correct answer is (D).** A frequency of 375 MHz is in the UHF range, which is 300–3,000 MHz. A frequency of 155 MHz (A) is in the VHF range of 30–175 MHz, while 155 GHz (B) is in the infrared range and 375 Hz (C) is in the very low frequency range.

4. **The correct answer is (A).** The *S* in SBAR stands for *Situation*. (The full acronym stands for "Situation, Background, Assessment, Recommendation.") Situation may include a description of the scene from EMS; however, it also includes age, gender, and chief complaint.

5. **The correct answer is (B).** Compensatory damages are awarded to the plaintiff if the defendant is found liable for the wrongdoing alleged by the lawsuit. These fines compensate the plaintiff for loss, lost wages, hospital bills, pain and suffering, or any demonstrable cost resulting from the wrongdoing. Accidental damages (A) would not be assessed in a neglect lawsuit. Suit is filed for neglect in civil court, so criminal damages (C) would not be assessed. Punitive damages (D) are sometimes awarded in civil lawsuits as punishment to the defendant. In this case, however, nothing indicates that the monetary award is punishment for wrongdoing; the question stem describes compensation only for actual losses.

6. **The correct answer is (C).** Since this minor is no longer pregnant, she is no longer considered emancipated. Despite being a parent and having been pregnant in the past (A), she is legally a minor now and requires a parent, guardian, or in loco parentis to sign and take responsibility for the refusal. (She would be able to make decisions for her child, however.) Taking this patient to the hospital against her will (B) is not kidnapping or false imprisonment, because the patient is legally a minor; in the absence of a responsible adult, such transport would be covered under implied consent. Consent is the key issue in this scenario, not the patient's possible injuries (D).

7. **The correct answer is (C).** Since you were not on duty at the time, you are generally covered under the good Samaritan laws. Despite your higher level of training, you are not equipped to the same degree as a paramedic on a medic unit, and you did not have a duty to act. (Legally, you could have stood by and watched the medical emergency, though that may be considered unethical.) Therefore, there cannot be a breach of duty. Answer choice (A) is incorrect because the survival rate of people who undergo cardiac arrest is very low even with rapid provision of CPR; extensive injury of a kind not commonly seen in cardiac arrest patients would have to be present for resultant harm to be considered. Answer option (B) is also incorrect; even if you identified yourself as a paramedic, you are not legally held to the standard of care of an on-duty paramedic, provided you do not perform *outside the scope* of a paramedic. Answer choice (D) is incorrect because it is possible (though unlikely) that a lack of ventilation during a cardiac arrest could cause the cardiac arrest to continue.

8. **The correct answer is (D).** An advance directive is any document that communicates the wishes of a person who is competent prior to a decline in health or sudden event. All of the options listed (DNR order, living will, organ donor card) are examples of advance directives.

9. **The correct answer is (B).** Water rescues begin with attempts that are least risky for the rescuer and proceed to greater risk levels only when safer efforts fail. The proper order is: first, *Reach* out to the person if close to shore; then *Throw* a life ring to the person; next, *Row* (or motor) a boat to the person; and finally, tether yourself and *Go* out to the person on foot.

10. **The correct answer is (A).** The caliber of bullet is not needed for documentation or treatment by the paramedic. Documentation of the furniture you moved or touched (B) will help crime scene investigators return the room to its layout during the shooting. It is important to document the missed IV stick (C) to account for this wound; in the event of the patient's death, the wound may require explanation on postmortem. Location of wounds (D) is always important because it can shed light on the bodily structures affected.

Appendix: Medications

Acetaminophen	
Class	Analgesic/antipyretic
Mechanism	Acts on hypothalamus to reduce fever; blocks pain impulse generation
Indications	Fever >100.2 F (>37.9 C), febrile seizure, pediatric pain relief
Contraindications	Inability to swallow or lack of gag reflex; risk of seizure
Interactions	Rarely interacts with other medications
Form	Liquid suspension (oral)
Dosage	15 mg/kg to a maximum of 1,000 mg
Considerations	Use with caution in patients with liver failure, hepatitis, or cirrhosis

Activated Charcoal	
Class	Adsorbent
Mechanism	Toxic substances in the GI tract attached to it
Indications	Oral poisonings and overdoses within about an hour of ingestion
Contraindications	Unresponsive patient or patient unable to protect their own airway; ingestion of acids, bases, or petroleum products
Interactions	Aspiration can be fatal
Form	25 g suspended in 125 mL liquid
Dosage	1–2 g/kg
Considerations	Mix and shake well

Adenosine

Class	Antidysrhythmic
Mechanism	Slows conduction through the AV node, disrupting reentry pathways
Indications	Paroxysmal SVT, SVT unresponsive to vagal maneuver
Contraindications	Sick sinus syndrome, junctional rhythms, 2nd- and 3rd-degree blocks, bronchoconstrictive lung disease
Interactions	Methylxanthines antagonize; carbamazepine potentiates
Form	3 mg/mL in 2 mL vials, 12 mg prefilled syringes
Dosage	1st dose: 6 mg rapid intravenous bolus followed by a 10 mL flush; 2nd and 3rd doses: 12 mg rapid intravenous bolus followed by flush
Considerations	Short half-life and duration of action; patient may pass out

Albuterol

Class	Sympathomimetic
Mechanism	Beta-2 agonist
Indications	Bronchospasm in COPD and patients with asthma
Contraindications	Hypersensitivity
Interactions	Beta-blockers may antagonize effects; tricyclic antidepressants may potentiate vascular effects
Form	2.5 mg in 3 mL solution for nebulization or MDI
Dosage	2.5 mg diluted to 3 mL in a nebulizer with 6–10 LPM O_2
Considerations	May cause tachycardia and feelings of anxiety

Alteplase

Class	Fibrinolytic
Mechanism	Converts plasminogen to plasmin, which digests fibrin strands in a clot
Indications	AMI, PE, and CVA
Contraindications	Active bleeding; recent surgery; previous CVA, CPR, AVM or aneurysm; uncontrolled hypertension
Interactions	Anticoagulants increase risk of bleeding
Form	50 mg and 100 mg powders that need to be reconstituted to 1 mg/mL
Dosage	15 mg bolus over 2 minutes, followed by 0.75 mg/kg infusion over 30 minutes to a maximum of 50 mg/kg
Considerations	Monitor vital signs and watch for bleeding

Amiodarone	
Class	Antidysrhythmic
Mechanism	Blocks cardiac Na^+ and K^+ channels, delaying repolarization
Indications	VF, VT
Contraindications	Hypersensitivity and STs with aberrancy
Interactions	May precipitate digitalis toxicity; beta-blockers and calcium channel blockers may cause sinus arrest; AV blocks
Form	50 mg/mL vials and prefilled syringes
Dosage	VF/pulseless VT: 300 mg as intravenous bolus; 150 mg after 3–5 minutes if no response; stable VT with pulses: 150 mg over 10 minutes
Considerations	Foams when shaken; may increase hypotension

Amyl Nitrite	
Class	Cyanide poisoning antidote
Mechanism	Prevents cyanide's toxic effects by converting hemoglobin to methemoglobin
Indications	Cyanide poisoning
Contraindications	None
Interactions	Antihypertensives, beta-blockers, and alcohol will worsen hypotension
Form	0.3 mg ampules for inhalation
Dosage	1–2 ampules crushed and inhaled for 30–60 seconds; repeat every 5 minutes until conscious
Considerations	Highly flammable; psychoactive recreational use; 1st step of 3-step treatment, followed by sodium nitrite and sodium thiosulfate

Aspirin	
Class	Antiplatelet and anti-inflammatory
Mechanism	Prevents platelets from aggregating
Indications	Chest pain of a cardiac origin
Contraindications	Hypersensitivity, active bleeding, or ulcers
Interactions	None
Form	81 mg chewable tablets
Dosage	162–324 mg, chewed
Considerations	Not recommended for children

Atenolol	
Class	Beta-1 selective antagonist
Mechanism	Decreases HR, cardiac contractility, and cardiac output
Indications	Hypertension, SVT, AF, atrial flutter; reduces myocardial damage during AMI
Contraindications	Heart failure, cardiogenic shock, bradycardia, lung disease, and hypotension
Interactions	Potentiates antihypertensive effects of calcium channel blockers and monoamine oxidase inhibitors (MAOIs)
Form	5 mg in 10 mL ampules
Dosage	5 mg for 5 minutes; repeat dose in 10 minutes
Considerations	Use with caution in patients with liver and renal dysfunction and patients with COPD

Atropine	
Class	Anticholinergic
Mechanism	Inhibits ACH at postsynaptic receptors; increases HR in sinus bradydysrhythmias
Indications	Hemodynamically significant bradycardia and organophosphate poisoning
Contraindications	AMI and myocardial ischemia
Interactions	Effects enhanced by antihistamines, procainamide, antipsychotics, and benzodiazepines
Form	1 mg in 10 mL prefilled syringes
Dosage	0.5–1 mg as intravenous bolus; repeatable to a maximum of 3 mg
Considerations	None

Benzocaine	
Class	Topical anesthetic
Mechanism	Blocks initiation and conduction of nerve impulses
Indications	Suppression of gag reflex during intubation
Contraindications	Hypersensitivity
Interactions	None
Form	Aerosol can of 20% benzocaine
Dosage	1-second long spray; repeated as needed
Considerations	Topical only

Bumetanide

Class	Loop diuretic
Mechanism	Inhibits reabsorption of sodium and chloride ions in the ascending limb of the loop of Henle
Indications	Pulmonary edema and CHF
Contraindications	Hypersensitivity and renal failure
Interactions	May increase risk of lithium poisoning
Form	0.25 mg/mL vials
Dosage	0.5–1 mg intravenously for 1–2 minutes
Considerations	1 mg bumetanide is equal to 40 mg furosemide

Calcium Chloride

Class	Electrolyte
Mechanism	Positive inotrope and ventricular automaticity
Indications	Hypocalcemia, hyperkalemia, hypermagnesemia, and beta-blocker and calcium channel blocker overdose
Contraindications	VF and digitalis toxicity
Interactions	Do not administer in the same intravenous line as sodium bicarbonate
Form	1 g in 10 mL prefilled syringe
Dosage	1 g, repeated as needed
Considerations	Do not use routinely in cardiac arrest

Calcium Gluconate

Class	Electrolyte
Mechanism	Positive inotrope and ventricular automaticity
Indications	Hypocalcemia, hyperkalemia, hypermagnesemia, and beta-blocker and calcium channel blocker overdose
Contraindications	VF and digitalis toxicity
Interactions	Do not administer in the same intravenous as sodium bicarbonate
Form	1 g in 10 mL prefilled syringe
Dosage	1 g, repeated as needed
Considerations	Do not use routinely in cardiac arrest

Clopidogrel

Class	Antiplatelet
Mechanism	Glycoprotein IIb/IIIa inhibitor
Indications	AMI and acute coronary syndromes
Contraindications	Active bleeding and ICH
Interactions	Should not be taken with proton pump inhibitors
Form	75 mg and 300 mg tablets
Dosage	300–600 mg loading dose
Considerations	None

Dexamethasone

Class	Corticosteroid
Mechanism	Suppresses acute and chronic inflammation
Indications	Anaphylaxis, asthma, COPD, and spinal cord injury
Contraindications	Hypersensitivity and uncontrolled infection
Interactions	Calcium
Form	100 mg/5 mL vials
Dosage	1 mg/kg as intravenous bolus
Considerations	Protect from heat

Dextrose (D50)

Class	Carbohydrate
Mechanism	Increased serum glucose levels
Indications	Hypoglycemia
Contraindications	Intracranial hemorrhage
Interactions	Sodium bicarbonate
Form	25 g in 50 mL prefilled syringe
Dosage	12.5–25 g
Considerations	Dilute for pediatric patients

Diazepam

Class	Benzodiazepine
Mechanism	Induces amnesia and sedation
Indications	Severe anxiety, seizures, and alcohol withdrawal
Contraindications	Hypersensitivity, glaucoma, myasthenia gravis, and head injury
Interactions	Incompatible with most drugs
Form	10 mg in 2 mL prefilled syringes
Dosage	5–10 mg slowly via intravenous administration
Considerations	Seizures may reoccur

Digoxin

Class	Inotropic agent
Mechanism	Positive inotrope; increases AV node refractory period
Indications	CHF, AF with rapid ventricular response, and atrial flutter
Contraindications	VF, VT, and hypersensitivity
Interactions	Amiodarone, verapamil, and quinidine
Form	0.25 mg/mL vials
Dosage	4–6 mcg/kg for 5 minutes
Considerations	Keep patient on a monitor

Diltiazem

Class	Calcium channel blocker
Mechanism	Reduces preload and afterload; blocks cardiac calcium channels during depolarization
Indications	AF with rapid ventricular response and SVT
Contraindications	Hypotension, sick sinus syndrome with no pacemaker, cardiogenic shock, and VT
Interactions	Avoid in patients on beta-blockers
Form	5 mg/mL (refrigerated)
Dosage	0.25 mg/kg for 2 minutes
Considerations	Caution in renal and hepatic insufficiency

Diphenhydramine

Class	Antihistamine and anticholinergic
Mechanism	Blocks histamine receptors; vasoconstricts
Indications	Allergic reactions and anaphylaxis
Contraindications	Asthma, pregnancy, glaucoma, hypertension, children, and MAOIs
Interactions	Potentiates alcohol and other anticholinergics; MAOIs prolong effects
Form	50 mg/mL vials
Dosage	25–50 mg either intramuscularly or as intravenous bolus
Considerations	None

Dobutamine

Class	Sympathomimetic
Mechanism	Increases myocardial stroke volume, contractility, and output without increasing HR
Indications	CHF and cardiogenic shock
Contraindications	Tachydysrhythmias and severe hypotension
Interactions	Incompatible with furosemide and bicarbonate
Form	1 mg/mL intravenous infusion
Dosage	2–20 mcg/kg/min, titrated to effect
Considerations	May increase infarct in patients with active AMI

Dopamine

Class	Sympathomimetic
Mechanism	Increases myocardial stroke volume, contractility, HR, and cardiac output; increases peripheral vascular resistance and preload while maintaining renal and mesenteric blood flow
Indications	CHF and cardiogenic shock
Contraindications	Tachydysrhythmias, severe hypotension, and pheochromocytoma
Interactions	MAOIs potentiate; beta-blockers and bicarbonate inhibit
Form	200 mg/5 mL vials
Dosage	Dilute 200 mg in 250 mL D5W; 2–20 mcg/kg/min, titrated to effect
Considerations	May increase infarct in patients with active AMI

Epinephrine, 1:1,000

Class	Sympathomimetic
Mechanism	Alpha, beta-1, and beta-2 agonist
Indications	Anaphylaxis and asthma
Contraindications	None in emergency setting
Interactions	MAOIs potentiate; beta-blockers and bicarbonate inhibit
Form	1 mg in 1 mL ampule
Dosage	0.3 mg intramuscularly or subcutaneously
Considerations	Increases myocardial O_2 demand

Epinephrine, 1:10,000

Class	Sympathomimetic
Mechanism	Alpha, beta-1, and beta-2 agonist
Indications	Cardiac arrest
Contraindications	None in emergency setting
Interactions	MAOIs potentiate; beta-blockers and bicarbonate inhibit
Form	1 mg in 10 mL prefilled syringe
Dosage	1 mg as intravenous bolus every 3–5 minutes during the arrest; double dose for ETT
Considerations	Increases myocardial O_2 demand

Epinephrine, Racemic

Class	Sympathomimetic
Mechanism	Alpha, beta-1, and beta-2 agonist
Indications	Anaphylaxis, asthma, croup
Contraindications	Epiglottitis and hypertension
Interactions	MAOIs potentiate; beta-blockers and bicarbonate inhibit
Form	0.16 mg in MDI
Dosage	2–3 puffs every 3–5 minutes as needed
Considerations	Increases myocardial O_2 demand

Eptifibatide	
Class	Glycoprotein IIb/IIIa inhibitor
Mechanism	Inhibits platelet aggregation and prevents binding of fibrinogen and von Willebrand factors
Indications	Angina, ACS, and Percutaneous Transluminal Coronary Angioplasty (PTCA)
Contraindications	Prior ICH, AAA, active bleeding or bleeding disorder, recent head or facial trauma, or ischemic stroke within past 3 months
Interactions	Incompatible with furosemide
Form	2 mg/mL vials
Dosage	180 mcg/kg as intravenous bolus over 1–2 minutes
Considerations	Avoid invasive procedures with risk of bleeding; must be administered directly from the glass bottle with vented intravenous setup

Etomidate	
Class	Hypnotic
Mechanism	Acts on reticular activating system
Indications	Premedication for intubation or cardioversion
Contraindications	Hypersensitivity
Interactions	None
Form	2 mg/mL vials
Dosage	0.2–0.6 mg/kg intravenously infused over 30–60 seconds
Considerations	Consider decreasing dose in older adults

Fentanyl	
Class	Opiate analgesic
Mechanism	Binds to opiate receptors
Indications	Pain management
Contraindications	Hypersensitivity
Interactions	None
Form	100 mcg/2 mL ampules
Dosage	1 mcg/kg slowly
Considerations	Chest wall rigidity with rapid high dose

Flumazenil	
Class	Benzodiazepine antagonist
Mechanism	Reverses sedative effects
Indications	Respiratory depression because of benzodiazepines
Contraindications	Hypersensitivity and tricyclic antidepressant overdose
Interactions	Tricyclic antidepressants
Form	0.1 mg/mL vials
Dosage	First dose: 0.2 mg intravenously or intraosseously; 2nd dose: 0.3 mg intravenously or intraosseously; 3rd dose: 0.5 mg intravenously or intraosseously
Considerations	May precipitate seizures in patients who take benzodiazepines regularly

Fosphenytoin	
Class	Anticonvulsant
Mechanism	Inhibits calcium movement across neuronal membrane; increases neuronal excitability
Indications	Seizures
Contraindications	Hypersensitivity and bradycardias
Interactions	Dopamine can cause severe hypotension; additive effect with other CNS depressants
Form	75 mg/mL vials
Dosage	15–20 mg PE/kg intravenously; infuse at 100–150 mg PE/min
Considerations	Use caution in patients with renal and hepatic insufficiency. Dosing is expressed in Phenytoin Equivalents (PE) to avoid dose conversions between products.

Furosemide	
Class	Loop diuretic
Mechanism	Inhibits reabsorption of sodium and chloride ions in the ascending limb of the loop of Henle
Indications	Pulmonary edema and CHF
Contraindications	Hypersensitivity, renal failure, and hypovolemia
Interactions	May increase risk of lithium poisoning
Form	10 mg/mL vials
Dosage	0.5–1 mg/kg intravenously over 1–2 minutes
Considerations	Ototoxic; projectile vomiting can occur with rapid infusion

Glucagon	
Class	Pancreatic hormone
Mechanism	Increased blood glucose level by releasing glycogen stores in the liver
Indications	Hypoglycemia and beta-blocker overdose
Contraindications	Hyperglycemia
Interactions	None
Form	1 mg powder requiring reconstitution with 1 mL saline
Dosage	Hypoglycemia: 1 mg intramuscularly; beta-blocker overdose: 3–10 mg intravenously over 10 minutes
Considerations	Ineffective with no glycogen stores

Haloperidol	
Class	Tranquilizer
Mechanism	Inhibits CNS catecholamine receptors and ascending reticular activating system
Indications	Acute psychosis
Contraindications	Parkinson disease; agitation from shock, hypoxia, or other source
Interactions	Alcohol potentiates; amphetamines and epinephrine antagonize
Form	5 mg/mL vials and ampules
Dosage	2–5 mg every 30–60 minutes
Considerations	Treat resulting hypotension with fluids and norepinephrine

Heparin	
Class	Anticoagulant
Mechanism	Prevents conversion of fibrinogen to fibrin
Indications	AMI and prophylaxis of clotting issues
Contraindications	Hypersensitivity, active bleeding, recent surgery, and thrombocytopenia
Interactions	None
Form	25,000 units/500 mL
Dosage	60 units/kg up to 4,000 units
Considerations	Does not lyse existing clots

Hydrocortisone

Class	Corticosteroid
Mechanism	Suppresses acute and chronic inflammation
Indications	Anaphylaxis, asthma, COPD, and spinal cord injury
Contraindications	Hypersensitivity, fungal infection, and premature infants
Interactions	Incompatible with heparin
Form	500 mg powder with reconstituting diluent
Dosage	4 mg/kg slowly
Considerations	None

Hydroxocobalamin

Class	Cyanide antidote
Mechanism	Binds with cyanide to form cyanocobalamin
Indications	Cyanide poisoning
Contraindications	None
Interactions	Avoid using the same intravenous line as other medications
Form	2.5 g in 250 mL glass vial
Dosage	5 g over 15 minutes
Considerations	Patient may become hypertensive (180/110 common)

Hydroxyzine

Class	Antihistamine, antiemetic, and anxiolytic
Mechanism	Potentiates analgesics
Indications	Nausea and vomiting
Contraindications	Hypersensitivity and early pregnancy
Interactions	Potentiates CNS depressants
Form	50 mg/mL vials
Dosage	25–100 mg intramuscularly only
Considerations	Injection site burning

Ipratropium

Class	Anticholinergic, bronchodilator
Mechanism	Inhibits ACH receptor sites of bronchial smooth muscle
Indications	Asthma and COPD
Contraindications	Hypersensitivity to atropine, alkaloids, and peanuts
Interactions	None
Form	0.5 mg/mL for nebulizer
Dosage	0.5 mg/mL for nebulizer
Considerations	Use after at least 1 dose of nebulized beta-agonist

Ketamine

Class	General anesthetic
Mechanism	Produces dissociative anesthesia by blocking NMDA receptors
Indications	Excited delirium; analgesia
Contraindications	Hypersensitivity; use with caution in schizophrenic patients, patients experiencing hallucinations or delusions, intoxicated patients, and chronic alcoholics
Interactions	May intensify the effects of other sedatives and pain medications
Form	10 mg/mL vials, 50 mg/mL vials, 100 mg/mL vials
Dosage	Excited delirium: 4 mg/kg intramuscularly or 2 mg/kg intravenously; analgesia: 0.2 mg/kg in 100 mL normal saline solution infused over 10 minutes
Considerations	Can increase HR, blood pressure, cardiac output, and myocardial oxygen demand

Ketorolac

Class	NSAID
Mechanism	Analgesic that does not sedate
Indications	Moderate to severe pain
Contraindications	Allergies to severe pain or other NSAIDs; patients with asthma, renal failure, or GI bleeding
Interactions	None
Form	30 mg/mL vials
Dosage	30–60 mg intramuscularly
Considerations	None

Labetalol

Class	Selective alpha blocker; nonselective beta-blocker
Mechanism	Total peripheral vascular resistance reduced without altering cardiac output
Indications	Hypertension
Contraindications	Asthma, CHF, cardiogenic shock, and bradycardias
Interactions	May inhibit bronchodilator effects of other beta-agonists
Form	5 mg/mL vials
Dosage	10 mg as intravenous bolus
Considerations	Closely monitor vital signs and ECG for signs of cardiogenic shock, bradycardias, and bronchospasm

Lidocaine

Class	Antidysrhythmic
Mechanism	Slows the rate of spontaneous phase 4 depolarization
Indications	VT and VF
Contraindications	Hypersensitivity
Interactions	Potentiates succinylcholine; procainamide exacerbates CNS depression
Form	20 mg/mL in prefilled syringe
Dosage	Initial: 1.5 mg/kg; repeat doses 0.75 mg/kg every 10 minutes until 3 mg/kg total
Considerations	High doses can result in seizures, coma, or death

Lorazepam

Class	Benzodiazepine
Mechanism	Anxiolytic, anticonvulsant, and sedative
Indications	Seizures and anxiety
Contraindications	Glaucoma and drug abuse
Interactions	Additive effects with other CNS depressants
Form	2 mg/mL prefilled syringes
Dosage	2–4 mg intramuscularly or intravenously; may be repeated
Considerations	Monitor respiratory rate and blood pressure

Magnesium Sulfate	
Class	Electrolyte
Mechanism	Reduces ACH release at the neuromuscular junction for smooth muscles
Indications	Hypomagnesemia, torsade de pointes, and eclampsia
Contraindications	Heart blocks
Interactions	Changes in cardiac function with cardiac glycosides
Form	0.5 mg/mL vials
Dosage	Seizures: 1–4 g over 3 minutes; torsade: 1–2 g for 5 minutes; asthma: 1–2 g over 3 minutes
Considerations	Calcium should be available as an antagonist if needed

Mannitol	
Class	Osmotic diuretic
Mechanism	Promotes movement of fluid from intracellular space to extracellular space
Indications	Cerebral edema, ICH, and rhabdomyolysis
Contraindications	CHF, hypotension, and pulmonary edema
Interactions	Digitalis
Form	200 mg/mL solution for intravenous piggyback bolus
Dosage	1 g/kg over 10 minutes
Considerations	May crystallize in cold; have ventilatory support available

Meperidine	
Class	Opiate analgesic
Mechanism	Binds to opiate receptors
Indications	Pain management
Contraindications	Hypersensitivity, undiagnosed head injury, or abdominal pain
Interactions	Do not give with current or recent MAOI use
Form	100 mg/mL prefilled syringes
Dosage	50–100 mg intramuscularly or subcutaneously; 25–50 mg intravenously
Considerations	May precipitate seizures in those with a history

Metaproterenol	
Class	Beta-2 agonist
Mechanism	Bronchial smooth muscle relaxant
Indications	Asthma and COPD
Contraindications	Hypersensitivity and tachydysrhythmias
Interactions	Additive effects with other sympathomimetics; beta-blockers antagonize
Form	MDI: 0.65 mg/puff
Dosage	2–3 puffs every 3 hours
Considerations	May cause hypotension and tachycardia

Methylprednisolone	
Class	Corticosteroid
Mechanism	Suppresses acute and chronic inflammation
Indications	Anaphylaxis, asthma, COPD, and spinal cord injury
Contraindications	Hypersensitivity, fungal infection, and premature infants
Interactions	Incompatible with heparin
Form	250 mg powder with reconstituting diluent
Dosage	Spinal: 30 mg/kg over 30 minutes; respiratory: 1–2 mg/kg as intravenous bolus
Considerations	Crosses placental barrier

Metoprolol	
Class	Beta-1 selective
Mechanism	Negative inotrope and dromotrope
Indications	SVT, AF, atrial flutter, and AMI
Contraindications	Heart failure, cardiogenic shock, and bradydysrhythmias
Interactions	MAOIs and calcium channel blockers potentiate
Form	1 mg/mL ampules
Dosage	Three 5 mg doses at 5-minute intervals
Considerations	Concurrent intravenous calcium channel blocker use may cause severe hypotension

Midazolam

Class	Benzodiazepine
Mechanism	Binds with GABA receptors in brain to produce sedation
Indications	Sedation for procedures
Contraindications	Glaucoma
Interactions	CNS depressants
Form	1 mg/mL vials
Dosage	2–5 mg as intravenous bolus
Considerations	Monitor cardiac and respiratory function

Morphine Sulfate

Class	Opiate analgesic
Mechanism	Binds to opiate receptors
Indications	Pain management
Contraindications	Hypersensitivity, undiagnosed head injury, or abdominal pain
Interactions	Do not give with current or recent MAOI use
Form	100 mg/mL prefilled syringes
Dosage	2–4 mg as intravenous bolus, repeatable
Considerations	Crosses placental barrier

Naloxone

Class	Opiate antagonist
Mechanism	Competitive inhibition at opiate receptors
Indications	Opiate overdose
Contraindications	Use with caution in patients who are narcotic dependent
Interactions	Incompatible with bisulfite and alkaline solutions
Form	1 mg/mL vials and prefilled syringes
Dosage	0.4–2 mg intravenously, intramuscularly, intranasally, subcutaneously, or via ETT
Considerations	May need to readminister because of short half-life; may cause vomiting; patient may be violent after receiving

Nifedipine	
Class	Calcium channel blocker
Mechanism	Inhibits movement of calcium ions across cell membrane
Indications	Hypertensive crisis and angina
Contraindications	Compensatory HTN, cardiogenic shock
Interactions	Beta-blockers potentiate
Form	10 and 20 mg liquid-filled capsules
Dosage	10 mg sublingually or buccally; have the patient bite the capsule and swallow
Considerations	Have beta-blocker available for reflex tachycardia

Nitroglycerine	
Class	Vasodilator
Mechanism	Relaxes vascular, GI, and uterine smooth muscle; reduces preload
Indications	Chest pain, AMI, CHF, and pulmonary edema
Contraindications	Hypotension, hypovolemia, emergency department medications within the last 48 hours
Interactions	Additive effects with other vasodilators
Form	0.4 mg tablets, 6 g tubes
Dosage	0.4 mg sublingually for angina; 0.4–1.2 mg for CHF; 1/2–1-inch paste
Considerations	Avoid giving in a right-sided MI until fluid can be administered; keep in a dark container

Nitrous Oxide	
Class	Gaseous analgesic
Mechanism	Unknown
Indications	Pain relief
Contraindications	Decreased level of consciousness, head injury, unable to follow instructions, and abdominal pain
Interactions	None
Form	D&E cylinders
Dosage	Have patient inhale deeply until pain is relieved
Considerations	Causes spontaneous abortion; ventilate area well

Norepinephrine	
Class	Sympathomimetic
Mechanism	Potent alpha agonist results in peripheral vasoconstriction; positive chronotrope and inotrope
Indications	Cardiogenic shock and significant hypotension
Contraindications	Hypotension caused by hypovolemia
Interactions	Sympathomimetics exacerbate dysrhythmias
Form	1 mg/mL vials
Dosage	Dilute 8 mg in 500 mL bag and infuse as intravenous piggyback at 0.1–2 mcg/kg/min, titrated to effect
Considerations	May cause fetal anoxia

Ondansetron	
Class	Antiemetic
Mechanism	Blocks action of serotonin, which causes vomiting
Indications	For prevention of vomiting
Contraindications	Allergy to medication or other similar medications
Interactions	None in the emergency situation
Form	2 mg/mL vials
Dosage	4 mg as intravenous bolus or intramuscularly; repeatable
Considerations	None

Oral Glucose	
Class	Carbohydrate
Mechanism	Increases blood glucose levels
Indications	Hypoglycemia
Contraindications	Decreased level of consciousness, nausea, and vomiting
Interactions	None
Form	15 g tubes of gel
Dosage	15–45 g by mouth
Considerations	Must be swallowed, so it is slow to act

Oxygen	
Class	Gas
Mechanism	Reverses hypoxemia
Indications	Hypoxemia and shock
Contraindications	High concentrations for patients with COPD and premature infants
Interactions	None
Form	O_2 cylinders
Dosage	1–15 LPM
Considerations	None

Oxytocin	
Class	Hormone
Mechanism	Increases uterine contractions
Indications	Postpartum hemorrhage
Contraindications	2nd fetus
Interactions	None
Form	10 units/mL
Dosage	10 units intramuscularly
Considerations	Monitor vital signs

Pancuronium	
Class	Paralytic
Mechanism	Blocks ACH receptors at the neuromuscular junction
Indications	Induction or maintenance of paralysis
Contraindications	Hypersensitivity and inability to control airway once given
Interactions	Positive chronotropes potentiate effects
Form	2 mg/mL vials and ampules
Dosage	0.1 mg/kg as slow intravenous bolus
Considerations	Prepare intubation equipment and have ventilatory support available prior to giving

Phenobarbital

Class	Barbiturate
Mechanism	Generally unknown
Indications	Seizures
Contraindications	Patients with a history of sedative or hypnotic addiction
Interactions	Additive effects with other CNS depressants, anticonvulsants, and MAOIs
Form	60 mg/mL vials and ampules
Dosage	100–250 mg as intravenous bolus
Considerations	Use with caution in older adults; decrease dosage

Phenytoin

Class	Anticonvulsant
Mechanism	Moves sodium out of the neuron, which reduces excitability; does the same in the ventricles
Indications	Seizures and digitalis-induced dysrhythmias
Contraindications	Hypersensitivity and bradydysrhythmias
Interactions	Sulfonamides anticoagulant; salicylates potentiate; may precipitate
Form	50 mg/mL vials
Dosage	10–20 mg/kg a slow intravenous bolus to a max of 1 g
Considerations	None

Pralidoxime

Class	Cholinesterase reactivator
Mechanism	Reactivates cholinesterase in the neuromuscular junction
Indications	Organophosphate poisoning
Contraindications	None
Interactions	Avoid concurrent use with respiratory depressants
Form	1 g powder for reconstitution
Dosage	1–2 g infusion over 30 minutes
Considerations	None

Procainamide	
Class	Antidysrhythmic
Mechanism	Reduces ectopic pacemaker's automaticity and intraventricular conduction
Indications	Monomorphic VT, reentry SVT refractory to adenosine, and AF with rapid ventricular response
Contraindications	Torsade de pointes and bradycardias
Interactions	Increases plasma levels of amiodarone and quinidine
Form	500 mg vials
Dosage	50 mg/min to a max of 17 mg/kg; stop administration if QRS widens by >50% over baseline; dysrhythmia suppressed
Considerations	Potent vasodilator and negative inotrope

Propofol	
Class	Sedative
Mechanism	Rapid onset sedation and anesthesia
Indications	Induction and maintenance of anesthesia and sedation
Contraindications	Hypovolemia and sensitivities to soy, peanuts, and eggs
Interactions	None
Form	10 mg/mL intravenous emulsion
Dosage	Induction: 1.5–3 mg/kg intravenous or intraosseously; maintenance: 25–75 mcg/kg/min as intravenous piggyback
Considerations	None

Propranolol	
Class	Beta-blocker
Mechanism	Nonselective blocker and negative chronotrope and inotrope
Indications	Hypertension, chest pain, VT, and VF
Contraindications	Bradydysrhythmias, cardiogenic shock, and CHF
Interactions	Effects reversed by norepinephrine and dopamine
Form	1 mg/mL vials
Dosage	1–3 mg diluted in 10–30 mL D5W, given at a max of 1 mg/min, with max total 5 mg
Considerations	Keep atropine available

Rocuronium

Class	Paralytic
Mechanism	Blocks ACH receptors at the neuromuscular junction
Indications	Induction or maintenance of paralysis
Contraindications	Hypersensitivity and inability to control airway once given
Interactions	Positive chronotropes potentiate effects
Form	10 mg/mL vials
Dosage	0.1 mg/kg as slow intravenous bolus
Considerations	Prepare intubation equipment and have ventilatory support available prior to giving

Sodium Bicarbonate

Class	Alkalinizing agent
Mechanism	Buffers metabolic acidosis
Indications	Metabolic acidosis in cardiac arrest and tricyclic antidepressant and aspirin overdoses
Contraindications	Alkalosis and hypokalemia
Interactions	Should not be used in the same intravenous line as calcium
Form	1 mEq/mL in 50 mL prefilled syringe
Dosage	1 mEq/kg as intravenous bolus
Considerations	Repeat as needed in tricyclic antidepressant overdose

Sodium Nitrate

Class	Cyanide antidote
Mechanism	Reacts with hemoglobin to form methemoglobin
Indications	Cyanide poisoning
Contraindications	None
Interactions	None
Form	30 mg/mL vials
Dosage	300 mg for 10 minutes
Considerations	Potent vasodilator will cause significant hypotension if given too rapidly; 2nd drug in 3-step treatment after amyl nitrite

Sodium Thiosulfate

Class	Cyanide antidote
Mechanism	Converts cyanide to nontoxic thiocyanate
Indications	Cyanide poisoning
Contraindications	None
Interactions	None
Form	12.5 g/50 mL vial
Dosage	12.5 g for 10 minutes
Considerations	3rd step in 3-step treatment after sodium nitrite

Streptokinase

Class	Fibrinolytic
Mechanism	Converts plasminogen to plasmin, which digests fibrin strands in a clot
Indications	AMI, PE, and CVA
Contraindications	Active bleeding; recent surgery; previous CVA, CPR, AVM or aneurysm; and uncontrolled hypertension
Interactions	Anticoagulants increase risk of bleeding
Form	250,000; 750,000; and 1.5 million unit powders that need to be reconstituted
Dosage	0.5–1.5 million units diluted to 45 mL, given over 1 hour
Considerations	Monitor vital signs and watch for bleeding

Succinylcholine Chloride

Class	Depolarizing paralytic
Mechanism	Attaches to ACH receptors in the neuromuscular junction, depolarizing the muscle
Indications	Rapid sequence intubation
Contraindications	Glaucoma, eye injuries, malignant hyperthermia, multisystem trauma, and major burns
Interactions	Oxytocin, beta-blockers, and organophosphates potentiate
Form	20 mg/mL vials
Dosage	1.5 mg/kg rapid as intravenous bolus
Considerations	Premedication with lidocaine may blunt increase in ICP; benzodiazepines should be used 1st in the conscious patient

Terbutaline

Class	Beta-2 selective agonist
Mechanism	Smooth muscle relaxant in bronchioles
Indications	Asthma and COPD
Contraindications	Hypersensitivity
Interactions	MAOIs and other sympathomimetics potentiate; beta-blockers antagonize
Form	1 mg/mL vials
Dosage	0.25 mg subcutaneously; repeatable once
Considerations	Use with caution in patients diagnosed with diabetes or hypertension and have had a seizure

Thiamine

Class	Vitamin
Mechanism	Necessary for carbohydrate metabolism
Indications	Coma of unknown origin, delirium tremens, beri-beri, and Wernicke encephalopathy
Contraindications	None
Interactions	Always give thiamine before dextrose
Form	100 mg/mL vials
Dosage	100 mg intravenous or intramuscularly
Considerations	Large doses associated with respiratory issues and hypotension

Tirofiban

Class	Glycoprotein IIb/IIIa inhibitor
Mechanism	Inhibits platelet aggregation and prevents binding of fibrinogen
Indications	Angina, ACS, and PTCA
Contraindications	Prior ICH, AAA, active bleeding or bleeding disorder, recent head or facial trauma, and ischemic stroke within past 3 months
Interactions	None
Form	50 mcg/mL vials
Dosage	0.4 mcg/kg/min intravenously over 30 minutes
Considerations	Avoid invasive procedures with risk of bleeding; must be administered directly from the glass bottle with vented intravenous setup

Vasopressin	
Class	Vasopressor
Mechanism	Potent vasoconstrictor in high doses
Indications	Alternative to 1st or 2nd dose of epinephrine in cardiac arrest
Contraindications	None in emergency setting
Interactions	None
Form	20 units/mL vials
Dosage	40 units
Considerations	None

Vecuronium	
Class	Paralytic
Mechanism	Blocks ACH receptors at the neuromuscular junction
Indications	Induction or maintenance of paralysis
Contraindications	Hypersensitivity and inability to control airway once given
Interactions	Positive chronotropes potentiate effects
Form	2 mg/mL vials and ampules
Dosage	20 mg powder
Considerations	Prepare intubation equipment and have ventilatory support available prior to giving

Verapamil	
Class	Calcium channel blocker
Mechanism	Selectively blocks calcium channels in cardiac and arterial smooth muscles
Indications	SVT, AF, and atrial flutter
Contraindications	Wolff-Parkinson-White syndrome, Lown-Ganong-Levine syndrome, bradycardias without pacemaker, cardiogenic shock, LV EF <30%
Interactions	Additive effects with beta-blockers; potentiates antihypertensives
Form	2.5 mg/mL vials
Dosage	2.5–5 mg as intravenous bolus over 2 minutes
Considerations	Be prepared to resuscitate; AV blocks and asystole may occur

Index

Supine hypotension syndrome, 309
Suppository dosage form, 20
Suppressor T-cells, 210, 211
Supraglottic airways, 74
Supraventricular tachycardia, 118
Surfactant, 63
Surgical cricothyrotomy, 76–77
Suspension dosage form, 20
Sutures of immovable joints, 366, 374
Swallowing, 240
S waves, 108
    cardiac conduction system, 104
    conduction disturbances, 136–141
Sympathetic nervous system
    anatomy, 169, 170
    cardiac control, 105
    digestion, 239
Sympathomimetics
    albuterol, 442
    dobutamine, 448
    dopamine, 448
    epinephrine (1:1,000), 449
    epinephrine (1:10,000), 449
    epinephrine (racemic), 449
    norepinephrine, 460
    toxidromes, 228
Symptoms, in patient assessment, 48
Synapse, 179, 183
Synaptic boutons, 179
Synchronized cardioversion, 159–161
Syncope, 192
    vasovagal reactions, 36
Synergism of drugs, 229
Synovial capsule, 366
    synovial fluid, 366
    synovium, 366
Synthetic cannabinoids, 236–237
Synthetic marijuana, 236
Syphilis, 220, 302–303
Syringes, prefilled, 30
Systemic inflammatory response
        syndrome (SIRS), 224, 225
Systemic lupus erythematosus, 215
Systole, 99
Systolic blood pressure (SBP), 12

T

Tablet dosage form, 20
Tachycardia
    junctional tachycardia, 121
    multifocal atrial tachycardia, 115
    polymorphic ventricular tachycardia,
        130
    septic shock, 36
    sinus tachycardia, 111
    supraventricular tachycardia, 118
    synchronized cardioversion, 159–161
    thyrotoxicosis, 198
    ventricular tachycardia, 128
Tamponade. *See* Cardiac tamponade
T-bone impact trauma, 338

T-cells, 199, 204, 205, 209
    cytotoxic response, 210–212
    negative selection, 210, 212
    regulatory or suppressor, 210, 211
Tears (eyes), 376
Technical rescue awareness, 432
Technical rescue operations, 432
Technical rescue technicians, 432
Teenagers. *See* Adolescents
Telegraphic speech, 186
Telemetry, communication, 418
Temperature
    body (*See* Core body temperature)
    and burns, 354
        thermal burns, 354–359
    and oxyhemoglobin dissociation,
        66–67
Temporal bones, 375
Temporal lobe, 170, 172, 186
Temporal summation, 181
Tendinitis, 374
Tendons, 365
    overuse syndromes, 374
    strains, 371
Tension headaches, 192
Tension pneumothorax, 389
Terbutaline, 466
Terrorism, 428–430
Testes, 200
    orchitis, 265
    testicular torsion, 265
Testimonial evidence, 304, 436
Testosterone, 200
Tetralogy of Fallot, 329
Thalamus, 173–174
Therapeutic effect, 23
Therapeutic index, 23
Thermal burns, 354–359
Thermoregulation, 279–280
    newborn, 328
    skin function, 347–348
    thermogenesis, 279
    thermolysis, 279–280
Thiamine, 466
    Wernicke encephalopathy, 231
Third-degree AV block on ECG, 125
Thoracic aortic aneurysm, 152
Thoracic duct, 213, 246
Thoracic vertebrae, 384, 385
Thought broadcasting, 272
Thought insertion, 272
Thought withdrawal, 272
Threatened abortion, 311
Threshold of medication, 23
Threshold value of action potential,
    178, 180–181
Thrombic strokes, 186
Thrombocytes, 267
Thrombophlebitis, 36
Thrombosis, and cardiac arrest, 157
Thrombus, and acute myocardial
    infarction, 142

Thymosin, 199, 210
Thymus gland, 199, 204, 205, 209, 210,
    212
Thyroid cartilage, 61, 62
Thyroid gland, 197
    hyperthyroidism, 197–198
    hypothyroidism, 197–199
Thyroid-stimulating hormone (TSH),
    197
Thyroid storm, 198
Thyronines, 197
Thyrotoxicosis, 198
Thyroxine, 197
Tidal volume, 65
    physiology of breathing, 64
    pregnancy, 308
Tirofiban, 466
Tobacco use, 416
Toddlers
    development, 400
    vital signs, 399
Tolerance to medications, 23, 229
Toll-like receptors (TLRs), 208
Tongue
    airway obstruction, 68, 70
    lower airway, 62
    sublingual route of administration,
        25
Tonic-clonic seizures, 189, 190
Topical anesthetic medication, 444
Topical dosage form, 20
Torsade de pointes. *See* Polymorphic
    ventricular tachycardia
Torus fractures, 368
Total lung volume, 64, 65
Toxicological emergencies, 227–237
    assessment, 229–230
    Poison Control Centers, 228
    routes of absorption, 228–229
    specific toxins, 230–236
    term definitions, 227–229
Toxic shock syndrome, 303
Toxidromes, 228
Toxoplasmosis, 310
Trabeculae, 365
Trace evidence, 436
Trachea
    deviation and pneumothorax, 286,
        389
    lower airway, 61, 62
    neck injuries, 383
    upper airway, 60, 61
Tracheobronchial injuries, 393
Tracheostomy tubes
    tracheostomy mask, 78
    ventilatory assistance, 77–78
Traction splints, 373
Tracts of axons, 179
Trade name of medication, 20
Traffic accidents, 417
Tranquilizers, 452
Transcellular passage, 246

Notes

Notes

Notes

Notes

Notes

Notes